EPR Effect-Based Tumor Targeted Nanomedicine

EPR Effect-Based Tumor Targeted Nanomedicine

Editor

Hiroshi Maeda

MDPI • Basel • Beijing • Wuhan • Barcelona • Belgrade • Manchester • Tokyo • Cluj • Tianjin

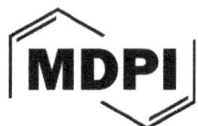

Editor
Hiroshi Maeda
BioDynamics Research Foundation
Kumamoto
Japan

Editorial Office
MDPI
St. Alban-Anlage 66
4052 Basel, Switzerland

This is a reprint of articles from the Special Issue published online in the open access journal *Journal of Personalized Medicine* (ISSN 2075-4426) (available at: www.mdpi.com/journal/jpm/special_issues/EPR_Nanomedicine).

For citation purposes, cite each article independently as indicated on the article page online and as indicated below:

LastName, A.A.; LastName, B.B.; LastName, C.C. Article Title. *Journal Name* **Year**, *Volume Number*, Page Range.

ISBN 978-3-0365-5428-0 (Hbk)
ISBN 978-3-0365-5427-3 (PDF)

© 2022 by the authors. Articles in this book are Open Access and distributed under the Creative Commons Attribution (CC BY) license, which allows users to download, copy and build upon published articles, as long as the author and publisher are properly credited, which ensures maximum dissemination and a wider impact of our publications.

The book as a whole is distributed by MDPI under the terms and conditions of the Creative Commons license CC BY-NC-ND.

Contents

Jun Fang
EPR Effect-Based Tumor Targeted Nanomedicine: A Promising Approach for Controlling Cancer
Reprinted from: *J. Pers. Med.* **2022**, *12*, 95, doi:10.3390/jpm12010095 1

Xin Wu, Yuhki Yokoyama, Hidekazu Takahashi, Shihori Kouda, Hiroyuki Yamamoto and Jiaqi Wang et al.
Improved In Vivo Delivery of Small RNA Based on the Calcium Phosphate Method
Reprinted from: *J. Pers. Med.* **2021**, *11*, 1160, doi:10.3390/jpm11111160 5

Yoshitaka Matsumoto, Nobuyoshi Fukumitsu, Hitoshi Ishikawa, Kei Nakai and Hideyuki Sakurai
A Critical Review of Radiation Therapy: From Particle Beam Therapy (Proton, Carbon, and BNCT) to Beyond
Reprinted from: *J. Pers. Med.* **2021**, *11*, 825, doi:10.3390/jpm11080825 23

Jun Wu
The Enhanced Permeability and Retention (EPR) Effect: The Significance of the Concept and Methods to Enhance Its Application
Reprinted from: *J. Pers. Med.* **2021**, *11*, 771, doi:10.3390/jpm11080771 55

Mohamed Haider, Amr Elsherbeny, Valeria Pittalà, Antonino N. Fallica, Maha Ali Alghamdi and Khaled Greish
The Potential Role of Sildenafil in Cancer Management through EPR Augmentation
Reprinted from: *J. Pers. Med.* **2021**, *11*, 585, doi:10.3390/jpm11060585 63

Md Abdus Subhan, Satya Siva Kishan Yalamarty, Nina Filipczak, Farzana Parveen and Vladimir P. Torchilin
Recent Advances in Tumor Targeting via EPR Effect for Cancer Treatment
Reprinted from: *J. Pers. Med.* **2021**, *11*, 571, doi:10.3390/jpm11060571 81

Shun'ichiro Taniguchi
In Situ Delivery and Production System (*i*DPS) of Anti-Cancer Molecules with Gene-Engineered *Bifidobacterium*
Reprinted from: *J. Pers. Med.* **2021**, *11*, 566, doi:10.3390/jpm11060566 109

Fatemah Bahman, Valeria Pittalà, Mohamed Haider and Khaled Greish
Enhanced Anticancer Activity of Nanoformulation of Dasatinib against Triple-Negative Breast Cancer
Reprinted from: *J. Pers. Med.* **2021**, *11*, 559, doi:10.3390/jpm11060559 129

Waliul Islam, Shintaro Kimura, Rayhanul Islam, Ayaka Harada, Katsuhiko Ono and Jun Fang et al.
EPR-Effect Enhancers Strongly Potentiate Tumor-Targeted Delivery of Nanomedicines to Advanced Cancers: Further Extension to Enhancement of the Therapeutic Effect
Reprinted from: *J. Pers. Med.* **2021**, *11*, 487, doi:10.3390/jpm11060487 141

Hiroshi Maeda
The 35th Anniversary of the Discovery of EPR Effect: A New Wave of Nanomedicines for Tumor-Targeted Drug Delivery—Personal Remarks and Future Prospects
Reprinted from: *J. Pers. Med.* **2021**, *11*, 229, doi:10.3390/jpm11030229 155

Shanghui Gao, Rayhanul Islam and Jun Fang
Tumor Environment-Responsive Hyaluronan Conjugated Zinc Protoporphyrin for Targeted Anticancer Photodynamic Therapy
Reprinted from: *J. Pers. Med.* **2021**, *11*, 136, doi:10.3390/jpm11020136 . . . . **173**

Dong Huang, Lingna Sun, Leaf Huang and Yanzuo Chen
Nanodrug Delivery Systems Modulate Tumor Vessels to Increase the Enhanced Permeability and Retention Effect
Reprinted from: *J. Pers. Med.* **2021**, *11*, 124, doi:10.3390/jpm11020124 . . . . **189**

Petr Chytil, Libor Kostka and Tomáš Etrych
HPMA Copolymer-Based Nanomedicines in Controlled Drug Delivery
Reprinted from: *J. Pers. Med.* **2021**, *11*, 115, doi:10.3390/jpm11020115 . . . . **215**

Babita Shashni and Yukio Nagasaki
Newly Developed Self-Assembling Antioxidants as Potential Therapeutics for the Cancers
Reprinted from: *J. Pers. Med.* **2021**, *11*, 92, doi:10.3390/jpm11020092 . . . . **237**

Nithya Subrahmanyam and Hamidreza Ghandehari
Harnessing Extracellular Matrix Biology for Tumor Drug Delivery
Reprinted from: *J. Pers. Med.* **2021**, *11*, 88, doi:10.3390/jpm11020088 . . . . **263**

Editorial

EPR Effect-Based Tumor Targeted Nanomedicine: A Promising Approach for Controlling Cancer

Jun Fang

Laboratory of Microbiology and Oncology, Faculty of Pharmaceutical Sciences, Sojo University, Kumamoto 860-0082, Japan; fangjun@ph.sojo-u.ac.jp; Tel.: +81-09-326-4137

Cancer remains the major threat to human health in most advanced countries in the world. Among the three major standard cancer treatments, i.e., surgery, radiation therapy, and chemotherapy, to date surgical removal is still the most effective therapeutic; however, cancer patients who could benefit from surgery are limited. For many cancer patients, chemotherapy is the final and important option. Although there is more than 70-year history of chemotherapy, conventional chemotherapy is far from successful. The major problem derives mostly from the lack of tumor selectivity; anticancer drugs are distributed not only in cancer but also in normal tissues. At the same time when they kill cancer cells, they also do harm to normal cells. The non-selective delivery of cytotoxic drugs induces severe adverse side effects that many cancer patients suffer from, which will also limit the usage/dosing for anticancer drugs, resulting in less antitumor effects. Thus, the development of therapeutic strategies with high tumor selectivity is urgently needed, and targeted anticancer therapy has become a focus of cancer research.

In this concern, molecular-target drugs have been extensively developed in the past two decades, which usually focus on essential kinases or receptors highly expressed in tumors. However, with the deepening of research, many limitations and drawbacks of molecular-target drugs have been recognized, and the major concern is the intrinsic heterogeneity of human solid tumors. Thus, anticancer spectra of molecular-target drugs are very narrow, and personalized medicine or precision medicine is necessary to achieve satisfactory effects, which results in enormous expenses of these drugs, including their toxic effects. More recently, immunotherapy has received extensive attention by focusing on immune escape mechanisms; however, similar problems to those of molecular-target drugs exist, which may become a hurdle of this anticancer strategy.

While molecular-target drugs target cancer at the molecular level, at a much earlier period of time, a more general tumor-targeting strategy had been depicted and developed by focusing on unique anatomical and pathophysiological features of solid tumors [1]. Compared to normal blood vessels, tumor blood vessels are very leaky due to the defected architecture of endothelial cells and high vascular permeability due to the highly expressed vascular mediators such as bradykinin (BK), nitric oxide (NO), and vascular endothelial growth factor (VEGF), by which the accumulation of macromolecules (i.e., larger than 40 kDa) selectively into tumor tissues could be achieved with very little distribution in normal tissues [1,2]. This unique phenomenon is coined the enhanced permeability and retention (EPR) effect, and it was first recovered by Matsumura and Maeda in 1986 [1], which is a landmark principle in the development of targeted anticancer drugs.

Based on the concept of the EPR effect, macromolecular anticancer strategy, i.e., nanomedicine, has been developed. Tumor-targeted drug delivery systems using nanoplatforms including liposome, polymeric micelles, polymer conjugate, and nanoparticles have become a promising fusion area for nanotechnology and medicine. In the past two decades, many researchers have been working on EPR effect-based nanomedicine, taking an enormous step forward. In 1980s, the founder of EPR effect, Professor Maeda, developed styrene maleic acid copolymer conjugated neocarzinostatin (SMANCS), which was approved in Japan in 1990s [1]. Recently, more nanomedicines have been used in clinic, for example, Doxil is an FDA approved liposomal drug for the treatment of Kaposi sarcoma and other cancers. Other clinically approved nanomedicine includes liposomal daunorubicin (DaunoXome), liposomal cytarabine (DepoCyt), nonpegylated liposomal doxorubicin (Myocet), pegylated L-asparaginase (Oncaspar), albumin-based paclitaxel nanoparticles Abraxane, and paclitaxel-containing polymeric micelles (Genexol-PM). More nanomedicines are in pre-clinical stage of development [3–9], all of which show superior tumor selectivity by taking advantage of the EPR effect, resulting in improved antitumor effects with less adverse effects [3–9].

A critical issue should be addressed is that the EPR effect is the phenomenon of blood vessels, which is largely dependent on tumor blood flow. While most animal solid tumor models that are rich in blood flow exhibit good EPR effect, many clinical cancers, especially advanced late-stage cancers and refractor cancers, are poor in tumor blood flow due to high coagulation activity and thrombi formation, thus showing unsatisfactory EPR effect [1,2,10–13]. Thus, further augmentation of the EPR effect is of great importance and necessity. In this regard, we should understand that the EPR effect is not a static phenomenon, it is a dynamic event, which could be enhanced by modulating vascular mediators in tumor such as using angiotensin II, NO/nitroglycerin, and angiotensin II, converting enzyme inhibitors and carbon monoxide [1,2,10,11]. A combination of vascular mediators with nanomedicines may become useful strategies for more effective antitumor nanomedicine. Other strategies, for example, by modulating tumor vessels [12] or by targeting tumor stroma and extracellular matrix [13], have also been extensively investigated and proven effective in improving the therapeutic effect of EPR effect-based nanomedicine.

This Special Issue of "EPR effect-based tumor targeted nanomedicine" includes 14 papers from experts working on the EPR effect and nanomedicines of a diverse range of areas. The discoverer of EPR effect, Professor Hiroshi Maeda, and his former students and colleagues summarized the history; principle; the progress and prospects of EPR effect-based tumor targeting strategies; and the application of nanomedicines [1,2,6,8], in which the concept of EPR effect is not only applied to the development of targeted anticancer drugs [3,4,9] but is also applicable for radiation therapy [5], bacterial therapy of cancer [7], and nucleic acid medicine [14]. Moreover, more papers in the Special Issue emphasized the significance of EPR enhancement, discussing the usefulness of potential EPR enhancers [1,2,10–13], which I believe to be an essential issue for successful anticancer therapy using nanomedicine.

The aim of targeted anticancer research is to develop anticancer drugs with high anticancer effects while showing low side effects, to provide patient friendly service, and to benefit most cancer patients. We believe EPR-based nanomedicine will be a promising paradigm to reach this goal and will be a solution for cancer in the future.

Funding: This research received no external funding.

Institutional Review Board Statement: Not applicable.

Informed Consent Statement: Not applicable.

Data Availability Statement: Not applicable.

Conflicts of Interest: The authors declare no conflict of interest.

References

1. Maeda, H. The 35th Anniversary of the Discovery of EPR Effect: A New Wave of Nanomedicines for Tumor-Targeted Drug Delivery—Personal Remarks and Future Prospects. *J. Pers. Med.* **2021**, *11*, 229. [CrossRef] [PubMed]
2. Wu, J. The Enhanced Permeability and Retention (EPR) Effect: The Significance of the Concept and Methods to Enhance Its Application. *J. Pers. Med.* **2021**, *11*, 771. [CrossRef] [PubMed]
3. Bahman, F.; Pittala, V.; Haider, M.; Greish, K. Enhanced Anticancer Activity of Nanoformulation of Dasatinib against Triple-Negative Breast Cancer. *J. Pers. Med.* **2021**, *11*, 559. [CrossRef] [PubMed]

4. Gao, S.; Islam, R.; Fang, J. Tumor Environment-Responsive Hyaluronan Conjugated Zinc Protoporphyrin for Targeted Anticancer Photodynamic Therapy. *J. Pers. Med.* **2021**, *11*, 136. [CrossRef] [PubMed]
5. Matsumoto, Y.; Fukumitsu, N.; Ishikawa, H.; Nakai, K.; Sakurai, H. A Critical Review of Radiation Therapy: From Particle Beam Therapy (Proton, Carbon, and BNCT) to Beyond. *J. Pers. Med.* **2021**, *11*, 825. [CrossRef] [PubMed]
6. Subhan, M.A.; Yalamarty, S.S.K.; Filipczak, N.; Parveen, F.; Torchilin, V.P. Recent Advances in Tumor Targeting via EPR Effect for Cancer Treatment. *J. Pers. Med.* **2021**, *11*, 571. [CrossRef]
7. Taniguchi, S. In Situ Delivery and Production System (iDPS) of Anti-Cancer Molecules with Gene-Engineered Bifidobacterium. *J. Pers. Med.* **2021**, *11*, 566. [CrossRef]
8. Chytil, P.; Kostka, L.; Etrych, T. HPMA Copolymer-Based Nanomedicines in Controlled Drug Delivery. *J. Pers. Med.* **2021**, *11*, 115. [CrossRef] [PubMed]
9. Shashni, B.; Nagasaki, Y. Newly Developed Self-Assembling Antioxidants as Potential Therapeutics for the Cancers. *J. Pers. Med.* **2021**, *11*, 92. [CrossRef] [PubMed]
10. Islam, W.; Kimura, S.; Islam, R.; Harada, A.; Ono, K.; Fang, J.; Nidome, T.; Sawa, T.; Maeda, H. EPR-Effect Enhancers Strongly Potentiate Tumor-Targeted Delivery of Nanomedicines to Advanced Cancers: Further Extension to Enhancement of the Therapeutic Effect. *J. Pers. Med.* **2021**, *11*, 487. [CrossRef] [PubMed]
11. Haider, M.; Elsherbeny, A.; Pittala, V.; Fallica, A.N.; Alghamdi, M.A.; Greish, H. The Potential Role of Sildenafil in Cancer Management through EPR Augmentation. *J. Pers. Med.* **2021**, *11*, 585. [CrossRef] [PubMed]
12. Huang, D.; Sun, L.; Huang, L.; Chen, Y. Nanodrug Delivery Systems Modulate Tumor Vessels to Increase the Enhanced Permeability and Retention Effect. *J. Pers. Med.* **2021**, *11*, 124. [CrossRef] [PubMed]
13. Subrahmanyam, N.; Ghandehari, H. Harnessing Extracellular Matrix Biology for Tumor Drug Delivery. *J. Pers. Med.* **2021**, *11*, 88. [CrossRef] [PubMed]
14. Wu, X.; Yokoyama, Y.; Takahashi, H.; Kouda, S.; Yamamoto, H.; Wang, J.; Morimoto, Y.; Minami, K.; Hata, T.; Shamma, A.; et al. Improved In Vivo Delivery of Small RNA Based on the Calcium Phosphate Method. *J. Pers. Med.* **2021**, *11*, 1160. [CrossRef] [PubMed]

Article

Improved In Vivo Delivery of Small RNA Based on the Calcium Phosphate Method

Xin Wu [1], Yuhki Yokoyama [1], Hidekazu Takahashi [2], Shihori Kouda [1], Hiroyuki Yamamoto [1], Jiaqi Wang [1], Yoshihiro Morimoto [2], Kazumasa Minami [3], Tsuyoshi Hata [2], Awad Shamma [1], Akira Inoue [2], Masahisa Ohtsuka [2], Satoshi Shibata [1], Shogo Kobayashi [2], Shuji Akai [4] and Hirofumi Yamamoto [1,2,*]

[1] Department of Molecular Pathology, Division of Health Sciences, Graduate School of Medicine, Osaka University, Yamadaoka 1-7, Suita, Osaka 565-0871, Japan; skure@nano-b.co.jp (X.W.); yokoyama.y2011@gmail.com (Y.Y.); s.kouda.c@gmail.com (S.K.); h.yamamoto1911@gmail.com (H.Y.); jiaqiwang4012@yahoo.com (J.W.); shamawad@sahs.med.osaka-u.ac.jp (A.S.); sshibata@sahs.med.osaka-u.ac.jp (S.S.)

[2] Department of Gastroenterological Surgery, Graduate School of Medicine, Osaka University, Yamadaoka 2-2, Suita, Osaka 565-0871, Japan; hide_tak77@yahoo.co.jp (H.T.); tamtam.hiro@gmail.com (Y.M.); tsuyoshihata1983@gmail.com (T.H.); inoue_medical@yahoo.co.jp (A.I.); masboenigma@gmail.com (M.O.); skobayashi@gesurg.med.osaka-u.ac.jp (S.K.)

[3] Department of Radiation Oncology, Graduate School of Medicine, Osaka University, Yamadaoka 2-2, Suita, Osaka 565-0871, Japan; k.minami@sahs.med.osaka-u.ac.jp

[4] Graduate School of Pharmaceutical Sciences, Osaka University, Yamadaoka 1-6, Suita, Osaka 565-0871, Japan; akai@phs.osaka-u.ac.jp

* Correspondence: hyamamoto@sahs.med.osaka-u.ac.jp; Tel.: +81-6-6879-2591; Fax: +81-6-6879-2591

Abstract: In the past few years, we have demonstrated the efficacy of a nanoparticle system, super carbonate apatite (sCA), for the in vivo delivery of siRNA/miRNA. Intravenous injection of sCA loaded with small RNAs results in safe, high tumor delivery in mouse models. To further improve the efficiency of tumor delivery and avoid liver toxicity, we successfully developed an inorganic nanoparticle device (iNaD) via high-frequency ultrasonic pulverization combined with PEG blending during the production of sCA. Compared to sCA loaded with 24 µg of miRNA, systemic administration of iNaD loaded with 0.75 µg of miRNA demonstrated similar delivery efficiency to mouse tumors with little accumulation in the liver. In the mouse therapeutic model, iNaD loaded with 3 µg of the tumor suppressor small RNA MIRTX resulted in an improved anti-tumor effect compared to sCA loaded with 24 µg. Our findings on the bio-distribution and therapeutic effect of iNaD provide new perspectives for future nanomedicine engineering.

Keywords: iNaD; siRNA; microRNA; calcium phosphate; PEG blending; cancer treatment

1. Introduction

Cancer is the second leading cause of death, with an estimated 18.1 million new cancer cases and 9.6 million deaths in 2018 worldwide [1]. The development of novel and effective cancer therapy is urgently needed. One of the most important therapeutic advances is nanotechnology-based medicine, which has the potential to surmount the limitations of cancer therapeutics [2]. Nanoparticles with a size of 10–100 nm are considered optimal for the passive targeting of tumors in vivo [3] due to the enhanced permeability and retention (EPR) effect, which is characterized by increased microvasculature leakage and impaired lymphatic function in tumors [4]. Thus, systemic administration of engineered nanoparticles provides an opportunity to deliver reagents more precisely to tumor tissues, reducing the toxicity to normal organs and enhancing the anti-cancer effects compared to incorporated reagents alone. Based on the EPR effect, remarkable advances have been made recently in engineering nanoparticles for clinical application [5], including RNA-based gene therapy (e.g., siRNA, microRNA), which has shown a tremendous anti-cancer effect [6,7]. siRNAs can silence any gene with a known sequence [8], whereas microRNAs (miRNAs) regulate the expression of multiple target genes [9].

Previously, we introduced a nanoparticle system, super carbonate apatite (sCA) consisting of inorganic ions (CO_3^{2-}, Ca^{2+}, and PO_4^{3-}), as an in vivo delivery system for siRNA/miRNA (Figure 1A) [10]. The nanoparticles enter the cells via endocytosis and quickly degrade at acidic pH in the endosomal compartments of tumor cells (Figure 1B). Intravenous injection of sCA achieves higher colorectal tumor delivery efficiency and less accumulation in normal tissues compared to two currently available systemic in vivo siRNA delivery systems, Invivofectamine 2.0 and AteloGene. Using this systematic delivery system, we have reported several siRNA- or miRNA-based cancer therapeutics in colorectal tumor mouse models [11–16]. Besides cancer treatment, sCA also systemically delivers miRNA to inflammatory lesions in vivo, treating inflamed colitis [17]. Local delivery of sCA incorporating plasmid DNA or siRNA to skin wounds can accelerate wound healing and reduce scar formation, demonstrating an effective approach for treating intractable abnormal scars [18,19]. sCA also exhibits significant efficiency as a CpG adjuvant for influenza vaccination [20] and near-infrared ray irradiation therapy for ICG [21]. In addition to the well-known RNA delivery methods, such as liposomes and micelles, our sCA system has been recognized as a new inorganic nanoparticle for siRNA/miRNA [22–25].

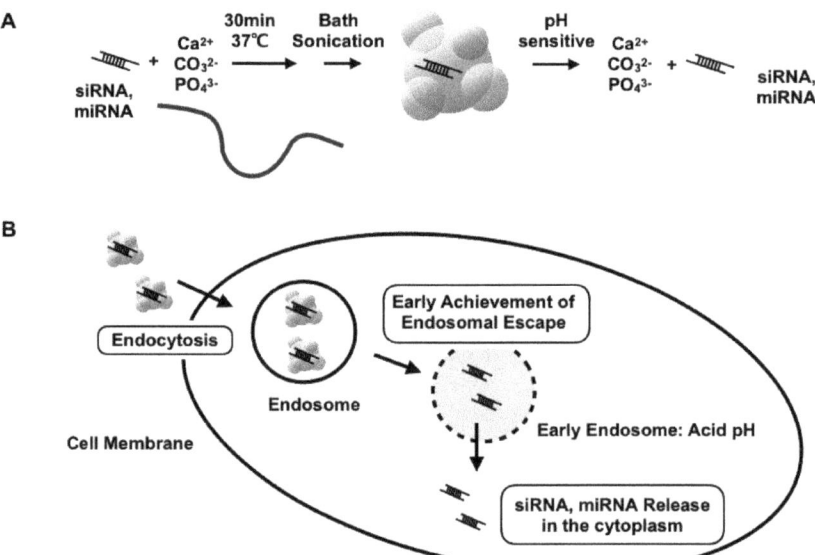

Figure 1. Schematic presentation of sCA-siRNA/miRNA. (A) Production of sCA nanoparticles involves mixing inorganic ions (CO_3^{2-}, Ca^{2+}, and PO_4^{3-}) with siRNA or miRNA and incubating at 37 °C for 30 min. After bath sonication, the sCA nanoparticles can be degraded at acidic pH to release the incorporated siRNA/miRNA compounds. (B) sCA nanoparticles enter the cell via endocytosis and are degradable in the acidic pH of endosomes, indicating quick achievement of endosomal escape.

Some notable hurdles still exist for RNA delivery systems. Non-viral vectors, such as polymeric, lipid-based, and inorganic vectors, are inefficient for miRNA transfer, with even lower efficacy in target gene repression than viral delivery [24,25]. In the case of the sCA system, unfavorable accumulation of siRNA/miRNA in the liver is still a major challenge, which is a common issue with viral vectors and lipid-based, polymeric, or inorganic nanoparticles [5,26,27]. Therefore, improving the efficiency of tumor delivery and reducing accumulation in the liver are necessary for the clinical application of sCA as a new inorganic nanoparticle for siRNA/miRNA.

As described in our first report of the sCA system [10], dynamic light scattering (DLS) analysis has demonstrated that the larger nanoparticles are 653 nm, whereas atomic force microscopy (AFM) revealed that the smaller nanoparticles range from 7 to 50 nm in size. The smaller nanoparticles comprised 99.7% of the particle numbers. Furthermore, laser microscopy confirmed the existence of microparticles. It has also become clear that intravenously injected particles > 100 nm in diameter are trapped by the reticuloendothelial system in the liver and spleen, leading to degradation by activated monocytes and macrophages [26]. As for tumor delivery, particles < 30 nm in diameter can penetrate tumor tissue better than larger nanoparticles [28,29]. Thus, we hypothesized that the reduction of large particles into smaller nanoparticles might decrease accumulation in the liver and increase tumor delivery.

In this study, we describe how we initially performed mechanical pulverization using wet jet-milling or adaptive focused acoustics (AFA) technology. As a wet jet-milling device, Star Burst causes materials in a slurry state to collide in an oblique direction at ultra-high pressure, thereby pulverizing and dispersing the materials. AFA is an advanced acoustics technology enabling the mechanical pulverization of samples through focused ultrasonication in a temperature-controlled and non-contact environment. AFA technology is well-known for shearing DNA and RNA for next-generation sequencing. This technology has also been used in the formation of liposomes [30]. To further improve the pulverization efficiency, we applied poly(ethylene glycol) (PEG) blending during sCA production, followed by pulverization. Interestingly, this approach produced a new size of nanoparticles, 600–700 nm. After purification and concentration using two kinds of hollow-fiber membranes with a pore size of 1 μm and 50 nm, we defined this new nanoparticle as an inorganic nanoparticle device (iNaD). With bio-distribution imaging and anti-tumor effects, we show that the iNaD results in less accumulation in normal tissues while highly improving tumor delivery efficiency compared to sCA. Taken together, our findings provide new insights for engineering nanomedicines.

2. Materials and Methods

2.1. Materials

Human colon cancer cell lines HCT116 and HT29, and human pancreatic cancer cell line Panc-1 were purchased from the American Type Culture Collection. HCT116 and Panc-1 cells were grown in DMEM, and HT29 cells were grown in RPMI supplemented with 10% fetal bovine serum (FBS). All cells were grown in a 5% CO_2 atmosphere at 37 °C. Methoxy-PEG-CO$(CH_2)_2$COO-NHS (Mw 10,000) was purchased from NOF Corporation (Tokyo, Japan). The miRNAs were purchased from GeneDesign, Inc. (Osaka, Japan) (miRNA34a: 5′-UGGCAGUGUCUUAGCUGGUUGU-3′; Alexa Flour 750-labeled at 5′ side of negative control miRNA: 5′-AUCCGCGCGAUAGUACGUA-3′; MIRTX: 5′-UCUAAACCACCAUAUGAAACCAGC-3′; negative control miRNA: 5′-AUCCGCGCGAU AGUACGUA-3′).

2.2. Production of sCA and iNaD

To produce sCA nanoparticles incorporating siRNA/miRNA, 4 μL of 1 M $CaCl_2$ was mixed with 2 μg of siRNA/miRNA in 1 mL of an inorganic solution (44 mM $NaHCO_3$, 0.9 mM NaH_2PO_4, 1.8 M $CaCl_2$, pH 7.5) and incubated at 37 °C for 30 min. The solution was centrifuged at 12,000 rpm for 3 min and the pellet was dissolved in saline containing 0.5% albumin. The products in the solution were sonicated (38 kHz, 80 W) in a water bath for 10 min. The solution was intravenously injected within 10 min. For the production of iNaD, methoxy-PEG-CO$(CH_2)_2$COO-NHS (Mw 10,000) was initially mixed during sCA production. AFA (Covaris S220, Woburn, MA, USA) was performed, followed by purification and concentration using 1 μm and 50 nm hollow-fiber membranes.

2.3. Assaying Nanoparticle Features

The particle size distribution was determined using a DLS analyzer, the nanoPartica SZ-100 (Horiba, Kyoto, Japan) or the Zetasizer (Malvern Panalytical, Worcestershire, UK). The zeta potential of the particles was measured using the Zetasizer.

2.4. miRNA Electrophoresis

The sCA-miRNA pellet was dissolved in 100 µL of 0.02 M EDTA. The collected miRNA sample was mixed with loading dye (Thermo Fisher Scientific, Waltham, MA, USA) and loaded in a 4.5% NuSieve GTG agarose gel (Lonza, Basel, Switzerland). Imaging was performed using ChemiDoc Touch (Bio-rad, Hercules, CA, USA).

2.5. Cell Proliferation Assay

HCT116 cells were uniformly seeded into 96-well plates (1×10^4 cells/well). Cell viability was evaluated by the Cell Counting Kit-8 (Dojindo, Kumamoto, Japan).

2.6. Quantitative Real-Time RT-PCR Analysis of mRNA Expression

Total RNA was collected from cultured cells or tumor tissues using TRIzol Reagent (Thermo Fisher Scientific), and complementary DNA was synthesized from 1.0 µg of total RNA using oligo dT primer and a Reverse Transcription System (Promega, Madison, WI, USA) according to the manufacturer's instructions. Real-time RT-PCR was carried out using LightCycler FastStart DNA Master SYBR Green I (Roche, Basel, Switzerland) on a LightCycler 2.0 II (Roche). Expression of the target gene was normalized relative to GAPDH mRNA expression using the $2^{-\Delta\Delta Ct}$ method. Primers are shown in Supplementary Table S1.

2.7. Western Blot Analysis

Tumor tissues were homogenized on ice with a homogenizer (Tissue Lyser, QIAGEN, Venlo, Netherlands). Protein samples were loaded onto Mini-Protean TGX 4–15% gels (Bio-Rad) and transferred using the Trans-Blot Turbo Blotting System (Bio-Rad). After blocking with Blocking One (Nacalai Tesque, Kyoto, Japan), the membrane was incubated overnight with primary antibodies against PIK3R1 (Cell Signaling Technology, Danvers, MA, USA), CXCR2 (Abcam, Cambridge, UK), and actin (Sigma-Aldrich, St. Louis, MO, USA). Secondary antibodies were incubated with ECL substrate (Bio-Rad), and bands were visualized using the ChemiDoc Touch Imaging System (Bio-Rad). Images were processed with Image Lab 5.2.1 software (Bio-rad).

2.8. Animals

Female BALB/cAJcl-nu/nu nude mice aged 6–8 weeks and female SKG/Jcl mice aged 6–7 weeks were purchased from CLEA Japan, Inc. (Tokyo, Japan). Studies using mouse models were conducted in strict accordance with the recommendations of the Guide for the Care and Use of Laboratory Animals of the Graduate School of Medicine, Osaka University. The protocol was approved by the Committee for the Ethics of Animal Experiments of Osaka University (Permit Number: 27-085-017).

2.9. Cell Line-Derived Xenograft Models

Human colon cancer HT29 cells or human pancreatic Panc-1 cells were inoculated subcutaneously into both the left and right flanks of mice to establish solid tumors. Imaging using IVIS lumina (PerkinElmer, Waltham, MA, USA) was performed when the tumor volume reached approximately 250 mm^3. For the anti-tumor activity study, treatment started when the tumors reached approximately 80 mm^3. Anti-tumor activity was evaluated in terms of tumor size, which was estimated using the following equation: $V = a \times b^2/2$, where a and b represent the major and minor axes of the tumor, respectively. In vivo functional validation on the effect of MIRTX was performed when the tumor volume reached approximately 200 mm^3.

2.10. Rheumatoid Arthritis Models

Female SKG/Jcl mice aged 8 weeks were given intraperitoneal injections (20 mg) of mannan (Sigma-Aldrich) suspended in 500 mL of saline or 500 mL of saline alone as a control. Joint swelling was monitored by inspection and scored as follows: 0, no joint swelling; 0.5, mild swelling of the ankle; 1.0, severe swelling of the ankle.

2.11. Statistical Analysis

All statistical analyses were carried out in GraphPad Prism 6 software (San Diego, CA, USA). The two-tailed *t*-test or one-way analysis of variance (ANOVA) followed by Tukey's multiple comparisons test were used as appropriate.

3. Results

3.1. Mechanical Pulverization of sCA-miRNA34a

miRNA34a functions as a mediator of tumor suppression via p53, inducing apoptosis, cell cycle arrest, and senescence [31]. As a first-in-human miRNA clinical study, the liposome-formulated mimic of miRNA-34a provided proof-of-concept for miRNA-based cancer therapy [32]. Here, we manufactured sCA nanoparticles incorporating miRNA34a (sCA-miRNA34a), followed by three kinds of mechanical pulverization (Figure 2). DLS analysis of the sCA-miRNA34a solution treated with bath sonication showed a peak size of 1289 ± 157 nm (mean ± SD), with a considerable amount of larger particles. Though wet jet-milling of sCA-miRNA34a reduced the particle size to 490 ± 150 nm (mean ± SD), the autocorrelation function revealed the existence of larger particles that were beyond the measurable range (>8000 nm). AFA treatment of sCA-miRNA34a resulted in a peak size of 935 ± 230 nm (mean ± SD) and the autocorrelation function had nothing particular to note.

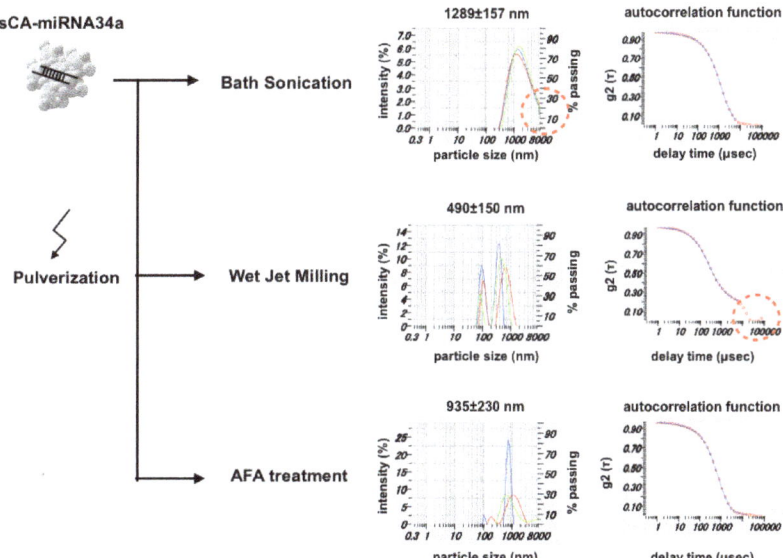

Figure 2. Pulverization of sCA-miRNA34a. The high-concentration sCA-miRNA34a solution for intravenous injection was analyzed by DLS. Three kinds of pulverization, bath sonication (38 kHz), wet jet-milling (30 pass), and adaptive focused acoustics (AFA) treatment (1 MHz), were performed to reduce the sCA-miRNA34a microparticles. Both particle size distribution and autocorrelation function are shown for each sample.

3.2. Production of PEG-Blended sCA Followed by Mechanical Pulverization

Next, we added PEG to the constitute mixture (i.e., 'PEG blending') to produce particles of sCA-miRNA34a plus PEG, and then performed mechanical pulverization. This procedure largely reduced the particle size. Bath sonication of sCA-miRNA34a + PEG contributed to reducing the microparticle formation. Wet jet-milling reduced the massive microparticles indicated by the autocorrelation function to a particle size of 562 ± 175 nm (mean ± SD). AFA treatment resulted in a particle size of 640 ± 55 nm (mean ± SD) at one peak (Figure 3A). When we examined the effect of mechanical pulverization on RNA degradation, wet jet-milling (20 pass and 30 pass) degraded the incorporated miRNA34a compared to bath sonication and AFA treatment (Figure 3B). We loaded 1 μg of intact miRNA34a on the same gel, which serves as an indicator of the molecular weight of miRNA34a. Bath sonication and AFA treatment maintained 2 μg of miRNA34a in the particles, while wet jet-milling treatment degraded miRNA34a. Among the three treatments, AFA could reduce the size of particles without damaging the miRNA34a. The proliferation assay of HCT116 cells showed that sCA-miRNA34a or AFA of sCA-miRNA34a + PEG could inhibit growth at 20% and 40% of control cells at 48 and 72 h, respectively (Figure 3C). To further investigate functional validation on the effect of miRNA34a, we performed quantitative real-time RT-PCR analysis on the target genes such as Survivin, Bcl-2, or E2F1 [33,34]. As shown in Figure 3D, downregulation of Survivin, Bcl-2, or E2F1 was confirmed in sCA-miRNA34a or AFA of sCA-miRNA34a + PEG-treated cells. When we applied atomic force microscopy (AFM) to the sCA-miRNA34a solution prepared for intravenous injection (without dilution), we observed that the particle image was hardly recognized, except for sCA-miRNA34a + PEG nanoparticles treated with AFA (Zmax size: 605 nm, Supplementary Figure S1).

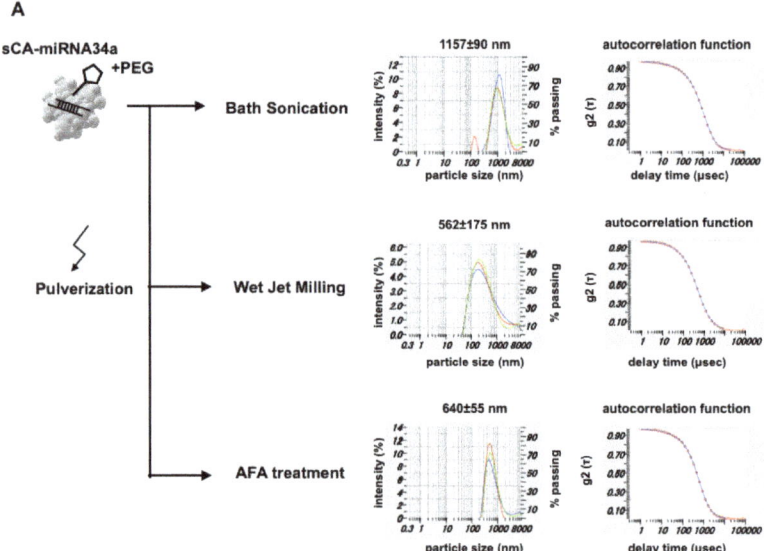

Figure 3. *Cont.*

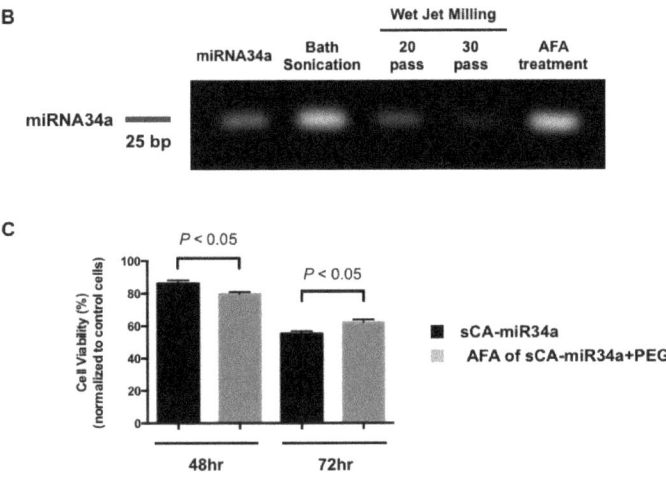

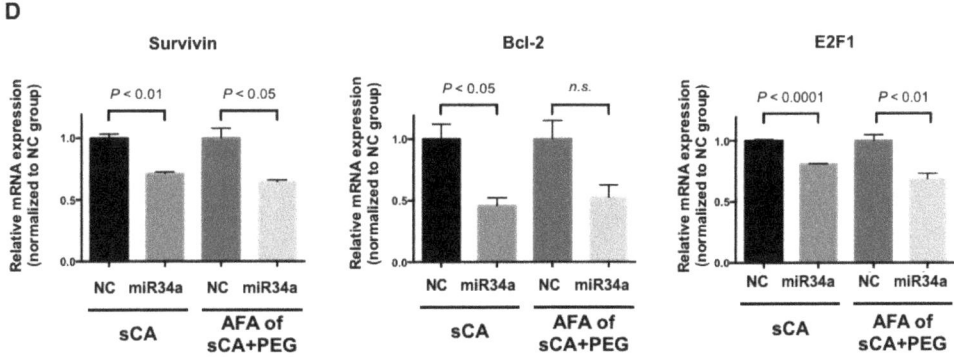

Figure 3. Pulverization of sCA-miRNA34a with PEG blending. (**A**) During sCA-miRNA34a production, methoxy-PEG-CO(CH$_2$)$_2$COO-NHS (Mw 10,000) targeting the OH group of sCA ([Ca$_{10}$(PO$_4$)$^{6-X}$(CO$_3$)^X(OH)$_2$]) was initially mixed with the constituents and three kinds of pulverization, bath sonication (38 kHz), wet jet-milling (30 pass), and AFA (1 MHz), performed after generation of the particles. The solution prepared for intravenous injection was directly (without dilution) analyzed by DLS, and both particle size distribution and autocorrelation function are shown for each sample. (**B**) Degradation of miRNA34a after the pulverization. (**C**) Proliferation assay of HCT116 human colon cancer cells at 48 and 72 h. (**D**) The mRNA expression of Survivin, Bcl-2, and E2F1 in HCT116 at 36 h after treatment. Data represent mean ± SEM (n = 4). *p*-values were obtained using the two-tailed *t* test.

3.3. Purification and Concentration

AFA treatment of sCA-miRNA blended with PEG produced nanoparticles of approximately 640 nm, with some fraction > 1 µm (Figure 3A). We collected these nanoparticles by removing microparticles using a 1 µm hollow-fiber membrane and concentrating the nanoparticles with a 50 nm hollow-fiber membrane (Figure 4A). In this experiment, we incorporated Alexa Fluor 750-labeled miRNA, which is visibly blue. As shown in Figure 4A, the four samples (bath sonication of sCA-miRNA, AFA of sCA-miRNA, bath sonication of sCA-miRNA + PEG, and AFA of sCA-miRNA + PEG) were purified and concentrated by the hollow-fiber membranes.

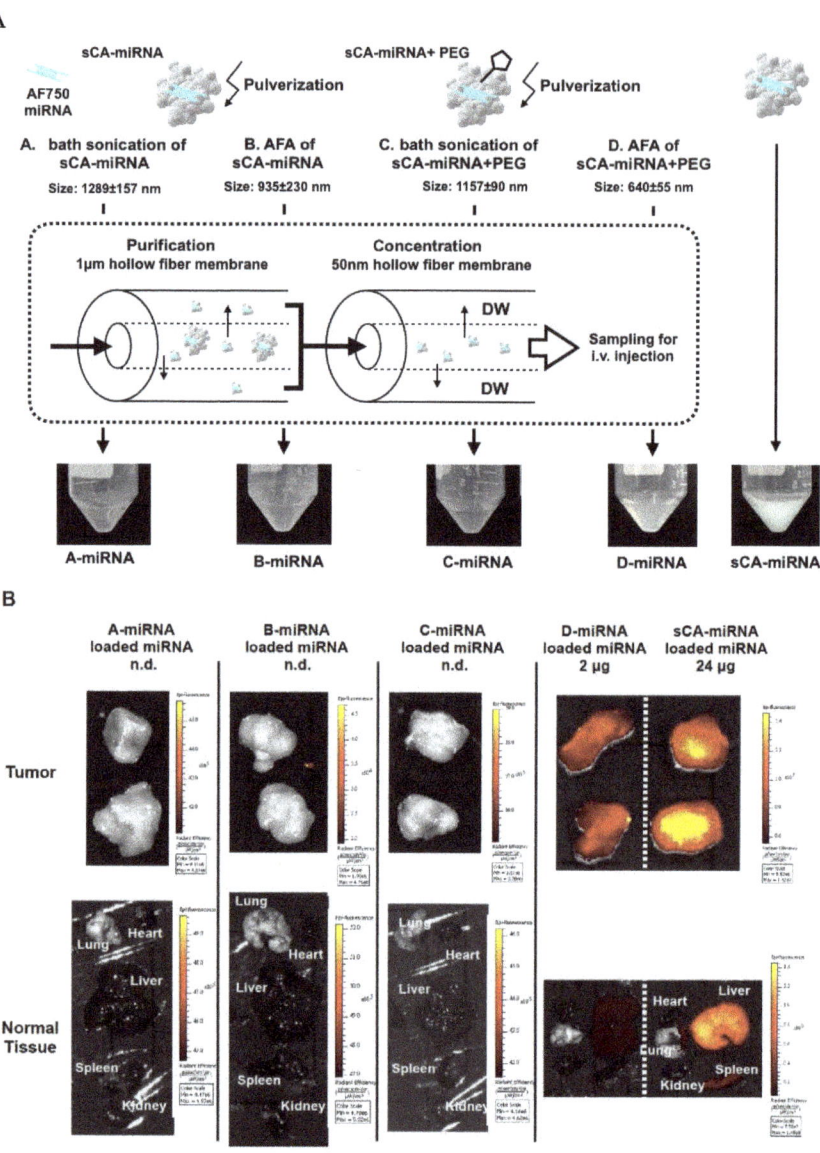

Figure 4. Purification and concentration followed by IVIS imaging. (**A**) The four samples (A: bath sonication of sCA-miRNA, B: AFA of sCA-miRNA, C: bath sonication of sCA-miRNA+PEG, and D: AFA of sCA-miRNA+PEG) were purified and concentrated using the 1 μm and 50 nm hollow-fiber membranes, resulting in A-miRNA, B-miRNA, C-miRNA, and D-miRNA. A-miRNA, B-miRNA, and C-miRNA looked transparent, whereas D-miRNA was cloudy blue and the sCA-miRNA sample for injection was a deep turquoise blue in color. (**B**) The four processed samples and sCA-miRNA were intravenously injected into mice bearing HT29 tumors. Ex vivo IVIS imaging of tumor and normal tissues (heart, lung, liver, spleen, and kidney) 1 h after the injection. The miRNA on processed samples A-miRNA, B-miRNA, and C-miRNA was not detectable (n.d.). The miRNA loading of D-miRNA was 2 μg, and that of sCA-miRNA was 24 μg.

Next, we examined the in vivo delivery of four fractions separated from the original sCA-miRNA using a subcutaneous tumor model (Figure 4B). Mice bearing HT29 tumors were intravenously injected with the processed miRNA from Figure 4A or sCA-miRNA (24 µg of Alexa Fluor 750-labeled miRNA). Ex vivo IVIS imaging 1 h after intravenous injection revealed that the fluorescence of sCA-miRNA accumulated in the tumors, liver, and spleen, whereas little fluorescence was detected in the tumors and normal tissues treated with miRNA processed by bath sonication of sCA-miRNA, AFA of sCA-miRNA, or bath sonication of sCA-miRNA + PEG. However, miRNA processed by AFA of sCA-miRNA + PEG (D-miRNA) retained high fluorescent intensity in tumors, with lower intensity in the liver than sCA-miRNA. Notably, this processed miRNA contained only one-twelfth the amount of miRNA (2 µg) as the sCA-miRNA (24 µg).

3.4. Bio-Distribution of New Nanoparticles as iNaD

Recent RNA carriers, such as liposomes, micelles, inorganic vectors, and atelocollagen, range in size from 30 to 300 nm [5,7,25]. Lipid- or polymer-based nanoparticles for systemic RNA delivery targeting tumors in clinical trials are approximately 80 to 200 nm, whereas bacterially derived 400 nm particles packaging miRNA16 mimics have completed phase I trials [8,24,25,35–37]. Therefore, we are currently conducting the first miRNA-based therapy in an animal model using 700 nm particles for systemic delivery to solid tumors. We defined the new nanoparticles as an iNaD system.

To confirm the reproducibility, we performed a repeat experiment using HT29 tumor-bearing mice by intravenously administering iNaD-miRNA (miRNA loading: 0.75 µg) or sCA-miRNA (miRNA loading: 24 µg). Compared to sCA-miRNA, iNaD-miRNA exhibited little fluorescence intensity in the liver but sustained accumulation in tumors (Figure 5A). Quantitative analyses revealed that the group treated with iNaD-miRNA had a significant decrease in fluorescence from Alexa Fluor 750-labeled miRNA in normal tissues (liver, spleen, lung, heart, kidney). Regarding delivery to tumors, the relative intensity of the tumors treated with sCA-miRNA was 1.54 ± 0.08 (mean ± SEM), whereas iNaD-miRNA with only 1/32 loaded miRNA had an intensity of 1.28 ± 0.04 (mean ± SEM) (Figure 5B).

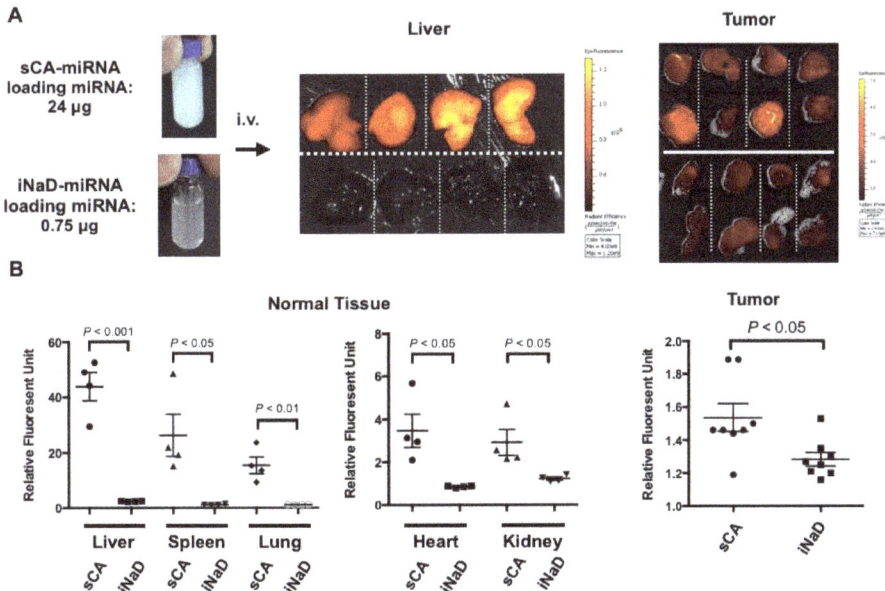

Figure 5. Bio-distribution of iNaD-miRNA. We defined the processed D-miRNA as the inorganic nanoparticle device (iNaD)

system. (**A**) sCA-miRNA (miRNA loading: 24 µg) or iNaD-miRNA (miRNA loading: 0.75 µg) was intravenously injected into HT29 tumor-bearing mice (tumors = 8 from 4 mice). Ex vivo IVIS imaging of the tumor and liver was performed 1 h after the injection. (**B**) Quantitative analyses of tumor and normal tissues (liver, spleen, lung, heart, kidney). Data represent mean ± SEM (n = 4 normal tissues from 4 mice, n = 8 tumors from 4 mice). *p*-values were obtained using the two-tailed *t* test.

3.5. Anti-Tumor Effect of iNaD-MIRTX

We reported a novel small RNA sequence, MIRTX, that significantly inhibits KRAS-mutant colorectal cancer cell growth in vitro and in vivo by suppressing NF-kB signaling pathways via direct inhibition of CXCR2 and PIK3R1 [15]. As shown in Figure 6A, we prepared sCA-MIRTX and iNaD-MIRTX for one intravenous injection. The iNaD-MIRTX was loaded with 3 µg of MIRTX, which is only one-eighth the loading of sCA-MIRTX (24 µg). In an aqueous solution, sCA-MIRTX had an average particle size of 1039 nm by DLS (Figure 6A) and the zeta potential was −37.9 mV, whereas iNaD-MIRTX had an average size of 666 nm with a zeta potential of −6.68 mV. In the mouse therapeutic model of Panc-1 tumors, sCA-MIRTX (MIRTX loading: 24 µg/injection), sCA-NC (negative control miRNA loading: 24 µg/injection), or iNaD-MIRTX (MIRTX loading: 3 µg/injection) was intravenously administered on days 0, 1, 3, 4, 5, 6, 7, 8, and 10. The tumors treated with iNaD-MIRTX were significantly smaller than those treated with sCA-NC or no treatment on day 11 (Figure 6B). Although sCA-MIRTX treatment resulted in a smaller tumor volume than sCA-NC or no treatment, the difference was not significant. The iNaD-MIRTX treatment resulted in a significant decrease in tumor weight on day 11 compared to no treatment and sCA-NC treatment (Figure 6C). To further verify the in vivo efficacy of MIRTX, we produced Panc-1 tumors on mice and administered sCA-NC (negative control miRNA loading: 24 µg/injection), sCA-MIRTX (MIRTX loading: 24 µg/injection), or iNaD-MIRTX (MIRTX loading: 3 µg/injection) on days 0, 1, and 2, followed by quantitative real-time RT-PCR and western blot analysis of CXCR2 and PIK3R1 on day 3 (Figure 6D), which we reported as targets of MIRTX [15]. The three repeated injections of iNaD-MIRTX led to a considerable decrease in the CXCR2 and PIK3R1 protein expression compared to sCA-MIRTX (Figure 6D). Although CXCR2 and PIK3R1 mRNA expression in tumors treated with iNaD-MIRTX was significantly decreased compared with control, they had no statistical significance when compared with those treated with sCA-NC (Supplementary Figure S2). These findings suggest that MIRTX suppressed translation of CXCR2 and PIK3R1 mRNA to the proteins.

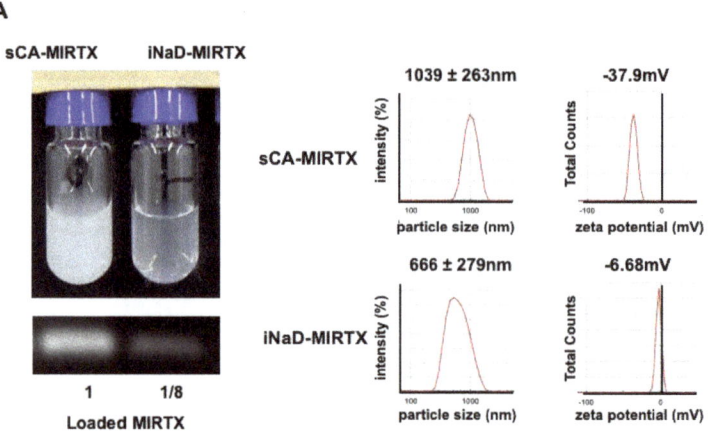

Figure 6. *Cont.*

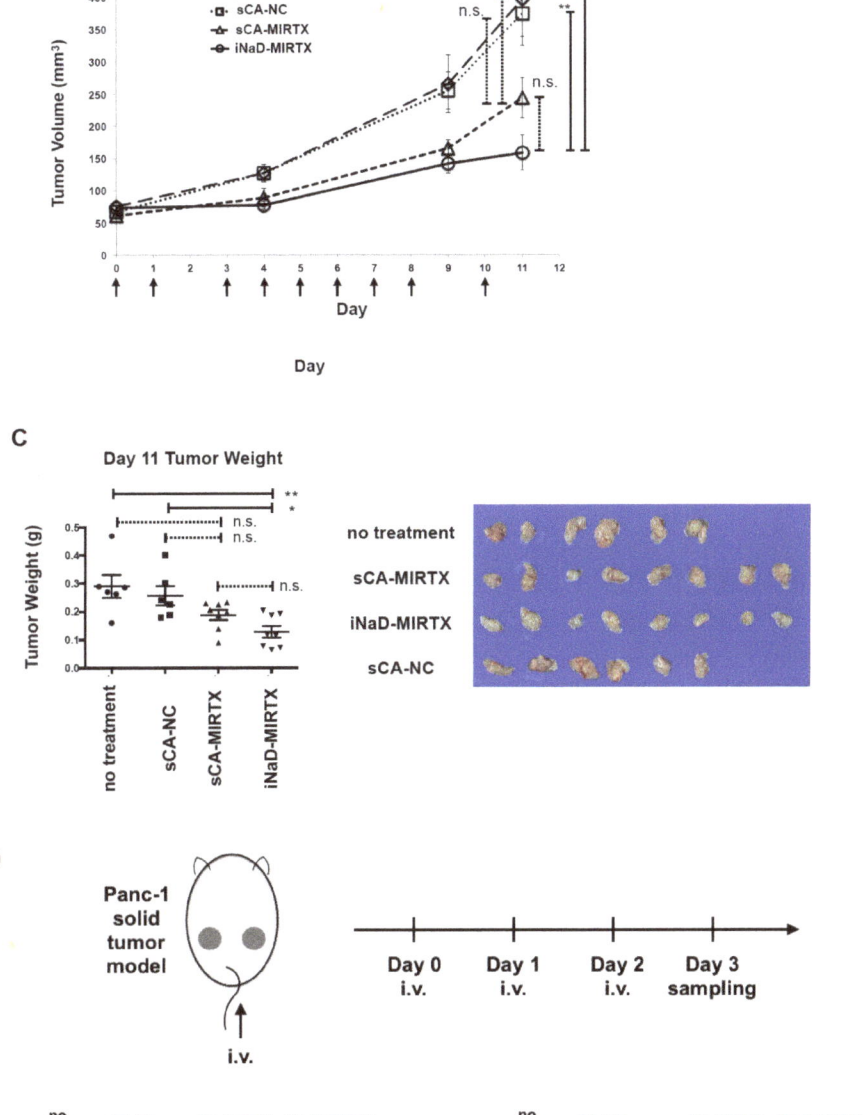

Figure 6. Anti-tumor effect of iNaD-MIRTX. (**A**) sCA-MIRTX and iNaD-MIRTX were prepared for one intravenous injection, followed by measurement of loaded MIRTX, DLS, and zeta potential analysis. The MIRTX loading of sCA-MIRTX was 24 µg,

and that of iNaD-MIRTX was 8 µg. (**B**) Therapeutic model of Panc-1 tumors. sCA-MIRTX (MIRTX loading: 24 µg/injection), sCA-NC (negative control miRNA loading: 24 µg/injection), or iNaD-MIRTX (MIRTX loading: 3 µg/injection) was intravenously administered on days 0, 1, 3, 4, 5, 6, 7, 8, and 10. Data represent mean ± SEM (n = 6–8 tumors from 3–4 mice). ** $p < 0.01$, n.s. = not significant, one-way ANOVA with Tukey's multiple comparisons test. (**C**) Tumor weight on day 11. Data represent mean ± SEM (n = 6–8 tumors from 3–4 mice). * $p < 0.05$, ** $p < 0.01$, n.s. = not significant, one-way ANOVA with Tukey's multiple comparisons test. (**D**) Mice were administered with sCA-MIRTX (MIRTX loading: 24 µg/injection) or iNaD-MIRTX (MIRTX loading: 3 µg/injection) on days 0, 1, and 2. Tumors were removed on day 3, and western blot analysis for CXCR2 and PIK3R1 was performed (n = 1–2 tumors from 2 mice for each group).

3.6. Bio-Distribution in Rheumatoid Arthritis Mice

Vascular permeability is an essential part of EPR and was first discovered through research on inflammation [38], raising the possibility of iNaD as a delivery vector to inflammatory lesions. To investigate whether iNaD has this ability, we performed an imaging experiment on inflammatory lesions using SKG/Jcl mice, a well-established genetic model of rheumatoid arthritis (RA) [39]. Mannan-injected SKG/Jcl mice exhibit many features of RA, beginning with joint swelling and developing into chronic destructive arthritis at the ankles and tail base, including joint ankylosis and deformity. Joint swelling was monitored by inspection and scored (Figure 7A). sCA-miRNA (24 µg of Alexa Fluor 750-labeled miRNA) or iNaD-miRNA (3 µg of Alexa Fluor 750-labeled miRNA) was intravenously administered to the tail tips of high arthritis score RA mice (severe swelling of the left and right ankles, RA score = 1 + 1; Figure 7B). iNaD-miRNA-treated mice exhibited more fluorescence at the swelling wrists, ankles, and tail base than mice treated with sCA-miRNA 40 min after intravenous injection (Figure 7C). iNaD-miRNA exhibited little fluorescence in the liver, whereas sCA-miRNA exhibited high liver accumulation, which is the substantial problem with sCA (Figure 7D).

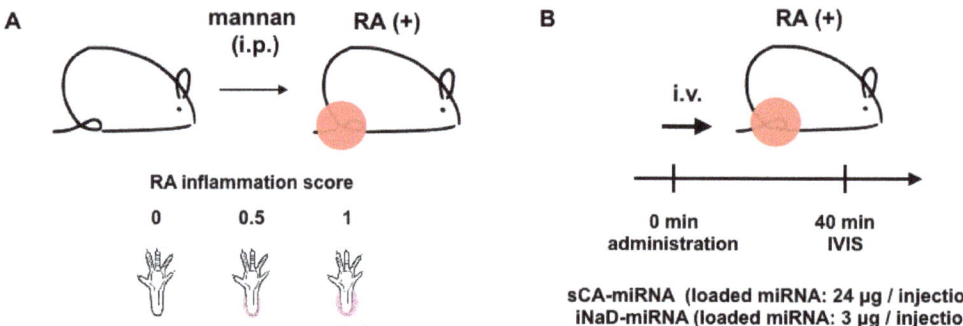

Figure 7. *Cont.*

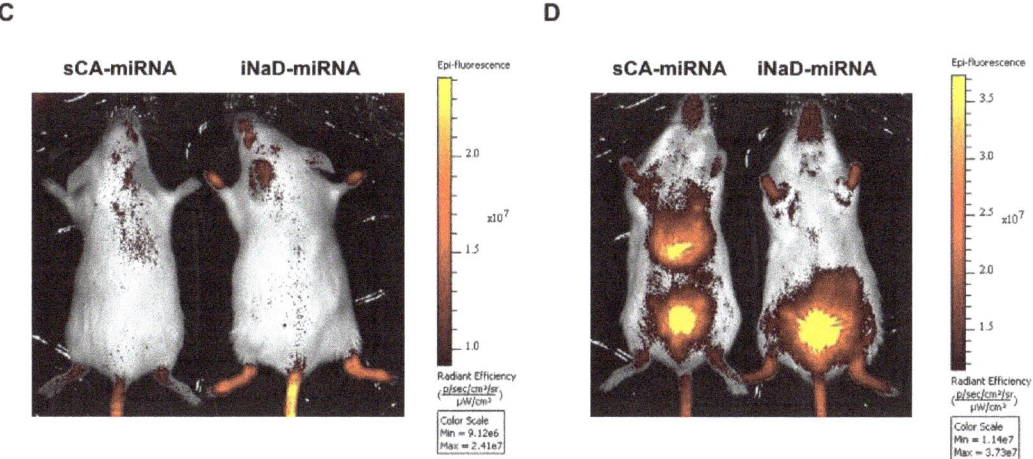

Figure 7. Bio-distribution in rheumatoid arthritis mice. (**A**) Female SKG/Jcl mice aged 8 weeks were given intraperitoneal injections (20 mg) of mannan suspended in 500 mL saline. Joint swelling was monitored by inspection and scored as 0 (no joint swelling), 0.5 (mild swelling of the ankle), or 1.0 (severe swelling of the ankle). (**B**) sCA-miRNA (loading: 24 µg of Alexa Fluor 750-labeled miRNA/injection) or iNaD-miRNA (loading: 3 µg of Alexa Fluor 750-labeled miRNA/injection) was intravenously administered into the tail tips of high arthritis score RA mice (severe swelling of the left and right ankles, RA score = 1 + 1). (**C**,**D**) IVIS imaging 40 min after the injection (C: back, D: abdomen). Left: sCA-miRNA-injected mouse. Right: iNaD-miRNA-injected mouse. Fluorescence from the miRNA accumulated in the liver of sCA-miRNA mice and was noted in the urine (bladder) of both mice.

4. Discussion

Aggregation at an early stage of crystallization is a common problem with the calcium phosphate (CaP) precipitation method, and microparticles are inevitably formed during the process. Instead of using PEGylation or complex modifications, we have disrupted the aggregation of carbonate apatite particles using bath sonication (38 kHz), resulting in the generation of 10 to 20 nm sCA nanoparticles for in vivo use [10]. To reduce microparticles, we demonstrated a novel combination method of PEG blending during the particle generation process followed by ultrasonic pulverization using high-frequency (1 MHz) AFA technology. Generally, PEGylation improves drug bioavailability, providing targeting ability by binding biologics. To control the growth of CaP-based nanoparticles, several studies have reported strategies to control the size by coating them with PEG [40–42]. However, the PEG blending alone was insufficient to reduce the particle size (Supplementary Figure S3). Furthermore, we failed to increase the uptake of Alexa 750-conjugate pegylated sCA-siRNA complex in the mouse xenograft model, which is different from that given by the iNaD-siRNA complex (data not shown).

Another feature of PEG is its sensitivity to degradation upon ultrasound sonication [43,44], which generates cavitation bubbles that collapse, producing pressures and shear forces [45]. Micelles of a di-block copolymer composed of poly(ethylene oxide) and poly(2-tetrahydropyranyl methacrylate) in aqueous solution are disrupted by high-frequency ultrasound (1.1 MHz) [46]. Thus, we hypothesized that AFA treatment with high-frequency (1 MHz) ultrasonic acoustic energy would improve the pulverization efficiency for sCA nanoparticles in concordance with the destruction of PEG, turning microparticles into nanoparticles. We added methoxy-PEG-CO(CH$_2$)$_2$COO-NHS (Mw 10,000), which is supposed to target the OH group of sCA ($[Ca_{10}(PO_4)^{6-X}(CO_3)^X(OH)_2]$) during the production process, and subsequent AFA treatment dramatically reduced the particle size without damaging the incorporated miRNA (Figure 3B and Supplementary Figure S1). When we measured the amount of PEG blended by ^{1}H NMR using di-sodium fumarate as the internal control, 1.2–1.8% (w/w) of methoxy-PEG-CO(CH$_2$)$_2$COO-NHS was contained in the iNaD particles (Supplementary Table S2). With this new approach, we have successfully reduced the microparticles of sCA into 600 to 700 nm nanoparticles with one peak.

Nanoparticles < 100 nm in diameter are thought to be optimal for tumor delivery [8,26]. The size of lipid- or polymer-based nanoparticles for systemic RNA delivery to tumors in clinical trials is almost 100 nm [8,35]. We had anticipated that smaller particles (<100 nm) would be produced from microparticles, but we found that the iNaD nanoparticles of approximately 700 nm in diameter can efficiently deliver siRNA/miRNA to tumors with little accumulation in normal tissues compared to the sCA system [11–20,22–25].

Recent nanomedicines designed to be 10–100 nm in diameter are expected to increase the accumulation of drugs in tumor tissues by utilizing the EPR effect. On the other hand, EnGeneIC Dream Vectors (EDVs) are bacterially derived 400 nm minicells [36]. In 2014, TargomiRs (EnGeneIC Dream Vectors) loaded with miR-16-based mimic miRNA underwent a phase I clinical trial in patients with malignant pleural mesothelioma and non-small-cell lung cancer who had failed standard therapies (ClinicalTrials.gov Identifier NCT02369198) [37]. This study provided important safety data, with an encouraging response and survival in patients with malignant pleural mesothelioma, and is expected to continue to a phase II study. Furthermore, bacteria of 1–2 μm in diameter (e.g., *Lactobacillus* sp. and *Salmonella typhimurium*) have also been reported to accumulate in tumors by virtue of the EPR effect [47–49]. Therefore, the EPR effect concept never limits the size of nanoparticles suitable for tumor delivery. The concept results from the extravasation of macromolecules through the vascular tumor, explaining the unique anatomical architecture surrounded by the dynamic pathophysiological reaction caused by vascular mediators (NO, kinin, PGs, cytokines, etc.) [38,50]. Thus, the optimal nanoparticle size could dynamically fluctuate due to the vascular mediators. Though 100 nm nanoparticles represent the majority of nanotechnology for cancer therapy, the larger nanoparticles may have a promising advantage. Compared to 100 nm particles, 700 nm particles should load much more siRNA/miRNA. According to the clinicaltrial.gov database, through the year 2019, 75 cancer nanomedicines were under clinical investigation in 190 clinical trials [51]. The success of phase 1 trials has been as high as 94%. However, the success rate drops to ~48% among completed phase 2 trials and slumps to a mere ~14% in phase 3 trials. The analyses have indicated that the main reasons for these failures are poor efficacy rather than toxicity. Enhancing the EPR effect allows more nanoparticles to be delivered to tumors, which can improve the therapeutic effects [38,52], whereas engineering larger nanoparticles, such as EDVs or iNaD, increases RNA loading efficiency and results in a successful outcome of cancer therapy. As shown in Figure 6, our in vivo functional validation findings on the effect of iNaD-MIRTX are consistent with a potent in vivo tumor inhibitory effect by iNaD-MIRTX, even though the loaded amount of MIRTX is much less on iNaD compared with sCA-MIRTX (3 μg vs. 24 μg).

Considering laboratory practice, the use of AFA may be a limitation in this study. In this regard, liposome-based delivery is easy to use. However, a common feature of recent RNA carriers, which include liposomes and polymers, is that in vivo systemic administration often results in accumulation in the liver, spleen, kidney, or lung [53–55]. The CaP-based system can avoid immunogenic reaction and is safe [24]. Indeed, carbonate apatite is utilized in dental clinics [56,57]. Nanomedicines with positive surface charges are easily bound to the vascular endothelial cells [58], whereas highly negatively charged nanoparticles tend to be taken up by the reticuloendothelial system in the liver and spleen [59]. Accordingly, the ideal surface charge of nanomedicines should be neutral or slightly negative [50]. Thus, the slightly negative zeta potential of iNaD may contribute to its lack of accumulation in the liver. This study firstly advocated a basic concept about 'PEG blending' to establish a clinically applicable CaP-based system. To make this system more simplified, we are currently underway to develop the second iNaD system that maintains PEG blending but does not necessitate an AFA device.

5. Conclusions

We successfully established a novel method for generating 700 nm CaP-based particles via high-frequency ultrasonic pulverization combined with PEG blending. This method has high disruption ability with little damage to loaded miRNA. This study is the first to demonstrate that 700 nm nanoparticles achieve high miRNA delivery efficiency to tumors and less accumulation in normal tissues. The findings provide new insights for engineering RNA nanoparticles and promote clinical translation of cancer nanomedicines.

Supplementary Materials: The following are available online at https://www.mdpi.com/article/10.3390/jpm11111160/s1, Figure S1: Atomic force microscopy analysis, Figure S2: Quantitative real-time RT-PCR analysis of mRNA expression in tumors, Figure S3: PEG blending during the production of sCA-miRNA. Table S1: Human specific Forward (F) and Reverse (R) primer sequences used for quantitative real-time RT-PCR analysis, Table S2: Quantification of PEG of sCA blended with PEG by ^{1}H NMR.

Author Contributions: Conceptualization, X.W. and H.Y. (Hirofumi Yamamoto); Investigation, X.W., Y.Y., S.K. (Shihori Kouda), H.Y. (Hiroyuki Yamamoto), J.W., Y.M., T.H., A.S., A.I., M.O. and S.S.; Methodology, K.M., S.K. (Shogo Kobayashi) and S.A.; Supervision, H.T., S.K. (Shogo Kobayashi), S.A. and H.Y. (Hirofumi Yamamoto); Validation, S.K. (Shihori Kouda), H.Y. (Hiroyuki Yamamoto), J.W., A.S. and S.S.; Writing–original draft, X.W.; Writing–review & editing, X.W. and H.Y. (Hirofumi Yamamoto). All authors have read and agreed to the published version of the manuscript.

Funding: This research was funded by Kagoshima Shinsangyo Sousei Investment Limited Partnership, grant number CST14001 and Grant-in-Aid for Scientific Research (A), JSPS KAKENHI Grant Number 18H04059.

Institutional Review Board Statement: Studies using mouse models were conducted in strict accordance with the recommendations of the Guide for the Care and Use of Laboratory Animals of the Graduate School of Medicine, Osaka University. The protocol was approved by the Committee for the Ethics of Animal Experiments of Osaka University (Permit Number: 27-085-017).

Informed Consent Statement: Not applicable.

Data Availability Statement: Not applicable.

Conflicts of Interest: The authors declare no conflict of interest.

References

1. Bray, F.; Ferlay, J.; Soerjomataram, I.; Siegel, R.L.; Torre, L.A.; Jemal, A. Global cancer statistics 2018: GLOBOCAN estimates of incidence and mortality worldwide for 36 cancers in 185 countries. *CA Cancer J. Clin.* **2018**, *68*, 394–424. [CrossRef]
2. Petros, R.A.; DeSimone, J.M. Strategies in the design of nanoparticles for therapeutic applications. *Nat. Rev. Drug Discov.* **2010**, *9*, 615–627. [CrossRef]
3. Davis, M.E.; Chen, Z.G.; Shin, D.M. Nanoparticle therapeutics: An emerging treatment modality for cancer. *Nat. Rev. Drug Discov.* **2008**, *7*, 771–782. [CrossRef]
4. Matsumura, Y.; Maeda, H. A new concept for macromolecular therapeutics in cancer chemotherapy: Mechanism of tumoritropic accumulation of proteins and the antitumor agent smancs. *Cancer Res.* **1986**, *46 Pt 1*, 6387–6392.
5. Mitchell, M.J.; Billingsley, M.M.; Haley, R.M.; Wechsler, M.E.; Peppas, N.A.; Langer, R. Engineering precision nanoparticles for drug delivery. *Nat. Rev. Drug Discov.* **2021**, *20*, 101–124. [CrossRef]
6. Roberts, T.C.; Langer, R.; Wood, M.J.A. Advances in oligonucleotide drug delivery. *Nat. Rev. Drug Discov.* **2020**, *19*, 673–694. [CrossRef]
7. Roma-Rodrigues, C.; Rivas-García, L.; Baptista, P.V.; Fernandes, A.R. Gene Therapy in Cancer Treatment: Why Go Nano? *Pharmaceutics* **2020**, *12*, 233. [CrossRef] [PubMed]
8. Mainini, F.; Eccles, M.R. Lipid and Polymer-Based Nanoparticle siRNA Delivery Systems for Cancer Therapy. *Molecules* **2020**, *25*, 2692. [CrossRef] [PubMed]
9. O'Neill, C.P.; Dwyer, R.M. Nanoparticle-Based Delivery of Tumor Suppressor microRNA for Cancer Therapy. *Cells* **2020**, *9*, 521. [CrossRef] [PubMed]
10. Wu, X.; Yamamoto, H.; Nakanishi, H.; Yamamoto, Y.; Inoue, A.; Tei, M.; Hirose, H.; Uemura, M.; Nishimura, J.; Hata, T.; et al. Innovative delivery of siRNA to solid tumors by super carbonate apatite. *PLoS ONE* **2015**, *10*, e0116022. [CrossRef]
11. Takeyama, H.; Yamamoto, H.; Yamashita, S.; Wu, X.; Takahashi, H.; Nishimura, J.; Haraguchi, N.; Miyake, Y.; Suzuki, R.; Murata, K.; et al. Decreased miR-340 expression in bone marrow is associated with liver metastasis of colorectal cancer. *Mol. Cancer Ther.* **2014**, *13*, 976–985. [CrossRef] [PubMed]

12. Takahashi, H.; Nishimura, J.; Kagawa, Y.; Kano, Y.; Takahashi, Y.; Wu, X.; Hiraki, M.; Hamabe, A.; Konno, M.; Haraguchi, N.; et al. Significance of Polypyrimidine Tract-Binding Protein 1 Expression in Colorectal Cancer. *Mol. Cancer Ther.* **2015**, *14*, 1705–1716. [CrossRef] [PubMed]
13. Ogawa, H.; Wu, X.; Kawamoto, K.; Nishida, N.; Konno, M.; Koseki, J.; Matsui, H.; Noguchi, K.; Gotoh, N.; Yamamoto, T.; et al. MicroRNAs Induce Epigenetic Reprogramming and Suppress Malignant Phenotypes of Human Colon Cancer Cells. *PLoS ONE* **2015**, *10*, e0127119. [CrossRef] [PubMed]
14. Hiraki, M.; Nishimura, J.; Takahashi, H.; Wu, X.; Takahashi, Y.; Miyo, M.; Nishida, N.; Uemura, M.; Hata, T.; Takemasa, I.; et al. Concurrent Targeting of KRAS and AKT by MiR-4689 Is a Novel Treatment Against Mutant KRAS Colorectal Cancer. *Mol. Ther. Nucleic Acids* **2015**, *4*, e231. [CrossRef]
15. Inoue, A.; Mizushima, T.; Wu, X.; Okuzaki, D.; Kambara, N.; Ishikawa, S.; Wang, J.; Qian, Y.; Hirose, H.; Yokoyama, Y.; et al. A miR-29b Byproduct Sequence Exhibits Potent Tumor-Suppressive Activities via Inhibition of NF-kappaB Signaling in KRAS-Mutant Colon Cancer Cells. *Mol. Cancer Ther.* **2018**, *17*, 977–987. [CrossRef]
16. Morimoto, Y.; Mizushima, T.; Wu, X.; Okuzaki, D.; Yokoyama, Y.; Inoue, A.; Hata, T.; Hirose, H.; Qian, Y.; Wang, J.; et al. miR-4711-5p regulates cancer stemness and cell cycle progression via KLF5, MDM2 and TFDP1 in colon cancer cells. *Br. J. Cancer* **2020**, *122*, 1037–1049. [CrossRef] [PubMed]
17. Fukata, T.; Mizushima, T.; Nishimura, J.; Okuzaki, D.; Wu, X.; Hirose, H.; Yokoyama, Y.; Kubota, Y.; Nagata, K.; Tsujimura, N.; et al. The Supercarbonate Apatite-MicroRNA Complex Inhibits Dextran Sodium Sulfate-Induced Colitis. *Mol. Ther. Nucleic Acids* **2018**, *12*, 658–671. [CrossRef]
18. Aoki, M.; Aoki, H.; Mukhopadhyay, P.; Tsuge, T.; Yamamoto, H.; Matsumoto, N.M.; Toyohara, E.; Okubo, Y.; Ogawa, R.; Takabe, K. Sphingosine-1-Phosphate Facilitates Skin Wound Healing by Increasing Angiogenesis and Inflammatory Cell Recruitment with Less Scar Formation. *Int. J. Mol. Sci.* **2019**, *20*, 3381. [CrossRef]
19. Aoki, M.; Matsumoto, N.M.; Dohi, T.; Kuwahawa, H.; Akaishi, S.; Okubo, Y.; Ogawa, R.; Yamamoto, H.; Takabe, K. Direct Delivery of Apatite Nanoparticle-Encapsulated siRNA Targeting TIMP-1 for Intractable Abnormal Scars. *Mol. Ther. Nucleic Acids* **2020**, *22*, 50–61. [CrossRef]
20. Takahashi, H.; Misato, K.; Aoshi, T.; Yamamoto, Y.; Kubota, Y.; Wu, X.; Kuroda, E.; Ishii, K.J.; Yamamoto, H.; Yoshioka, Y. Carbonate Apatite Nanoparticles Act as Potent Vaccine Adjuvant Delivery Vehicles by Enhancing Cytokine Production Induced by Encapsulated Cytosine-Phosphate-Guanine Oligodeoxynucleotides. *Front. Immunol.* **2018**, *9*, 783. [CrossRef]
21. Tamai, K.; Mizushima, T.; Wu, X.; Inoue, A.; Ota, M.; Yokoyama, Y.; Miyoshi, N.; Haraguchi, N.; Takahashi, H.; Nishimura, J.; et al. Photodynamic Therapy Using Indocyanine Green Loaded on Super Carbonate Apatite as Minimally Invasive Cancer Treatment. *Mol. Cancer Ther.* **2018**, *17*, 1613–1622. [CrossRef] [PubMed]
22. Merhautova, J.; Demlova, R.; Slaby, O. MicroRNA-Based Therapy in Animal Models of Selected Gastrointestinal Cancers. *Front. Pharmacol.* **2016**, *7*, 329. [CrossRef] [PubMed]
23. Takahashi, R.U.; Prieto-Vila, M.; Kohama, I.; Ochiya, T. Development of miRNA-based therapeutic approaches for cancer patients. *Cancer Sci.* **2019**, *110*, 1140–1147. [CrossRef]
24. Abd-Aziz, N.; Kamaruzman, N.I.; Poh, C.L. Development of MicroRNAs as Potential Therapeutics against Cancer. *J. Oncol.* **2020**, *2020*, 8029721. [CrossRef] [PubMed]
25. Forterre, A.; Komuro, H.; Aminova, S.; Harada, M. A Comprehensive Review of Cancer MicroRNA Therapeutic Delivery Strategies. *Cancers* **2020**, *12*, 1852. [CrossRef] [PubMed]
26. Pecot, C.V.; Calin, G.A.; Coleman, R.L.; Lopez-Berestein, G.; Sood, A.K. RNA interference in the clinic: Challenges and future directions. *Nat. Rev. Cancer* **2011**, *11*, 59–67. [CrossRef]
27. Blanco, E.; Shen, H.; Ferrari, M. Principles of nanoparticle design for overcoming biological barriers to drug delivery. *Nat. Biotechnol.* **2015**, *33*, 941–951. [CrossRef]
28. Perrault, S.D.; Walkey, C.; Jennings, T.; Fischer, H.C.; Chan, W.C. Mediating tumor targeting efficiency of nanoparticles through design. *Nano Lett.* **2009**, *9*, 1909–1915. [CrossRef]
29. Cabral, H.; Matsumoto, Y.; Mizuno, K.; Chen, Q.; Murakami, M.; Kimura, M.; Terada, Y.; Kano, M.R.; Miyazono, K.; Uesaka, M.; et al. Accumulation of sub-100 nm polymeric micelles in poorly permeable tumours depends on size. *Nat. Nanotechnol.* **2011**, *6*, 815–823. [CrossRef]
30. Tejera-Garcia, R.; Ranjan, S.; Zamotin, V.; Sood, R.; Kinnunen, P.K. Making unilamellar liposomes using focused ultrasound. *Langmuir* **2011**, *27*, 10088–10097. [CrossRef]
31. Hermeking, H. p53 enters the microRNA world. *Cancer Cell* **2007**, *12*, 414–418. [CrossRef]
32. Hong, D.S.; Kang, Y.K.; Borad, M.; Sachdev, J.; Ejadi, S.; Lim, H.Y.; Brenner, A.J.; Park, K.; Lee, J.L.; Kim, T.Y.; et al. Phase 1 study of MRX34, a liposomal miR-34a mimic, in patients with advanced solid tumours. *Br. J. Cancer* **2020**, *122*, 1630–1637. [CrossRef] [PubMed]
33. Agostini, M.; Knight, R.A. miR-34: From bench to bedside. *Oncotarget* **2014**, *5*, 872–881. [CrossRef] [PubMed]
34. Tazawa, H.; Tsuchiya, N.; Izumiya, M.; Nakagama, H. Tumor-suppressive miR-34a induces senescence-like growth arrest through modulation of the E2F pathway in human colon cancer cells. *Proc. Natl. Acad. Sci. USA* **2007**, *104*, 15472–15477. [CrossRef]
35. Setten, R.L.; Rossi, J.J.; Han, S.P. The current state and future directions of RNAi-based therapeutics. *Nat. Rev. Drug Discov.* **2019**, *18*, 421–446. [CrossRef]

36. MacDiarmid, J.A.; Mugridge, N.B.; Weiss, J.C.; Phillips, L.; Burn, A.L.; Paulin, R.P.; Haasdyk, J.E.; Dickson, K.A.; Brahmbhatt, V.N.; Pattison, S.T.; et al. Bacterially derived 400 nm particles for encapsulation and cancer cell targeting of chemotherapeutics. *Cancer Cell* **2007**, *11*, 431–445. [CrossRef]
37. van Zandwijk, N.; Pavlakis, N.; Kao, S.C.; Linton, A.; Boyer, M.J.; Clarke, S.; Huynh, Y.; Chrzanowska, A.; Fulham, M.J.; Bailey, D.L.; et al. Safety and activity of microRNA-loaded minicells in patients with recurrent malignant pleural mesothelioma: A first-in-man, phase 1, open-label, dose-escalation study. *Lancet Oncol.* **2017**, *18*, 1386–1396. [CrossRef]
38. Maeda, H.; Nakamura, H.; Fang, J. The EPR effect for macromolecular drug delivery to solid tumors: Improvement of tumor uptake, lowering of systemic toxicity, and distinct tumor imaging in vivo. *Adv. Drug Deliv. Rev.* **2013**, *65*, 71–79. [CrossRef]
39. Yoshitomi, H.; Sakaguchi, N.; Kobayashi, K.; Brown, G.D.; Tagami, T.; Sakihama, T.; Hirota, K.; Tanaka, S.; Nomura, T.; Miki, I.; et al. A role for fungal {beta}-glucans and their receptor Dectin-1 in the induction of autoimmune arthritis in genetically susceptible mice. *J. Exp. Med.* **2005**, *201*, 949–960. [CrossRef]
40. Kakizawa, Y.; Furukawa, S.; Kataoka, K. Block copolymer-coated calcium phosphate nanoparticles sensing intracellular environment for oligodeoxynucleotide and siRNA delivery. *J. Control. Release* **2004**, *97*, 345–356. [CrossRef]
41. Giger, E.V.; Puigmartí-Luis, J.; Schlatter, R.; Castagner, B.; Dittrich, P.S.; Leroux, J.C. Gene delivery with bisphosphonate-stabilized calcium phosphate nanoparticles. *J. Control. Release* **2011**, *150*, 87–93. [CrossRef]
42. Pittella, F.; Miyata, K.; Maeda, Y.; Suma, T.; Watanabe, S.; Chen, Q.; Christie, R.J.; Osada, K.; Nishiyama, N.; Kataoka, K. Pancreatic cancer therapy by systemic administration of VEGF siRNA contained in calcium phosphate/charge-conversional polymer hybrid nanoparticles. *J. Control. Release* **2012**, *161*, 868–874. [CrossRef]
43. Wang, R.; Murali, V.S.; Draper, R. Detecting Sonolysis of Polyethylene Glycol Upon Functionalizing Carbon Nanotubes. *Methods Mol. Biol.* **2017**, *1530*, 147–164.
44. Kawasaki, H.; Takeda, Y.; Arakawa, R. Mass spectrometric analysis for high molecular weight synthetic polymers using ultrasonic degradation and the mechanism of degradation. *Anal. Chem.* **2007**, *79*, 4182–4187. [CrossRef]
45. Suslick, K.S. Sonochemistry. *Science* **1990**, *247*, 1439–1445. [CrossRef]
46. Wang, J.; Pelletier, M.; Zhang, H.; Xia, H.; Zhao, Y. High-frequency ultrasound-responsive block copolymer micelle. *Langmuir* **2009**, *25*, 13201–13205. [CrossRef] [PubMed]
47. Zhao, M.; Yang, M.; Li, X.M.; Jiang, P.; Baranov, E.; Li, S.; Xu, M.; Penman, S.; Hoffman, R.M. Tumor-targeting bacterial therapy with amino acid auxotrophs of GFP-expressing Salmonella typhimurium. *Proc. Natl. Acad. Sci. USA* **2005**, *102*, 755–760. [CrossRef]
48. Zhao, M.; Yang, M.; Ma, H.; Li, X.; Tan, X.; Li, S.; Yang, Z.; Hoffman, R.M. Targeted therapy with a Salmonella typhimurium leucine-arginine auxotroph cures orthotopic human breast tumors in nude mice. *Cancer Res.* **2006**, *66*, 7647–7652. [CrossRef] [PubMed]
49. Fang, J.; Liao, L.; Yin, H.; Nakamura, H.; Shin, T.; Maeda, H. Enhanced bacterial tumor delivery by modulating the EPR effect and therapeutic potential of Lactobacillus casei. *J. Pharm. Sci.* **2014**, *103*, 3235–3243. [CrossRef] [PubMed]
50. Fang, J.; Islam, W.; Maeda, H. Exploiting the dynamics of the EPR effect and strategies to improve the therapeutic effects of nanomedicines by using EPR effect enhancers. *Adv. Drug Deliv. Rev.* **2020**, *157*, 142–160. [CrossRef]
51. He, H.; Liu, L.; Morin, E.E.; Liu, M.; Schwendeman, A. Survey of Clinical Translation of Cancer Nanomedicines-Lessons Learned from Successes and Failures. *Acc. Chem. Res.* **2019**, *52*, 2445–2461. [CrossRef]
52. Islam, W.; Fang, J.; Imamura, T.; Etrych, T.; Subr, V.; Ulbrich, K.; Maeda, H. Augmentation of the Enhanced Permeability and Retention Effect with Nitric Oxide-Generating Agents Improves the Therapeutic Effects of Nanomedicines. *Mol. Cancer Ther.* **2018**, *17*, 2643–2653. [CrossRef] [PubMed]
53. Kim, S.H.; Jeong, J.H.; Lee, S.H.; Kim, S.W.; Park, T.G. Local and systemic delivery of VEGF siRNA using polyelectrolyte complex micelles for effective treatment of cancer. *J. Control. Release* **2008**, *129*, 107–116. [CrossRef]
54. Zuckerman, J.E.; Choi, C.H.; Han, H.; Davis, M.E. Polycation-siRNA nanoparticles can disassemble at the kidney glomerular basement membrane. *Proc. Natl. Acad. Sci. USA* **2012**, *109*, 3137–3142. [CrossRef] [PubMed]
55. Takeshita, F.; Minakuchi, Y.; Nagahara, S.; Honma, K.; Sasaki, H.; Hirai, K.; Teratani, T.; Namatame, N.; Yamamoto, Y.; Hanai, K. Efficient delivery of small interfering RNA to bone-metastatic tumors by using atelocollagen in vivo. *Proc. Natl. Acad. Sci. USA* **2005**, *102*, 12177–12182. [CrossRef] [PubMed]
56. Kudoh, K.; Fukuda, N.; Kasugai, S.; Tachikawa, N.; Koyano, K.; Matsushita, Y.; Ogino, Y.; Ishikawa, K.; Miyamoto, Y. Maxillary Sinus Floor Augmentation Using Low-Crystalline Carbonate Apatite Granules With Simultaneous Implant Installation: First-in-Human Clinical Trial. *J. Oral Maxillofac. Surg.* **2019**, *77*, 985.e1–985.e11. [CrossRef]
57. Nakagawa, T.; Kudoh, K.; Fukuda, N.; Kasugai, S.; Tachikawa, N.; Koyano, K.; Matsushita, Y.; Sasaki, M.; Ishikawa, K.; Miyamoto, Y. Application of low-crystalline carbonate apatite granules in 2-stage sinus floor augmentation: A prospective clinical trial and histomorphometric evaluation. *J. Periodontal Implant Sci.* **2019**, *49*, 382–396. [CrossRef]
58. Campbell, R.B.; Fukumura, D.; Brown, E.B.; Mazzola, L.M.; Izumi, Y.; Jain, R.K.; Torchilin, V.P.; Munn, L.L. Cationic charge determines the distribution of liposomes between the vascular and extravascular compartments of tumors. *Cancer Res.* **2002**, *62*, 6831–6836.
59. Li, S.D.; Huang, L. Pharmacokinetics and biodistribution of nanoparticles. *Mol. Pharm.* **2008**, *5*, 496–504. [CrossRef]

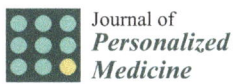

Review

A Critical Review of Radiation Therapy: From Particle Beam Therapy (Proton, Carbon, and BNCT) to Beyond

Yoshitaka Matsumoto [1,2,*], Nobuyoshi Fukumitsu [3], Hitoshi Ishikawa [4], Kei Nakai [1,2] and Hideyuki Sakurai [1,2]

1. Department of Radiation Oncology, Clinical Medicine, Faculty of Medicine, University of Tsukuba, Tsukuba 305-8575, Japan; knakai@pmrc.tsukuba.ac.jp (K.N.); hsakurai@pmrc.tsukuba.ac.jp (H.S.)
2. Proton Medical Research Center, University of Tsukuba Hospital, Tsukuba 305-8576, Japan
3. Department of Radiation Oncology, Kobe Proton Center, Kobe 650-0047, Japan; fukumitsun@yahoo.co.jp
4. National Institute of Quantum and Radiological Science and Technology Hospital, Chiba 263-8555, Japan; ishikawa.hitoshi@qst.go.jp
* Correspondence: ymatsumoto@pmrc.tsukuba.ac.jp; Tel.: +81-29-853-7100

Abstract: In this paper, we discuss the role of particle therapy—a novel radiation therapy (RT) that has shown rapid progress and widespread use in recent years—in multidisciplinary treatment. Three types of particle therapies are currently used for cancer treatment: proton beam therapy (PBT), carbon-ion beam therapy (CIBT), and boron neutron capture therapy (BNCT). PBT and CIBT have been reported to have excellent therapeutic results owing to the physical characteristics of their Bragg peaks. Variable drug therapies, such as chemotherapy, hormone therapy, and immunotherapy, are combined in various treatment strategies, and treatment effects have been improved. BNCT has a high dose concentration for cancer in terms of nuclear reactions with boron. BNCT is a next-generation RT that can achieve cancer cell-selective therapeutic effects, and its effectiveness strongly depends on the selective ^{10}B accumulation in cancer cells by concomitant boron preparation. Therefore, drug delivery research, including nanoparticles, is highly desirable. In this review, we introduce both clinical and basic aspects of particle beam therapy from the perspective of multidisciplinary treatment, which is expected to expand further in the future.

Keywords: particle beam therapy; proton beam therapy; carbon-ion beam therapy; boron neutron capture therapy; combination therapy; drug delivery

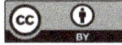

1. Background: Particle Beam Therapy as a Novel Radiotherapy

1.1. Promotion and Expansion of Particle Therapy Facilities

Particle beam therapy is a type of radiotherapy (RT). Particle beam therapy delivers a high radiation dose to tumors and as technology has improved, enables antitumor effects. The application of drug therapy is an integral part of development. We review the present status and future aspects of particle beam therapy in terms of drug therapy. Proton beam therapy (PBT) and carbon-ion beam therapy (CIBT) are common particle beam therapies. In 1946, Wilson suggested for the first time the use of accelerated protons in radiation therapy (RT) [1]. He investigated the depth-dose profile of protons accelerated at the cyclotron in Berkeley (CA, USA) and observed a steep increase in energy deposition at the end of the particle range, which is known as the Bragg peak. In 1958, the first clinical use of accelerated protons in the pituitary gland of 26 patients with advanced breast cancer was reported by the Lawrence Radiation Laboratory in Berkeley [2]. Several clinical studies have been conducted in the following decades. However, they were performed in a physics laboratory; thus, they had little beam time, and beam lines were not necessarily designed for medical use. The first medical treatment facilities to use PBT were constructed at the Clatterbridge Oncology Center (UK) in 1989, which uses a cyclotron and at Loma Linda University (CA, USA) in 1990, which uses a synchrotron. The first medical treatment facility for CIBT was initiated in HIMAC in Chiba (Japan), in 1994. As of 2019, over

250,000 patients have been treated with particle therapy (proton and carbon-ion [C-ion] beams). The number of treatment facilities has rapidly increased in recent years. Currently, treatment is provided at 100 facilities worldwide. The United States has the highest number with 40 facilities, followed by Japan with 24 facilities, Germany with seven facilities, and Russia with five facilities. There are 95 PBT facilities and 12 CIBT facilities [3]. Japan has more than 20 particle therapy facilities on its small land area and is one of the countries where particle therapy is becoming increasingly popular (Figure 1).

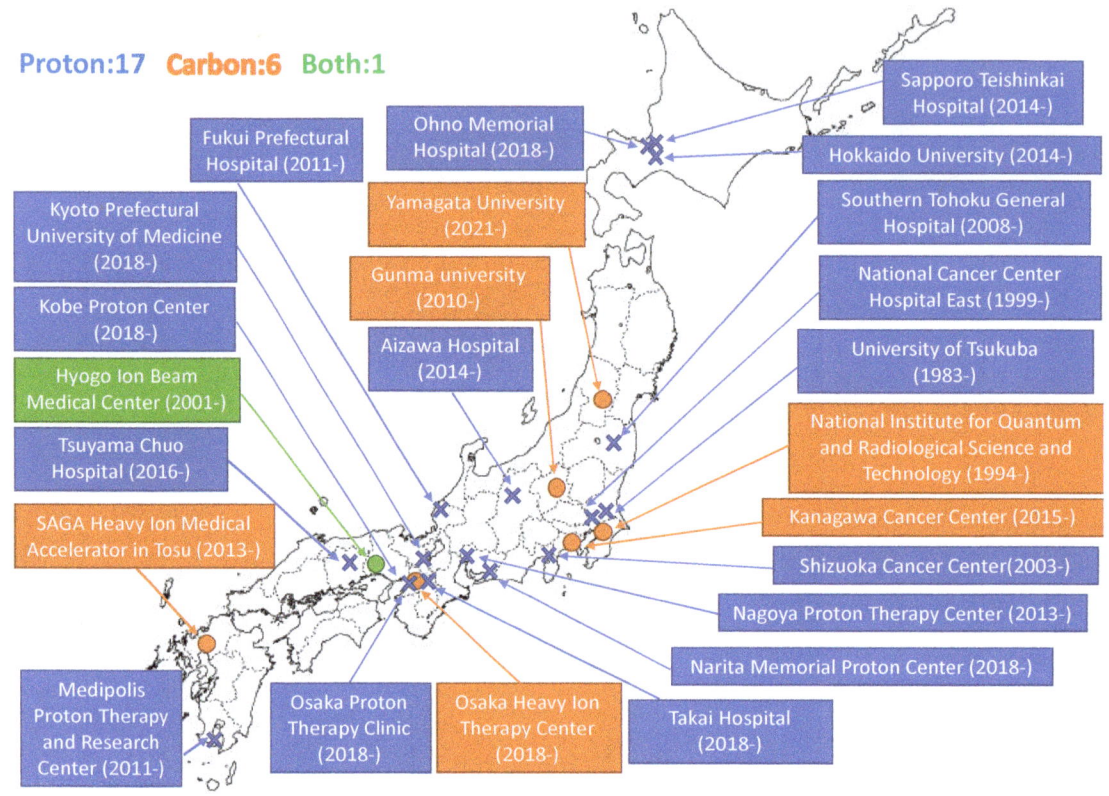

Figure 1. Expansion of particle beam therapy facility in Japan.

1.2. Physical Aspects of Particle Therapy

The dose distributions of protons and C-ions largely differ from those of photons, which are used in conventional RT. The biggest difference in physical characteristics is the existence of depth-dose distribution, the so-called Bragg peak, and by having this characteristic, particle beam therapy can give the maximum energy to the surroundings near the stop (cancer part) (Figure 2a). Although the dose distributions of protons and C-ions are very similar, the difference is that C-ion beams have narrower penumbra and longer fragmentation tails than proton beams [4].

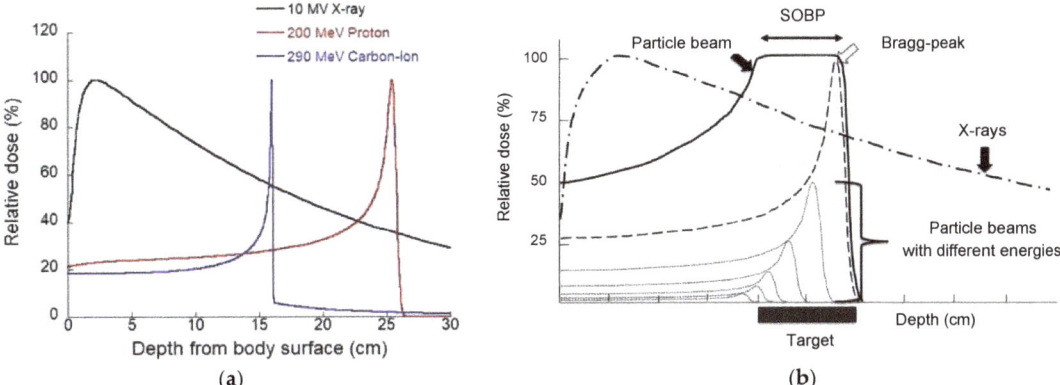

Figure 2. (a) Depth-dose distributions of clinical X-ray, proton, and carbon-ion beams and (b) the spread-out Bragg peak (SOBP).

In particle therapy, an extended Bragg peak (spread-out Bragg peak; SOBP) is formed to fit this Bragg peak to the size of the cancer (Figure 2b). Beam formation technology has evolved dramatically in recent years, and an increasing number of facilities are introducing an active scanning system (ASS) in addition to the conventional passive scattering system (PSS). PSS uses a rotating scatterer to expand the beam vertically and horizontally, and a collimator and bolus are used to optimize the beam to the cancer shape in front of the patient [5]. In contrast, the ASS uses a thin pencil beam, which is deflected vertically and horizontally by electromagnets, and the depth can be adjusted by changing the energy of the accelerator [6]. The advantage of the active scanning technique is its application in complexly shaped target volumes and reduction in the cost of manufacturing patient-specific devices, such as compensators, and the disadvantage is its larger lateral penumbra [7–11].

1.3. Biological Aspects of Particle Therapy

The concept of quality and quantity is important to understand the biological effects of PBT. The quality of PBT is defined as the amount of energy transferred per track (linear energy transfer; LET). Radiation with high LET can cause more severe damage to cells, represented by complex DNA damage that is difficult to repair. A parameter that quantitatively expresses the difference in biological effects due to this difference in LET is the relative biological effectiveness (RBE), which is defined as the dose ratio between the reference photon radiation and the particle radiation that produces the same biological effect. The international standard for proton RBE is 1.1; however, recent studies have shown that the distal end of a proton-SOBP shows a slightly higher RBE value depending on the increase in LET [12]. In contrast, carbon lines with high LET show high RBE values, with approximately 1.5 as the biological RBE and 3.0 as the clinical RBE [4,13,14]. Furthermore, it is important to recognize that although RBE is a useful parameter for expressing relative effects, its value may vary depending on the biological endpoint and the level of biological effect [15]. In addition, it is known that C-ions with higher LET radiation have a killing effect on hypoxic and generally radioresistant tumors [16]. The biological effect of radiation is enhanced in the presence of oxygen (oxygen effect) [17]. The oxygen enhancement ratio (OER) is a parameter that indicates the difference in biological effects depending on the presence or absence of oxygen. The OER is expressed as the ratio of the absorbed doses required to induce the same biological effect with and without oxygen. RBE and OER are LET-dependent variables (Figure 3), and the higher the LET, the higher the RBE, which reaches its maximum at approximately 100–200 keV/μm and then decreases (overkill effect). The OER shows a value of approximately 2.5–3.0 at low LET and asymptotically approaches 1 at high LET. High RBE [15,18–21] and low OER [16,22–24] values are characteristic biological properties of heavy-ion beams with high LETs.

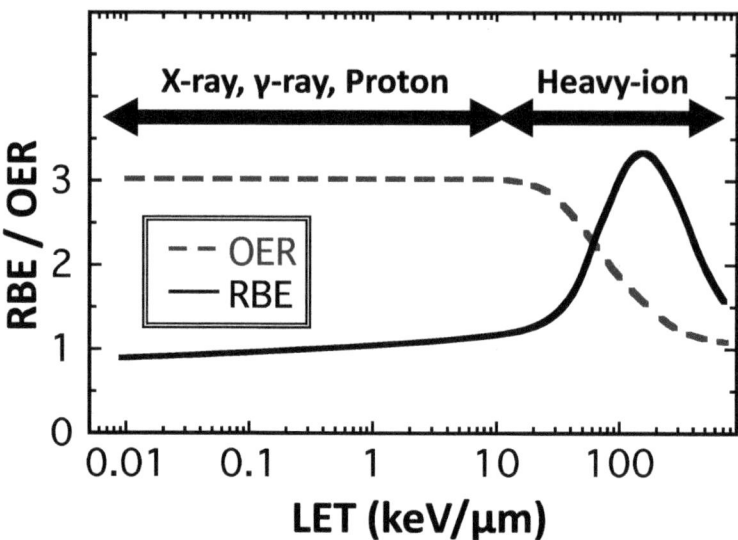

Figure 3. Relationship between RBE, OER, and LETs.

2. The Role of Particle Beam Therapy in Multidisciplinary Treatments in Clinics

This chapter outlines particle beam therapy, which is often used in combination with drug therapy.

2.1. Esophageal Cancer

In 2020, it was estimated that 18,440 new patients developed esophageal cancer and 16,170 died in the United States [25]. Hence, the case fatality risk of esophageal cancer is still high, and the disease is currently the sixth leading cause of cancer-related deaths [26]. The gold standard treatment for localized esophageal cancer is surgery. However, some patients are unfit for surgery because of their advanced tumors (unresectable), poor general conditions (medically inoperable), refusal to undergo surgery, and concurrent chemoradiotherapy (CCRT) is considered for them as an alternative curative treatment to surgery [27]. However, cardiopulmonary toxicities after CCRT using photon beams are still associated with late adverse effects and would disturb the administration of high-dose chest irradiation in the treatments for esophageal and lung cancers [28,29]. Especially, a standard total irradiation dose in the treatment for esophageal cancer (50.4 Gy in 28 fractions) is less than that for lung cancer (60 Gy in 30 fractions) because larger irradiation fields are necessary to entirely cover the primary tumor and regional lymph nodes of thoracic esophageal cancers [30]. It is known that local and/or regional recurrences are the most frequent failure patterns after CCRT for esophageal cancer [31] and there are significant relationships between cardiopulmonary toxicity and irradiated volumes and doses in the lung and heart [32,33]. Therefore, dose escalation to the target while avoiding unnecessary doses to the lung and heart is a reasonable approach to improve treatment outcomes for esophageal cancer.

PBT offers advantageous physical properties to RT for the treatment of various cancers and can reduce the radiation dose and irradiated volume in organs at risk, such as the lung and heart, in RT for esophageal cancer compared with photon therapy [34,35]. We initially reported the usefulness of PBT alone or a PBT boost following photon RT without concurrent chemotherapy for patients with unresectable esophageal cancer [36]. In the case of PBT alone, the median total dose was 80 Gy RBE (Gy [RBE]), but patients were given a median dose of 46 Gy using photons with a boost to 80 Gy (RBE) using protons. Thereafter, CCRT using cisplatin/5 fluorouracil added to a median dose of 60 Gy (RBE) using PBT alone was performed in 40 patients, and no grade 3 cardiopulmonary toxicities were observed in our recent study [37]. In a Japanese multicenter retrospective study, clinical outcomes obtained from 202 patients (195 with squamous cell carcinoma and seven with adenocarcinoma) treated between 2009 and 2013 at four institutes were investigated. The 5-year rates of overall survival (OS) and local control of patients with stages I and II were 75.4% and 74.0%, respectively, and the corresponding rates of stages III and IV were 36.8% and 53.8%, respectively. Furthermore, grade 3 cardiopulmonary toxicities were observed in only three (1.5%) patients [38]. Table 1 shows that the incidence of cardiopulmonary toxicities in CCRT for esophageal cancer after PBT was less than that after photon RT [39–43]. A recent randomized study compared the total toxicity burden (TTB) and progression-free survival (PFS) between intensity-modulated radiotherapy (IMRT) and PBT and revealed that there was no significant difference in PFS between the two arms. However, the mean TTB, which was the other primary endpoint of the study, was 2.3 times higher for IMRT (39.9; 95% highest posterior density interval, 26.2–54.9) than for PBT (17.4; 10.5–25.0) and the PBT arm experienced numerically fewer cardiopulmonary toxicities and postoperative complications [43].

Table 1. Cardiopulmonary toxicities of photon RT and PBT for esophageal cancer.

Author	N	RT Modality	Treatment	Endpoint	Late Toxicity Rate	
					Heat	Lung
DeCesaris [15]	36	Photon RT	Preope/definitive	Perioperative death	13.9%	
	18	Proton			0%	
Wang [6]	320	IMRT	Preope/definitive	Grade 3 (2y/5y)	18%/21%	NA
	159	Proton			11%/13%	NA
Wang [17]	208	3DCRT	Preoperative	Perioperative complication	15.9%	30.3%
	164	IMRT			17.1%	23.8%
	72	Proton			9.7%	13.9%
Makishima [10]	19	3DCRT	Definitive	Grade 3	0%	10.3%
	25	Proton			0%	0%
Xi [18]	211	IMRT	Preope/definitive	Grade 3	2.4%	4.7%
	132	Proton			0.8%	2.3%
Lin [19]	61	IMRT	Preope/definitive	Grade 3	5 *	11 *
	46	Proton			3 *	5 *

RT, radiotherapy; IMRT, intensity-modulated radiotherapy; 3DCRT, three-dimensional conformal radiotherapy; NA, not assessed; *, number of events.

Recently, the impact of maintaining host immunity on patient survival has brought focus on CCRT for esophageal cancer, and lymphocyte count during CCRT may be a representative landmark for predicting survival [44,45]. Since PBT avoids unnecessary doses to the body of patients compared with photon RT, the studies showed that lymphocyte counts during PBT were well maintained and OS after PBT tended to be better than that after photon RT [45,46]. A pencil beam scanning method that provides a better dose distribution than passive scattering, which reduces the doses to the normal tissues close to the target, is currently available at most institutes, and future prospective studies may further confirm the true efficacy including survival outcomes of PBT for esophageal cancer.

2.2. Pancreatic Cancer

Pancreatic cancer is well known as one of the cancers with a poor prognosis and remains challenging to treat. According to a survey, there are an estimated 57,600 new patients and 47,050 deaths worldwide annually [26]. Surgery is the gold standard for the curative treatment of pancreatic cancer, and chemotherapy for pancreatic cancer has made great strides in the last few decades. The role of RT is to control local lesions, such as original tumors and locoregional lymph node metastases. Since the pancreas is surrounded by organs that are at risk, such as the stomach and duodenum, it is difficult to deliver a higher radiation dose for conventional photon RT. Therefore, particle beam therapy, which has an excellent dose concentration, is highly recommended for the treatment of pancreatic cancer and is mainly used for curative therapy of unresectable diseases and preoperative therapy for resectable diseases.

There have been few reports of particle beam therapy for pancreatic cancer before 2010, but it has been increasing rapidly since then. This is largely due to advances in chemotherapy and technological advances in particle beam therapy. Table 2 shows a review of concurrent PBT combined with chemotherapy for pancreatic cancer. Hong et al. conducted preoperative CCRT using proton beams and capecitabine in 25 patients with resectable pancreatic cancer and reported a 75% 1-year OS rate in 2011 [47]. After that, some clinical studies using proton beams commonly combined with capecitabine, gemcitabine, 5-FU, and S-1, have been reported, and Hong et al. reported a 2-year OS rate of 42% in their subsequent report in 2014 [48]. In the curative treatment for the unresectable or borderline resectable disease, the 1- and 2-year OS rates after PBT were 62–77.5% and 40–50.8%, respectively [49–52]. Maemura et al. performed induction chemotherapy followed by CCRT using proton beams. In their study, gemcitabine was used for induction therapy, and S-1 was concurrently combined. The irradiation dose was either a standard dose of 50 Gy or escalated dose of 67.5 Gy (RBE) with 25 fractions and achieved a 1-year OS rate of 80% [53]. Regarding toxicity, gastrointestinal ulcers have been reported as a late adverse event in some studies [48,49,53]. Pancreatic cancer using CIBT has been reported at several institutions in Japan, and Kawashiro et al. summarized the data as a retrospective multi-institutional study [54]. They investigated 72 patients whose irradiation dose was 52.8 and 55.2 Gy (RBE) with 12 fractions and concurrent chemotherapy was performed in 56 patients using gemcitabine or S-1. The OS rates were 73% and 46% at 1 and 2 years, respectively, and late adverse events (ulcers) were found in one patient. Using in vitro and in vivo studies, Sai et al. demonstrated that C-ion beam combined with gemcitabine had a superior potential to kill pancreatic cancer stem-like cells [55]. Chemotherapy for pancreatic cancer has improved prognosis with the advent of gemcitabine and has since been further improved with the combination of other drugs, such as nab-paclitaxel [56,57]. In addition, FOLFIRINOX has been demonstrated to have a higher antitumor effect than gemcitabine [58]. To date, the use of FOLFIRINOX in combination with particle beam therapy has been uncertain due to its strong side effects, however, in Europe, a prospective study on the combination of FOLFIRINOX as induction therapy for preoperative CIBT was conducted [59]. With regard to the technical progress of particle beam therapy, the concomitant boost [49,50,52,60], active scanning [61], and layer-stacking boost techniques [62] have been attempted.

Table 2. Concurrent particle beam therapy combined with chemotherapy for pancreatic cancer.

Author	N	RT	Dose	Chemotherapy	Treatment	Outcome
Hong [46]	25	proton	30GyRBE/10fr 25GyRBE/5fr	capecitabine	preoperative	OS: 75%/1Y
Terashima [48]	50	proton	50GyRBE/25fr 70.2GyRBE/26fr 67.5GyRBE/25fr	gemcitabine	curative	OS: 76.8%/1Y, PFS: 64.3%/1Y
Hong [47]	50	proton	25GyRBE/5fr	capecitabine	preoperative	OS: 42%/2Y
Maemura [52]	10	proton	50GyRBE/25fr 67.5GyRBE/25fr	gemcitabine, S-1	curative	OS: 80, 45, 22.5%/1, 2, 3Y
Kim [49]	37	proton	45GyRBE/10fr	capecitabine, 5-FU	curative	OS: 75.7%/1Y, PFS: 64.8%/1Y, 19.3M
Jethea [50]	13	proton	50GyRBE/25fr	capecitabine, 5-FU	curative	OS: 62, 40%/1, 2Y, 16M
Hiroshima [51]	42	proton	50–67.5GyRBE/25-33fr	gemcitabine, S-1	curative	OS: 77.5, 50.8%/1, 2Y, 25.6M
Kawashiro [53]	72	carbon	52.8GyRBE/12fr 55.2GyRBE/12fr	gemcitabine, S-1 (n = 56)	curative	OS: 73, 46%/1, 2Y, 21.5M
Vitolo [58]		carbon	38.4GyRBE/4fr	FOLFIRINOX, gemcitabine	preoperative	

Value in outcome represents overall survival rate, progression-free survival rate, and median survival time. OS: overall survival, PFS: progression-free survival.

2.3. Prostate Cancer

Prostate cancer (PC) screening and early diagnosis using prostate-specific antigen have indicated that there are approximately 192,000 new patients per year in the US [26]. In Japan, the annual number of newly diagnosed patients also increases every year, and over 12,500 PC-related deaths were estimated in 2019 [63]. Furthermore, almost half of Japanese patients with PC are over 75 years old, and RT plays an important role as a representative nonsurgical and curative treatment, especially for elderly patients. Since PC control after RT is dose-dependent [64], recent advances in modern RT techniques, including IMRT and brachytherapy, under image guidance can provide successful treatment outcomes by allowing delivery of higher doses to the prostate with less toxicity to the organs at risk, such as the rectum and bladder, compared with conventional three-dimensional conformal RT [65,66].

Protons and C-ions are charged particles and have been used for PC treatment through particle therapy for several decades. PBT was initially used as a tool for dose escalation after photon RT. The first randomized study compared the results between photon RT and PBT in patients with advanced PC. In the study, patients in the standard-dose and high-dose groups were treated with pelvic RT at 50.4 Gy/28 fr, followed by local photon RT at 16.8 Gy/8 fr (total dose: 67.2 Gy/36 fr) and local PBT at 25.2 Gy equivalents (GyRBE)/12 fr (total dose: 75.6 GyRBE/40 fr), respectively, and a better local control was achieved in the high-dose PBT group than in the standard-dose photon RT group (8-year local control rate: 73% vs. 59%) [67]. In addition, the incidence of grade 3 rectal bleeding was recorded in only 2.9% of the patients in the high-dose PBT group, although the corresponding rate of RTOG9413 using pelvic RT followed by local photon boost was 4.3% despite using a 70.2 Gy dose (5.4 Gy lower than the abovementioned 75.6 Gy PBT dose in the randomized study) [68].

The PROG95-09 trial tested a prostate PBT boost of either 19.8 GyRBE/11 fr (standard-dose group) or 28.8 GyRBE/16 fr (high-dose group) following 50.4 Gy/28 fr by local photon RT without regional irradiation for patients with stage T1–2 PC; the 10-year biochemical failures were observed in 32.4% and 16.7% of patients in the standard-dose and high-dose groups, respectively ($p < 0.0001$) [69]. Regarding toxicity, there were no significant differences between the standard-dose and high-dose groups; grade 3 gastrointestinal (GI) and genitourinary (GU) events were only noted in 1% and 2% of patients in the high-dose group, respectively, and 0% and 2% in the standard-dose group, respectively. At almost the same time, a randomized trial was conducted to determine the effectiveness of dose escalation using photon RT. The 10-year recurrence-free rates in the standard-dose group (70 Gy/35 fr) and in the high-dose group (78 Gy/39 fr) were 50% and 73%, respectively ($p = 0.004$); however, grade 3 GI and GU adverse events in the high-dose group were observed in 3.3% and 6.6% of patients, respectively, suggesting higher event rates compared with those in the 79.2 GyRBE dose of the high-dose group in the PROG95-09 trial described above [70] (Table 3).

Table 3. Clinical outcomes of photon and PBT trials for prostate cancer.

Author	N	RT Modality	Total Dose (Gy)	Photon (Gy)	Proton (GyRBE)	Efficacy (%)	Late toxicity (Grade 3) (%)	
							GI	GU
Shipley [67]	202	Photon +Proton	75.6 67.2	50.4 (pelvis) 50.4 (pelvis) + 16.8 (local)	25.2 (local)	8y-LC:73	2.9	NA
		Photon			-	59	0	NA
Roach [68]	440	Photon	70.2 70.2	50.4 (pelvis) + 19.8 (local) 70.2 (local)		7y-PFS:40	4.3	3
		Photon				27	0	0
Local prostate irradiation								
Zeitman [69]	393	Photon +Proton	79.2 70.2	50.4 (local) 50.4 (local)	28.8 (local)	10y-bRF:83	1	2
		Photon +Proton			19.8 (local)	67	0	2
Kuban [70]	301	Photon	78.0 70.0	78.0 (local) 78.0 (local)		10y-FFF:73	7	3
		Photon				50	1	5

GI, gastrointestinal; GU, genitourinary; LC, local control; PFS, progression-free survival; bRF, biochemical relapse-free; FFF, freedom from any failures.

In the same period, the efficacy of a combination of androgen deprivation therapy (ADT) with RT for intermediate- and high-risk patients with PC on not only disease control but also overall survival was shown in a randomized trial [71] and high-dose local PBT without photon RT yielded favorable outcomes regarding both PC control and adverse effects [72]. The clinical outcomes of local high-dose PBT combined with ADT were equal to or superior to those of local high-dose photon RT or PBT combined with pelvic or prostate RT. Furthermore, C-ions have been used for patients with PC as a local RT since 1995 at the National Institute of Quantum and Radiological Science and Technology Hospital, and the optimal RT dose and appropriate use of ADT in CIBT for PC have been investigated through several clinical trials [73]. At present, ADT is combined with CIBT for 2–6 months in intermediate-risk PC patients and for 2 years in high-risk PC patients based on previous phase I/II and II clinical trials; however, the appropriate indication criteria and duration of ADT use for PC in combination with high-dose RT, including PBT and CIBT, remains unknown.

Multi-institutional cohort studies involving four Japanese institutes were conducted to determine the appropriate use of ADT combined with PBT, and 520 intermediate-risk and 555 high-risk PC patients treated with PBT between 2008 and 2011 were analyzed [74]. Overall, the use of short-term ADT for ≤6 months improved the biochemical recurrence-free survival (bRFS), but no benefit of ADT for> 6 months was observed. The effectiveness of short-term ADT on bRFS was more evident in patients with two or three intermediate-risk factors than in those with a single factor. In contrast, short-term ADT for ≤6 months did not improve bRFS in the high-risk group. The study revealed that ADT for 12 and 21 months is preferable for patients with single and multiple risk factors, respectively, with high-dose PBT. Since ADT may cause dysfunction in lipid, glucose, and mineral metabolisms, especially in the elderly, prospective studies are necessary to determine the optimal ADT use and avoid unnecessary ADT administration in combination with high-dose RT for patients with PC.

2.4. Pediatric Cancer

The large difference between radiation therapy for aged patients and pediatric patients is the possibility of several complications. The following are typical complications and various complications that have been studied using photon RT: (1) Reproductive dysfunction: Sex cells are highly radiosensitive, and it is said that sperm cell depletion and morphological abnormalities can occur even at 10 cGy or less. Sanders et al. reported that 463 boys received total body irradiation of 10, 12, 14, and 15.5 Gy, and only five (1%) became fathers [75]. The Childhood Cancer Survivor Study (CCSS) examined 1915 patients after treatment for pediatric cancers, and the rate of miscarriage increased 3.6 times in cases with whole-brain and whole-spinal irradiation and 1.7 times in cases with pelvic irradiation [76]. (2) Cardiac complications: According to a CCSS, the relative risk of death from cardiac complications was as high as 11.9 (95% confidence interval (CI): 9.1–15. (3) in 2717 five-year-old or older survivors after chemotherapy for pediatric Hodgkin lymphoma. In cases where the mediastinum was irradiated with 42 Gy or more, it was reported to be 41.5 (95% CI: 18.1–82.1) [77]. PBT has a superior dose concentration with cytotoxicity equivalent to photons; thus, it is expected to be utilized for the treatment of patients with pediatric cancer. Moreover, although there are few clinical reports because secondary cancers develop years–decades later, PBT is expected to reduce secondary cancers. In Japan, PBT for patients with pediatric cancer became the first medical insurance coverage for all cancer diseases in 2016, which indicates high expectations for pediatric cancer treatment.

PBT is used for the treatment of cancers, such as brain tumors, neuroblastoma, and soft tissue tumors. PBT is not often administered alone and is often multidisciplinary with surgery or chemotherapy. Glioma, medulloblastoma, ependymoma, germinoma, and craniopharyngioma make up a lot of brain tumors. Eaton et al. compared the treatment results of photon RT and PBT for pediatric medulloblastoma. Both treatment protocols were the same as craniospinal and focal irradiation, with vincristine, cisplatin, cyclophosphamide, and lomustine. Second cancers were found in three of 43 patients in the photon RT group and none of the 45 in the PBT group [78]. They also investigated the endocrine result of photon RT and PBT in 77 patients and reported hypothyroidism as 69% and 23%, sex hormone deficiency as 19% and 3%, and any endocrine replacement therapy as 78% and 55%, respectively, and concluded that PBT may reduce the risk of some endocrine abnormalities [79]. Rhabdomyosarcoma (RMS) is a high-grade tumor characterized by local invasiveness and is the most common soft tissue sarcoma in pediatric patients. RMS can occur all over the body; however, the most common sites are the head and neck, followed by the pelvis. RMS is treated using a multidisciplinary approach. Clinical experiences in the treatment of pediatric RMS with PBT indicated safety and effectiveness with low acute toxicities and disease control comparable to photon irradiation [80–82]. Mizumoto et al. retrospectively summarized data from a multicenter study in Japan and reported the clinical outcome of 55 children aged 0–19 years (median, 5 years) who received PBT for RMS with doses ranging from 36–60 Gy (RBE). Surgical resection before PBT was performed in 41 patients (75%), and 53 patients (96%) received chemotherapy. The number of patients that enrolled during pre-PBT, pre- PBT and during PBT, and only during PBT was 17, 34, and two patients, respectively. The median follow-up time was 24.5 months. Acute toxicity of more than grade 3 was found in 16% of the patients, but they recovered well after PBT. A total of 87% of the patients experienced hematologic toxicities more than grade 3, which were very likely to be related to PBT [83].

3. Current Basic Research on Combination with Particle Therapy

3.1. Combination Therapy

In recent years, the content and quality of cancer treatment have been greatly developed along with advancements in science and technology. In other words, the introduction of new therapeutic concepts and methods into clinical practice through the invention and improvement in medical devices that enable high-precision RT, such as particle beam therapy, has brought progress in the cancer treatment. Early detection of early-stage cancers using modern diagnostic imaging technologies contributes to the improvement in survival rates of cancer patients; however, the clinical outcomes of many advanced-stage cancers using a single treatment method remain disappointing. Therefore, a multidisciplinary treatment combining RT with surgery, chemotherapy, molecular targeted therapy, or immunotherapy has been tested, especially for advanced-stage cancers, for a long period. How can a combined protocol be adapted for particle beam therapy? Recent basic biological studies have reported the possibility that higher sensitization effects can be demonstrated with proton beams, which have similar biological effects to photon beams. However, it is expected that combination experiments with C-ions, rather than protons, will show unexpected results. In this section, we summarize the latest findings on the combined effects of particle RT and various cancer treatment modalities.

3.2. Chemotherapy

Chemotherapy is often combined with RT for advanced-stage cancers, given before (neoadjuvant), at the same time (concomitant), and after (adjuvant) RT, and the efficacy and feasibility of the combination therapy have been confirmed in most of them. Many of the goals of RT and chemotherapy combinations are to treat locally and systemically distributed cancers, respectively.

However, it is well known that a combination of drugs and radiation can have local synergistic effects. As a typical example, concurrent chemoradiotherapy consisting of photon RT combined with platinum compounds for head and neck squamous cell carcinoma had a significant benefit of OS with a 10% reduction, but neoadjuvant or adjuvant chemotherapy did not [84]. In contrast, heavy particle beams with a high LET have a smaller sensitizing effect by various chemotherapeutic agents than photon beams. The sensitizing effect of camptothecin, cisplatin, gemcitabine, and paclitaxel, which are frequently used in the field of RT, is remarkable for X-rays, but extremely small for C-ions of 103 keV/μm [85]. Similarly, when glioblastoma (GBM) cells were treated with carbon wire and temozolomide (TMZ), only additive effects were observed [86]. In contrast, a remarkable synergistic effect with a decrease in the shoulder of the cell survival curve was observed in S-phase human colon cancer-derived cells when antimetabolite gemcitabine (2′,2′-difluoro-2′-deoxycytidine, dFdCyd) was combined with C-ions [87]. Proton beams, which exhibit biological effects similar to those of photon beams, can be expected to be more effective in combination with chemotherapeutic agents than C-ions, and concurrent chemoradiotherapy using protons is widespread in clinical practice. However, in recent years, differences between X-rays and proton beams have been reported, such as in gene expression and protein levels due to various double-helix DNA cleavages and DNA responses and disorders in the process of cell death [88,89]. It has been reported that overall DNA damage differs to some extent after proton and X-ray irradiation and that proton-irradiated cells preferentially undergo homologous recombination [90]. This result suggests that the distribution of DNA repair types differs between protons and X-rays. Our research also confirmed that the recovery phenomenon is less likely to occur after proton irradiation than after X-ray irradiation [91]. Furthermore, it has been reported that the sensitizing effect of CDDP may differ between X-rays and protons [92]. The combination index for CDDP in the three types of cells was 0.82–1.00 by X-ray, whereas it was 0.73–0.89 by proton beam, indicating that the proton beam has a stronger sensitizing effect. Analysis using the Cell Cycle Indicator System (fluorescent ubiquitination-based cell cycle indicator or FUCCI) also showed that CDDP and proton beam increased apoptotic cells and G2/M arrest induction more significantly than X-rays. This difference was particularly pronounced in radiation-resistant cells, suggesting that chemoradiotherapy with X-rays and protons may have different effects on radiation-resistant cancers.

3.3. Molecular Targeted Therapy

The toxicity of normal tissues is often increased by chemoradiotherapy, limiting the amount of drug or radiation that can be administered [93]. This fact is far from ideal, and more effective and less toxic combination therapies are needed for the systemic therapy combined with radiation. Against this background, research and development of molecular-targeted drugs are underway. It specifically inhibits cell survival, information exchange with surrounding tissues, and signal transduction associated with responses to internal and external stresses, including radiation. Recent developments in the fields of biotechnology and cell biology have revealed and rapidly elucidated signal transduction and intracellular crosstalk.

A suitable target molecule for a drug used for RT should be overexpressed in many tumors to be treated and not in the normal tissue surrounding the tumor [94,95]. Molecules involved in the mechanism of radioresistance are also ideal. Given these conditions, good examples of reasonable targets related to RT include epidermal growth factor receptor (EGFR), vascular endothelial growth factor (VEGF), phosphatidylinositol-3-kinase/protein kinase B/mammalian target of rapamycin (PI3K/Akt/mTOR) pathway, Ras pathway, and histone deacetylation. The efficacy of these molecular-targeted drugs in combination with photon therapy has been demonstrated in both basic research and clinically, for example, with EGFR inhibitors.

Although there is insufficient clinical data on the use of particle beams in combination with molecularly targeted drugs and the efficacy of these drugs is not yet clear, many interesting data have been reported from basic biological experiments using cells and mice. The number of relevant studies has increased from approximately 30 in 2010 to over 140 in 2020. The combination of the proton beam and a VEGF inhibitor, bevacizumab, decreased cell survival, increased apoptosis levels, and cell cycle arrest in melanoma cells [96]. The EGFR inhibitor gefitinib preferentially sensitized non-small cell lung cancer cells (H460 and H1299) to proton radiation compared to gamma radiation [97]. Cetuximab (Cmab) also preferentially sensitizes cancer stem cells (SQ-20B/CSCs) isolated from head and neck squamous cell carcinoma (SQ-20B) to carbon beam irradiation compared to photon irradiation [98]. Furthermore, C-ions + Cmab strongly inhibits the enhanced invasion ability of SQ-20B/CSCs, and it has been suggested that the combination therapy is a very promising treatment that suppresses the migration and infiltration process of all cancers as well as CSCs. A PARP inhibitor (PARPi), AZD2281, enhanced the effect of protons on human lung cancer cells (A549) and pancreatic cancer cells (MIAPaCa-2), inducing an increase in γ-H2AX counts and an increase in G2/M arrest [99]. Another PARPi, olaparib and niraparib, sensitized the cytotoxic effects of protons on lung, pancreatic, esophageal, and head and neck cancer cells as well as on X-rays [100–102]. These inhibitors have sustained DNA damage from irradiation, delayed apoptosis, prolonged cell cycle arrest, promoted aging, and had more synergistic effects on cells with high proliferation rates. In addition, PARP inhibitors have been effective against C-ions, and the PARPi ADZ2281 enhances the cell-killing effect of carbon rays on pancreatic cancer cells [103]. The combination of talazoparib and carbon beams dramatically reduced the number of GBM stem cells (GSCs), induced prominent and long-term G2/M block, and reduced GSC proliferation [104]. Owing to its multifunctional role and low expression in normal cells, Hsp90 inhibitors are considered a good target for cancer therapy; however, there are few reports on its effects in combination with particle therapy, and we found two reports on its combination with carbon beams [105,106]. 17AAG enhanced the cytotoxic effect on lung cancer cells and the antitumor effect on lung cancer transplanted tumors after C-ions to the same extent as X-rays [105]. This sensitizing effect was due to the inhibition of homologous recombination repair by 17AAG, and as a result, the strong induction of G2 arrest was confirmed. The combination of C-ions with different LET (14 and 50 keV/μm) and another Hsp90 inhibitor, PU-H71, showed higher or similar enhancement ratios compared to X-rays [106]. This result suggests a dependence of the enhancement ratio of molecular-targeted drugs on LET. Valproic acid, a histone deacetylase inhibitor

(HDACi), sensitizes hepatocellular carcinoma cells to proton beams more strongly than photon beams by prolonging DNA damage and enhancing apoptosis [107]. In addition, Tsuboi et al. reported that another HDACi, suberoylanilide hydroxamic acid, enhanced the cell-killing effect of C-ions [108]. The combination of novel molecularly targeted drugs and particle radiotherapy has great potential to improve patient outcomes. However, the basic biological knowledge of this combination therapy is scarce, and further research is needed both in vitro and in vivo.

3.4. Nanoparticles

Metal nanoparticles (MNPs), such as gold and platinum, have been reported to exhibit radiosensitizing effects in photon-irradiated cells and animal models [109–111]. Experiments have shown that the mechanism is largely due to the interaction of photons with high-Z metal atoms to produce low-energy electrons (especially Auger electrons) [112,113], which in turn promotes the production of reactive oxygen species [114]. Currently, several attempts are being made to introduce nanoparticles into clinical practice.

However, because the interaction of charged particles is largely independent of the atomic number Z of the target, the sensitization of particle beams by MNPs is expected to be even smaller than that of photon beams. However, several experiments have confirmed the large sensitizing effect of the combination of proton beams with MNPs [114,115]. C-ions with high LET, in combination with magnetic nanoparticles, reduce the fluence per unit dose, making the probability of direct interaction at therapeutic doses unrealistic.

Furthermore, in recent years, the application of biomaterials, such as polymer nanofibers, for cancer treatment and drug delivery systems has increased [116,117]. Polymeric nanofibers are an exciting new class of materials and have attracted great attention because of their remarkable properties, such as high specific surface area, high porosity, high molecular alignment, and nano-size effects [118–120]. Additionally, many different types of molecules can be easily incorporated into nanofibers to greatly expand their drug-loading capacity or to provide a sustained release of the embedded drug molecules [121,122]. Nanofibers with continuous drug release properties that can enhance the efficacy of anticancer drugs, molecularly targeted drugs, and hyperthermia are being developed [116,123–125], and we believe that developments in this field will greatly benefit the sensitization of radiation.

3.5. Immunotherapy

The idea of using immunotherapy in combination with particle beam therapy is completely different from the combination of anticancer drugs and molecular-targeted drugs. It has been shown that local irradiation of tumors acts as an immune adjuvant and can elicit a systemic tumor immune response by killing tumor cells in situ [126–128]. Its basic mechanism is the induction of immunogenic cell death in the tumor microenvironment and the sequential activation of systemic cell-mediated immunity [129,130]. Danger signals and the release of tumor-specific antigens after ionizing radiation can turn the irradiated tumor into an in-situ vaccine. Recently, important angiogenic and immunosuppressive factors, such as vascular endothelial growth factor, interleukin 6 and 8, and hypoxia-inducing factor 1α, have been significantly downregulated after high-energy proton irradiation [131]. It has also been reported that proton irradiation mediates cell surface expression of calreticulin on tumor cells and increases susceptibility to cytotoxic T lymphocyte killing [132]. These findings suggest that PBT can inhibit angiogenesis and has an immunosuppressive mechanism, and thus, its therapeutic use can be expanded [133]. The C-ions correlated more with immune activation and prevention of metastasis in mouse models when used in combination with dendritic cell infusion [134–136]. In addition, in clinical cases, abscopal reactions have been reported in patients who received topical C-ion treatment [137,138].

In clinical studies using PBT, a phase I study in which an intratumoral injection of hydroxyapatite was used as an immune adjuvant after PBT was locally advanced or recurrent to prevent local or distant recurrence due to the activation of the immune system. It was performed in patients with hepatocellular carcinoma. The conditions of four of the nine patients were reported to have exacerbated [139]. Regarding C-ions, abscopal reactions have been reported in patients receiving topical C-ion treatment [137,138]. A promising approach to using this strategy to remove cancer cells that have spread to unirradiated areas is to combine particle therapy with immune system regulators, such as immune checkpoint inhibitors and cytokines. In addition, tumor-specific immune responses can be obtained by converting the tumor into an effective in situ vaccine using particle therapy.

4. Relationship between Boron Neutron Capture Therapy (BNCT) and Boron Compounds

4.1. The Principle of BNCT

The principle of boron neutron capture therapy was proposed four years after the discovery of neutrons by Chadwick in 1932 [140,141]. It uses ^{10}B, which has a large absorbable cross section for thermal neutrons. It is one of the RT classified as particle beam RT and is characterized by the external irradiation of thermal neutrons, which have no electric charge, and the use of high-LET particle beams (alpha rays and lithium nuclei) produced by the reaction of neutrons with ^{10}B in the body for cellular damage (treatment of malignant tumors). In principle, if boron can be directed to the target area, the reaction will occur only in that area and shows a cell-killing effect.

Briefly, it is common to use ^{10}B as a compound that reacts easily with thermal neutrons, that is, a compound with a large absorbable cross section (3850 barns, 1 barn = 10^{-24} cm^2). A ^{10}B compound with tumor-accumulating properties is administered intravenously to the organism beforehand. When ^{10}B has accumulated in the tumor, thermal neutrons are injected into the affected area by external irradiation. The neutrons react with ^{10}B to produce alpha rays (helium nuclei) and lithium nuclei (Figure 4). Both of these have a short range of approximately 10 microns (about the size of a cell) and can provide high energy without exceeding the diameter of the cell. The principle is that the more selective the distribution of ^{10}B to tumor cells, the less the damage to normal tissues and the higher the antitumor effect.

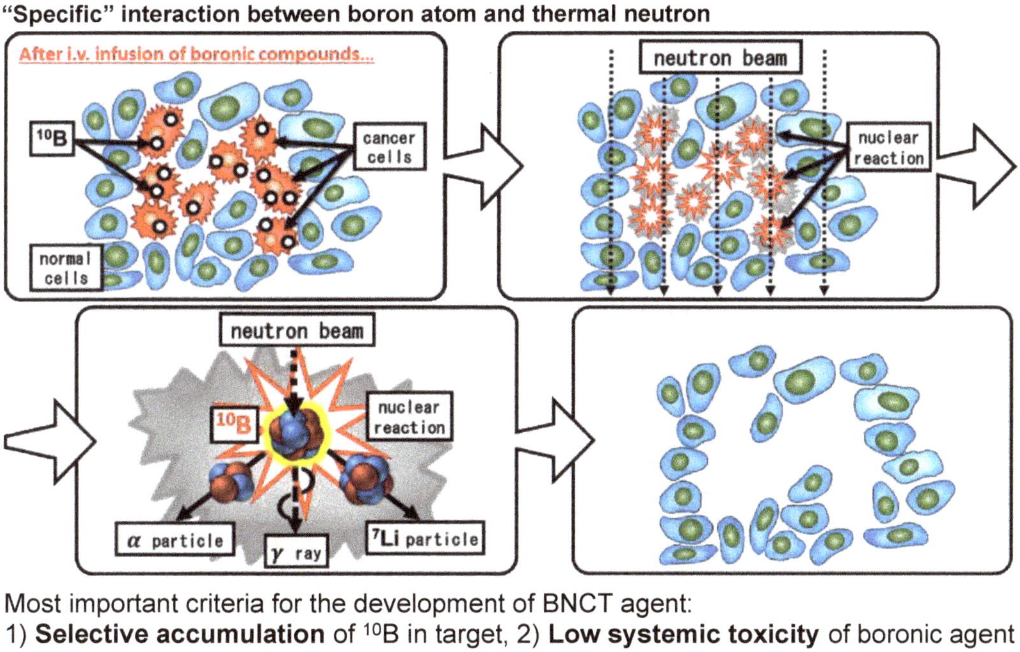

Figure 4. Selective cell destruction using boron neutron capture therapy (BNCT).

In RT, the accuracy of spatial positioning has been improved by increasing the accuracy of the treatment device and body sides. These techniques include respiratory synchronization, image-guided RT, and stereotactic RT. However, BNCT is a bimodal therapy, which is different from conventional RT in that it utilizes the difference in drug distribution, especially drug uptake between normal and tumor tissues, to achieve an effect. Thus, BNCT consists of two steps: the drug is responsible for tumor selectivity and the external irradiation of thermal neutrons is used to produce the effect. Therefore, it was necessary to develop a boron-containing compound with tumor-accumulating properties and a high-intensity thermal neutron source capable of delivering a sufficient dose (flux) for the treatment.

4.2. The History of BNCT

In the early days of research and development, the necessary thermal neutrons could only be obtained from experimental reactors. Clinical studies using experimental reactors were initiated in the United States in the 1960s, but the inadequate performance of ^{10}B compounds prevented the discovery of promising results [142–144].

Since then, basic and clinical research has been conducted in Japan and Europe [145–148]. Neutron sources have generally been used through beam shaping, in which the beam from the core of a research reactor is attenuated to increase the proportion of low-energy thermal neutrons [149–152]. However, in recent years, as the use of nuclear reactors has become increasingly difficult for both commercial and research purposes, high-power neutron sources, such as the Japan Proton Accelerator Research Complex (J-PARK, Tokai, Japan), have been developed in the field of physics, and research on thermal neutron sources for therapeutic use without using nuclear reactors has become popular as a spin-out of these sources [153–156]. Accelerator neutron sources can be installed in hospitals for medical use, and they have a higher potential for medical applications than the use of nuclear reactors because they are not subject to the strict regulations of nuclear reactors.

Japan was the first country to begin its clinical application. An accelerator-based BNCT clinical study in Japan was developed based on the previous BNCT treatment in nuclear reactors, that is, malignant brain tumors and head and neck cancers were the first targets [157–159]. In June 2020, Stella Pharma's L-*p*-boronophenylalanine (BPA) agents and Sumitomo Heavy Industries' NeuCure were the first drugs and devices for BNCT to be covered by health insurance in Japan. As a result, BNCT has become a medical treatment option that utilizes drugs and medical devices, and its use as a full-fledged treatment for a limited number of indications has started. In addition, several research institutes and companies in the United States or China have succeeded in producing thermal neutron beams that can be installed in hospitals [160,161].

4.3. Reactor and Accelerator-Based Neutron Source

In terms of the medical use of nuclear reactors, the research reactor (JRR-4) at the Japan Atomic Energy Research Institute (the Japan Atomic Energy Agency) was modified for medical use in collaboration with the Department of Neurosurgery at the University of Tsukuba, with an operating room, simulation room, irradiation room, remote anesthesia equipment, and even experimental equipment [162,163]. With the development of a simulation calculation code, noncircumferential irradiation using epithermal neutrons can now be handled [164–167]. Epithermal neutrons are slightly higher in energy than thermal neutrons, and after entering the body, they become thermal neutrons and cause a neutron capture reaction, which has the advantage of allowing treatment of brain tumors with external irradiation [168,169]. While thermal neutrons themselves can only treat superficial lesions with a depth of approximately 2 cm, epithermal neutrons can treat lesions with a depth of approximately 6 cm, and the clinical application of epithermal neutrons will shift from intraoperative irradiation by craniotomy to external irradiation without anesthesia. The clinical application of thermal external neutrons has shifted from intraoperative irradiation by craniotomy to external irradiation without anesthesia.

In addition, unlike charged particles, neutron beams cannot be directly accelerated because they do not have an electric charge, and their handling is more difficult than charged particles [170].

4.4. Head and Neck Cancers

In head and neck cancer, the involvement of the human papilloma virus and the introduction of IMRT have reduced complications, and nivolumab has been introduced to treat recurrence. Head and neck cancer BNCT was used as a salvage treatment for patients who had already been irradiated and were at the time of recurrence or inoperable. It has attracted attention as a new treatment option for patients who have no other choice but palliative treatment, and because of the large number of cases compared to malignant brain tumors, it is thought to have been approved ahead of other treatments. The clinical study cases of head and neck cancer treated with BNCT are summarized in Table 4.

Table 4. The summary of the clinical study cases of head and neck cancer treated using BNCT.

Facility	Neutron Source	Year	Tumor	Patients No.	Boron Agents	Clinical Course
Osaka University [171,172]	KUR JRR4	2001–2014	Rec H&N	45	BSH, BPA	5y 32% 10y 21% PR 29% CR 51%
Kawasaki Medical College [173]	KUR JRR4	2003–2011	Rec H&N	20	BPA	PR 35% CR 55%
Kawasaki Medical College	KUR JRR4	2006–2012	H&N preop.	7	BPA	5y 42% PR 1/7 CR 5/7
Helsinki University Central Hospital [174]	FiR-1	2003–2008	Rec H&N	30	BPA	MST 13mo PR 31% CR 45%
Taipei Veterans General Hospital [175]	THOR	2010–2011	Rec H&N	10	BPA	PR 40% CR 30%

KUR: Kyoto Research Reactor, Kumatori, Osaka, Japan; JRR4: Japan Research Reactor No.4; Tokai, Ibaraki, Japan; FiR-1: Finland Reactor 1, Otaniemi, Finland, THOR: Tsing Hua open-pool Reactor, Hsinchu Taiwan, Rec H&N: recurrent head and neck cancer, H&N preoperative: head and neck cancer patients of preoperative state, BSH: disodium mercaptoundecahydrododecaborate, BPA: L-*p* boronophenylalanine, 5y: 5 year survival rate, 10y: 10 year survival rate, PR: Partial response rate, CR: Complete response rate, MST: Median overall survival time.

4.5. Malignant Brain Tumor

For malignant brain tumors, especially GBM, the combination of TMZ and radiation after maximum possible resection has been the standard of care since the breakthrough of TMZ [176], however, there has been no major technological innovation since then.

Malignant brain tumor BNCT has been used as the postoperative RT of choice in newly diagnosed cases or as salvage therapy in cases of recurrence [177]. The University of Tsukuba conducted a clinical study on newly diagnosed malignant glioma and showed that several protocols, including intraoperative irradiation of the craniotomy, prolonged survival by about two times compared to the standard treatment at that time using photon RT [178]. Chemotherapy at that time was in transition from nitrosoureas to TMZ. The median survival of 27 months was an epoch-making figure at that time, although the total number of patients was only a few dozen and there was selection bias, such as a lack of deep-seated disease. Similar to the head and neck region, clinical trials have been conducted for previously irradiated malignant gliomas that have recurred and are awaiting approval. Recent clinical studies on GBM treated using BNCT are summarized in Table 5. Malignant meningioma is another candidate for BNCT [179].

Table 5. The summary of the recent clinical study cases of glioblastoma treated using BNCT.

Facility	Neutron Source	Year	Tumor	Patients No.	Boron Agents	Clinical Course (Month)
University of Tsukuba [178]	JRR4	1998–2007	GBM	15	BPA, BSH	MST 23.3 27.1
Tokusima University [180,181]	KUR JRR4	1998–2008	GBM	23	BSH	MST 15.5 19.5 26.2
Osaka Medical College [182–184]	KUR	2002–2006 2002–2007	GBM rGBM	21 19	BPA, BSH BSH, BPA	MST 14.5 23.5 MST 10.8

KUR: Kyoto Research Reactor, Kumatori, Osaka, Japan; JRR4: Japan Research Reactor No.4, Tokai, Ibaraki, Japan; GBM: glioblastoma multiforme; rGBM: recurrent glioblastoma; BSH: disodium mercaptoundecahydrododecaborate; BPA L-p boronophenylalanine; MST, median overall survival time.

4.6. Requirements for Drugs for BNCT and Current Boron Compounds

Research and development of boron compounds for BNCT continues; however, the number of clinically available agents is very limited, with only two compounds, BPA and mercaptoundecahydro-closo-dodecaborate (BSH). The ideal BNCT drug would be able to accumulate ^{10}B only in tumors and would not have any toxicity or effect on its own. The concentration required for the treatment depends on the intensity of the neutron beam.

BPA is the main component of borofalan, a newly approved drug for BNCT in Japan (Figure 5a). BPA is composed of the amino acid phenylalanine bound to a single atom of boron. The boron content is thus not high (approximately 5% by weight). It is believed to be absorbed into the cytoplasm via amino acid transporters in tumor cells with an active metabolism. Since tyrosine is a substrate of melanin, it was first used in BNCT for malignant melanoma [146], and its accumulation effect was later found in many histological types of tumors; it was also used for head and neck cancer and malignant brain tumors [185,186]. BSH is a low molecular weight compound with a molecular weight of approximately 200 and has been used for malignant brain tumors (Figure 5b) [187,188]. They do not accumulate in tumors and penetrate tissues by diffusion, and they do not cross the blood-brain barrier in normal brain tissues. This point was reversed in a BNCT clinical study using BSH for malignant brain tumors, which utilized the fact that malignant brain tumors normally diffuse into the interstitium only around disrupted tumor blood vessels. Inevitably, there are also studies using protocols that expect additive effects by combining multiple drugs, that is, BPA and BSH in a two-drug combination, but at present, BSH alone is not used because of the complexity of the procedure and the low tumor/blood ratio.

In addition, as a technological development for diagnosis, fluorine-labeled BPA (^{18}FBPA) has been developed for positron emission tomography (PET) examination [189–191]. The advantage of being able to determine the accumulation of boron drugs before BNCT treatment has been found to reliably predict the therapeutic effect of BNCT.

BNCT is a single-irRT, and the thermal neutron fluence (n/cm^2: the number of particles passing through a unit area) required for a single treatment is approximately 1×10^{13} (within one hour of treatment), which can be generated by current accelerators. To achieve tumor control with this neutron fluence dose, a tissue or intracellular ^{10}B concentration of 20–40 µg/mL is required. To maintain this concentration for the duration of irradiation, the dose of drug administered to the body must be extremely high and must be administered for a short period, and for BPA, a dose of 500 mg/kg is required. According to the dosage and administration approved in Japan, 30 g of the compound was administered in 3 h to a human weighing 60 kg. Compared to anticancer drugs and antibiotics, where the dosage ranges from a few hundred milligrams to a few grams at most, 30 g is a huge amount. Of course, the boron drug alone does not have an antitumor effect, but it does need to accumulate in the tumor.

The ideal conditions for a boron compound for BNCT are:

- The concentration of ^{10}B in the tumor tissue or cells must be at least 20 µg/mL during neutron irradiation.

- It must be safely administered and excreted.
- No toxicity is observed in bolus doses of several tens of grams.
- It must be water-soluble
- The tumor/normal tissue (T/N) ratio or tumor/blood (T/B) ratio should be as high as possible. The result is a drug with high therapeutic efficacy and reduced damage to normal tissues.

Attempts to develop new boron compounds that are more effective and safer have been ongoing for a long time, and applications of nanoparticles using drug delivery systems, antibody drugs, low-molecular-weight boron compounds have been studied and attempts to improve the tumor/normal tissue ratio as a standard have been ongoing for a long time.

4.7. Development of New Boron Compounds

4.7.1. Problems with Existing Boron Compounds and New Drug Development

While general low-molecular-weight anticancer drugs show cell-killing effects at extremely low concentrations of 10^{-6} to 10^{-9} M in tumors, the concentration of boron agents that show therapeutic effects in BNCT is extremely high, at 10^{-3} M in the tumor (Figure 5c). Therefore, according to the guidelines for the development of BNCT irradiation systems, it is desirable to have a T/B ratio and a T/N ratio of ≥ 3.0, from the viewpoint of safety [192]. However, BPA, which is currently widely used in BNCT, is rapidly excreted from the tumor by transporters, and its retention in the tumor is low. In May 2020, steboronin was launched as the world's first boron drug for BNCT in Japan, but its dosage is extremely high at 9000 mg/300 mL. In addition, to achieve excellent therapeutic effects in BNCT, it is important not only to maintain high concentrations of boron drugs in the tumor but also to distribute them homogeneously. Masunaga et al. have shown that quiescent cancer cells have reduced BPA uptake compared with proliferating cancer cells [193,194]. Since it has been reported that quiescent cells include hypoxic cells and CSCs that are resistant to various cancer therapies, including radiation [195–197], it can be inferred that the heterogeneous uptake distribution greatly affects the therapeutic effect of BPA-BNCT. Therefore, it is highly desirable to develop a delivery technology that enables tumor-selective and efficient delivery of boron drugs in BNCT therapy.

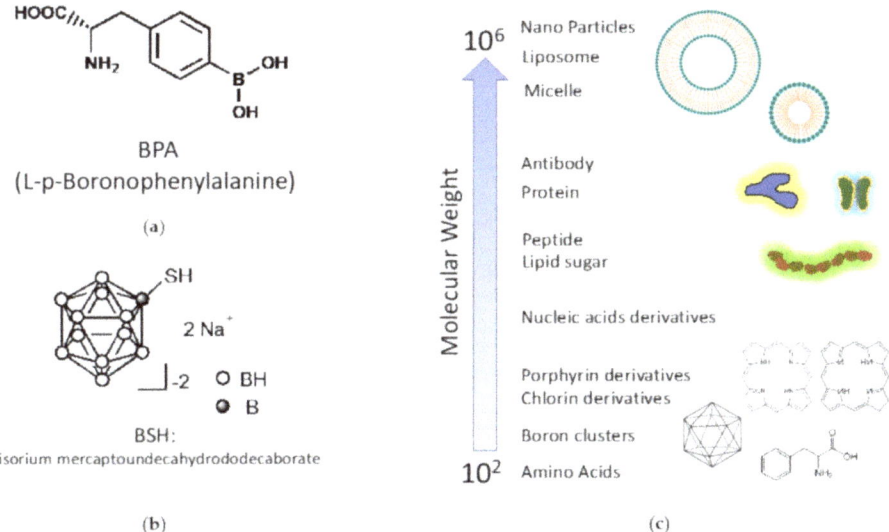

Figure 5. Chemical structures of (**a**) BPA and (**b**) BSH, and (**c**) molecular weight of various compounds.

4.7.2. Drug Development Using Existing Boron Compounds

As a method for the highly efficient delivery of boron drugs, investigations using liposomes [198], antibody modification [199], and dendrimers [200] have been reported. Kueffer et al. reported that tumor accumulation could be improved by encapsulating BSH in liposomes and improving blood retention, but since BSH also accumulated in normal cells, a strategy to add tumor cell selectivity is necessary [201]. Kang et al. reported that BSH was efficiently taken up by cancer cells by encapsulating it in liposomes modified with a peptide that has a high affinity for integrin $\alpha v \beta 3$, which is highly expressed in neovascularization and GBM [202]. Maruyama et al. found that boron drugs encapsulated in PEGylated liposomes improved tumor retention and maintained tumor BPA levels at 30 µg/g tissue for at least 72 h after intravenous administration [203]. Furthermore, Nomoto et al. reported that BPA gel formed by mixing polyvinyl alcohol (PVA) and BPA could inhibit the excretion of BPA from tumors by allowing BPA to enter cells through endocytosis [204]. We also tried to improve the active accumulation of one of the existing boron compounds, BSH, to cancer using ND201, which is cyclodextrin modified with folic acid (Figure 6) [205]. As a result, ND201 induced active cancer accumulation and high retention of BSH depending on the expression level of folic acid receptors in cancer cells and succeeded in obtaining excellent antitumor effects using neutron irradiation.

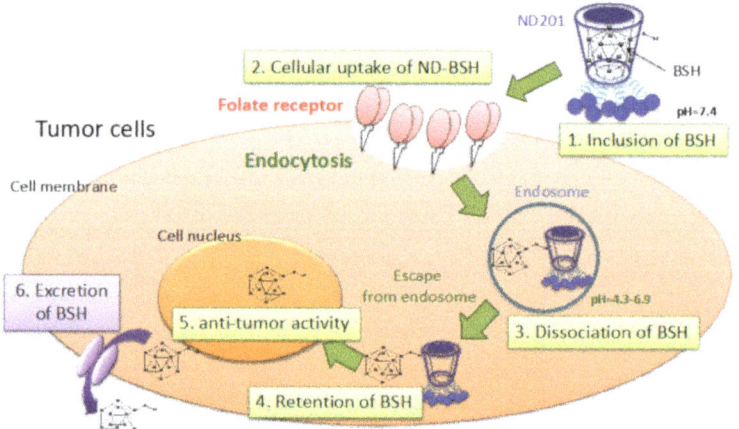

Figure 6. The mechanism of action of ND-BSH. BSH is included in the lumen of ND201 and recognizes cancer cells targeting the folate receptor.

4.7.3. Development of Next-Generation Boron Drug for Fusion with Drug Delivery System Technology

As mentioned above, a drug delivery system (DDS) that can control the intracellular uptake pathway and intracellular retention must be developed for BNCT. There are two concepts of DDS in solid tumor therapy: active targeting and passive targeting. Active targeting utilizes the specific binding ability of molecules for targeting. Passive targeting utilizes the characteristics of the tumor vascular system to achieve selective tumor accumulation. In general, macromolecules do not easily leak from normal blood vessels. However, in solid tumors, macromolecules tend to leak from tumor blood vessels because of characteristics, such as increased neovascularization and vascular permeability. In addition, because of the immaturity of the lymphatic system and other reasons, macromolecules that leak locally in the tumor remain there for a long time. As a result, high-molecular-weight anticancer drugs that are highly stable in the blood can be passively targeted [206,207]. This is the enhanced permeability and retention (EPR) effect. The EPR effect, first announced in 1986, has been accepted worldwide and has contributed to the development of methods to deliver anticancer drugs, nucleic acids, genes, and peptides to cancer tissues in polymeric polymers, liposome preparations, and micelle preparations at the animal experimental level.

Nakamura et al. focused on the structure of lipids that form liposomes and developed boron lipids, distearoyl boron lipid (DSBL), and boron cholesterol with chlossodecaborate [208], and confirmed the long-term survival after thermal neutron irradiation in a mouse colon cancer CT26 cell transplantation model with an intratumor boron concentration of more than 170 ppm [209]. Nishiyama et al. synthesized PEG-b-P (Glu-SSH), a biodegradable poly(ethylene glycol)-poly(glutamic acid) block copolymer containing BSH disulfide bonded to mercaptoethylamine, and developed nanomicelles by self-assembly [210]. After administration of 50 mg B/kg to mice implanted with CT26 mouse colon tumor, the intratumor boron concentration reached 69 ppm after 24 h, indicating a T/B concentration ratio of more than 20 and a strong BNCT antitumor effect. In addition, Nakamura et al. developed a boron compound, maleimide-functionalized closo-dodecaborate (MID), which can be introduced into cysteine [211], and focused on the phenomenon that stained serum albumin accumulates in tumor tissue (EPR effect), maleimide-functionalized closo-dodecaborate albumin conjugates (MID-AC) was prepared by binding MID to serum albumin and verified the antitumor effect of BNCT using cancer transplant mice [212]. Nagasaki et al. developed nanomicelles (PM micelles) in which vinylcarborane was polymerized in biodegradable polyethylene glycol-polylactic acid block copolymer micelles [213]. In an experiment using tumor-bearing mice, PM micelles reached 14 ppm after 24 h of administration, and the tumors disappeared in two out of five mice after 25 days of thermal neutron irradiation. More recently, a collaboration between our group and the Nagasaki laboratory has led to the development of PBA-modified polymeric nanoparticles (Nano^{PBA}) with sialic acid orientation as a boron preparation that has different targeting properties from LAT1 and can maintain ^{10}B levels in tumors for a long time [214]. Nano^{PBA} has a supramolecular structure consisting of a core and shell composed of poly(lactic acid) (PLA) and poly(ethylene glycol) (PEG) segments (Figure 7). PBA is located at the hydrophilic end of the polymer, and a large number of PBAs are exposed on the surface of the nanoparticles and bind to the membranes of cancer cells in multiple ways, resulting in a very strong targeting effect. In this study, the efficacy and safety of Nano^{PBA} were verified by administering Nano^{PBA} to a B16 melanoma-bearing mouse model that highly expresses sialic acid, followed by irradiation with thermal neutron radiation. The results showed that Nano^{PBA} showed a longer intratumor accumulation time than BPA and showed a potent antitumor effect by efficient tumor targeting even at a low dose of 1/100. Furthermore, focusing on the anaerobic glycolytic system, which is characteristic of cancer, a collaboration between our group and Maeda laboratory has developed a multifunctional boron compound, styrene-maleic acid (SMA)-glucosamine borate complex, [215]. The complex is a novel boron compound with multiple functions that can induce changes in the metabolic system and suppress the growth of cancer by the contained boric acid and glucosamine and can also induce cell lethality by BNCT (Figure 8). A remarkable cancer growth inhibitory effect was confirmed by irradiating a cancer-bearing mouse model transplanted with Chinese hamster squamous cell SCCVII with thermal neutrons by administering 125 mg/kg of SMA-glucosamine borate complex. This was an antitumor effect equivalent to that of the 500 mg/kg BPA-administered group, and the SMA-glucosamine borate complex was able to show efficacy at ^{10}B, which is 1/70 of that of BPA.

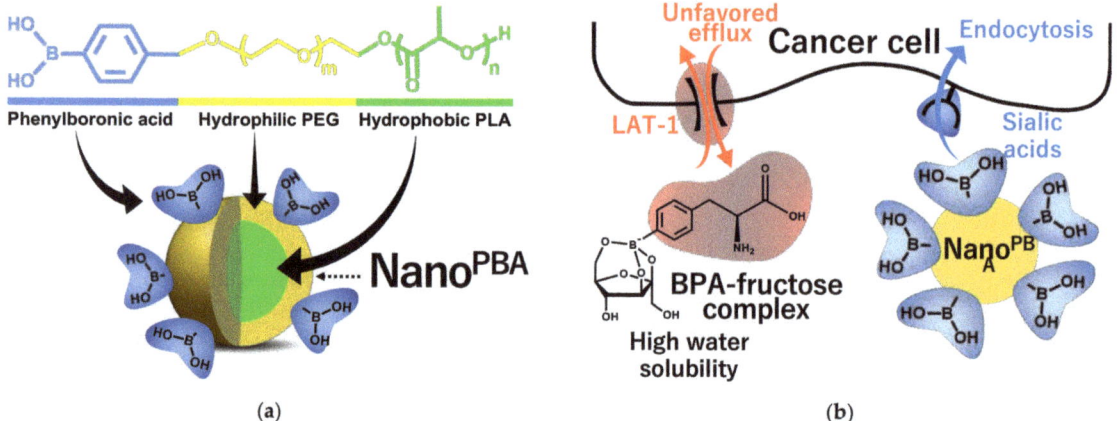

Figure 7. (**a**) Schematic illustration of molecular design for PBA-decorated polymeric nanoparticle as a novel BNCT agent and (**b**) different accumulation mechanism from BPA-f.

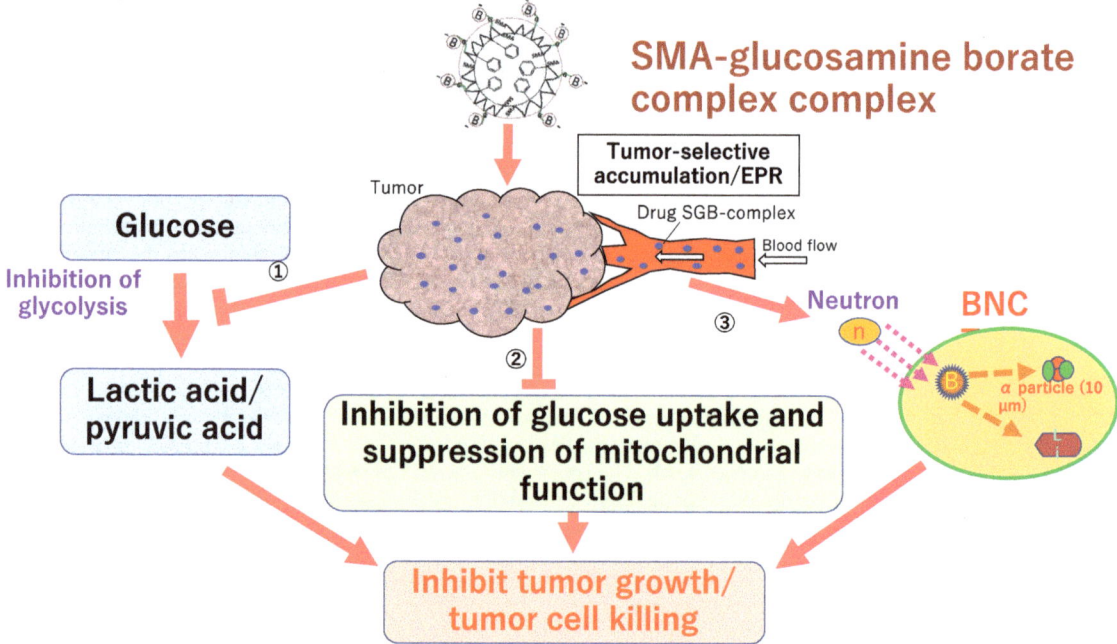

Figure 8. Multifunctional cancer growth inhibitory effect by SMA-glucosamine borate complex targeting treatment-resistant cancer cells.

4.7.4. Challenges in Conducting BNCT Research

At present, there are no clinical studies using these new compounds, except for phase II studies conducted on boronated porphyrin. In Japan, recurrent head and neck cancers are covered by public insurance, and the number of BNCT treatment facilities is expected to increase, as well as the number of applicable diseases and patients. As a result, the number of researchers involved in the development of new boron agents is expected to increase.

Further focus on the development of new drugs is desirable, with the understanding that the doses of boron compounds are orders of magnitude higher than those of conventional drugs, and that they do not need to have their drug effects, and therefore require tumor accumulation and more stringent safety evaluation. In other words, as mentioned above, it is clear that the development of new boron preparations is urgently needed in addition to the radiobiological research of BNCT to further expand the indications for BNCT. However, the number of neutron sources that can be used for BNCT is limited, and there are only a few facilities in the world where biological and chemical experiments using cells and especially laboratory animals are possible. We at the University of Tsukuba have been developing a new Linac accelerator BNCT device for several years and have already completed a device that can withstand the practical level (Figure 9). The facility also has a biological laboratory where basic research on cells and small animals (mouse and rat) irradiated with an accelerator BNCT device is possible, and animal experiments can be performed with a GLP-compliant grade. In the near future, we plan to publish a large number of research results on new boron drug candidates using this facility.

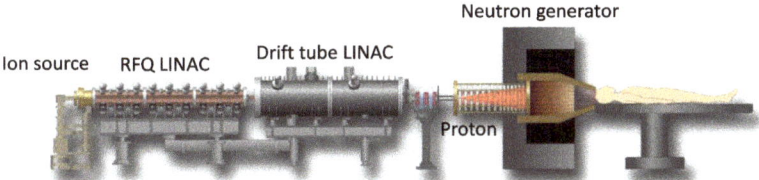

Accelerator based neutron source developed by University of Tsukuba and High Energy Accelerator Research Organization (KEK)

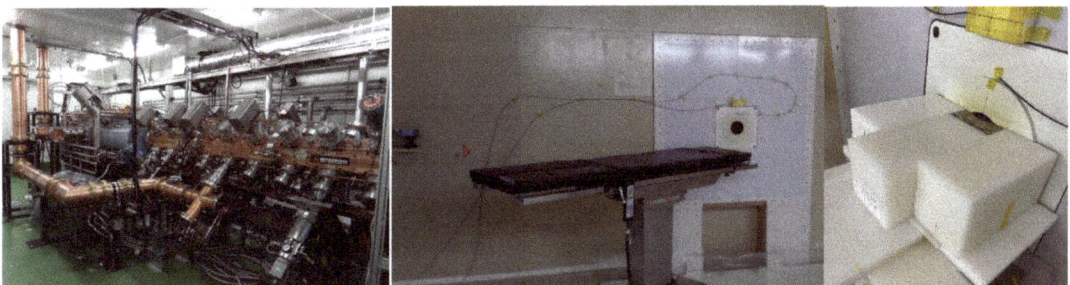

8MeV Linac   Beam port : Patient setup and cell sample irradiation

Figure 9. Newly developed accelerator-based neutron source (Tsukuba model).

5. Concluding Remarks

The main purpose of combination therapy using existing therapies such as chemotherapy, molecular targeted agents, and radiation is to control the local area using radiation and to suppress metastasis, including micrometastasis, using chemotherapy and molecular targeted agents. In recent years, this trend has been changing, and combination protocols aimed at synergistically increasing the effect on the local area have been considered but have not been established. Owing to the limited number of facilities for particle therapy, there have been few results from both basic and clinical applications, and in principle, it has been considered to follow the conventional combination method in photon RT. However, with the recent remarkable development in the field of nanoparticles and biomaterials, the possibility of proposing new drugs and new combination therapies that better match the characteristics of particle RT is being demonstrated. In this review, we summarized the status of combination therapies in clinical practice with a focus on particle RT and summarized the latest findings on various combination therapies that are being clarified from basic biology, to provide an opportunity to consider combination therapies that should contribute to the next generation of particle RT for cancer.

The current particle therapy has achieved sufficient progress in the field of physical engineering, such as the miniaturization of accelerators and freedom of irradiation direction using gantries. However, the biological benefits are not yet fully understood, leaving the potential for clinical contributions. One of the reasons for this is that the uncertainty of biological problems is much greater than that of physical problems. Therefore, from a clinical point of view, in addition to the biological effects of particle beams, it is highly desirable to clarify the advantages and limitations of using particle beams in combination with other biological therapies. The expected benefits of combined RT include: (1) radiosensitization of tumor tissue (ideally tumor-specific), (2) protection of normal tissue, and (3) induction of bystander or abscopal effects in distant regions.

In PBT, combination therapy has been attempted based on the experience of photon RT, and the combination of radiation and cytotoxic chemotherapy has become the standard treatment for most locally advanced cancers. Because of its excellent dose distribution and mild biological effects, PBT can reduce the exposure dose of normal tissues, which may have side effects when used in combination with other therapies (Cox 2007). In contrast, the physical and biological properties of carbon ions are very different from those of photons, and while they can produce unexpected results, as in the immunotherapy described above, the risks are undeniably greater than expected.

Finally, BNCT, which is now covered by health insurance in Japan, is a different type of RT that must be used in combination with drugs. In recent years, researchers in the fields of drug development and drug delivery have become interested in radiation cancer therapy, probably because of the development and awareness of BNCT. In addition to the accelerator-based BNCT, our facility is equipped with experimental facilities for physics, chemistry, biology, and medicine, and we promise to make a significant contribution to future BNCT research. We hope that drug research in the field of BNCT will have a significant impact on the development of combination therapies for other types of particle therapies.

Author Contributions: Y.M. wrote Section 1, Section 3, Section 4.7, and Section 5. N.F. wrote Sections 2.3 and 2.4. H.I. wrote Sections 2.1 and 2.2. K.N. wrote Sections 4.1–4.6. H.S. supervised the manuscript. All authors have read and agreed to the published version of the manuscript.

Funding: This research was funded by JSPS KAKENHI, Grant Numbers JP15K09986 and JP18K07256, Takeda Science Foundation, Grant Number DLQC0004J, and Japan Agency for Medical Research and Development (AMED), Grant Number JP20lm0203010.

Institutional Review Board Statement: All animal experimental procedures were performed based on submitted animal experimental plans (approval number: 18-190, 19-154, 19-199 and 20-233), which were inspected and approved by the animal research committee of the University of Tsukuba and Kumamoto University.

Informed Consent Statement: Not applicable.

Data Availability Statement: The data that support the findings in this article are available from the corresponding author, Y.M., upon reasonable request.

Acknowledgments: We wish to acknowledge the exceptional work of the Proton Medical Research Center at the University of Tsukuba in the field of particle radiobiology. The corresponding author would like to express special thanks to Hiroshi Maeda for giving him this opportunity to write a special issue about particle radiobiology.

Conflicts of Interest: The authors declare no conflict of interest.

References

1. Wilson, R.R. Radiological use of fast protons. *Radiology* **1946**, *47*, 487–491. [CrossRef] [PubMed]
2. Lawrence, J.H.; Tobias, C.A.; Born, J.L.; Mc, C.R.; Roberts, J.E.; Anger, H.O.; Low-Beer, B.V.; Huggins, C.B. Pituitary irradiation with high-energy proton beams: A preliminary report. *Cancer Res.* **1958**, *18*, 121–134.

3. Particle Therapy Co-Operative Group. 2021. Available online: https://www.ptcog.ch/ (accessed on 22 July 2021).
4. Suit, H.; DeLaney, T.; Goldberg, S.; Paganetti, H.; Clasie, B.; Gerweck, L.; Niemierko, A.; Hall, E.; Flanz, J.; Hallman, J.; et al. Proton vs carbon ion beams in the definitive radiation treatment of cancer patients. *Radiother. Oncol. J. Eur. Soc. Ther. Radiol. Oncol.* **2010**, *95*, 3–22. [CrossRef]
5. Mohan, R.; Grosshans, D. Proton therapy—Present and future. *Adv. Drug Deliv. Rev.* **2017**, *109*, 26–44. [CrossRef]
6. Lomax, A. Intensity modulation methods for proton radiotherapy. *Phys. Med. Biol.* **1999**, *44*, 185–205. [CrossRef]
7. Bert, C.; Durante, M. Motion in radiotherapy: Particle therapy. *Phys. Med. Biol.* **2011**, *56*, R113–R144. [CrossRef]
8. DeLaney, T.F. Proton therapy in the clinic. *Front. Radiat Oncol.* **2011**, *43*, 465–485.
9. Engelsman, M.; Schwarz, M.; Dong, L. Physics controversies in proton therapy. *Semin. Radiat. Oncol.* **2013**, *23*, 88–96. [CrossRef]
10. Hyer, D.E.; Hill, P.M.; Wang, D.; Smith, B.R.; Flynn, R.T. A dynamic collimation system for penumbra reduction in spot-scanning proton therapy: Proof of concept. *Med. Phys.* **2014**, *41*, 091701. [CrossRef]
11. Schippers, J.M.; Lomax, A.J. Emerging technologies in proton therapy. *Acta Oncol.* **2011**, *50*, 838–850. [CrossRef]
12. Durante, M.; Debus, J. Heavy charged particles: Does improved precision and higher biological effectiveness translate to better outcome in patients? *Semin. Radiat. Oncol.* **2018**, *28*, 160–167. [CrossRef]
13. Weyrather, W.K.; Kraft, G. RBE of carbon ions: Experimental data and the strategy of RBE calculation for treatment planning. *Radiother. Oncol. J. Eur. Soc. Ther. Radiol. Oncol.* **2004**, *73*, S161. [CrossRef]
14. Kanai, T.; Matsufuji, N.; Miyamoto, T.; Mizoe, J.; Kamada, T.; Tsuji, H.; Kato, H.; Baba, M.; Tsujii, H. Examination of GyE system for HIMAC carbon therapy. *Int. J. Radiat. Oncol. Biol. Phys.* **2006**, *64*, 650–656. [CrossRef] [PubMed]
15. Ando, K.; Kase, Y. Biological characteristics of carbon-ion therapy. *Int. J. Radiat. Biol.* **2009**, *85*, 715–728. [CrossRef] [PubMed]
16. Furusawa, Y.; Fukutsu, K.; Aoki, M.; Itsukaichi, H.; Eguchi-Kasai, K.; Ohara, H.; Yatagai, F.; Kanai, T.; Ando, K. Inactivation of aerobic and hypoxic cells from three different cell lines by accelerated (3)He-, (12)C- and (20)Ne-ion beams. *Radiat. Res.* **2000**, *154*, 485–496. [CrossRef]
17. Gray, L.H.; Green, F.O.; Hawes, C.A. Effect of nitric oxide on the radiosensitivity of tumour cells. *Nature* **1958**, *182*, 952–953. [CrossRef]
18. Ito, A.; Nakano, H.; Kusano, Y.; Hirayama, R.; Furusawa, Y.; Murayama, C.; Mori, T.; Katsumura, Y.; Shinohara, K. Contribution of indirect action to radiation-induced mammalian cell inactivation: Dependence on photon energy and heavy-ion LET. *Radiat. Res.* **2006**, *165*, 703–712. [CrossRef]
19. Hirayama, R.; Ito, A.; Tomita, M.; Tsukada, T.; Yatagai, F.; Noguchi, M.; Matsumoto, Y.; Kase, Y.; Ando, K.; Okayasu, R.; et al. Contributions of direct and indirect actions in cell killing by high-LET radiations. *Radiat. Res.* **2009**, *171*, 212–218. [CrossRef] [PubMed]
20. Aoki-Nakano, M.; Furusawa, Y. Misrepair of DNA double-strand breaks after exposure to heavy-ion beams causes a peak in the LET-RBE relationship with respect to cell killing in DT40 cells. *J. Radiat. Res.* **2013**, *54*, 1029–1035. [CrossRef]
21. Takahashi, A.; Kubo, M.; Ma, H.; Nakagawa, A.; Yoshida, Y.; Isono, M.; Kanai, T.; Ohno, T.; Furusawa, Y.; Funayama, T.; et al. Nonhomologous end-joining repair plays a more important role than homologous recombination repair in defining radiosensitivity after exposure to high-LET radiation. *Radiat. Res.* **2014**, *182*, 338–344. [CrossRef]
22. Blakely, E.A.; Tobias, C.A.; Yang, T.C.; Smith, K.C.; Lyman, J.T. Inactivation of human kidney cells by high-energy monoenergetic heavy-ion beams. *Radiat. Res.* **1979**, *80*, 122–160. [CrossRef]
23. Hirayama, R.; Furusawa, Y.; Fukawa, T.; Ando, K. Repair kinetics of DNA-DSB induced by X-rays or carbon ions under oxic and hypoxic conditions. *J. Radiat. Res.* **2005**, *46*, 325–332. [CrossRef]
24. Wenzl, T.; Wilkens, J.J. Theoretical analysis of the dose dependence of the oxygen enhancement ratio and its relevance for clinical applications. *Radiat. Oncol.* **2011**, *6*, 171. [CrossRef]
25. Bray, F.; Ferlay, J.; Soerjomataram, I.; Siegel, R.L.; Torre, L.A.; Jemal, A. Global cancer statistics 2018: GLOBOCAN estimates of incidence and mortality worldwide for 36 cancers in 185 countries. *CA Cancer J. Clin.* **2018**, *68*, 394–424. [CrossRef]
26. Siegel, R.L.; Miller, K.D.; Jemal, A. Cancer statistics, 2020. *CA Cancer J. Clin.* **2020**, *70*, 7–30. [CrossRef]
27. Kitagawa, Y.; Uno, T.; Oyama, T.; Kato, K.; Kato, H.; Kawakubo, H.; Kawamura, O.; Kusano, M.; Kuwano, H.; Takeuchi, H.; et al. Esophageal cancer practice guidelines 2017 edited by the Japan Esophageal Society: Part 1. *Esophagus* **2019**, *16*, 1–24. [CrossRef] [PubMed]
28. Morota, M.; Gomi, K.; Kozuka, T.; Chin, K.; Matsuura, M.; Oguchi, M.; Ito, H.; Yamashita, T. Late toxicity after definitive concurrent chemoradiotherapy for thoracic esophageal carcinoma. *Int. J. Radiat. Oncol. Biol. Phys.* **2009**, *75*, 122–128. [CrossRef] [PubMed]
29. Bradley, J.D.; Paulus, R.; Komaki, R.; Masters, G.; Blumenschein, G.; Schild, S.; Bogart, J.; Hu, C.; Forster, K.; Magliocco, A.; et al. Standard-dose versus high-dose conformal radiotherapy with concurrent and consolidation carboplatin plus paclitaxel with or without cetuximab for patients with stage IIIA or IIIB non-small-cell lung cancer (RTOG 0617): A randomised, two-by-two factorial phase 3 study. *Lancet Oncol.* **2015**, *16*, 187–199.
30. Minsky, B.D.; Pajak, T.F.; Ginsberg, R.J.; Pisansky, T.M.; Martenson, J.; Komaki, R.; Okawara, G.; Rosenthal, S.A.; Kelsen, D.P. INT 0123 (Radiation Therapy Oncology Group 94-05) phase III trial of combined-modality therapy for esophageal cancer: High-dose versus standard-dose radiation therapy. *J. Clin. Oncol. Off. J. Am. Soc. Clin. Oncol.* **2002**, *20*, 1167–1174. [CrossRef] [PubMed]

31. Kato, K.; Muro, K.; Minashi, K.; Ohtsu, A.; Ishikura, S.; Boku, N.; Takiuchi, H.; Komatsu, Y.; Miyata, Y.; Fukuda, H.; et al. Phase II study of chemoradiotherapy with 5-fluorouracil and cisplatin for Stage II-III esophageal squamous cell carcinoma: JCOG trial (JCOG 9906). *Int. J. Radiat. Oncol. Biol. Phys.* **2011**, *81*, 684–690. [CrossRef]
32. Shirai, K.; Tamaki, Y.; Kitamoto, Y.; Murata, K.; Satoh, Y.; Higuchi, K.; Nonaka, T.; Ishikawa, H.; Katoh, H.; Takahashi, T.; et al. Dose-volume histogram parameters and clinical factors associated with pleural effusion after chemoradiotherapy in esophageal cancer patients. *Int. J. Radiat. Oncol. Biol. Phys.* **2011**, *80*, 1002–1007. [CrossRef] [PubMed]
33. Wei, X.; Liu, H.H.; Tucker, S.L.; Wang, S.; Mohan, R.; Cox, J.D.; Komaki, R.; Liao, Z. Risk factors for pericardial effusion in inoperable esophageal cancer patients treated with definitive chemoradiation therapy. *Int. J. Radiat. Oncol. Biol. Phys.* **2008**, *70*, 707–714. [CrossRef] [PubMed]
34. Makishima, H.; Ishikawa, H.; Terunuma, T.; Hashimoto, T.; Yamanashi, K.; Sekiguchi, T.; Mizumoto, M.; Okumura, T.; Sakae, T.; Sakurai, H. Comparison of adverse effects of proton and X-ray chemoradiotherapy for esophageal cancer using an adaptive dose-volume histogram analysis. *J. Radiat. Res.* **2015**, *56*, 568–576. [CrossRef] [PubMed]
35. Hirano, Y.; Onozawa, M.; Hojo, H.; Motegi, A.; Zenda, S.; Hotta, K.; Moriya, S.; Tachibana, H.; Nakamura, N.; Kojima, T.; et al. Dosimetric comparison between proton beam therapy and photon radiation therapy for locally advanced esophageal squamous cell carcinoma. *Radiat. Oncol.* **2018**, *13*, 23. [CrossRef]
36. Mizumoto, M.; Sugahara, S.; Nakayama, H.; Hashii, H.; Nakahara, A.; Terashima, H.; Okumura, T.; Tsuboi, K.; Tokuuye, K.; Sakurai, H. Clinical results of proton-beam therapy for locoregionally advanced esophageal cancer. *Strahlenther. Onkol.* **2010**, *186*, 482–488. [CrossRef] [PubMed]
37. Ishikawa, H.; Hashimoto, T.; Moriwaki, T.; Hyodo, I.; Hisakura, K.; Terashima, H.; Ohkohchi, N.; Ohno, T.; Makishima, H.; Mizumoto, M.; et al. Proton beam therapy combined with concurrent chemotherapy for esophageal cancer. *Anticancer Res.* **2015**, *35*, 1757–1762. [CrossRef]
38. Ono, T.; Wada, H.; Ishikawa, H.; Tamamura, H.; Tokumaru, S. Clinical results of proton beam therapy for esophageal cancer: Multicenter retrospective study in Japan. *Cancers* **2019**, *11*, 993. [CrossRef]
39. DeCesaris, C.M.; Berger, M.; Choi, J.I.; Carr, S.R.; Burrows, W.M.; Regine, W.F.; Simone, C.B., 2nd; Molitoris, J.K. Pathologic complete response (pCR) rates and outcomes after neoadjuvant chemoradiotherapy with proton or photon radiation for adenocarcinomas of the esophagus and gastroesophageal junction. *J. Gastrointest. Oncol.* **2020**, *11*, 663–673. [CrossRef]
40. Wang, X.; Palaskas, N.L.; Yusuf, S.W.; Abe, J.I.; Lopez-Mattei, J.; Banchs, J.; Gladish, G.W.; Lee, P.; Liao, Z.; Deswal, A.; et al. Incidence and onset of severe cardiac events after radiotherapy for esophageal cancer. *J. Thorac. Oncol.* **2020**, *15*, 1682–1690. [CrossRef]
41. Wang, J.; Wei, C.; Tucker, S.L.; Myles, B.; Palmer, M.; Hofstetter, W.L.; Swisher, S.G.; Ajani, J.A.; Cox, J.D.; Komaki, R.; et al. Predictors of postoperative complications after trimodality therapy for esophageal cancer. *Int. J. Radiat. Oncol. Biol. Phys.* **2013**, *86*, 885–891. [CrossRef] [PubMed]
42. Xi, M.; Xu, C.; Liao, Z.; Chang, J.Y.; Gomez, D.R.; Jeter, M.; Cox, J.D.; Komaki, R.; Mehran, R.; Blum, M.A.; et al. Comparative outcomes after definitive chemoradiotherapy using proton beam therapy versus intensity modulated radiation therapy for esophageal cancer: A retrospective, single-institutional analysis. *Int. J. Radiat. Oncol. Biol. Phys.* **2017**, *99*, 667–676. [CrossRef]
43. Lin, S.H.; Hobbs, B.P.; Verma, V.; Tidwell, R.S.; Smith, G.L.; Lei, X.; Corsini, E.M.; Mok, I.; Wei, X.; Yao, L.; et al. Randomized phase IIB trial of proton beam therapy versus intensity-modulated radiation therapy for locally advanced esophageal cancer. *J. Clin. Oncol. Off. J. Am. Soc. Clin. Oncol.* **2020**, *38*, 1569–1579. [CrossRef]
44. Davuluri, R.; Jiang, W.; Fang, P.; Xu, C.; Komaki, R.; Gomez, D.R.; Welsh, J.; Cox, J.D.; Crane, C.H.; Hsu, C.C.; et al. Lymphocyte nadir and esophageal cancer survival outcomes after chemoradiation Therapy. *Int. J. Radiat. Oncol. Biol. Phys.* **2017**, *99*, 128–135. [CrossRef] [PubMed]
45. Fang, P.; Shiraishi, Y.; Verma, V.; Jiang, W.; Song, J.; Hobbs, B.P.; Lin, S.H. Lymphocyte-sparing effect of proton therapy in patients with esophageal cancer treated with definitive chemoradiation. *Int. J. Part.* **2018**, *4*, 23–32. [CrossRef] [PubMed]
46. Routman, D.M.; Garant, A.; Lester, S.C.; Day, C.N.; Harmsen, W.S.; Sanheuza, C.T.; Yoon, H.H.; Neben-Wittich, M.A.; Martenson, J.A.; Haddock, M.G.; et al. A Comparison of grade 4 lymphopenia with proton versus photon radiation therapy for esophageal cancer. *Adv. Radiat. Oncol.* **2019**, *4*, 63–69. [CrossRef]
47. Hong, T.S.; Ryan, D.P.; Blaszkowsky, L.S.; Mamon, H.J.; Kwak, E.L.; Mino-Kenudson, M.; Adams, J.; Yeap, B.; Winrich, B.; DeLaney, T.F.; et al. Phase I study of preoperative short-course chemoradiation with proton beam therapy and capecitabine for resectable pancreatic ductal adenocarcinoma of the head. *Int. J. Radiat. Oncol. Biol. Phys.* **2011**, *79*, 151–157. [CrossRef]
48. Hong, T.S.; Ryan, D.P.; Borger, D.R.; Blaszkowsky, L.S.; Yeap, B.Y.; Ancukiewicz, M.; Deshpande, V.; Shinagare, S.; Wo, J.Y.; Boucher, Y.; et al. A phase 1/2 and biomarker study of preoperative short course chemoradiation with proton beam therapy and capecitabine followed by early surgery for resectable pancreatic ductal adenocarcinoma. *Int. J. Radiat. Oncol. Biol. Phys.* **2014**, *89*, 830–838. [CrossRef] [PubMed]
49. Terashima, K.; Demizu, Y.; Hashimoto, N.; Jin, D.; Mima, M.; Fujii, O.; Niwa, Y.; Takatori, K.; Kitajima, N.; Sirakawa, S.; et al. A phase I/II study of gemcitabine-concurrent proton radiotherapy for locally advanced pancreatic cancer without distant metastasis. *Radiother. Oncol. J. Eur. Soc. Ther. Radiol. Oncol.* **2012**, *103*, 25–31. [CrossRef]
50. Kim, T.H.; Lee, W.J.; Woo, S.M.; Kim, H.; Oh, E.S.; Lee, J.H.; Han, S.S.; Park, S.J.; Suh, Y.G.; Moon, S.H.; et al. Effectiveness and safety of simultaneous integrated boost-proton beam therapy for localized pancreatic cancer. *Technol. Cancer Res. Treat.* **2018**, *17*, 1533033818783879. [CrossRef]

51. Jethwa, K.R.; Tryggestad, E.J.; Whitaker, T.J.; Giffey, B.T.; Kazemba, B.D.; Neben-Wittich, M.A.; Merrell, K.W.; Haddock, M.G.; Hallemeier, C.L. Initial experience with intensity modulated proton therapy for intact, clinically localized pancreas cancer: Clinical implementation, dosimetric analysis, acute treatment-related adverse events, and patient-reported outcomes. *Adv. Radiat. Oncol.* **2018**, *3*, 314–321. [CrossRef]
52. Hiroshima, Y.; Fukumitsu, N.; Saito, T.; Numajiri, H.; Murofushi, K.N.; Ohnishi, K.; Nonaka, T.; Ishikawa, H.; Okumura, T.; Sakurai, H. Concurrent chemoradiotherapy using proton beams for unresectable locally advanced pancreatic cancer. *Radiother. Oncol. J. Eur. Soc. Ther. Radiol. Oncol.* **2019**, *136*, 37–43. [CrossRef]
53. Maemura, K.; Mataki, Y.; Kurahara, H.; Kawasaki, Y.; Iino, S.; Sakoda, M.; Ueno, S.; Arimura, T.; Higashi, R.; Yoshiura, T.; et al. Comparison of proton beam radiotherapy and hyper-fractionated accelerated chemoradiotherapy for locally advanced pancreatic cancer. *Pancreatology* **2017**, *17*, 833–838. [CrossRef] [PubMed]
54. Kawashiro, S.; Yamada, S.; Okamoto, M.; Ohno, T.; Nakano, T.; Shinoto, M.; Shioyama, Y.; Nemoto, K.; Isozaki, Y.; Tsuji, H.; et al. Multi-institutional study of carbon-ion radiotherapy for locally advanced pancreatic cancer: Japan carbon-ion radiation oncology study group (J-CROS) study 1403 pancreas. *Int. J. Radiat. Oncol. Biol. Phys.* **2018**, *101*, 1212–1221. [CrossRef]
55. Sai, S.; Wakai, T.; Vares, G.; Yamada, S.; Kamijo, T.; Kamada, T.; Shirai, T. Combination of carbon ion beam and gemcitabine causes irreparable DNA damage and death of radioresistant pancreatic cancer stem-like cells in vitro and in vivo. *Oncotarget* **2015**, *6*, 5517–5535. [CrossRef]
56. McGuigan, A.; Kelly, P.; Turkington, R.C.; Jones, C.; Coleman, H.G.; McCain, R.S. Pancreatic cancer: A review of clinical diagnosis, epidemiology, treatment and outcomes. *World J. Gastroenterol.* **2018**, *24*, 4846–4861. [CrossRef] [PubMed]
57. Zhan, H.X.; Xu, J.W.; Wu, D.; Wu, Z.Y.; Wang, L.; Hu, S.Y.; Zhang, G.Y. Neoadjuvant therapy in pancreatic cancer: A systematic review and meta-analysis of prospective studies. *Cancer Med.* **2017**, *6*, 1201–1219. [CrossRef]
58. Blazer, M.; Wu, C.; Goldberg, R.M.; Phillips, G.; Schmidt, C.; Muscarella, P.; Wuthrick, E.; Williams, T.M.; Reardon, J.; Ellison, E.C.; et al. Neoadjuvant modified (m) FOLFIRINOX for locally advanced unresectable (LAPC) and borderline resectable (BRPC) adenocarcinoma of the pancreas. *Ann. Surg. Oncol* **2015**, *22*, 1153–1159. [CrossRef]
59. Vitolo, V.; Cobianchi, L.; Brugnatelli, S.; Barcellini, A.; Peloso, A.; Facoetti, A.; Vanoli, A.; Delfanti, S.; Preda, L.; Molinelli, S.; et al. Preoperative chemotherapy and carbon ions therapy for treatment of resectable and borderline resectable pancreatic adenocarcinoma: A prospective, phase II, multicentre, single-arm study. *BMC Cancer* **2019**, *19*, 922. [CrossRef]
60. Fukumitsu, N.; Okumura, T.; Hiroshima, Y.; Ishida, T.; Numajiri, H.; Murofushi, K.N.; Ohnishi, K.; Aihara, T.; Ishikawa, H.; Tsuboi, K.; et al. Simulation study of dosimetric effect in proton beam therapy using concomitant boost technique for unresectable pancreatic cancers. *Jpn. J. Radiol.* **2018**, *36*, 456–461. [CrossRef]
61. Chuong, M.; Badiyan, S.N.; Yam, M.; Li, Z.; Langen, K.; Regine, W.; Morris, C.; Snider, J., 3rd; Mehta, M.; Huh, S.; et al. Pencil beam scanning versus passively scattered proton therapy for unresectable pancreatic cancer. *J. Gastrointest. Oncol.* **2018**, *9*, 687–693. [CrossRef] [PubMed]
62. Mori, S.; Shinoto, M.; Yamada, S. Four-dimensional treatment planning in layer-stacking boost irradiation for carbon-ion pancreatic therapy. *Radiother. Oncol. J. Eur. Soc. Ther. Radiol. Oncol.* **2014**, *111*, 258–263. [CrossRef]
63. *Cancer Registry and Statistics*; Cancer Information Service, National Cancer Center: Tokyo, Japan, 2021; (Vital Statistics of Japan).
64. Fowler, J.F.; Ritter, M.A.; Chappell, R.J.; Brenner, D.J. What hypofractionated protocols should be tested for prostate cancer? *Int. J. Radiat. Oncol. Biol. Phys.* **2003**, *56*, 1093–1104. [CrossRef]
65. Michalski, J.M.; Yan, Y.; Watkins-Bruner, D.; Bosch, W.R.; Winter, K.; Galvin, J.M.; Bahary, J.P.; Morton, G.C.; Parliament, M.B.; Sandler, H.M. Preliminary toxicity analysis of 3-dimensional conformal radiation therapy versus intensity modulated radiation therapy on the high-dose arm of the Radiation Therapy Oncology Group 0126 prostate cancer trial. *Int. J. Radiat. Oncol. Biol. Phys.* **2013**, *87*, 932–938. [CrossRef]
66. Fellin, G.; Mirri, M.A.; Santoro, L.; Jereczek-Fossa, B.A.; Divan, C.; Mussari, S.; Ziglio, F.; La Face, B.; Barbera, F.; Buglione, M.; et al. Low dose rate brachytherapy (LDR-BT) as monotherapy for early stage prostate cancer in Italy: Practice and outcome analysis in a series of 2237 patients from 11 institutions. *Br. J. Radiol.* **2016**, *89*, 20150981. [CrossRef] [PubMed]
67. Shipley, W.U.; Verhey, L.J.; Munzenrider, J.E.; Suit, H.D.; Urie, M.M.; McManus, P.L.; Young, R.H.; Shipley, J.W.; Zietman, A.L.; Biggs, P.J.; et al. Advanced prostate cancer: The results of a randomized comparative trial of high dose irradiation boosting with conformal protons compared with conventional dose irradiation using photons alone. *Int. J. Radiat. Oncol. Biol. Phys.* **1995**, *32*, 3–12. [CrossRef]
68. Roach, M., 3rd; DeSilvio, M.; Valicenti, R.; Grignon, D.; Asbell, S.O.; Lawton, C.; Thomas, C.R., Jr.; Shipley, W.U. Whole-pelvis, "mini-pelvis", or prostate-only external beam radiotherapy after neoadjuvant and concurrent hormonal therapy in patients treated in the Radiation Therapy Oncology Group 9413 trial. *Int. J. Radiat. Oncol. Biol. Phys.* **2006**, *66*, 647–653. [CrossRef] [PubMed]
69. Zietman, A.L.; Bae, K.; Slater, J.D.; Shipley, W.U.; Efstathiou, J.A.; Coen, J.J.; Bush, D.A.; Lunt, M.; Spiegel, D.Y.; Skowronski, R.; et al. Randomized trial comparing conventional-dose with high-dose conformal radiation therapy in early-stage adenocarcinoma of the prostate: Long-term results from proton radiation oncology group/american college of radiology 95-09. *J. Clin. Oncol. Off. J. Am. Soc. Clin. Oncol.* **2010**, *28*, 1106–1111. [CrossRef]
70. Kuban, D.A.; Tucker, S.L.; Dong, L.; Starkschall, G.; Huang, E.H.; Cheung, M.R.; Lee, A.K.; Pollack, A. Long-term results of the M. D. Anderson randomized dose-escalation trial for prostate cancer. *Int. J. Radiat. Oncol. Biol. Phys.* **2008**, *70*, 67–74. [CrossRef]

71. D'Amico, A.V.; Manola, J.; Loffredo, M.; Renshaw, A.A.; DellaCroce, A.; Kantoff, P.W. 6-month androgen suppression plus radiation therapy vs radiation therapy alone for patients with clinically localized prostate cancer: A randomized controlled trial. *JAMA* **2004**, *292*, 821–827. [CrossRef] [PubMed]
72. Schulte, R.W.; Slater, J.D.; Rossi, C.J., Jr.; Slater, J.M. Value and perspectives of proton radiation therapy for limited stage prostate cancer. *Strahlenther. Onkol.* **2000**, *176*, 3–8. [CrossRef]
73. Ishikawa, H.; Tsuji, H.; Kamada, T.; Akakura, K.; Suzuki, H.; Shimazaki, J.; Tsujii, H.; Working Group for Genitourinary Tumors. Carbon-ion radiation therapy for prostate cancer. *Int. J. Urol. Off. J. Jpn. Urol. Assoc.* **2012**, *19*, 296–305. [CrossRef] [PubMed]
74. Murakami, M.; Ishikawa, H.; Shimizu, S.; Iwata, H.; Okimoto, T.; Takagi, M.; Murayama, S.; Akimoto, T.; Wada, H.; Arimura, T.; et al. Optimal androgen deprivation therapy combined with proton beam therapy for prostate cancer: Results from a multi-institutional study of the japanese radiation oncology study group. *Cancers* **2020**, *12*, 1690. [CrossRef] [PubMed]
75. Sanders, J.E.; Hawley, J.; Levy, W.; Gooley, T.; Buckner, C.D.; Deeg, H.J.; Doney, K.; Storb, R.; Sullivan, K.; Witherspoon, R.; et al. Pregnancies following high-dose cyclophosphamide with or without high-dose busulfan or total-body irradiation and bone marrow transplantation. *Blood* **1996**, *87*, 3045–3052. [CrossRef]
76. Green, D.M.; Whitton, J.A.; Stovall, M.; Mertens, A.C.; Donaldson, S.S.; Ruymann, F.B.; Pendergrass, T.W.; Robison, L.L. Pregnancy outcome of female survivors of childhood cancer: A report from the childhood cancer survivor study. *Am. J. Obs. Gynecol.* **2002**, *187*, 1070–1080. [CrossRef] [PubMed]
77. Mertens, A.C.; Liu, Q.; Neglia, J.P.; Wasilewski, K.; Leisenring, W.; Armstrong, G.T.; Robison, L.L.; Yasui, Y. Cause-specific late mortality among 5-year survivors of childhood cancer: The Childhood Cancer Survivor Study. *J. Natl. Cancer Inst.* **2008**, *100*, 1368–1379. [CrossRef]
78. Eaton, B.R.; Esiashvili, N.; Kim, S.; Weyman, E.A.; Thornton, L.T.; Mazewski, C.; MacDonald, T.; Ebb, D.; MacDonald, S.M.; Tarbell, N.J.; et al. Clinical Outcomes among children with standard-risk medulloblastoma treated with proton and photon radiation therapy: A comparison of disease control and overall survival. *Int. J. Radiat. Oncol. Biol. Phys.* **2016**, *94*, 133–138. [CrossRef]
79. Eaton, B.R.; Esiashvili, N.; Kim, S.; Patterson, B.; Weyman, E.A.; Thornton, L.T.; Mazewski, C.; MacDonald, T.J.; Ebb, D.; MacDonald, S.M.; et al. Endocrine outcomes with proton and photon radiotherapy for standard risk medulloblastoma. *Neuro-Oncol.* **2016**, *18*, 881–887. [CrossRef]
80. Cotter, S.E.; Herrup, D.A.; Friedmann, A.; Macdonald, S.M.; Pieretti, R.V.; Robinson, G.; Adams, J.; Tarbell, N.J.; Yock, T.I. Proton radiotherapy for pediatric bladder/prostate rhabdomyosarcoma: Clinical outcomes and dosimetry compared to intensity-modulated radiation therapy. *Int. J. Radiat. Oncol. Biol. Phys.* **2011**, *81*, 1367–1373. [CrossRef] [PubMed]
81. Ladra, M.M.; Szymonifka, J.D.; Mahajan, A.; Friedmann, A.M.; Yong Yeap, B.; Goebel, C.P.; MacDonald, S.M.; Grosshans, D.R.; Rodriguez-Galindo, C.; Marcus, K.J.; et al. Preliminary results of a phase II trial of proton radiotherapy for pediatric rhabdomyosarcoma. *J. Clin. Oncol. Off. J. Am. Soc. Clin. Oncol.* **2014**, *32*, 3762–3770. [CrossRef]
82. Weber, D.C.; Ares, C.; Albertini, F.; Frei-Welte, M.; Niggli, F.K.; Schneider, R.; Lomax, A.J. Pencil beam scanning proton therapy for pediatric parameningeal rhabdomyosarcomas: Clinical outcome of patients treated at the paul scherrer institute. *Pediatr. Blood Cancer* **2016**, *63*, 1731–1736. [CrossRef] [PubMed]
83. Mizumoto, M.; Murayama, S.; Akimoto, T.; Demizu, Y.; Fukushima, T.; Ishida, Y.; Oshiro, Y.; Numajiri, H.; Fuji, H.; Okumura, T.; et al. Preliminary results of proton radiotherapy for pediatric rhabdomyosarcoma: A multi-institutional study in Japan. *Cancer Med.* **2018**, *7*, 1870–1874. [CrossRef]
84. Pignon, J.P.; Bourhis, J.; Domenge, C.; Designe, L. Chemotherapy added to locoregional treatment for head and neck squamous-cell carcinoma: Three meta-analyses of updated individual data. MACH-NC Collaborative Group. Meta-Analysis of Chemotherapy on Head and Neck Cancer. *Lancet* **2000**, *355*, 949–955. [CrossRef]
85. Schlaich, F.; Brons, S.; Haberer, T.; Debus, J.; Combs, S.E.; Weber, K.J. Comparison of the effects of photon versus carbon ion irradiation when combined with chemotherapy in vitro. *Radiat. Oncol.* **2013**, *8*, 260. [CrossRef]
86. Harrabi, S.; Combs, S.E.; Brons, S.; Haberer, T.; Debus, J.; Weber, K.J. Temozolomide in combination with carbon ion or photon irradiation in glioblastoma multiforme cell lines—Does scheduling matter? *Int. J. Radiat. Biol.* **2013**, *89*, 692–697. [CrossRef] [PubMed]
87. Harrabi, S.B.; Adeberg, S.; Winter, M.; Haberer, T.; Debus, J.; Weber, K.J. S-phase-specific radiosensitization by gemcitabine for therapeutic carbon ion exposure in vitro. *J. Radiat. Res.* **2016**, *57*, 110–114. [CrossRef]
88. Carter, R.J.; Nickson, C.M.; Thompson, J.M.; Kacperek, A.; Hill, M.A.; Parsons, J.L. Complex DNA damage induced by high linear energy transfer alpha-particles and protons triggers a specific cellular DNA damage response. *Int. J. Radiat. Oncol. Biol. Phys.* **2018**, *100*, 776–784. [CrossRef]
89. Luhr, A.; von Neubeck, C.; Krause, M.; Troost, E.G.C. Relative biological effectiveness in proton beam therapy—Current knowledge and future challenges. *Clin. Transl. Radiat. Oncol.* **2018**, *9*, 35–41. [CrossRef]
90. Grosse, N.; Fontana, A.O.; Hug, E.B.; Lomax, A.; Coray, A.; Augsburger, M.; Paganetti, H.; Sartori, A.A.; Pruschy, M. Deficiency in homologous recombination renders Mammalian cells more sensitive to proton versus photon irradiation. *Int. J. Radiat. Oncol. Biol. Phys.* **2014**, *88*, 175–181. [CrossRef]
91. Matsumoto, Y.; Ando, K.; Kato, T.A.; Sekino, Y.; Ishikawa, H.; Sakae, T.; Tsuboi, K.; Sakurai, H. Difference in degree of sub-lethal damage recovery between clinical proton beams and X-Rays. *Radiat. Prot. Dosim.* **2019**, *183*, 93–97. [CrossRef]

92. Iwata, H.; Shuto, T.; Kamei, S.; Omachi, K.; Moriuchi, M.; Omachi, C.; Toshito, T.; Hashimoto, S.; Nakajima, K.; Sugie, C.; et al. Combined effects of cisplatin and photon or proton irradiation in cultured cells: Radiosensitization, patterns of cell death and cell cycle distribution. *J. Radiat. Res.* **2020**, *61*, 832–841. [CrossRef]
93. Krause, M.; Zips, D.; Thames, H.D.; Kummermehr, J.; Baumann, M. Preclinical evaluation of molecular-targeted anticancer agents for radiotherapy. *Radiother. Oncol. J. Eur. Soc. Ther. Radiol. Oncol.* **2006**, *80*, 112–122. [CrossRef]
94. Chae, Y.K.; Pan, A.P.; Davis, A.A.; Patel, S.P.; Carneiro, B.A.; Kurzrock, R.; Giles, F.J. Path toward precision oncology: Review of targeted therapy studies and tools to aid in defining "actionability" of a molecular lesion and patient management support. *Mol. Cancer* **2017**, *16*, 2645–2655. [CrossRef]
95. Falzone, L.; Salomone, S.; Libra, M. Evolution of cancer pharmacological treatments at the turn of the third millennium. *Front. Pharm.* **2018**, *9*, 1300. [CrossRef]
96. Koricanac, L.B.; Zakula, J.J.; Petrovic, I.M.; Valastro, L.M.; Cirrone, G.A.; Cuttone, G.; Ristic-Fira, A.M. Anti-tumour activity of fotemustine and protons in combination with bevacizumab. *Chemotherapy* **2010**, *56*, 214–222. [CrossRef]
97. Park, H.J.; Oh, J.S.; Chang, J.W.; Hwang, S.G.; Kim, J.S. Proton irradiation sensitizes radioresistant non-small cell lung cancer cells by modulating epidermal growth factor receptor-mediated DNA repair. *Anticancer. Res.* **2016**, *36*, 205–212.
98. Moncharmont, C.; Guy, J.B.; Wozny, A.S.; Gilormini, M.; Battiston-Montagne, P.; Ardail, D.; Beuve, M.; Alphonse, G.; Simoens, X.; Rancoule, C.; et al. Carbon ion irradiation withstands cancer stem cells' migration/invasion process in Head and Neck Squamous Cell Carcinoma (HNSCC). *Oncotarget* **2016**, *7*, 47738–47749. [CrossRef]
99. Hirai, T.; Saito, S.; Fujimori, H.; Matsushita, K.; Nishio, T.; Okayasu, R.; Masutani, M. Radiosensitization by PARP inhibition to proton beam irradiation in cancer cells. *Biochem. Biophys. Res. Commun.* **2016**, *478*, 234–240. [CrossRef]
100. Wera, A.C.; Lobbens, A.; Stoyanov, M.; Lucas, S.; Michiels, C. Radiation-induced synthetic lethality: Combination of poly(ADP-ribose) polymerase and RAD51 inhibitors to sensitize cells to proton irradiation. *Cell Cycle* **2019**, *18*, 1770–1783. [CrossRef]
101. Kageyama, S.I.; Junyan, D.; Hojo, H.; Motegi, A.; Nakamura, M.; Tsuchihara, K.; Akimoto, T. PARP inhibitor olaparib sensitizes esophageal carcinoma cells to fractionated proton irradiation. *J. Radiat. Res.* **2020**, *61*, 177–186. [CrossRef]
102. Wang, L.; Cao, J.; Wang, X.; Lin, E.; Wang, Z.; Li, Y.; Li, Y.; Chen, M.; Wang, X.; Jiang, B.; et al. Proton and photon radiosensitization effects of niraparib, a PARP-1/-2 inhibitor, on human head and neck cancer cells. *Head Neck* **2020**, *42*, 2244–2256. [CrossRef]
103. Hirai, T.; Shirai, H.; Fujimori, H.; Okayasu, R.; Sasai, K.; Masutani, M. Radiosensitization effect of poly(ADP-ribose) polymerase inhibition in cells exposed to low and high liner energy transfer radiation. *Cancer Sci.* **2012**, *103*, 1045–1050. [CrossRef] [PubMed]
104. Lesueur, P.; Chevalier, F.; El-Habr, E.A.; Junier, M.P.; Chneiweiss, H.; Castera, L.; Muller, E.; Stefan, D.; Saintigny, Y. Radiosensitization effect of talazoparib, a parp inhibitor, on glioblastoma stem cells exposed to low and high linear energy transfer radiation. *Sci. Rep.* **2018**, *8*, 3664. [CrossRef] [PubMed]
105. Hirakawa, H.; Fujisawa, H.; Masaoka, A.; Noguchi, M.; Hirayama, R.; Takahashi, M.; Fujimori, A.; Okayasu, R. The combination of Hsp90 inhibitor 17AAG and heavy-ion irradiation provides effective tumor control in human lung cancer cells. *Cancer Med.* **2015**, *4*, 426–436. [CrossRef]
106. Li, H.K.; Matsumoto, Y.; Furusawa, Y.; Kamada, T. PU-H71, a novel Hsp90 inhibitor, as a potential cancer-specific sensitizer to carbon-ion beam therapy. *J. Radiat. Res.* **2016**, *57*, 572–575. [CrossRef]
107. Yu, J.I.; Choi, C.; Shin, S.W.; Son, A.; Lee, G.H.; Kim, S.Y.; Park, H.C. Valproic acid sensitizes hepatocellular carcinoma cells to proton therapy by suppressing NRF2 activation. *Sci. Rep.* **2017**, *7*, 14986. [CrossRef] [PubMed]
108. Gerelchuluun, A.; Maeda, J.; Manabe, E.; Brents, C.A.; Sakae, T.; Fujimori, A.; Chen, D.J.; Tsuboi, K.; Kato, T.A. Histone deacetylase inhibitor induced radiation sensitization effects on human cancer cells after photon and hadron radiation exposure. *Int. J. Mol. Sci.* **2018**, *19*, 496. [CrossRef]
109. Rosa, S.; Connolly, C.; Schettino, G.; Butterworth, K.T.; Prise, K.M. Biological mechanisms of gold nanoparticle radiosensitization. *Cancer Nanotechnol.* **2017**, *8*, 2. [CrossRef]
110. Wang, H.; Mu, X.; He, H.; Zhang, X.D. Cancer radiosensitizers. *Trends Pharm. Sci.* **2018**, *39*, 24–48. [CrossRef]
111. Klebowski, B.; Depciuch, J.; Parlinska-Wojtan, M.; Baran, J. Applications of noble metal-based nanoparticles in medicine. *Int. J. Mol. Sci.* **2018**, *19*, 4031. [CrossRef] [PubMed]
112. Jeremic, B.; Aguerri, A.R.; Filipovic, N. Radiosensitization by gold nanoparticles. *Clin. Transl. Oncol.* **2013**, *15*, 593–601. [CrossRef] [PubMed]
113. Schuemann, J.; Bagley, A.F.; Berbeco, R.; Bromma, K.; Butterworth, K.T.; Byrne, H.L.; Chithrani, B.D.; Cho, S.H.; Cook, J.R.; Favaudon, V.; et al. Roadmap for metal nanoparticles in radiation therapy: Current status, translational challenges, and future directions. *Phys. Med. Biol.* **2020**, *65*, 21RM02. [CrossRef]
114. Peukert, D.; Kempson, I.; Douglass, M.; Bezak, E. Metallic nanoparticle radiosensitisation of ion radiotherapy: A review. *Phys. Med.* **2018**, *47*, 121–128. [CrossRef]
115. Lacombe, S.; Porcel, E.; Scifoni, E. Particle therapy and nanomedicine: State of art and research perspectives. *Cancer Nanotechnol.* **2017**, *8*, 9. [CrossRef] [PubMed]
116. Chen, L.; Fujisawa, N.; Takanohashi, M.; Najmina, M.; Uto, K.; Ebara, M. A smart hyperthermia nanofiber-platform-enabled sustained release of doxorubicin and 17AAG for synergistic cancer therapy. *Int. J. Mol. Sci.* **2021**, *22*, 2542. [CrossRef] [PubMed]
117. Chen, W.; Wu, Z.; Yang, H.; Guo, S.; Li, D.; Cheng, L. In vitro and in vivo evaluation of injectable implants for intratumoral delivery of 5-fluorouracil. *Pharm. Dev. Technol.* **2014**, *19*, 223–231. [CrossRef]

118. Kim, Y.J.; Ebara, M.; Aoyagi, T. Temperature-responsive electrospun nanofibers for 'on-off' switchable release of dextran. *Sci. Technol. Adv. Mater.* **2012**, *13*, 064203. [CrossRef] [PubMed]
119. Wang, Y.; Kotsuchibashi, Y.; Liu, Y.; Narain, R. Study of bacterial adhesion on biomimetic temperature responsive glycopolymer surfaces. *ACS Appl. Mater. Interfaces* **2015**, *7*, 1652–1661. [CrossRef] [PubMed]
120. Wang, Y.; Kotsuchibashi, Y.; Uto, K.; Ebara, M.; Aoyagi, T.; Liu, Y.; Narain, R. pH and glucose responsive nanofibers for the reversible capture and release of lectins. *Biomater. Sci.* **2015**, *3*, 152–162. [CrossRef]
121. Okada, T.; Niiyama, E.; Uto, K.; Aoyagi, T.; Ebara, M. Inactivated sendai virus (HVJ-E) immobilized electrospun nanofiber for cancer therapy. *Materials* **2015**, *9*, 12. [CrossRef]
122. Suzuki, K.; Tanaka, H.; Ebara, M.; Uto, K.; Matsuoka, H.; Nishimoto, S.; Okada, K.; Murase, T.; Yoshikawa, H. Electrospun nanofiber sheets incorporating methylcobalamin promote nerve regeneration and functional recovery in a rat sciatic nerve crush injury model. *Acta Biomater.* **2017**, *53*, 250–259. [CrossRef] [PubMed]
123. Niiyama, E.; Uto, K.; Lee, C.M.; Sakura, K.; Ebara, M. Hyperthermia nanofiber platform synergized by sustained release of paclitaxel to improve antitumor efficiency. *Adv. Healthc Mater.* **2019**, *8*, e1900102. [CrossRef]
124. Niiyama, E.; Uto, K.; Lee, C.M.; Sakura, K.; Ebara, M. Alternating magnetic field-triggered switchable nanofiber mesh for cancer thermo-chemotherapy. *Polymers* **2018**, *10*, 1018. [CrossRef] [PubMed]
125. Fujisawa, N.; Takanohashi, M.; Chen, L.; Uto, K.; Matsumoto, Y.; Takeuchi, M.; Ebara, M. A Diels-Alder polymer platform for thermally enhanced drug release toward efficient local cancer chemotherapy. *Sci. Technol. Adv. Mater.* **2021**, *22*, 522–531. [CrossRef] [PubMed]
126. Formenti, S.C.; Demaria, S. Systemic effects of local radiotherapy. *Lancet Oncol.* **2009**, *10*, 718–726. [CrossRef]
127. Haikerwal, S.J.; Hagekyriakou, J.; MacManus, M.; Martin, O.A.; Haynes, N.M. Building immunity to cancer with radiation therapy. *Cancer Lett* **2015**, *368*, 198–208. [CrossRef] [PubMed]
128. Scheithauer, H.; Belka, C.; Lauber, K.; Gaipl, U.S. Immunological aspects of radiotherapy. *Radiat. Oncol.* **2014**, *9*, 185. [CrossRef]
129. Galluzzi, L.; Buque, A.; Kepp, O.; Zitvogel, L.; Kroemer, G. Immunogenic cell death in cancer and infectious disease. *Nat. Rev. Immunol.* **2017**, *17*, 97–111. [CrossRef]
130. Grass, G.D.; Krishna, N.; Kim, S. The immune mechanisms of abscopal effect in radiation therapy. *Curr. Probl. Cancer* **2016**, *40*, 10–24. [CrossRef]
131. Girdhani, S.; Lamont, C.; Hahnfeldt, P.; Abdollahi, A.; Hlatky, L. Proton irradiation suppresses angiogenic genes and impairs cell invasion and tumor growth. *Radiat. Res.* **2012**, *178*, 33–45. [CrossRef] [PubMed]
132. Gameiro, S.R.; Malamas, A.S.; Bernstein, M.B.; Tsang, K.Y.; Vassantachart, A.; Sahoo, N.; Tailor, R.; Pidikiti, R.; Guha, C.P.; Hahn, S.M.; et al. Tumor cells surviving exposure to proton or photon radiation share a common immunogenic modulation signature, rendering them more sensitive to T cell-mediated killing. *Int. J. Radiat. Oncol. Biol. Phys.* **2016**, *95*, 120–130. [CrossRef] [PubMed]
133. Girdhani, S.; Sachs, R.; Hlatky, L. Biological effects of proton radiation: What we know and don't know. *Radiat. Res.* **2013**, *179*, 257–272. [CrossRef] [PubMed]
134. Ando, K.; Fujita, H.; Hosoi, A.; Ma, L.; Wakatsuki, M.; Seino, K.I.; Kakimi, K.; Imai, T.; Shimokawa, T.; Nakano, T. Intravenous dendritic cell administration enhances suppression of lung metastasis induced by carbon-ion irradiation. *J. Radiat. Res.* **2017**, *58*, 446–455. [CrossRef]
135. Ogata, T.; Teshima, T.; Kagawa, K.; Hishikawa, Y.; Takahashi, Y.; Kawaguchi, A.; Suzumoto, Y.; Nojima, K.; Furusawa, Y.; Matsuura, N. Particle irradiation suppresses metastatic potential of cancer cells. *Cancer Res.* **2005**, *65*, 113–120. [PubMed]
136. Ohkubo, Y.; Iwakawa, M.; Seino, K.; Nakawatari, M.; Wada, H.; Kamijuku, H.; Nakamura, E.; Nakano, T.; Imai, T. Combining carbon ion radiotherapy and local injection of alpha-galactosylceramide-pulsed dendritic cells inhibits lung metastases in an in vivo murine model. *Int. J. Radiat. Oncol. Biol. Phys.* **2010**, *78*, 1524–1531. [CrossRef]
137. Durante, M.; Brenner, D.J.; Formenti, S.C. Does heavy ion therapy work through the immune system? *Int. J. Radiat. Oncol. Biol. Phys.* **2016**, *96*, 934–936. [CrossRef] [PubMed]
138. Durante, M.; Reppingen, N.; Held, K.D. Immunologically augmented cancer treatment using modern radiotherapy. *Trends Mol. Med.* **2013**, *19*, 565–582. [CrossRef]
139. Abei, M.; Okumura, T.; Fukuda, K.; Hashimoto, T.; Araki, M.; Ishige, K.; Hyodo, I.; Kanemoto, A.; Numajiri, H.; Mizumoto, M.; et al. A phase I study on combined therapy with proton-beam radiotherapy and in situ tumor vaccination for locally advanced recurrent hepatocellular carcinoma. *Radiat. Oncol.* **2013**, *8*, 239. [CrossRef]
140. Taylor, H.J.; Goldhaber, M. Detection of nuclear disintegration in a photographic emulsion. *Nature* **1935**, *135*, 341. [CrossRef]
141. GL, L. Biological effects and therapeutic possiblilities of neutron. *Am. J. Roentgenol.* **1936**, *36*, 1–13.
142. Farr, L.E.; Sweet, W.H.; Robertson, J.S.; Foster, C.G.; Locksley, H.B.; Sutherland, D.L.; Mendelsohn, M.L.; Stickley, E.E. Neutron capture therapy with boron in the treatment of glioblastoma multiforme. *Am. J. Roentgenol. Radium Nucl. Med.* **1954**, *71*, 279–293.
143. Slatkin, D.N. A history of boron neutron capture therapy of brain tumours. Postulation of a brain radiation dose tolerance limit. *Brain* **1991**, *114*, 1609–1629. [CrossRef] [PubMed]
144. Sweet, W.H. Early history of development of boron neutron capture therapy of tumors. *J. Neurooncol.* **1997**, *33*, 19–26. [CrossRef]
145. Hatanaka, H.; Nakagawa, Y. Clinical results of long-surviving brain tumor patients who underwent boron neutron capture therapy. *Int. J. Radiat. Oncol. Biol. Phys.* **1994**, *28*, 1061–1066. [CrossRef]

146. Mishima, Y.; Honda, C.; Ichihashi, M.; Obara, H.; Hiratsuka, J.; Fukuda, H.; Karashima, H.; Kobayashi, T.; Kanda, K.; Yoshino, K. Treatment of malignant melanoma by single thermal neutron capture therapy with melanoma-seeking 10B-compound. *Lancet* **1989**, *2*, 388–389. [CrossRef]
147. Sauerwein, W.; Zurlo, A.; Group, E.B.N.C.T. The EORTC Boron Neutron Capture Therapy (BNCT) Group: Achievements and future projects. *Eur. J. Cancer* **2002**, *38*, S31–S34. [CrossRef]
148. Wittig, A.; Moss, R.L.; Stecher-Rasmussen, F.; Appelman, K.; Rassow, J.; Roca, A.; Sauerwein, W. Neutron activation of patients following boron neutron capture therapy of brain tumors at the high flux reactor (HFR) Petten (EORTC Trials 11961 and 11011). *Strahlenther. Onkol.* **2005**, *181*, 774–782. [CrossRef]
149. Sakamoto, S.; Kiger, W.S., 3rd; Harling, O.K. Sensitivity studies of beam directionality, beam size, and neutron spectrum for a fission converter-based epithermal neutron beam for boron neutron capture therapy. *Med. Phys.* **1999**, *26*, 1979–1988. [CrossRef] [PubMed]
150. Kobayashi, T.; Kanda, K.; Ujeno, Y.; Ishida, M.R. Biomedical irradiation system for boron neutron capture therapy at the Kyoto University Reactor. *Basic Life Sci.* **1990**, *54*, 321–339.
151. Auterinen, I.; Kotiluoto, P.; Hippelainen, E.; Kortesniemi, M.; Seppala, T.; Seren, T.; Mannila, V.; Poyry, P.; Kankaanranta, L.; Collan, J.; et al. Design and construction of shoulder recesses into the beam aperture shields for improved patient positioning at the FiR 1 BNCT facility. *Appl. Radiat. Isot.* **2004**, *61*, 799–803. [CrossRef] [PubMed]
152. Nakamura, T.; Horiguchi, H.; Kishi, T.; Motohashi, J.; Sasajima, F.; Kumada, H. Resumption of JRR-4 and characteristics of neutron beam for BNCT. *Appl. Radiat. Isot.* **2011**, *69*, 1932–1935. [CrossRef] [PubMed]
153. Wang, C.K.; Blue, T.E.; Gahbauer, R.A. A design study of an accelerator-based epithermal neutron source for boron neutron capture therapy. *Strahlenther. Onkol.* **1989**, *165*, 75–78. [PubMed]
154. Kreiner, A.J.; Baldo, M.; Bergueiro, J.R.; Cartelli, D.; Castell, W.; Thatar Vento, V.; Gomez Asoia, J.; Mercuri, D.; Padulo, J.; Suarez Sandin, J.C.; et al. Accelerator-based BNCT. *Appl. Radiat. Isot.* **2014**, *88*, 185–189. [CrossRef]
155. Kumada, H.; Kurihara, T.; Yoshioka, M.; Kobayashi, H.; Matsumoto, H.; Sugano, T.; Sakurai, H.; Sakae, T.; Matsumura, A. development of beryllium-based neutron target system with three-layer structure for accelerator-based neutron source for boron neutron capture therapy. *Appl. Radiat. Isot.* **2015**, *106*, 78–83. [CrossRef]
156. Taskaev, S.; Berendeev, E.; Bikchurina, M.; Bykov, T.; Kasatov, D.; Kolesnikov, I.; Koshkarev, A.; Makarov, A.; Ostreinov, G.; Porosev, V.; et al. Neutron source based on vacuum insulated tandem accelerator and lithium target. *Biology* **2021**, *10*, 350.
157. Hirose, K.; Konno, A.; Hiratsuka, J.; Yoshimoto, S.; Kato, T.; Ono, K.; Otsuki, N.; Hatazawa, J.; Tanaka, H.; Takayama, K.; et al. Boron neutron capture therapy using cyclotron-based epithermal neutron source and borofalan ((10)B) for recurrent or locally advanced head and neck cancer (JHN002): An open-label phase II trial. *Radiother. Oncol. J. Eur. Soc. Ther. Radiol. Oncol.* **2021**, *155*, 182–187. [CrossRef] [PubMed]
158. Kanno, H.; Nagata, H.; Ishiguro, A.; Tsuzuranuki, S.; Nakano, S.; Nonaka, T.; Kiyohara, K.; Kimura, T.; Sugawara, A.; Okazaki, Y.; et al. Designation products: Boron neutron capture therapy for head and neck carcinoma. *Oncologist* **2021**, *26*, e1250–e1255. [CrossRef] [PubMed]
159. Miyatake, S.I.; Wanibuchi, M.; Hu, N.; Ono, K. Boron neutron capture therapy for malignant brain tumors. *J. Neurooncol.* **2020**, *149*, 1–11. [CrossRef]
160. Provenzano, L.; Koivunoro, H.; Postuma, I.; Longhino, J.M.; Boggio, E.F.; Farias, R.O.; Bortolussi, S.; Gonzalez, S.J. The essential role of radiobiological figures of merit for the assessment and comparison of beam performances in boron neutron capture therapy. *Phys. Med.* **2019**, *67*, 9–19. [CrossRef]
161. Lee, P.Y.; Tang, X.; Geng, C.; Liu, Y.H. A bi-tapered and air-gapped beam shaping assembly used for AB-BNCT. *Appl. Radiat. Isot.* **2021**, *167*, 109392. [CrossRef] [PubMed]
162. Yamamoto, T.; Matsumura, A.; Yamamoto, K.; Kumada, H.; Shibata, Y.; Nose, T. In-phantom two-dimensional thermal neutron distribution for intraoperative boron neutron capture therapy of brain tumours. *Phys. Med. Biol.* **2002**, *47*, 2387–2396. [CrossRef]
163. Kumada, H.; Yamamoto, K.; Matsumura, A.; Yamamoto, T.; Nakagawa, Y.; Nakai, K.; Kageji, T. Verification of the computational dosimetry system in JAERI (JCDS) for boron neutron capture therapy. *Phys. Med. Biol.* **2004**, *49*, 3353–3365. [CrossRef] [PubMed]
164. Wojnecki, C.; Green, S. A preliminary comparative study of two treatment planning systems developed for boron neutron capture therapy: MacNCTPlan and SERA. *Med. Phys.* **2002**, *29*, 1710–1715. [CrossRef]
165. Koivunoro, H.; Kumada, H.; Seppala, T.; Kotiluoto, P.; Auterinen, I.; Kankaanranta, L.; Savolainen, S. Comparative study of dose calculations with SERA and JCDS treatment planning systems. *Appl. Radiat. Isot.* **2009**, *67*, S126–S129. [CrossRef]
166. Li, H.S.; Liu, Y.W.; Lee, C.Y.; Lin, T.Y.; Hsu, F.Y. Verification of the accuracy of BNCT treatment planning system THORplan. *Appl. Radiat. Isot.* **2009**, *67*, S122–S125. [CrossRef] [PubMed]
167. Kumada, H.; Yamamoto, K.; Yamamoto, T.; Nakai, K.; Nakagawa, Y.; Kageji, T.; Matsumura, A. Improvement of dose calculation accuracy for BNCT dosimetry by the multi-voxel method in JCDS. *Appl. Radiat. Isot.* **2004**, *61*, 1045–1050. [CrossRef]
168. Nakagawa, Y.; Pooh, K.; Kobayashi, T.; Kageji, T.; Uyama, S.; Matsumura, A.; Kumada, H. Clinical review of the Japanese experience with boron neutron capture therapy and a proposed strategy using epithermal neutron beams. *J. Neurooncol.* **2003**, *62*, 87–99. [CrossRef] [PubMed]
169. Watanabe, K.; Yoshihashi, S.; Ishikawa, A.; Honda, S.; Yamazaki, A.; Tsurita, Y.; Uritani, A.; Tsuchida, K.; Kiyanagi, Y. First experimental verification of the neutron field of Nagoya University Accelerator-driven neutron source for boron neutron capture therapy. *Appl. Radiat. Isot.* **2021**, *168*, 109553. [CrossRef]

170. Nakamura, S.; Igaki, H.; Ito, M.; Imamichi, S.; Kashihara, T.; Okamoto, H.; Nishioka, S.; Iijima, K.; Chiba, T.; Nakayama, H.; et al. Neutron flux evaluation model provided in the accelerator-based boron neutron capture therapy system employing a solid-state lithium target. *Sci. Rep.* **2021**, *11*, 8090. [CrossRef] [PubMed]
171. Kato, I.; Ono, K.; Sakurai, Y.; Ohmae, M.; Maruhashi, A.; Imahori, Y.; Kirihata, M.; Nakazawa, M.; Yura, Y. Effectiveness of BNCT for recurrent head and neck malignancies. *Appl. Radiat. Isot.* **2004**, *61*, 1069–1073. [CrossRef]
172. Kato, I.; Fujita, Y.; Maruhashi, A.; Kumada, H.; Ohmae, M.; Kirihata, M.; Imahori, Y.; Suzuki, M.; Sakrai, Y.; Sumi, T.; et al. Effectiveness of boron neutron capture therapy for recurrent head and neck malignancies. *Appl. Radiat. Isot.* **2009**, *67*, S37–S42. [CrossRef]
173. Aihara, T.; Morita, N.; Kamitani, N.; Kumada, H.; Ono, K.; Hiratsuka, J.; Harada, T. BNCT for advanced or recurrent head and neck cancer. *Appl. Radiat. Isot.* **2014**, *88*, 12–15. [CrossRef]
174. Kankaanranta, L.; Seppala, T.; Koivunoro, H.; Saarilahti, K.; Atula, T.; Collan, J.; Salli, E.; Kortesniemi, M.; Uusi-Simola, J.; Valimaki, P.; et al. Boron neutron capture therapy in the treatment of locally recurred head-and-neck cancer: Final analysis of a phase I/II trial. *Int. J. Radiat. Oncol. Biol. Phys.* **2012**, *82*, e67–e75. [CrossRef] [PubMed]
175. Wang, L.W.; Wang, S.J.; Chu, P.Y.; Ho, C.Y.; Jiang, S.H.; Liu, Y.W.; Liu, Y.H.; Liu, H.M.; Peir, J.J.; Chou, F.I.; et al. BNCT for locally recurrent head and neck cancer: Preliminary clinical experience from a phase I/II trial at Tsing Hua Open-Pool Reactor. *Appl. Radiat. Isot.* **2011**, *69*, 1803–1806. [CrossRef] [PubMed]
176. Stupp, R.; Mason, W.P.; van den Bent, M.J.; Weller, M.; Fisher, B.; Taphoorn, M.J.; Belanger, K.; Brandes, A.A.; Marosi, C.; Bogdahn, U.; et al. Radiotherapy plus concomitant and adjuvant temozolomide for glioblastoma. *New Engl. J. Med.* **2005**, *352*, 987–996. [CrossRef]
177. Barth, R.F.; Yang, W.; Rotaru, J.H.; Moeschberger, M.L.; Boesel, C.P.; Soloway, A.H.; Joel, D.D.; Nawrocky, M.M.; Ono, K.; Goodman, J.H. Boron neutron capture therapy of brain tumors: Enhanced survival and cure following blood-brain barrier disruption and intracarotid injection of sodium borocaptate and boronophenylalanine. *Int. J. Radiat. Oncol. Biol. Phys.* **2000**, *47*, 209–218. [CrossRef]
178. Yamamoto, T.; Nakai, K.; Kageji, T.; Kumada, H.; Endo, K.; Matsuda, M.; Shibata, Y.; Matsumura, A. Boron neutron capture therapy for newly diagnosed glioblastoma. *Radiother. Oncol. J. Eur. Soc. Ther. Radiol. Oncol.* **2009**, *91*, 80–84. [CrossRef] [PubMed]
179. Takai, S.; Wanibuchi, M.; Kawabata, S.; Takeuchi, K.; Sakurai, Y.; Suzuki, M.; Ono, K.; Miyatake, S.I. Reactor-based boron neutron capture therapy for 44 cases of recurrent and refractory high-grade meningiomas with long-term follow-up. *Neuro-Oncol.* **2021**. [CrossRef]
180. Kageji, T.; Nagahiro, S.; Matsuzaki, K.; Mizobuchi, Y.; Toi, H.; Nakagawa, Y.; Kumada, H. Boron neutron capture therapy using mixed epithermal and thermal neutron beams in patients with malignant glioma-correlation between radiation dose and radiation injury and clinical outcome. *Int. J. Radiat. Oncol. Biol. Phys.* **2006**, *65*, 1446–1455. [CrossRef]
181. Kageji, T.; Mizobuchi, Y.; Nagahiro, S.; Nakagawa, Y.; Kumada, H. Clinical results of boron neutron capture therapy (BNCT) for glioblastoma. *Appl. Radiat. Isot.* **2011**, *69*, 1823–1825. [CrossRef] [PubMed]
182. Miyatake, S.; Kawabata, S.; Kajimoto, Y.; Aoki, A.; Yokoyama, K.; Yamada, M.; Kuroiwa, T.; Tsuji, M.; Imahori, Y.; Kirihata, M.; et al. Modified boron neutron capture therapy for malignant gliomas performed using epithermal neutron and two boron compounds with different accumulation mechanisms: An efficacy study based on findings on neuroimages. *J. Neurosurg.* **2005**, *103*, 1000–1009. [CrossRef]
183. Kawabata, S.; Miyatake, S.; Kuroiwa, T.; Yokoyama, K.; Doi, A.; Iida, K.; Miyata, S.; Nonoguchi, N.; Michiue, H.; Takahashi, M.; et al. Boron neutron capture therapy for newly diagnosed glioblastoma. *J. Radiat. Res.* **2009**, *50*, 51–60. [CrossRef] [PubMed]
184. Miyatake, S.; Kawabata, S.; Yokoyama, K.; Kuroiwa, T.; Michiue, H.; Sakurai, Y.; Kumada, H.; Suzuki, M.; Maruhashi, A.; Kirihata, M.; et al. Survival benefit of Boron neutron capture therapy for recurrent malignant gliomas. *J. Neurooncol.* **2009**, *91*, 199–206. [CrossRef] [PubMed]
185. Ono, K.; Masunaga, S.; Suzuki, M.; Kinashi, Y.; Takagaki, M.; Akaboshi, M. The combined effect of boronophenylalanine and borocaptate in boron neutron capture therapy for SCCVII tumors in mice. *Int. J. Radiat. Oncol. Biol. Phys.* **1999**, *43*, 431–436. [CrossRef]
186. Coderre, J.A.; Elowitz, E.H.; Chadha, M.; Bergland, R.; Capala, J.; Joel, D.D.; Liu, H.B.; Slatkin, D.N.; Chanana, A.D. Boron neutron capture therapy for glioblastoma multiforme using p-boronophenylalanine and epithermal neutrons: Trial design and early clinical results. *J. Neurooncol.* **1997**, *33*, 141–152. [CrossRef]
187. Finkel, G.C.; Poletti, C.E.; Fairchild, R.G.; Slatkin, D.N.; Sweet, W.H. Distribution of 10B after infusion of Na210B12H11SH into a patient with malignant astrocytoma: Implications for boron neutron capture therapy. *Neurosurgery* **1989**, *24*, 6–11. [CrossRef]
188. Kageji, T.; Nakagawa, Y.; Kitamura, K.; Matsumoto, K.; Hatanaka, H. Pharmacokinetics and boron uptake of BSH (Na2B12H11SH) in patients with intracranial tumors. *J. Neurooncol* **1997**, *33*, 117–130. [CrossRef] [PubMed]
189. Imahori, Y.; Ueda, S.; Ohmori, Y.; Sakae, K.; Kusuki, T.; Kobayashi, T.; Takagaki, M.; Ono, K.; Ido, T.; Fujii, R. Positron emission tomography-based boron neutron capture therapy using boronophenylalanine for high-grade gliomas: Part I. *Clin. Cancer Res.* **1998**, *4*, 1825–1832. [PubMed]
190. Imahori, Y.; Ueda, S.; Ohmori, Y.; Sakae, K.; Kusuki, T.; Kobayashi, T.; Takagaki, M.; Ono, K.; Ido, T.; Fujii, R. Positron emission tomography-based boron neutron capture therapy using boronophenylalanine for high-grade gliomas: Part II. *Clin. Cancer Res.* **1998**, *4*, 1833–1841. [PubMed]

191. Aihara, T.; Hiratsuka, J.; Morita, N.; Uno, M.; Sakurai, Y.; Maruhashi, A.; Ono, K.; Harada, T. First clinical case of boron neutron capture therapy for head and neck malignancies using 18F-BPA PET. *Head Neck* **2006**, *28*, 850–855. [CrossRef]
192. *Guidebook on Accelerator BPA-BNCT*; Japan Society for Neutron Capture Therapy, Osaka/Japan Society for Radiation Oncology: Tokyo, Japan, 2020.
193. Masunaga, S.; Ono, K.; Sakurai, Y.; Suzuki, M.; Takagaki, M.; Kobayashi, T.; Kinashi, Y.; Akaboshi, M. Responses of total and quiescent cell populations in solid tumors to boron and gadolinium neutron capture reaction using neutrons with two different energy spectra. *Jpn. J. Cancer Res.* **1998**, *89*, 81–88. [CrossRef]
194. Masunaga, S.; Ono, K.; Sakurai, Y.; Takagaki, M.; Kobayashi, T.; Suzuki, M.; Kinashi, Y.; Akaboshi, M. Response of quiescent and total tumor cells in solid tumors to neutrons with various cadmium ratios. *Int. J. Radiat. Oncol. Biol. Phys.* **1998**, *41*, 1163–1170. [CrossRef]
195. Abad, E.; Samino, S.; Yanes, O.; Potesil, D.; Zdrahal, Z.; Lyakhovich, A. Activation of glycogenolysis and glycolysis in breast cancer stem cell models. *Biochim. Biophys. Acta Mol. Basis Dis.* **2020**, *1866*, 165886. [CrossRef]
196. Bao, B.; Azmi, A.S.; Li, Y.; Ahmad, A.; Ali, S.; Banerjee, S.; Kong, D.; Sarkar, F.H. Targeting CSCs in tumor microinvironment: The potential role of ROS-associated miRNAs in tumor aggressiveness. *Curr. Stem. Cell Res.* **2014**, *9*, 22–35. [CrossRef]
197. Luo, M.; Wicha, M.S. Targeting cancer stem cell redox metabolism to enhance therapy responses. *Semin. Radiat. Oncol.* **2019**, *29*, 42–54. [CrossRef] [PubMed]
198. Nakamura, H. Boron lipid-based liposomal boron delivery system for neutron capture therapy: Recent development and future perspective. *Future Med. Chem.* **2013**, *5*, 715–730. [CrossRef] [PubMed]
199. Nakase, I.; Aoki, A.; Sakai, Y.; Hirase, S.; Ishimura, M.; Takatani-Nakase, T.; Hattori, Y.; Kirihata, M. Antibody-based receptor targeting using an fc-binding peptide-dodecaborate conjugate and macropinocytosis induction for boron neutron capture therapy. *ACS Omega* **2020**, *5*, 22731–22738. [CrossRef] [PubMed]
200. Yamagami, M.; Tajima, T.; Ishimoto, K.; Miyake, H.; Michiue, H.; Takaguchi, Y. Physical modification of carbon nanotubes with a dendrimer bearing terminal mercaptoundecahydrododecaborates (Na2B12H11S). *Heteroat. Chem.* **2018**, *29*, e21467. [CrossRef]
201. Kueffer, P.J.; Maitz, C.A.; Khan, A.A.; Schuster, S.A.; Shlyakhtina, N.I.; Jalisatgi, S.S.; Brockman, J.D.; Nigg, D.W.; Hawthorne, M.F. Boron neutron capture therapy demonstrated in mice bearing EMT6 tumors following selective delivery of boron by rationally designed liposomes. *Proc. Natl. Acad. Sci. USA* **2013**, *110*, 6512–6517. [CrossRef] [PubMed]
202. Kang, W.; Svirskis, D.; Sarojini, V.; McGregor, A.L.; Bevitt, J.; Wu, Z. Cyclic-RGDyC functionalized liposomes for dual-targeting of tumor vasculature and cancer cells in glioblastoma: An in vitro boron neutron capture therapy study. *Oncotarget* **2017**, *8*, 36614–36627. [CrossRef] [PubMed]
203. Maruyama, K.; Ishida, O.; Kasaoka, S.; Takizawa, T.; Utoguchi, N.; Shinohara, A.; Chiba, M.; Kobayashi, H.; Eriguchi, M.; Yanagie, H. Intracellular targeting of sodium mercaptoundecahydrododecaborate (BSH) to solid tumors by transferrin-PEG liposomes, for boron neutron-capture therapy (BNCT). *J. Control. Release* **2004**, *98*, 195–207. [CrossRef]
204. Nomoto, T.; Inoue, Y.; Yao, Y.; Suzuki, M.; Kanamori, K.; Takemoto, H.; Matsui, M.; Tomoda, K.; Nishiyama, N. Poly(vinyl alcohol) boosting therapeutic potential of p-boronophenylalanine in neutron capture therapy by modulating metabolism. *Sci. Adv.* **2020**, *6*, eaaz1722. [CrossRef] [PubMed]
205. Matsumoto, Y.; Hattori, K.; Arima, H.; Motoyama, K.; Higashi, T.; Ishikawa, H.; Fukumitsu, N.; Aihara, T.; Nakai, K.; Kumada, H.; et al. Folate-appended cyclodextrin improves the intratumoral accumulation of existing boron compounds. *Appl. Radiat. Isot.* **2020**, *163*, 109201. [CrossRef] [PubMed]
206. Maeda, H. The 35th anniversary of the discovery of EPR effect: A new wave of nanomedicines for tumor-targeted drug delivery-personal remarks and future prospects. *J. Pers. Med.* **2021**, *11*, 229. [CrossRef]
207. Matsumura, Y.; Maeda, H. A new concept for macromolecular therapeutics in cancer chemotherapy: Mechanism of tumoritropic accumulation of proteins and the antitumor agent smancs. *Cancer Res.* **1986**, *46*, 6387–6392.
208. Koganei, H.; Ueno, M.; Tachikawa, S.; Tasaki, L.; Ban, H.S.; Suzuki, M.; Shiraishi, K.; Kawano, K.; Yokoyama, M.; Maitani, Y.; et al. Development of high boron content liposomes and their promising antitumor effect for neutron capture therapy of cancers. *Bioconjug Chem.* **2013**, *24*, 124–132. [CrossRef] [PubMed]
209. Tachikawa, S.; Miyoshi, T.; Koganei, H.; El-Zaria, M.E.; Vinas, C.; Suzuki, M.; Ono, K.; Nakamura, H. Spermidinium closo-dodecaborate-encapsulating liposomes as efficient boron delivery vehicles for neutron capture therapy. *Chem. Commun.* **2014**, *50*, 12325–12328. [CrossRef]
210. Mi, P.; Yanagie, H.; Dewi, N.; Yen, H.C.; Liu, X.; Suzuki, M.; Sakurai, Y.; Ono, K.; Takahashi, Y.; Cabral, H.; et al. Block copolymer-boron cluster conjugate for effective boron neutron capture therapy of solid tumors. *J. Control. Release* **2017**, *254*, 1–9. [CrossRef] [PubMed]
211. Kikuchi, S.; Kanoh, D.; Sato, S.; Sakurai, Y.; Suzuki, M.; Nakamura, H. Maleimide-functionalized closo-dodecaborate albumin conjugates (MID-AC): Unique ligation at cysteine and lysine residues enables efficient boron delivery to tumor for neutron capture therapy. *J. Control. Release* **2016**, *237*, 160–167. [CrossRef] [PubMed]
212. Ishii, S.; Sato, S.; Asami, H.; Hasegawa, T.; Kohno, J.Y.; Nakamura, H. Design of S-S bond containing maleimide-conjugated closo-dodecaborate (SSMID): Identification of unique modification sites on albumin and investigation of intracellular uptake. *Org. Biomol. Chem.* **2019**, *17*, 5496–5499. [CrossRef]

213. Sumitani, S.; Oishi, M.; Yaguchi, T.; Murotani, H.; Horiguchi, Y.; Suzuki, M.; Ono, K.; Yanagie, H.; Nagasaki, Y. Pharmacokinetics of core-polymerized, boron-conjugated micelles designed for boron neutron capture therapy for cancer. *Biomaterials* **2012**, *33*, 3568–3577. [PubMed]
214. Kim, A.; Suzuki, M.; Matsumoto, Y.; Fukumitsu, N.; Nagasaki, Y. Non-isotope enriched phenylboronic acid-decorated dual-functional nano-assembles for an actively targeting BNCT drug. *Biomaterials* **2021**, *268*, 120551. [PubMed]
215. Islam, W.; Matsumoto, Y.; Fang, J.; Harada, A.; Niidome, T.; Ono, K.; Tsutsuki, H.; Sawa, T.; Imamura, T.; Sakurai, K.; et al. Polymer-conjugated glucosamine complexed with boric acid shows tumor-selective accumulation and simultaneous inhibition of glycolysis. *Biomaterials* **2021**, *269*, 120631. [CrossRef] [PubMed]

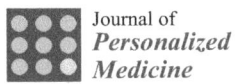

Review

The Enhanced Permeability and Retention (EPR) Effect: The Significance of the Concept and Methods to Enhance Its Application

Jun Wu

Center for Comparative Medicine, Beckman Research Institute of the City of Hope, 1500 East Duarte Rd, Duarte, CA 91010, USA; jwu@coh.org; Tel.: +1-626-218-3305

Abstract: Chemotherapy for human solid tumors in clinical practice is far from satisfactory. Despite the discovery and synthesis of hundreds of thousands of anticancer compounds targeting various crucial units in cancer cell proliferation and metabolism, the fundamental problem is the lack of targeting delivery of these compounds selectively into solid tumor tissue to maintain an effective concentration level for a certain length of time for drug-tumor interaction to execute anticancer activities. The enhanced permeability and retention effect (EPR effect) describes a universal pathophysiological phenomenon and mechanism in which macromolecular compounds such as albumin and other polymer-conjugated drugs beyond certain sizes (above 40 kDa) can progressively accumulate in the tumor vascularized area and thus achieve targeting delivery and retention of anticancer compounds into solid tumor tissue. Targeting therapy via the EPR effect in clinical practice is not always successful since the strength of the EPR effect varies depending on the type and location of tumors, status of blood perfusion in tumors, and the physical-chemical properties of macromolecular anticancer agents. This review highlights the significance of the concept and mechanism of the EPR effect and discusses methods for better utilizing the EPR effect in developing smarter macromolecular nanomedicine to achieve a satisfactory outcome in clinical applications.

Keywords: EPR effect; nanomedicine; drug delivery; arterial infusion; canine cancer

Citation: Wu, J. The Enhanced Permeability and Retention (EPR) Effect: The Significance of the Concept and Methods to Enhance Its Application. *J. Pers. Med.* **2021**, *11*, 771. https://doi.org/10.3390/jpm11080771

Academic Editor: Jun Fang

Received: 19 July 2021
Accepted: 4 August 2021
Published: 6 August 2021

Publisher's Note: MDPI stays neutral with regard to jurisdictional claims in published maps and institutional affiliations.

Copyright: © 2021 by the author. Licensee MDPI, Basel, Switzerland. This article is an open access article distributed under the terms and conditions of the Creative Commons Attribution (CC BY) license (https://creativecommons.org/licenses/by/4.0/).

1. Introduction

It is crucial to understand the pathophysiological characteristics of solid tumor growth, especially the compound transportation regulation of the tumor vasculature, in order to achieve selective drug delivery and therapeutic effects for cancer chemotherapy. It has been well observed that tumor vessels are highly permeable to macromolecular compounds. After entering tumor tissue, these macromolecular compounds are trapped inside the tumor tissue for a prolonged period of time. In 1986, Hiroshi Maeda and his colleagues from Kumamoto University School of Medicine coined the term enhanced permeability and retention effect (the EPR effect) to describe the unique pathophysiological phenomenon of the solid tumor vasculature [1]. Since this theory is very important for understanding tumor vessel transportation regulation, the EPR effect has been well accepted as one of the universal pathophysiological characteristics of solid tumors, and acts as a fundamental principle for designing and developing tumor-targeting delivery of anticancer drugs [2,3]. However, the development of nanomedicine has been frustrated for decades in achieving satisfactory therapeutic benefits in clinical practice. Therefore, the existence and intensity of the EPR effect in human solid tumor circumstances has been debated [4,5]. For example, it is considered that the EPR effect is more significant in experimental small animal tumor models than in human tumors. The delivery efficiency of nanoparticles into human tumor tissue is very low compared to that in animal tumor models. The extravasation mechanism for nanoparticles into tumors is not only via the gaps between endothelial cells in the tumor vasculature, but also via the transcellular pathways by vesiculo-vacuolar organelles

(VVOs) [6]. Therefore, it is crucial to recognize the significance of the EPR effects, its pathophysiological mechanism, its pitfalls, and strategies for better harnessing this concept in drug development and clinical application.

2. The EPR Effect: The Universal Pathophysiological Phenomena in Rodents, Other Mammalian Animals and Human Solid Tumors

The EPR effect has been well observed and documented in solid tumors of rodents, rabbits, canines, and human patients [1–3,7–13]. It is based on several pathophysiological characteristics of solid tumors:

(1) Massive irregular neovascularization in tumors with structural and functional abnormalities in tumor blood vessels. To meet urgent demands for nutrient and oxygen supplies, the tumor vasculature is very dense and tortuous, with deficient basement membranes and fenestrated structures of endothelial tubes in some immature vessels. The pericytes and smooth muscle cells surrounding tumor blood vessels are either deficient or malfunctional in smooth muscle alpha actin when responding to blood pressure regulation stimuli [14–16]. Recent studies have found that the gaps between endothelial cells in tumor vessels are at low frequency, and the transendothelial pathways are the dominant mechanism of nanoparticle extravasation in tumors [17]. This is consistent with the previous observation that macromolecules are highly permeable in the mature veins or venules, constructed by a continuous endothelium with closed interendothelial cell junctions [18]. These structures render them highly permeable to nutrients, especially macromolecules, to be extravasated from tumor blood vessels into the interstitial space of tumor tissue.

(2) Elevated expression of inflammatory factors such as prostaglandins, bradykinin, nitric oxide, peroxynitrite, interleukin 1 beta, interleukin 2, interleukin 6, proteases, interferon gamma, VEGF and HIF−1 alpha. All these factors coordinate in solid tumor tissues and sustain the EPR effect [7,19–21].

(3) Lack of efficient drainage of lymphatic systems in solid tumor tissue. This deficiency results in the retention of extravasated macromolecules in tumor tissues, which provides the opportunity for passive targeting delivery of macromolecular anticancer drugs [1,7,22].

3. The Significance and Challenges in Concept and Application of the EPR Effect in Human Cancer Therapy

One of the arguments for the EPR effect concerns the roles of interstitial fluid pressure [23,24] and solid stress [25] in solid tumor tissue. The interstitial fluid pressure and solid stress exist due to the expansion of the tumor mass against surrounding normal tissue. Different from interstitial fluid pressure, the solid stress in tumors is considered to be residual stress that compresses blood vessels in tumor tissues, causing hypoxia and impeding drug delivery [26]. It is believed that interstitial fluid pressure and solid stress are the major obstacles preventing efficient delivery of macromolecules into tumor tissue [27]. However, we have seen tremendous evidence that macromolecules do accumulate in both rodent and human solid tumor tissues in size-dependent and time-dependent manners. Interstitial fluid pressure or solid stress hinders drug penetration into the center of tumor tissue, but it does not prevent the macromolecular agents from extravasating and accumulating in the peripheral area of tumor tissue. The EPR effect occurs primarily in the peritumoral area [28]. Interstitial fluid pressure and solid stress provide the mechanism for the retention effect because under such pressure or stress the formation of functional lymphatic vessels is prevented due to their collapse from the pressure [22]. The interstitial fluid pressure and heterogeneous blood supply are both observed in rodent and human solid tumors; therefore, these are not valid reasons for rebuttals that assume the EPR effect won't function in human solid tumor tissue.

It is critical to understand and remember that the peripheral highly vascularized area is the most vigorously growing zone of tumors. The center of tumor tissues lacks blood flow and is necrotic or seminecrotic [28]. When suppressing the growing activities in peritumoral zones, tumors are restricted or eliminated. It is not necessary for an anticancer drug to penetrate into the center of a solid tumor to execute anticancer activities. For example, trastuzumab (Herceptin) is an antibody that is successful in treating Her2 positive breast cancer growth, and penetrates only into the vascularized area [29].

There are limited examples of successful nanomedicine treatments in cancer therapy. This is one of the biggest challenges for the application of the EPR effect in nanomedicine design and clinical practice. Some doubt the usefulness of the EPR effect in clinical practice by using the example of Doxil, a polyethylene glycol (PEG) modified-liposome formulation of doxorubicin, which does not appear to significantly improve the benefits of solid tumor treatment compared with parental free drug doxorubicin [4,5]. Pegylated liposomal doxorubicin does have a significantly longer half-life in blood circulation in patients and achieves about a 10~15-fold higher concentration in tumor tissues compared with surrounding normal tissues [30], which indicates that pegylated liposomal doxorubicin does accumulate into tumor tissue by the EPR effect. In a Phase III clinical trial, an overall response rate of 45.9% was achieved [31]. Pegylated liposomal doxorubicin exhibits better therapeutic benefit than that of free doxorubicin; however, the overall therapeutic outcome is still not satisfactory. The problem of therapeutic efficacy is probably due to compromised tumor cell killing properties by the pegylation of liposomes. An in vitro study found that pegylated liposomal doxorubicin had almost no cytotoxicity effect in the first 24 h, and only achieved about 12% cytotoxicity at 48 h in a colon cancer cell line HT29 [32]. Pegylation of liposomes significantly reduced the drug release rate, and also significantly reduced the cytotoxicity potency (25% vs. 75%) of anastrozole when compared with the free drug at the 72 h time point [33]. In another similar case, pegylation of liposomal cisplatin drastically decreased cytotoxic potency by increasing cytotoxicity IC50 from 2 μg/mL (free cisplatin) to 40 μg/mL (pegylated liposomal cisplatin) when compared to that at the 48 h time point [34]. Therefore, it is not the EPR effect that failed in clinical trials but the pegylation of liposomal chemo drugs that failed to achieve satisfactory cytotoxicity efficacy within 48-h period in clinical application.

The abnormality of tumor blood vessels obstructs the blood flow into tumor tissue. Since the tumor vascular formation is mainly attributed to the effects of vascular endothelial growth factor (VEGF), the application of VEGF antibodies antagonizes the effect of VEGF and temporarily normalizes tumor vasculature [35]. The tumor vascular normalization increased the uptake and penetration of fluorescent-labeled bovine serum albumin into tumor tissue, indicating that normalization of the tumor vasculature could increase the uptake of small particles (less than 20 nm in diameter) into tumor tissue, but hindered the uptake of larger particles above 125 nm in diameter [36]. The procedure of normalization could hamper the EPR effect because it decreases the permeability of large particles crossing the tumor vessel by reducing the gaps between endothelial cells in the tumor vessels. Many permeability factors like bradykinin, nitric oxide, prostaglandins are produced by infiltrating inflammatory cells and these factors may not be "corrected" by the anti-VEGF normalizing strategy. Thus, when attempting to normalize tumor vessels to improve the delivery of nanomedicine, the size of nanoparticles, the timing order of drug administration and vascular normalization could be critical to achieving the desired delivery results [36]. The normalization effect is therefore transient, limited, and highly heterogeneous in various tumor types or tumor locations. It should be combined with other modulation approaches such as hyperthermia, radiotherapy and sonoporation to enhance the EPR effect when applying vascular normalization [37].

4. Potential Solutions for Improving EPR Effect-Based Nanomedicine in Human Cancer Therapy

4.1. Better Design of Drug and Combination with EPR Effect Enhancing Modulators

The extent of the EPR effect varies between small animal tumors and human tumors by types and locations. To better utilize the EPR effect for human tumor therapy, the design of nanomedicine should be improved.

Size and physical-chemical properties such as surface charge and spatial configuration are crucial for a drug to achieve the EPR effect. Studies using serial molecular sizes of HPMA copolymers in solid tumor animal models indicated that the threshold of macromolecular molecules (drugs) to be retained and accumulated in tumor tissue is above 40 kDa [38]. Nanoparticles in the range of 100~200 nm are considered the optimal size for achieving the EPR effect in solid tumors while escaping the filtration traps of the liver and spleen [39]. Negative or neutral surface charges are also important for achieving excellent plasma half-lives longer than several hours in circulation in order to be accumulated in tumor tissue. Particles in worm-like shapes such as ellipsoidal, cylindrical and discoidal shapes, or filomicelles, can achieve better accumulation results within tumors [40]. Deformability and degradability are also important for a smarter drug to be released in the right environmental condition to execute a tumor-killing effect once it enters the tumor tissue [39,40]. As an example, HPMA copolymer-conjugated pirarubicin achieved very promising clinical therapeutic results in a patient with stage IV prostate cancer with extensive metastasis [41].

On the other hand, the delivery of macromolecular drugs can be enhanced by temporarily modulating the EPR effect in the targeted tumor tissues, such as applying adjuvants like nitric oxide donors to enhance the EPR effect to facilitate the drug delivery into tumor tissue. As mentioned before, many other inflammatory factors involved in the EPR effect can be utilized to modulate the intensity of this effect to facilitate drug extravasation, accumulation, and penetration into tumor tissue [42–46]. The EPR effect can also be markedly enhanced by photo-immunotherapy with antibody-photosensitizer conjugate pretreatment to achieve up to a 24-fold greater accumulation of nanomedicines in tumors. Such significant enhancement has been termed the super-enhanced permeability and retention effect [47].

4.2. Improving EPR Effect-Based Nanomedicine by Enhancing Blood Flow in Solid Tumor during Drug Administration

Blood flow in solid tumors is critical for the success of nanomedicine delivery via the EPR effect [44,46,48–51]. However, it is usually overlooked. One of the major differences between rodent solid tumors and human solid tumors is blood flow rate. Generally, the blood flow rate is about 800-fold higher in human normal organs than in mouse normal organs. For example, the normal flow rate for a mouse normal liver is about 1.8 mL/100 g/min, but it is about 1450 mL/100 g/mL in a typical human normal liver. The blood flow in mouse muscle is about 0.91 mL/100 g/mL, but it is about 750 mL/100 g/mL in a typical human muscle [52]. In 6 C3 HED lymphosarcoma in C3 H mice, the blood flow in large tumors was about 5.4 mL/100 g/min [51] while in human breast tumors, the mean blood flow was about 30~64.8 mL/100 g/min [53]. Higher blood flow means higher shear force in blood vessels and quicker wash off. The difference in blood flow rate between normal tissue and tumor tissue in rodents and humans may be important to explain why nanomedicines can accumulate better in rodent solid tumors than in human solid tumors.

The application of angiotensin II could be very efficient for drug delivery via increasing the blood flow into stagnated tumor blood vessels. Hori et al., demonstrated that when applying angiotensin II in rodent or human subjects, the blood flow in tumors was selectively increased up to 5.7-fold without increasing the blood flow in normal tissue [15]. This is because the systemic blood pressure increased but the tumor blood vessels remain relaxed due to a lack of response to angiotensin II. Such increases in blood flow in tumor tissue greatly improved the perfusion of blood into tumor tissue to achieve a higher magnitude of delivery of anticancer drugs into the solid tumor tissue [15,16]. Hori and his colleagues further demonstrated that tumor blood flow fluctuates due to circadian regulation. Tumor blood flow is increased during the night and the tumor doubling rate is also higher during the night. When they administered anticancer drugs during the night, the therapeutic efficacy was significantly improved [54]. Such brilliant discoveries have yet to be broadly recognized and applied in clinic settings by the nanomedicine drug developers and clinical oncologists.

4.3. Improving EPR Effect-Based Nanomedicine Therapeutic Effect by Arterial Infusion via Tumor Feeding Artery

Administration of nanomedicines via intravenous infusion could be problematic to achieve the desired amount of drug into tumor tissue because of high shear force to the endothelial wall brought by fast blood flow, as we discussed above. However, when administering nanomedicines via the tumor feeding artery, the strong blood flow brings more nanomedicine into tumor tissues if the size and stickiness of the nanomedicine are right for blood vessels in tumors. There are tremendous successful reports about using lipiodol for delivering SMANCS and other anticancer drugs [12,55,56] by infusion via the tumor feeding artery. However, very few other nanomedicines are designed for arterial infusion to solid tumors. It should be noted that nowadays imaging-guided catheter interventional therapy for solid tumors is very popular in clinics around the world. Radiologists are very skillful in performing interventional therapy via a tumor-feeding artery; however, the optimal nanomedicine fit for such arterial infusion is rarely available. Current low-molecular-weight drugs such as cisplatin for tumor arterial infusion are simply suspended in lipid vehicle solution. The drugs diffuse and wash out like they would in common intravenous infusion. They cannot achieve the retention effect in tumor tissue, which results in low therapeutic efficacy.

4.4. Improving EPR Effect-Based Nanomedicine Preclinical Development by Using Large Animal Tumor Models

The last but not least critical issue is the selection of better animal models for the preclinical development of nanomedicine. Most products of nanomedicine are developed in small rodent tumor models. The tumors in mice are either induced by carcinogens or created by genetic engineering such as knocking in or knocking out certain genes that are related to the tumor initiation. Transplantation of a tumor from donor to recipient is another major way to create syngeneic tumor models, or xenograft tumor models, by established cell lines or fresh tumor tissues. Patient-derived xenograft (PDX) models have featured in preclinical studies in recent years. However, there is a vast difference in size between mice and humans, and thus the drug absorption, metabolism, distribution and exclusion profiles, as well as the pharmacokinetic and pharmacodynamic properties of the drugs in tumor tissue, would be very different in mice and humans. The tumors induced by cell lines or tumor tissue might also result in extreme growth behavior, such as an extraordinarily large size or an abnormally fast-growing pattern that is rarely seen in human tumors. Although rodent solid tumors exhibit excellent results of the EPR effect, the strength of the EPR effect could be very different compared to that in solid tumors of human patients. Thus, the EPR effect of a nanomedicine candidate measured in rodent tumor models might not be correctly estimated for translating into human clinical application. Canine cancers are naturally occurring with full-spectrum heterogeneity of tumor cell populations, bona fide tumor microenvironments and spatial structures that faithfully reflect the intrinsic status of blood flow and interstitial pressures of tumors. Studies show that copper−64 liposomes exhibited excellent permeability and retention (tumor uptake levels at 24 h after injection achieved 3.68-fold higher than at 1 h after injection) in different canine cancers at various locations such as mammary glands, neck muscle, front paw and intranasal regions [13]. Using larger animals such as canine cancer models is, therefore, better for guiding the preclinical development of nanomedicine. Unfortunately, there are few publications featuring utilization of canine cancer models for nanomedicine development. Companion animals as translational models can provide more accurate measurements of therapeutic efficacy based on the EPR effect and, therefore, should be considered as major animal models for the development of nanomedicine.

5. Conclusions

The EPR effect is the fundamental pathophysiological phenomenon of solid tumors universally observed in solid tumors in rodents and humans, as well as in other mammalian species. It is also the guiding principle for developing nanomedicine (including polymer-conjugated macromolecular anticancer drugs) aimed at passive and progressive drug delivery and retention inside the tumor tissue to achieve selective and highly efficient anticancer outcomes. However due to the heterogeneous strength in various microenvironment situations, the EPR effect has been challenged for its existence and importance in nanomedicine design and application. As a matter of fact, the EPR effect has been observed in human tumor tissues for various macromolecular compounds. When discussing the heterogeneity of the EPR effect, it should be clear that the heterogeneity is confined to the strength of the accumulation and retention of the EPR effect that varies in different types of solid tumors under various tissue environments.

The real challenge is how to utilize the EPR effect in designing and improving the therapeutic efficacy of nanomedicine. There are several enhancing strategies to improve delivery and accumulation efficacies, such as optimal size and surface charge, smarter mechanism for drug release and administration kinetics. Due to their rigid structure property, the accumulation performance of nanoparticles in tumor tissues may not necessarily be the same as with other macromolecules such as linear polymers and biological macromolecules such as albumins. Therefore, further modification of nanoparticles with polymers to improve the affinity of the nanoparticles with tumor related endothelial cells may be necessary.

Blood flow plays a critical role in delivering nanomedicines into tumor tissues. Arterial infusion via a tumor-feeding artery, and the timing of using tumor blood flow enhancers or EPR effect modulators should be applied to nanomedicine to achieve better therapeutic effects. As the strength of the EPR effect is quite different between small animal tumor models and human tumors, the selection of big animal models is also critical for guiding the design of nanomedicine by properly estimating the efficacy of tumor-targeting delivery via the EPR effect. Companion animal tumor models such as canine cancer should be utilized to guide the development of nanomedicine.

When considering the EPR effect, retention efficacy is crucial because for a drug to execute anticancer activities it should maintain above a certain effective concentration level for a certain length of time in the tumor tissue to achieve a satisfactory result.

A better future of nanomedicine via the EPR effect is yet to come.

Funding: This research received no external funding.

Institutional Review Board Statement: Not applicable.

Informed Consent Statement: Not applicable.

Data Availability Statement: Not applicable.

Acknowledgments: The author thanks Jim Isbell and Yingyan Wu.

Conflicts of Interest: The authors declare no conflict of interest.

References

1. Matsumura, Y.; Maeda, H. A new concept for macromolecular therapeutics in cancer chemotherapy: Mechanism of tumoritropic accumulation of proteins and the antitumor agent smancs. *Cancer Res.* **1986**, *46 Pt 1*, 6387–6392.
2. Duncan, R. Polymer conjugates for tumour targeting and intracytoplasmic delivery. The EPR effect as a common gateway? *Pharm. Sci. Technol. Today* **1999**, *2*, 441–449. [CrossRef]
3. Torchilin, V. Tumor delivery of macromolecular drugs based on the EPR effect. *Adv. Drug Deliv. Rev.* **2011**, *63*, 131–135. [CrossRef]
4. Nichols, J.W.; Bae, Y.H. EPR: Evidence and fallacy. *J. Control. Release* **2014**, *190*, 451–464. [CrossRef]
5. Danhier, F. To exploit the tumor microenvironment: Since the EPR effect fails in the clinic, what is the future of nanomedicine? *J. Control. Release* **2016**, *244*, 108–121. [CrossRef] [PubMed]
6. Shi, Y.; Van Der Meel, R.; Chen, X.; Lammers, T. The EPR effect and beyond: Strategies to improve tumor targeting and cancer nanomedicine treatment efficacy. *Theranostics* **2020**, *10*, 7921–7924. [CrossRef]
7. Maeda, H.; Wu, J.; Sawa, T.; Matsumura, Y.; Hori, K. Tumor vascular permeability and the EPR effect in macromolecular therapeutics: A review. *J. Control. Release* **2000**, *65*, 271–284. [CrossRef]
8. Maeda, H. The enhanced permeability and retention (EPR) effect in tumor vasculature: The key role of tumor-selective macromolecular drug targeting. *Adv. Enzym. Regul.* **2001**, *41*, 189–207. [CrossRef]

9. Stylianopoulos, T. EPR-effect: Utilizing size-dependent nanoparticle delivery to solid tumors. *Ther. Deliv.* **2013**, *4*, 421–423. [CrossRef] [PubMed]
10. Wong, A.D.; Ye, M.; Ulmschneider, M.B.; Searson, P.C. Quantitative analysis of the enhanced permeation and retention (EPR) effect. *PLoS ONE* **2015**, *10*, e0123461. [CrossRef] [PubMed]
11. Kalyane, D.; Raval, N.; Maheshwari, R.; Tambe, V.; Kalia, K.; Tekade, R.K. Employment of enhanced permeability and retention effect (EPR): Nanoparticle-based precision tools for targeting of therapeutic and diagnostic agent in cancer. *Mater. Sci. Eng. C Mater. Biol. Appl.* **2019**, *98*, 1252–1276. [CrossRef]
12. Nagamitsu, A.; Konno, T.; Oda, T.; Tabaru, K.; Ishimaru, Y.; Kitamura, N. Targeted cancer chemotherapy for VX2 tumour implanted in the colon with lipiodol as a carrier. *Eur. J. Cancer* **1998**, *34*, 1764–1769. [CrossRef]
13. Hansen, A.E.; Petersen, A.L.; Henriksen, J.R.; Børresen, B.; Rasmussen, P.; Elema, D.R.; Rosenschold, P.M.A.; Kristensen, A.T.; Kjær, A.; Andresen, T.L. Positron emission tomography based elucidation of the enhanced permeability and retention effect in dogs with cancer using copper-64 liposomes. *ACS Nano* **2015**, *9*, 6985–6995. [CrossRef] [PubMed]
14. Benjamin, L.E.; Golijanin, D.; Itin, A.; Pode, D.; Keshet, E. Selective ablation of immature blood vessels in established human tumors follows vascular endothelial growth factor withdrawal. *J. Clin. Investig.* **1999**, *103*, 159–165. [CrossRef]
15. Suzuki, M.; Hori, K.; Saito, S.; Abe, I.; Sato, H. A new approach to cancer chemotherapy: Selective enhancement of tumor blood flow with angiotensin II. *J. Natl. Cancer Inst.* **1981**, *67*, 663–669.
16. Hori, K.; Zhang, Q.H.; Saito, S.; Tanda, S.; Li, H.C.; Suzuki, M. Microvascular mechanisms of change in tumor blood flow due to angiotensin II, epinephrine, and methoxamine: A functional morphometric study. *Cancer Res.* **1993**, *53*, 5528–5534.
17. Sindhwani, S.; Syed, A.M.; Ngai, J.; Kingston, B.R.; Maiorino, L.; Rothschild, J.; Macmillan, P.; Zhang, Y.; Rajesh, N.U.; Hoang, T.; et al. The entry of nanoparticles into solid tumours. *Nat. Mater.* **2020**, *19*, 566–575. [CrossRef]
18. Dvorak, H.F.; Nagy, J.A.; Dvorak, J.T.; Dvorak, A. Identification and characterization of the blood vessels of solid tumors that are leaky to circulating macromolecules. *Am. J. Pathol.* **1988**, *133*, 95–109. [PubMed]
19. Wu, J.; Akaike, T.; Hayashida, K.; Okamoto, T.; Okuyama, A.; Maeda, H. Enhanced vascular permeability in solid tumor involving peroxynitrite and matrix metalloproteinases. *Jpn. J. Cancer Res.* **2001**, *92*, 439–451. [CrossRef] [PubMed]
20. Wu, J.; Akaike, T.; Hayashida, K.; Miyamoto, Y.; Nakagawa, T.; Miyakawa, K.; Müller-Esterl, W.; Maeda, H. Identification of bradykinin receptors in clinical cancer specimens and murine tumor tissues. *Int. J. Cancer* **2002**, *98*, 29–35. [CrossRef]
21. Wu, J.; Akaike, T.; Maeda, H. Modulation of enhanced vascular permeability in tumors by a bradykinin antagonist, a cyclooxygenase inhibitor, and a nitric oxide scavenger. *Cancer Res.* **1998**, *58*, 159–165.
22. Leu, A.J.; Berk, D.; Lymboussaki, A.; Alitalo, K.; Jain, R.K. Absence of functional lymphatics within a murine sarcoma: A molecular and functional evaluation. *Cancer Res.* **2000**, *60*, 4324–4327. [PubMed]
23. Griffon-Etienne, G.; Boucher, Y.; Brekken, C.; Suit, H.D.; Jain, R.K. Taxane-induced apoptosis decompresses blood vessels and lowers interstitial fluid pressure in solid tumors: Clinical implications. *Cancer Res.* **1999**, *59*, 3776–3782.
24. Jain, R.K. Delivery of novel therapeutic agents in tumors: Physiological barriers and strategies. *J. Natl. Cancer Inst.* **1989**, *81*, 570–576. [CrossRef] [PubMed]
25. Nia, H.T.; Liu, H.; Seano, G.; Datta, M.; Jones, D.; Rahbari, N.; Incio, J.; Chauhan, V.; Jung, K.; Martin, J.D.; et al. Solid stress and elastic energy as measures of tumour mechanopathology. *Nat. Biomed. Eng.* **2017**, *1*, 0004. [CrossRef]
26. Jain, R.K. An indirect way to tame cancer. *Sci. Am.* **2014**, *310*, 46–53. [CrossRef] [PubMed]
27. Stylianopoulos, T.; Martin, J.; Chauhan, V.; Jain, S.R.; Diop-Frimpong, B.; Bardeesy, N.; Smith, B.L.; Ferrone, C.R.; Hornicek, F.J.; Boucher, Y.; et al. Causes, consequences, and remedies for growth-induced solid stress in murine and human tumors. *Proc. Natl. Acad. Sci. USA* **2012**, *109*, 15101–15108. [CrossRef] [PubMed]
28. Fang, J.; Nakamura, H.; Maeda, H. The EPR effect: Unique features of tumor blood vessels for drug delivery, factors involved, and limitations and augmentation of the effect. *Adv. Drug Deliv. Rev.* **2011**, *63*, 136–151. [CrossRef]
29. Baker, J.H.; Lindquist, K.E.; Huxham, L.A.; Kyle, A.H.; Sy, J.T.; Minchinton, A.I. Direct visualization of heterogeneous extravascular distribution of trastuzumab in human epidermal growth factor receptor type 2 overexpressing xenografts. *Clin. Cancer Res.* **2008**, *14*, 2171–2179. [CrossRef]
30. Gabizon, A.; Shmeeda, H.; Barenholz, Y. Pharmacokinetics of pegylated liposomal doxorubicin: Review of animal and human studies. *Clin. Pharmacokinet.* **2003**, *42*, 419–436. [CrossRef]
31. Northfelt, D.W.; Dezube, B.J.; Thommes, J.A.; Miller, B.J.; Fischl, M.A.; Kien, A.F.; Kaplan, L.D.; Du Mond, C.; Mamelok, R.D.; Henry, D.H. Pegylated-liposomal doxorubicin versus doxorubicin, bleomycin, and vincristine in the treatment of AIDS-related Kaposi's sarcoma: Results of a randomized phase III clinical trial. *J. Clin. Oncol.* **1998**, *16*, 2445–2451. [CrossRef]
32. Pham, T.M.H.; Le, P.L.; Nguyen, V.L.; Nguyen, T.H.; Ho, A.S.; Nguyen, L.T.; Bui, T.T. Developing and evaluating in vitroeffect of pegylated liposomal doxorubicin on human cancer cells. *J. Chem. Pharm. Res.* **2015**, *7*, 2239–2243.
33. Shavi, G.V.; Reddy, M.S.; Raghavendra, R.; Nayak, U.Y.; Kumar, A.R.; Deshpande, P.B.; Udupa, N.; Behl, G.; Dave, V.; Kushwaha, K. PEGylated liposomes of anastrozole for long-term treatment of breast cancer: In vitro and in vivo evaluation. *J. Liposome Res.* **2016**, *26*, 28–46. [CrossRef] [PubMed]
34. Marzban, E.; Alavizadeh, S.H.; Ghiadi, M.; Khoshangosht, M.; Khashyarmanesh, Z.; Abbasi, A.; Jaafari, M.R. Optimizing the therapeutic efficacy of cisplatin PEGylated liposomes via incorporation of different DPPG ratios: In vitro and in vivo studies. *Colloids Surf. B Biointerfaces* **2015**, *136*, 885–891. [CrossRef] [PubMed]

35. Jain, R.K. Normalization of tumor vasculature: An emerging concept in antiangiogenic therapy. *Science* **2005**, *307*, 58–62. [CrossRef] [PubMed]
36. Chauhan, V.P.; Stylianopoulos, T.; Martin, J.D.; Popović, Z.; Chen, O.; Kamoun, W.S.; Bawendi, M.G.; Fukumura, D.; Jain, R.K. Normalization of tumour blood vessels improves the delivery of nanomedicines in a size-dependent manner. *Nat. Nanotechnol.* **2012**, *7*, 383–388. [CrossRef]
37. Ojha, T.; Pathak, V.; Shi, Y.; Hennink, W.E.; Moonen, C.T.; Storm, G.; Kiessling, F.; Lammers, T. Pharmacological and physical vessel modulation strategies to improve EPR-mediated drug targeting to tumors. *Adv. Drug Deliv. Rev.* **2017**, *119*, 44–60. [CrossRef]
38. Noguchi, Y.; Wu, J.; Duncan, R.; Strohalm, J.; Ulbrich, K.; Akaike, T.; Maeda, H. Early phase tumor accumulation of macromolecules: A great difference in clearance rate between tumor and normal tissues. *Jpn. J. Cancer Res.* **1998**, *89*, 307–314. [CrossRef]
39. Longmire, M.; Choyke, P.L.; Kobayashi, H. Clearance properties of nano-sized particles and molecules as imaging agents: Considerations and caveats. *Nanomedicine* **2008**, *3*, 703–717. [CrossRef] [PubMed]
40. Blanco, E.; Shen, H.; Ferrari, M. Principles of nanoparticle design for overcoming biological barriers to drug delivery. *Nat. Biotechnol.* **2015**, *33*, 941–951. [CrossRef]
41. Dozono, H.; Yanazume, S.; Nakamura, H.; Etrych, T.; Chytil, P.; Ulbrich, K.; Fang, J.; Arimura, T.; Douchi, T.; Kobayashi, H.; et al. HPMA Copolymer-conjugated pirarubicin in multimodal treatment of a patient with stage IV prostate cancer and extensive lung and bone metastases. *Target. Oncol.* **2015**, *11*, 101–106. [CrossRef] [PubMed]
42. Seki, T.; Fang, J.; Maeda, H. Enhanced delivery of macromolecular antitumor drugs to tumors by nitroglycerin application. *Cancer Sci.* **2009**, *100*, 2426–2430. [CrossRef] [PubMed]
43. Maeda, H. Nitroglycerin enhances vascular blood flow and drug delivery in hypoxic tumor tissues: Analogy between angina pectoris and solid tumors and enhancement of the EPR effect. *J. Control Release* **2010**, *142*, 296–298. [CrossRef] [PubMed]
44. Maeda, H. The link between infection and cancer: Tumor vasculature, free radicals, and drug delivery to tumors via the EPR effect. *Cancer Sci.* **2013**, *104*, 779–789. [CrossRef]
45. Maeda, H.; Nakamura, H.; Fang, J. The EPR effect for macromolecular drug delivery to solid tumors: Improvement of tumor uptake, lowering of systemic toxicity, and distinct tumor imaging in vivo. *Adv. Drug Deliv. Rev.* **2013**, *65*, 71–79. [CrossRef]
46. Fang, J.; Islam, W.; Maeda, H. Exploiting the dynamics of the EPR effect and strategies to improve the therapeutic effects of nanomedicines by using EPR effect enhancers. *Adv. Drug Deliv. Rev.* **2020**, *157*, 142–160. [CrossRef]
47. Sano, K.; Nakajima, T.; Choyke, P.L.; Kobayashi, H. Markedly enhanced permeability and retention effects induced by photoimmunotherapy of tumors. *ACS Nano* **2012**, *7*, 717–724. [CrossRef]
48. Maeda, H.; Tsukigawa, K.; Fang, J. A retrospective 30 years after discovery of the enhanced permeability and retention effect of solid tumors: Next-generation chemotherapeutics and photodynamic therapy–Problems, solutions, and prospects. *Microcirculation* **2016**, *23*, 173–182. [CrossRef]
49. Maeda, H. Toward a full understanding of the EPR effect in primary and metastatic tumors as well as issues related to its heterogeneity. *Adv. Drug Deliv. Rev.* **2015**, *91*, 3–6. [CrossRef]
50. Islam, W.; Fang, J.; Imamura, T.; Etrych, T.; Subr, V.; Ulbrich, K.; Maeda, H. Augmentation of the enhanced permeability and retention effect with nitric oxide-generating agents improves the therapeutic effects of nanomedicines. *Mol. Cancer Ther.* **2018**, *17*, 2643–2653. [CrossRef]
51. Siracka, E.; Pappová, N.; Pípa, V.; Durkovský, J. Changes in blood flow of growing experimental tumor determined by the clearance of 133Xe. *Neoplasma* **1979**, *26*, 173–177. [PubMed]
52. Davies, B.; Morris, T. Physiological parameters in laboratory animals and humans. *Pharm. Res.* **1993**, *10*, 1093–1095. [CrossRef] [PubMed]
53. Wilson, C.B.; Lammertsma, A.A.; McKenzie, C.G.; Sikora, K.; Jones, T. Measurements of blood flow and exchanging water space in breast tumors using positron emission tomography: A rapid and noninvasive dynamic method. *Cancer Res.* **1992**, *52*, 1592–1597.
54. Hori, K.; Suzuki, M.; Tanda, S.; Saito, S.; Shinozaki, M.; Zhang, Q.H. Circadian variation of tumor blood flow in rat subcutaneous tumors and its alteration by angiotensin II-induced hypertension. *Cancer Res.* **1992**, *52*, 912–916. [PubMed]
55. Tabaru, K.; Konno, T.; Oda, T.; Nagamitsu, A.; Ishimaru, Y.; Kitamura, N. Treatment of VX2 carcinoma implanted in the liver with arterial and intraperitoneal administration of oily anticancer agents. *Cancer Chemother. Pharmacol.* **2001**, *47*, 149–154. [PubMed]
56. Konno, T.; Maeda, H.; Iwai, K.; Tashiroa, S.; Makia, S.; Morinaga, T.; Mochinaga, M.; Hiraoka, T.; Yokoyama, I. Effect of arterial administration of high-molecular-weight anticancer agent SMANCS with lipid lymphographic agent on hepatoma: A preliminary report. *Eur. J. Cancer Clin. Oncol.* **1983**, *19*, 1053–1065. [CrossRef]

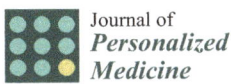

Review

The Potential Role of Sildenafil in Cancer Management through EPR Augmentation

Mohamed Haider [1,2,*], Amr Elsherbeny [3], Valeria Pittalà [4], Antonino N. Fallica [4], Maha Ali Alghamdi [5,6] and Khaled Greish [6,*]

1. Department of Pharmaceutics and Pharmaceutical Technology, College of Pharmacy, University of Sharjah, Sharjah 27272, United Arab Emirates
2. Research Institute of Medical & Health Sciences, University of Sharjah, Sharjah 27272, United Arab Emirates
3. Division of Molecular Therapeutics and Formulation, School of Pharmacy, University of Nottingham, Nottingham NG7 2RD, UK; amr.elsherbeny@nottingham.ac.uk
4. Department of Drug and Health Science, University of Catania, 95125 Catania, Italy; vpittala@unict.it (V.P.); antonio.fallica93@gmail.com (A.N.F.)
5. Department of Biotechnology, College of Science, Taif University, Taif 21974, Saudi Arabia; mahaasg@agu.edu.bh
6. Department of Molecular Medicine, Princess Al-Jawhara Centre for Molecular Medicine, School of Medicine and Medical Sciences Arabian Gulf University, Manama 329, Bahrain
* Correspondence: mhaider@sharjah.ac.ae (M.H.); khaledfg@agu.edu.bh (K.G.); Tel.: +97-156-761-5401 (M.H.); +973-1723-7393 (K.G.)

Citation: Haider, M.; Elsherbeny, A.; Pittalà, V.; Fallica, A.N.; Alghamdi, M.A.; Greish, K. The Potential Role of Sildenafil in Cancer Management through EPR Augmentation. *J. Pers. Med.* **2021**, *11*, 585. https://doi.org/10.3390/jpm11060585

Academic Editor: Jun Fang

Received: 25 April 2021
Accepted: 18 June 2021
Published: 21 June 2021

Publisher's Note: MDPI stays neutral with regard to jurisdictional claims in published maps and institutional affiliations.

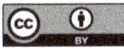

Copyright: © 2021 by the authors. Licensee MDPI, Basel, Switzerland. This article is an open access article distributed under the terms and conditions of the Creative Commons Attribution (CC BY) license (https://creativecommons.org/licenses/by/4.0/).

Abstract: Enhanced permeation retention (EPR) was a significant milestone discovery by Maeda et al. paving the path for the emerging field of nanomedicine to become a powerful tool in the fight against cancer. Sildenafil is a potent inhibitor of phosphodiesterase 5 (PDE-5) used for the treatment of erectile dysfunction (ED) through the relaxation of smooth muscles and the modulation of vascular endothelial permeability. Overexpression of PDE-5 has been reported in lung, colon, metastatic breast cancers, and bladder squamous carcinoma. Moreover, sildenafil has been reported to increase the sensitivity of tumor cells of different origins to the cytotoxic effect of chemotherapeutic agents with augmented apoptosis mediated through inducing the downregulation of Bcl-xL and FAP-1 expression, enhancing reactive oxygen species (ROS) generation, phosphorylating BAD and Bcl-2, upregulating caspase-3,8,9 activities, and blocking cells at G0/G1 cell cycle phase. Sildenafil has also demonstrated inhibitory effects on the efflux activity of ATP-binding cassette (ABC) transporters such as ABCC4, ABCC5, ABCB1, and ABCG2, ultimately reversing multidrug resistance. Accordingly, there has been a growing interest in using sildenafil as monotherapy or chemoadjuvant in EPR augmentation and management of different types of cancer. In this review, we critically examine the basic molecular mechanism of sildenafil related to cancer biology and discuss the overall potential of sildenafil in enhancing EPR-based anticancer drug delivery, pointing to the outcomes of the most important related preclinical and clinical studies.

Keywords: sildenafil; phosphodiesterase 5 inhibitors; drug repurposing; cancer; chemoadjuvant

1. Introduction

Sildenafil, (5-(2-ethoxy-5-((4-methylpiperazine-1-yl)sulfonyl)phenyl)-1-methyl-3-propyl-1H-pyrazolo[3,4-d]pyrimidin-7(6H)-one), sold as citrate salt, is a drug primarily prescribed for the treatment of ED (Figure 1). Sildenafil exerts its biological effects through the inhibition of PDE-5 [1,2]. Phosphodiesterases are a class of enzymes responsible for the degradation of cyclic AMP (cAMP) or GMP (cGMP) to their respective nucleotides 5′-AMP and 5′-GMP.

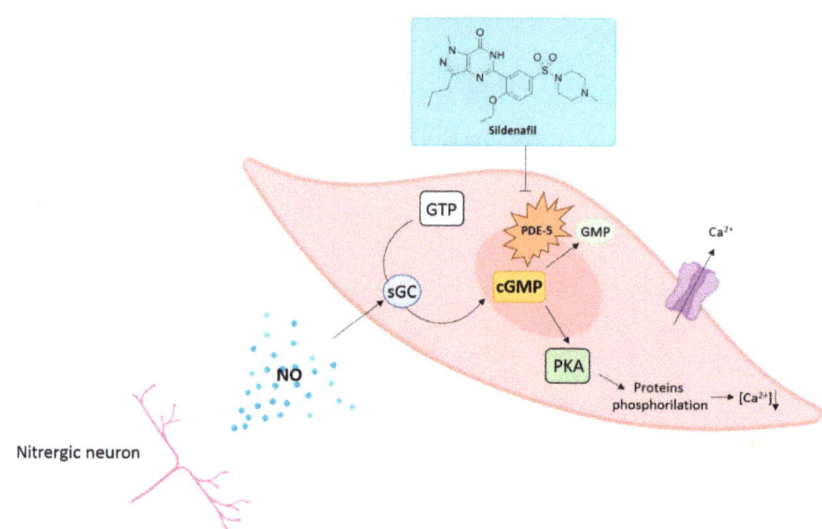

Figure 1. NO/sGC/cGMP pathway and sildenafil mechanism of action in erectile tissues and chemical structure of sildenafil.

Nowadays, 11 PDE isoforms have been identified [3]. These isozymes share an aminoacidic homology superior to 65% and differ for their tissue distribution and affinity toward cAMP or cGMP; the latter is specifically degraded by PDE-5, -6, and -9 [4–6]. PDEs exert their catalytic activity as homodimers [7,8]. In each monomer, it is possible to highlight the presence of a zinc-binding motif, a catalytic binding pocket, two allosteric sites able to bind cAMP or cGMP, and a residue of serine in position 92 whose phosphorylation enhances the enzymatic activity through the activation of protein kinases A and G (PKA and PKG) [7,9]. PDEs regulate in an isoform-dependent manner different physiological roles such as platelet aggregation, inflammation, immune system activation, hormone secretion, vision, cardiac contractility, and muscle metabolism, smooth muscle contractility, depression, calcium intracellular concentration, cell proliferation, and penile erection [10]. The latter is an event that originates from the release of the gasotransmitter nitric oxide (NO) by nitrergic neurons and endothelial cells in case of sexual stimulation [11]. The physicochemical properties of NO allow it to diffuse into cells activating the enzyme soluble guanylyl cyclase (sGC) that in turn converts GTP into cGMP. In erectile tissues, cGMP triggers the phosphorylation of specific proteins involved in the modulation of the intracellular calcium ions concentration. A decreased concentration of calcium ions through the activation of Ca^{2+}-ATPase dependent transporters and BKCa channels produces the vasodilation of blood vessels in the corpus cavernosum, leading to a penile erection [12]. cGMP binding to the allosteric sites of PDE-5 facilitates the binding of additional cGMP molecules to the active site of the enzyme and the consequent abolishment of cGMP activity (Figure 1) [9].

After an oral administration, sildenafil exerts its biological properties in few minutes, and its actions last around 12 h. The drug is metabolized by hepatic enzymes and possesses inhibitory properties toward CYP3A4, altering the metabolism of other classes of drugs such as antimycotic azoles and HIV protease inhibitors [13,14]. Common side effects are represented by rhinitis, headache, flushing, cardiovascular effects, and priapism. In addition, despite its selectivity towards the PDE-5 isozyme (IC50 = 3.5 nM), sildenafil possesses also the capability to bind PDE-6 (IC50 = 34 nM), an isoform specifically expressed in rod and cone cells of the retina determining visual side effects [15,16].

Sildenafil is characterized by the presence of a pyrazo-lo[4,3-d]pyrimidin-7(6H)-one nucleus that mimics the cGMP chemical structure. The pyrazole ring is decorated with alkyl substituents, whereas the pyrimidone ring is substituted with a phenyl ring bearing an ethoxy moiety and an N4-methylpiperazine-1-yl-sulfonyl moiety. Cocrystallization studies highlighted the binding mode of sildenafil to PDE-5 (Figure 2) [17]. The catalytic site of PDE-5 is characterized by the presence of four peculiar subsites. The M subsite (metal-binding subsite) possesses a zinc ion that takes interactions with histidine and aspartate amino acid residues and coordinates two water molecules. One aspartic residue and one water molecule coordinated by the zinc ion are also shared with a magnesium ion that takes interaction with four additional water molecules. The spatial disposition of the water molecules and amino acid residues involved in the interaction with zinc and magnesium ions retained an octahedral geometry [18]. The second water molecule coordinated by zinc and unbonded to magnesium is involved in a hydrogen bond with an additional water molecule whose spatial disposition is assured by hydrogen bonds with Tyr612 and the unsubstituted nitrogen atom of the pyrazole ring of sildenafil. This specific hydrogen bond network seems to play a pivotal role in the inhibition of the PDE-5; indeed, it is speculated that this water molecule acts as the nucleophile responsible for the hydrolysis of the phosphodiester bond of cGMP [19]. The Q pocket (core pocket) accommodates the heterocyclic ring of sildenafil. In this subsite, a Phe820 residue and the highly conserved Gln817 residue make a π-stacking interaction and a hydrogen bond with the amide function of the pyrimidinone ring, respectively. The hydrophobic subsite (H region) consists of a pocket in which highly lipophilic amino acid residues takes Van der Waals interactions with the ethoxyphenyl moiety linked to the heterocyclic core of sildenafil. Finally, a Tyr664 amino acid residue in the L region (lid pocket) undertakes a hydrogen bond with the N4 atom of the piperazine ring [18].

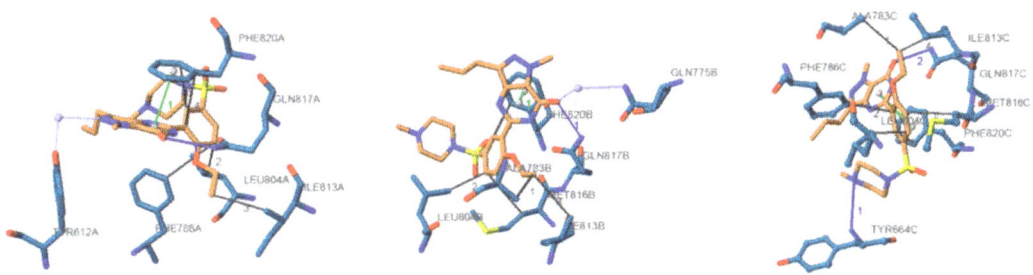

Figure 2. Docked position of sildenafil in the PDE-5 active site: ligand is represented in orange; amino acid residues in blue; hydrogen bonds are shown as solid blue lines; face-to-face stacking interaction in solid green lines; hydrogen bonds in dark solid grey lines; water bridges are represented in light solid grey lines. Image from the PLIP web service [20] using the PDB ID 2H42 [18].

The uncovering of sildenafil properties by Pfizer researchers represented one of the most resounding examples of serendipity in the drug discovery field (Figure 3) [11,21]. As a matter of fact, the cardiovascular research group operating in Pfizer in 1989 was looking for new drugs exploitable for the treatment of angina pectoris, a pathological condition caused by a temporary spasm of the coronary arteries with the consequent reduction of oxygen flow into the heart tissue [22]. The first clinical trials highlighted that UK-92,480 (sildenafil investigational code) did not possess any advantage when compared with other drugs commonly used for the treatment of angina pectoris, such as nitrates [23]. Indeed, doses of UK-92,480 administered intravenously or orally ranging from 20 to 200 mg weakly modified the hemodynamic parameters and potentiated the effects of nitrates. In response to these findings, UK-92,480 seemed to be not effective for the goal of the study, and

Pfizer researchers started to fear that the drug development of UK-92,480 could suffer a setback. Unexpectedly, among the limited number of side effects detected during these studies, penile erection resulted as the most surprising [24]. At the time of the research, ED was considered as a condition primarily originated by psychological disturbs and treated with invasive injections of vasodilating substances in the penile tissues [11]. Moreover, PDE-5 was known to be principally localized in platelets and vascular smooth muscle cells, whereas its localization in the erectile tissues was never properly investigated. A subsequent study brought to light the presence of this specific enzymatic isoform in erectile tissues [25], allowing a better comprehension of the physiological processes that regulate penile erection [26]. In addition, this discovery confirmed that ED could be treated with orally administrable PDE-5 inhibitors because of the specific expression of this isozyme in erectile tissues, paving the way for the potential placing on the market of a class of compounds exploitable for an unmet clinical need. After 21 separate additional clinical trials carried out from 1993 to 1996 performed on a total number of about 3000 men aged 19 to 87 years old [11], the efficacy and patient's compliance of UK-92,480, later named as sildenafil, was definitely confirmed. These results determined UK-92,480 approval by the FDA in March 1998 in the United States and by the EMA in September 1998 [27] under the trade name of Viagra. The placing on the market of this drug represented a global market breakthrough for the treatment of ED, with more than USD 400 million earned only in 1998 and more than USD 1 billion.

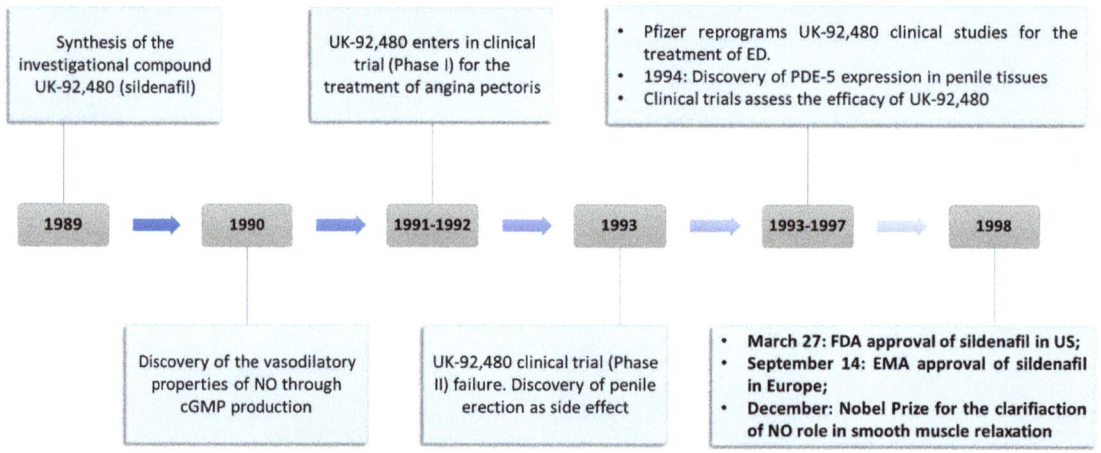

Figure 3. Timeline and milestones of sildenafil drug discovery.

In 2003, additional PDE-5 inhibitors entered the market (vardenafil and tadalafil), and in recent years, avanafil, mirodenafil, lodenafil, and udenafil have been approved in a limited number of countries (Figure 4) [28].

In 2010, sildenafil's patent expired, and several industries started the production of this drug under generic names. Nevertheless, several clinical trials have been carried out in order to assess the efficacy of sildenafil for the treatment of other disabling pathologies [29–32].

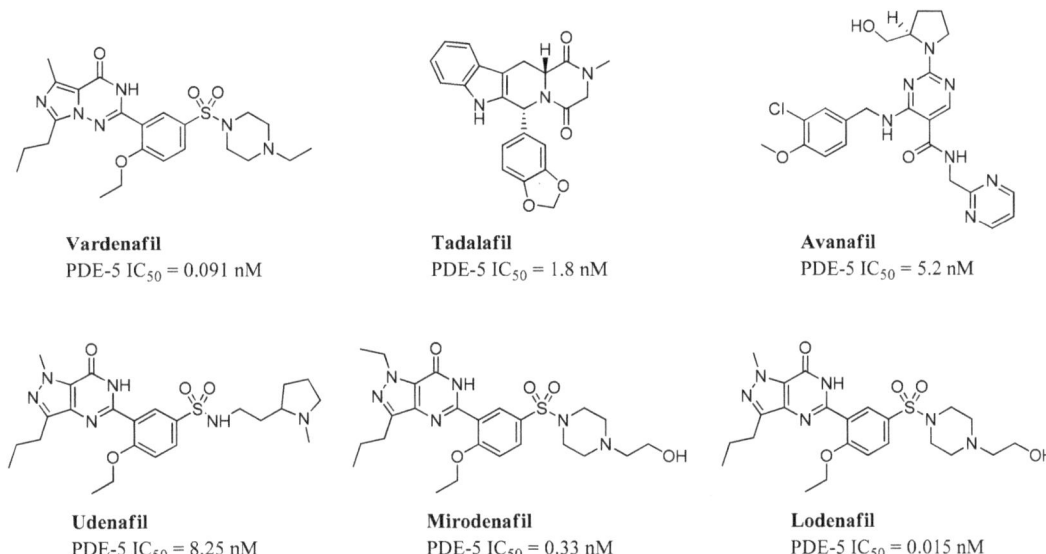

Figure 4. Chemical structures and IC$_{50}$ values of commercial PDE-5 inhibitor.

2. Drug Repurposing Approach for the Identification of New Therapeutic Application

In spite of the increased understanding of prevention, diagnosis, therapy, and prognosis of human maladies, translation of this whole set of knowledge into new drugs has been far slower than estimated. A new drug discovery project generally starts with an unmet clinical need as the primary driving motivation. Initial efforts often occur in academia producing data to support a hypothesis that may result in the identification of a new target or a new therapeutic approach in a specific disease. In our time, however, drug discovery and development processes are resource- and time intensive and highly multifaceted requiring multidisciplinary profiles and innovative approaches. The attrition rate is another relevant aspect that the global pharmaceutical industry has to take into serious consideration when approaching a new discovery project. The latest estimations suggest that it takes more than 10 years and around USD 2 billion for a new drug to reach the market. There is growing pressure to set up cheaper and more effective ways to bring safe and efficacious drugs to the market. Within this framework, the drug discovery process is unceasingly experiencing changes and adjustments to achieve improvements in efficiency, productivity, and profitability. In this context, the so-called drug repositioning (or repurposing) process is attracting growing interest [33]. This strategy implies the identification of new therapeutic applications different from the original regulatory indication for approved or investigational drugs. The benefits of this strategy include tremendous savings of time and money, low risk of failure since the majority of preclinical and clinical trials, safety assessment, and, sometimes, pharmaceutical formulation have been completed. Finally, yet importantly, repurposed drugs may highlight novel targets and pathways that can be further investigated. In the past, the most significant examples of drug repurposing have been mainly based on serendipity rather than on a systematic approach. Once an off-target or a new on-target effect was detected, it was the object of further investigation and/or commercial exploitation. An outstanding example is represented by Zidovudine, which was originally developed as an anticancer agent but later became the first FDA-approved drug for the treatment of HIV after being identified from an in vitro screening of compound libraries [34]. Other remarkable examples include thalidomide, which was originally developed for morning sickness, and later, on the basis of pharmacological analysis, was approved for the treatment of erythema nodosum leprosum and multiple myeloma [35]. Minoxidil, originally indicated for the treatment of hypertension, was discovered by means of a retrospective clinical analysis. However, sildenafil represents maybe the foremost example. Originally investigated for angina, it represents maybe a perfect example of retrospective clinical analysis. Sildenafil was repurposed by Pfizer for the first time in the late 1990s for the management of ED. By 2014 it held the market-lead with a 47% share of the ED drug market and a worldwide sales calculation of around USD 2 billion [36]. Soon after its approval as Viagra, the discovery of the upregulation of PDE5 gene expression in pulmonary hypertensive lungs boosted further preclinical and clinical studies on sildenafil to test the role of PDE5 selective inhibitors in lung diseases [37]. Later, in 2005, the drug was repurposed once more for the treatment of pulmonary arterial hypertension and approved under the trade name Revatio [12,38]. Recently, other indications for which sildenafil has been studied include Raynaud's disease, digital ulcer, heart failure, hypertensive cardiac hypertrophy, cerebral circulation, and different types of cancers including lung and colorectal malignancies [39,40].

3. In Vitro and In Vivo Applications of Sildenafil in Cancer Treatment

Many studies reported the use of sildenafil in combination with chemotherapeutic agents in the treatment of a variety of cancers (Table 1). Das et al. reported an increase in chemotherapeutic efficacy of DOX when coadministered with sildenafil in vitro on PC-3 and DU145 human prostate cancer cells. It was shown that combination therapy resulted in a relatively higher apoptotic rate on tumor cells by enhancing ROS generation, reducing B-cell lymphoma-extra large (Bcl-xL) expression, phosphorylating BAD, and upregulating caspase-3 and caspase-9 activities [41]. Further investigations on the molecular mechanisms involved in the sensitization of prostate cancer cells by sildenafil outlined the role of CD95 in DOX-mediated apoptosis [42]. The effect of sildenafil in enhancing the anticancer properties of DOX was eliminated when CD95 apoptosis-inducing death receptor was knocked down using siRNA. However, this was not the case when cells were treated with DOX alone. In addition, the combination therapy induced downregulation of Fas-associated phosphatase-1 (FAP-1) expression, a known inhibitor of CD95-mediated apoptosis, increasing cellular death and reducing tumor viability. Moreover, cells cotreated with sildenafil and DOX showed a reduced expression of both long and short forms of caspase-8 regulating enzymes Fas-associated death domain (FADD) interleukin-1-converting enzyme (FLICE)-like inhibitory protein (FLIP-L and -S), which are involved in the regulation of cellular apoptosis, compared to DOX-monotherapy [42]. Comparable results were reported for using the same therapeutic combination in the treatment of 4T1 murine breast cancer cells where synergistic activity was observed [43]. The outlined mechanisms clearly demonstrate the improved cytotoxic activity of DOX when combined with sildenafil, thereby potentially improving the clinical response and patient survival rate whilst ameliorating DOX toxic side effects. In vitro studies examining the potentiation of the antitumor activity of cisplatin when given in conjugation with sildenafil on MCF-7 human breast cancer cells showed a dose-dependent cytotoxic effect of sildenafil illustrating its potentiation effect on the chemotherapeutic agent [44]. Similar results were obtained upon cotreatment of MCF-7 and MDA-MB-468 human breast cancer cells with cisplatin and sildenafil, which was accompanied by a significant increase in accumulation of ROS into the extracellular environment in both breast adenocarcinomas cell lines [45].

The effect of coadministration of vincristine and sildenafil on PC-3 and DU145 human prostate cancer cell lines showed that a significant increase in vincristine-induced mitotic arrest and mitotic index [46]. The probability of cells being held in metaphase was dramatically increased in presence of sildenafil. This was particularly relevant in the tripolar spindle and multiple spindle poles. Nevertheless, a nonsignificant decrease in the level of cytokinesis was observed when cells responsive to vincristine were treated with sildenafil. Interestingly, the phosphorylation of Bcl-2 with caspase activation amplification including caspase-3, -8, and -9, and cleavage of poly [ADP-ribose] polymerase 1 (PARP-1), a caspase-3 substrate, was markedly increased when sildenafil was coadministered with vincristine; a similar feat previously demonstrated when sildenafil was combined with DOX on prostate cell lines incurring the coherence between the results reported between different studies. Additionally, sildenafil was shown to enhance vincristine-induced perturbation of microtubule–kinetochore interactions incurring higher apoptotic effects [46].

Roberts et al. reported that combination therapy of curcumin and sildenafil may induce gastrointestinal tumor cell death in HCT116, HT29, HuH7, HEP3B, and HEPG2 human gastrointestinal tumor cells through endoplasmic reticulum stress, reactive oxygen/nitrogen species, and increasing autophagosome and autolysosome levels prompting cancer cellular death [47]. Similar results were obtained when studying the effect of coadministration of curcumin and sildenafil on immunocompetent BALB/c mice implanted with CT26 murine colorectal cancer cells in which the use of sildenafil and curcumin as chemoadjuvants significantly enhanced the cytotoxic effect of 5-fluorouracil and anti-PD1 immunotherapy in vivo [48]. Such properties clearly express the ability of sildenafil to enhance cytotoxic properties of chemotherapeutic modalities as well as larger immunotherapeutic treating complexes.

The therapeutic efficacy of docetaxel and sildenafil in advanced prostate cancer was investigated by stimulating nitric oxide—cyclic guanosine-3′,5′-monophosphate (NO-cGMP) signaling. Human prostatic cancer (C4-2B) cells revealed overexpression of functional phosphodiesterase type 5 (PDE5) and its role with NO for aberrant cGMP accumulation. It was suggested that a subtherapeutic dose of docetaxel and a physiologically achievable sildenafil concentration could induce synergistic activity by increasing cGMP and blocking cells at G0/G1, inhibiting cell growth and inducing apoptosis. Similar results were observed in syngeneic cell lines and Pten cKO derived tumoroids where an increase in caspase-3 and PARP cleavage was detected [49]. The combination treatment demonstrated a significant decrease in tumoroid size and growth, with loss of integrity, apoptosis, condensed structure, and structural blebbing [50]. A demonstration between the 3D model translation, compared to the 2D line, further suggests an enhanced probability for in vivo studies and clinical application on patients.

The cytotoxicity of sildenafil/crizotinib loaded poly(ethylene glycol)-poly(DL-lactic acid) (PEG-PLA) polymeric micelles on MCF-7 human breast cancer cell lines was studied. Micelles with an average size between 93 and 127 nm and an encapsulation efficiency percentage (EE%) of both medications (>70%) were prepared using the solvent displacement method. In vitro cytotoxicity assays using crizotinib alone displayed 22% cellular viability, compared to 10% only upon coadministration of sildenafil, i.e., a 2.2-fold decrease in cell viability, after treatment for 48 hrs. This was attributed to previous reports on the wide inhibitory effect of sildenafil on several ATP-binding cassette (ABC) efflux transporters, henceforth overcoming cancer cell resistance and promoting their apoptosis [51]. Codelivery of these medications using nanoparticles further decreased the cell viability to 4%, illustrating the potential impact of formulation designs on enhancing the therapeutic outcomes of this regimen [52]. While these results suggest that the application of the dual-therapy in the nano form has shown a significant impact on the 2D tumor cells, issues regarding the formulation stability, pharmacokinetics, biodistribution, and in vitro 3D model and in vivo replication should be assessed before such formulations progress into the clinical phases.

Table 1. Examples of in vitro and in vivo studies for the effect of sildenafil in different types of cancer.

Cancer	Type of Study	Tumor Model	Therapy	Therapeutic Outcome	Ref.
Prostate Cancer	In vitro	PC-3 and DU145 prostate cancer cells	Sildenafil (10 μM)	No significant changes in % Cell death compared to control	[41]
			DOX (1.5 μM with PC-3 and 0.5 μM with DU145)	7.52% and 45.01% cell death in PC-3 and DU145 cells, respectively.	
			DOX (1.5 μM with PC-3 and 0.5 μM with DU145) + Sildenafil (10 μM)	18.71% and 56.82% cell death in PC-3 and DU145 cells, respectively.	
	In vivo	Athymic male BALB/cAnNCr-nu/nu mice injected with PC-3 cells and 50-μL matrigel matrices	DOX (1.5 mg/kg)	Tumor weight/Body weight ratio = 0.015	
			Intraperitoneal DOX (1.5 mg/kg) + Sildenafil (5 mg/kg) OR intraperitoneal DOX (3 mg/kg) + oral Sildenafil (10 mg/kg)	Tumor weight/Body weight ratio = 0.010	
Breast Cancer	In vitro	4T1 mammary carcinoma cells	DOX (1 μM)	50% cell death	[43]
			Sildenafil (10,30,100 μM)	No significant changes compared to control	
			DOX (1 μM) + Sildenafil (1 μM)	72.2% cell death	
			DOX (1 μM) + Sildenafil (30 μM)	91.9% cell death	
			DOX (1 μM) + Sildenafil (100 μM)	97.6% cell death	
	In vivo	Female Balb/c mice injected with 4T1 mammary carcinoma cells	DOX (5 mg/kg)	Tumor volume = 570%	
			Sildenafil (1 mg/kg)	Tumor volume = 400%	
			DOX (5 mg/kg) + Sildenafil (1 mg/kg)	Tumor volume = 121.3%	
Breast Cancer	In vitro	MCF-7 breast cancer cells	Sildenafil	IC$_{50}$ = 14 μg/mL	[44]
			Cisplatin	IC$_{50}$ = 4.43 μg/mL	
			Sildenafil + Cisplatin	IC$_{50}$ = 3.98 μg/mL	
	In vivo	Swiss albino female mice injected with Ehrlich ascites carcinoma (EAC) cells	Sildenafil (5 mg/kg)	30.4% decrease in tumor volume	
			Cisplatin (7.5 mg/kg)	58.8% decrease in tumor volume	
			Sildenafil (5 mg/kg) + Cisplatin (7.5 mg/kg)	79% decrease in tumor volume	
Colorectal Cancer	In vitro	HT-29, SW480, SW620, HCT116 and SW1116 colorectal cancer cells	Sildenafil	IC$_{50}$ (72hrs) = 190.91 μM in HT-29 217.27 μM SW480 206.68 μM SW620 246.20 μM HCT116 271.22 μM SW1116	[39]
	In vivo	Balb/c nude mice injected with SW480 or HCT116 colorectal cancer cells	Sildenafil (50 mg/kg) and (150 mg/kg)	In SW480, 40.1% and 57.8% tumor inhibition with 50 mg/kg and 150 mg/kg, respectively.	
				In HCT116, 13.3% and 61.4% tumor inhibition with 50 mg/kg and 150 mg/kg, respectively.	

Table 1. Cont.

Cancer	Type of Study	Tumor Model	Therapy	Therapeutic Outcome	Ref.
Prostate Cancer	In vivo	Nude mice were injected with PC-3 prostate cancer cells	Sildenafil (10 mg/kg)	Tumor weight = 969.9 ± 92.2 mg	[46]
			Vincristine (0.5 mg/kg)	Tumor weight = 623.5 ± 132.2 mg	
			Sildenafil (10 mg/kg) + Vincristine (0.5 mg/kg)	Tumor weight = 207.6 ± 36.7 mg	
Breast Cancer	In vitro	MCF-7 Breast cancer cells	Sildenafil	No significant changes in % cell viability compared to control	[52]
			Crizotinib	IC_{50} = 34.19 and 22% cell viability	
			Crizotinib + Sildenafil	IC_{50} = 3.34 and 10% cell viability	
			Blank PEG-PLA micelles	No significant changes in % cell viability compared to control	
			Crizotinib loaded PEG-PLA micelles	14% cell viability	
			Crizotinib (55.25 µM)/Sildenafil (40.33 µM)- coloaded PEG-PLA micelles	4% cell viability	
Lung Cancer	In vitro	A549 human lung carcinoma cells	DOX	29.87% cell death	[53]
			DOX + Sildenafil	34.69% cell death	
			DOX/Sildenafil-coloaded NLC	38.37% cell death	
			DOX/Sildenafil-coloaded NLC-RGD	44.32% cell death	

In a different study, nanostructured lipid carrier (NLCs) coloaded with DOX and sildenafil citrate and tagged with arginyl-glycyl-aspartic acid (RGD) were prepared and their effect on human lung carcinoma A549 cells was studied [53]. The drug-loaded NLCs were prepared by homogenization method producing an optimum formula having an average size, polydispersity index, zeta potential, and EE% for DOX and sildenafil of 80.5 nm, 0.23, −18.5, 56.04 ± 1.25% and 81.62 ± 3.14%, respectively. The use of coloaded NLCs induced higher cytotoxicity and cancer cell apoptosis, compared to the free drug. It was suggested that this may be due to the enhanced cellular uptake and accumulation of drugs associated with integrin-mediated endocytosis and ABC transporter inhibition. Real-time PCR also revealed that sildenafil reduced the expression of ABCC1 and nuclear factor erythroid 2 related factor 2 (Nrf2) proteins, which incurred an increased intracellular concentration of anticancer drugs, as previously reported. It would be interesting to further explore the effect of the DOX/sildenafil-loaded nanoparticle formulation on the degree of ROS production, caspases activation, and proapoptotic protein expression [53,54].

In vivo studies using athymic male BALB/cAnNCr-nu/nu mice bearing prostatic cancer showed that the coadministration of sildenafil increased the efficacy of DOX while reducing DOX-associated cardiac dysfunction [41]. Immunohistochemistry demonstrated that the active form of caspase-3 was induced in tumors from sildenafil- and DOX-treated mice, compared with DOX-treated or nontreated control groups, henceforth explaining the relatively higher tumor volume reduction with the cotreatment. Furthermore, Doppler echocardiography showed a marked improvement in the left ventricular fractional shortening (LVFS) and left ventricular ejection fraction (LVEF) with sildenafil–DOX cotreatment rather than DOX alone. These results suggest a relatively lower systemic cytotoxicity associated with the cotreatment compared to monotherapy [41].

Treatment of female Balb/c mice inoculated with 4T1 murine mammary carcinoma cells with sildenafil/DOX combination therapy also demonstrated a significant reduction of tumor growth [43]. It was suggested that this effect is due to a higher migration of effective immune cells to the tumor site due to the vasodilatory effects of sildenafil, rather than an inherent cytotoxic effect of the drug. The results were in correlation with in vitro studies which demonstrated the lack of anticancer properties of sildenafil. Animals treated with DOX–sildenafil combination showed a 4.7 reduction in tumor size with a 2.7-fold increase in drug concentrations in comparison to DOX alone. Interestingly, when DOX was loaded into styrene-maleic acid (SMA) micelles and administered to the mice after sildenafil treatment, it showed a statistically insignificant increase in tumor accumulation, compared to SMA–DOX alone. This was not the case when dioctadecyl-3,3,3′,3′-tetramethylindocarbocyanine perchlorate (DiI) was loaded in SMA micelles and codelivered with sildenafil, where a statistically significant threefold increase was observed, compared to SMA–DiI alone. This difference could be associated with the variable particle size and physicochemical characteristics associated between both formulations. It was reported that SMA–DOX had a much smaller size (14.59 nm), compared to SMA–DiI (134.12 nm), hence would be able to accumulate to a larger extent at the tumor site, compared to the larger SMA–DiI without the need of sildenafil as a chemoadjuvant. These results raise the question of whether the magnitude of sildenafil efficacy as a chemoadjuvant could be affected by varying the particle size and characteristics of the nanoparticles used. A more holistic comparison would be to use comparable particles with close physicochemical properties to overcome such limitations [43].

Similarly, other in vivo studies using a combination of sildenafil and cisplatin showed a significant decrease in tumor volume in mice bearing breast cancer tumor, compared to the control group. Investigation of the local tissue microenvironment, apoptosis, and proliferation of the tumor cells after treatment with combination therapy showed an increase in caspase-3 levels with a considerable decrease in tumor necrosis factor-α contents, angiogenin, and vascular endothelial growth factor expression. However, the expression of Ki-67 nuclear protein which is usually present during the late G1, S, G2, and M phases of the cell cycle failed to show any significant changes when compared to the control group [44].

Muniyan et al. orthotopically implanted luciferase-labeled C4-2B cells into the dorsolateral lobe of the prostate in immunodeficient mice to investigate the therapeutic efficacy of coadministration of docetaxel and sildenafil in advanced prostate cancer [50]. The therapeutic combination significantly lowered tumor weight, compared to docetaxel alone. Further exploration in the molecular pathways responsible for this phenomenon identified a lower percentage of Ki67-positive nuclei and a higher frequency of cleaved caspase-3 positive cells, compared to groups treated with monotherapy, thus promoting apoptosis and tumor regression [50]. Likewise, Hsu et al. reported the synergistic effects between vincristine and sildenafil in PC-3-derived cancer xenografts in nude mice, demonstrating a decrease in tumor weight, compared to the single chemotherapeutic agent [46].

4. The Role of Sildenafil in Circumventing Anticancer Drug Resistance

MDR is a complex process in which cancer cells evolve to evade the deleterious effects of anticancer chemotherapy. A plethora of biological strategies had been described in association with the development of MDR. Enhanced drug metabolism, gene amplification, increase in DNA damage repair, epigenetic regulation of the drug targets, and autophagy all have been described.

Among different processes of drug resistance, overexpression of active transporters that actively efflux substrates of different chemical/biological natures is the most studied pathway, notably, the increase of drug efflux pumps ATP-binding cassette (ABC) transporters [55–59]. ABC transporter comprises ABCs (multidrug resistance-associated proteins (MRPs)), ABCB1 (P-glycoprotein/MDR1), and ABCG2 (BCRP/MXR/ABCP)) all were reported to be overexpressed in cancer developing the MDR. This superfamily transporter system mainly consists of integral membrane proteins. These proteins convert the energy that comes from ATP hydrolysis into the translocation of substrates across the membrane's bilayer either into the cytoplasm or out of the cytoplasm. This movement is facilitated by a pair of transmembrane domains (TMDs), which when overexpressed in cancer cells, contribute to cell drug resistance by pumping out the intracellular drugs and therefore decreasing their cellular uptake and effect [60]. cGMP was implicated as a substrate for ATP-binding cassette (ABC) transporters in the multidrug resistance (MDR) cancer cells [58,59]. Accordingly, sildenafil was investigated as a potential player for reversing MDR in cancer cells.

Sildenafil increased the level of the second messenger's cGMP through inhibition of PDE5, which is considered to be substrates for ABCC4/human MDR protein 4 (MRP4) and ABCC5/human MDR protein5 (MRP5), resulting in inhibition of the efflux pump activity. Furthermore, it inhibited the activity of ABC transporters such as ABCB1 and ABCG2, thereby increasing the sensitivity of MDR cells to various drugs. Moreover, the suppression of PDE5 could activate the cGMP-PKG pathway that mediates many processes causing cellular apoptosis or growth suppression (cell cycle arrest) of cancer cells [61].

Shi et al. demonstrated the effect of sildenafil on ABC transporters using ABC-mediated MDR on cancer cells. The cytotoxicity assays and drug accumulation results showed that sildenafil remarkably sensitized the ABCB1-overexpressing cells to the ABCB1 substrates (colchicine, vinblastine, and paclitaxel) with a high accumulation rate of the paclitaxel inside the cells. A similar effect on ABCG2-overexpressing cells was noted in relation to the substrates (flavopiridol, mitoxantrone, and SN-38) with a significant accumulation of mitoxantrone. In contrast, sildenafil had no effect on ABCC1-overexpressing cells and its tested substrate (vincristine). Altogether, these data strongly suggest a potential role for sildenafil in reversing anticancer drug resistance [62].

5. Sildenafil and Anticancer Drug Delivery through EPR Augmentation

PDE5 inhibitors such as sildenafil had demonstrated their effect on smooth muscle layers of blood vessels leading to vasodilation in tissues that express the specific isoenzyme. Indeed, one known side effect of this class of drugs is systemic hypotension that denotes the susceptibility of normal vascular cell types to PDE5 inhibitors [63].

Smooth muscle relaxation thereby modulates vascular endothelial permeability that increases the inflow of blood to the normal and pathological tissues such as inflamed tissues and tumor tissues, leading to the accumulation of nanoparticles of molecular weight exceeding 40 kD and augmenting preferential drug targeting in the diseased tissues such as tumors. This accumulation normally occurs due to the abnormalities in tumor vascularity due to poorly aligned and faulty vascular endothelial cells that have wide fenestrations of up to 4 μm [64–66]. Traditionally, the EPR effect involves two aspects. First, the drug preferential biodistribution is related to the size of the drug and the delivery vehicle applied to achieve the differential accumulation of the drug in tumor tissues. As the size of the drug and the delivery vehicle is more than the limit of the renal excretion threshold, nanoparticles usually exhibit increased plasma half-life. Second, the EPR effect involves retention of the nano-based system due to the lack of efficient lymphatic clearance [67–69].

Unfortunately, a very slim volume of existing literature examines the response of tumor vasculature to PDE5 inhibitors. PDE inhibition could potentially result in improvement of blood supply to the tumor tissues through similar mechanisms employed for ED.

In order to augment the EPR effect of macromolecular drugs, sildenafil needs to be preferentially applied locally to the tumor site. Relevant work had been pioneered by Maeda et al., in which they applied the nitric oxide donor Lipiodol® through the arterial catheter to the tumor feeding artery with reported success in the management of clinically advanced cases of primary and secondary liver tumors [70]. This early experience proved that in order to selectively utilize a vasodilating agent to improve the EPR effect, the vasodilation needs to be restricted to the blood supply in the close vicinity of the tumor tissues, otherwise widespread vasodilation can enhance the delivery of the nanoconstructs to other off-target tissues and induce systemic hypotension.

Greish et al. demonstrated that using sildenafil in conjunction with DOX increased the concentration of the anticancer drug in tumor tissues by 2.7 folds, and eventually resulted in 4.7 folds improved anticancer activity against the 4T1 breast cancer in mice. This work suggests a positive effect of PDE5 inhibitors to further augment enhanced permeability and retention (EPR) effect on EPR effect [43]. A relevant study by Black et al. demonstrated the effect of PDE5 inhibitors on enhancing tumor vascular permeability in the brain tumor model of 9L gliosarcoma-bearing in rats. Sildenafil administration increased the tumor capillary permeability in comparison to the normal brain capillaries, which showed no significant increase in vascular permeability. Additionally, the study proved a synergistic effect of the use of anthracycline chemotherapy combined with the sildenafil and further improved the survival by nearly twofold longer than the group treated with the chemotherapeutic agent alone [71]. Another work by Zhang et al. provided further direct evidence of the potential of PDE 5 inhibitors in augmenting EPR-mediated anticancer chemotherapy in vivo. In their study, the team employed a combined micelle incorporating both cisplatin and sildenafil. The team proposed that tumor acidity can preferentially release the PDE5 inhibitor from the micelle, further augmenting its concentration in tumor tissues. This strategy was proved effective in increasing both drug accumulation and anticancer activity in the tested cancer model of B16F10 melanoma in C57BL/6 mice, altogether indicating a potential and promising rule for PDE5 inhibitors in augmenting EPR-based anticancer drug delivery [72].

It is noteworthy to mention that sildenafil application for augmenting local tumor tissue concentrations of chemotherapy is not exclusive to nanosized molecules. It can similarly increase the local concentration of conventional chemotherapeutic agents [43]. However, small molecules traverse barriers freely into the tumor or the normal tissue and immediately disappear from the tumor or the normal tissue by diffusion primarily into blood capillaries. Therefore, the residence time of conventional small molecular drugs in cancer tissue is usually counted in minutes, while that of nanosized molecules by days to weeks, owing to the retention aspect in the EPR effect. Accordingly, since tumor tissues lack functional lymphatics, the enhanced delivery of bioactive nanosize molecules in the tumor is usually retained for considerable durations.

6. Clinical Studies

The use of sildenafil in the management of different types of cancer has been the subject of various clinical trials (http://www.clinicaltrials.gov accessed on 1 March 2021) (Table 2). A number of clinical trials such as NCT00142506, NCT00544076, NCT00057759, and NCT00511498, evaluated the use of sildenafil alone or in combination with alprostadil or hyperbaric oxygen therapy in the management of ED. Those trials focused on restoring the erectile function for patients with prostate cancer after radiotherapy or nerve-sparing prostatectomy. Clinical trial NCT02106871 was designed to assess the use of sildenafil monotherapy in the treatment of fatigue in patients with pancreatic cancer. It is suggested that sildenafil increases protein synthesis, alters protein expression and nitrosylation, and reduces fatigue in human skeletal muscle especially in patients with reduced skeletal muscle functions [73]. The concept has yet to be clinically tested as the study was terminated due to a lack of funds. The ability of sildenafil monotherapy to improve renal functions in patients with kidney cancer after partial nephrectomy and protect the kidney from the side effects of surgery was investigated in clinical trial NCT01950923. The study involved the oral administration of sildenafil to 30 patients prior to surgery, followed by assessment of kidney functions. The trial was completed but the results have yet to be reported. In clinical trial NCT00165295, sildenafil was tested in the treatment of Waldenstrom's Macroglobulinemia (WM), a rare and incurable type of non-Hodgkin lymphoma. It was suggested that sildenafil blocks the function of several proteins necessary to the survival of cancer cells, and laboratory tests have shown that it can destroy WM cells [74]. The study involved 30 patients who received incremental doses of sildenafil orally for 2 years. The clinical trial has been completed with no reported side effects, but the complete results of the study are not published yet. Sildenafil was also tested for the treatment of Lymphangioma in pediatric patients in clinical trial NCT01290484. The results showed a significant decrease of lymphatic malformation in four out of seven patients included in the study after oral administration of sildenafil for 20 weeks with no observed complications in any subject [75].

Table 2. Examples of clinical trials using sildenafil in treatment of different types of cancers *.

Types of Cancer	Treatment	Objective	Stage
Pancreatic Cancer	Sildenafil	Management of fatigue in cancer patient undergoing chemotherapy	Phase I
Non-small Cell Lung Cancer	Sildenafil, Paclitaxel, Carboplatin	Improvement in distribution and efficacy of cytotoxic anticancer agents	Phase II, III
Prostate Cancer	Sildenafil	Management of ED during and after radiotherapy with or without hormone Therapy	Phase III
	Sildenafil, Alprostadil	Management of ED post-operatively in patients undergoing nerve-sparing robotic-assisted radical prostatectomy	Phase III
	Sildenafil	Investigate the effect of dosage regimen on ED in patients after nerve-sparing laparoscopic radical prostatectomy	Not applicable
	Sildenafil, Hyperbaric oxygen therapy	Management of ED in patients after nerve-sparing radical retropubic prostatectomy	Phase IV
Solid Tumor	Regorafenib Sildenafil	Investigation of the antitumor effects of the regorafenib and sildenafil combination, the pre-treatment expression of phosphodiesterase type 5 (PDE5) in tumor samples, and the impact of sildenafil on the pharmacokinetics of regorafenib	Phase I
Kidney Tumor	Sildenafil	Improving Postoperative Kidney Function in Patients With Kidney Cancer undergoing Robotic Partial Nephrectomy	Phase I
Colorectal Cancer	Sildenafil Vacuum erection device (VED)	Management of ED After Laparoscopic Resection	Phase IV
Breast Cancer	Sildenafil Doxorubicin	Improving antitumor effects of DOX and protection from cardiac toxicity	Phase I
Brain Cancer and Glioblastoma	Sildenafil Sorafenib Tosylate Valproic Acid	Increase the concentration of anticancer drug in the brain and stop the growth of tumor cells by blocking BCG2 drug efflux pump in the blood–brain barrier	Phase II
Waldenstrom Macroglobulinemia	Sildenafil	Treatment by blocking the function of several proteins necessary to the survival of cancer cells	Phase II
Myelodysplastic Syndrome (MDS)	Nivolumab Cytarabine Sildenafil	Studying the pathogenesis and resistance of myelodysplastic syndrome using combination therapy	Phase I, II

* Source: https://clinicaltrials.gov/ (accessed on 1 March 2021).

The use of sildenafil as a chemoadjuvant in the treatment of different types of cancers was investigated. The clinical trial NCT01375699 investigated the use of sildenafil as a cardioprotective agent in female patients primarily with breast cancer treated with DOX against the cardiotoxic effects of the drug. Patients were given oral sildenafil daily for one week prior to the scheduled first dose of DOX. The treatment continued until 2 weeks after the last scheduled dose of DOX and multiple biomarkers for cardiotoxicity were measured [76]. The results showed that adding sildenafil to DOX chemotherapy is safe and well tolerated but did not significantly improve cardiac protection during chemotherapy when compared to the control group. The trial NCT00752115 used sildenafil combination with chemotherapeutic agents such as carboplatin and paclitaxel in patients with advanced non-small-cell lung cancer to improve the biodistribution and efficacy of the chemotherapeutic agents. Patients received a weekly dose of 50 mg sildenafil orally and progression-free survival was monitored. The phase I clinical trial NCT02466802 assessed the use of regorafenib in combination with sildenafil in patients with progressive advanced solid tumors. The study results showed that the drug combination is safe and that the lethality of this combination could be enhanced in vitro and in vivo by the addition of neratinib to the treatment regimen in a colorectal cancer model. Accordingly, it was further recommended to perform a phase I trial in colorectal cancer patients using the combination of the three drugs [77]. The phase II clinical study NCT01817751 is currently investigating the use of sildenafil as a chemoadjuvant in the treatment of patients with recurrent high-grade glioma. Orally administered sildenafil twice a day for four weeks is used in combination with sorafenib and valproic acid to test its ability to increase the concentration of the chemotherapeutic agents in the brain and preventing the growth of tumor cells by blocking BCG2 drug efflux pump in the blood–brain barrier.

It is very clear that most of the clinical trials focused on using sildenafil as a chemoadjuvant to reverse side effects associated with chemotherapy such as ED or cardiotoxicity. This means that much of the potential for the use of sildenafil in the treatment of different types of cancer remains theoretical, lacking solid clinical evidence. More clinical trials are still required to test the possibility to use sildenafil in circumventing anticancer drug resistance and as an EPR augmentation tool for enhancement of anticancer drug delivery.

7. Conclusions and Future Recommendations

The paradigm of drug repurposing remains of significant interest for the pharmaceutical and health care communities. A deeper understanding of the molecular pathology and pharmacology of the current therapeutic entities in the market plays an important role in the utilization of current resources in the management of various diseases. Further to Meade's visionary discovery of EPR, he recommended further augmentation of this key biological effect by manipulating vascular dynamics at macro- and micro-organizational levels. Sildenafil has demonstrated its ability in enhancing anticancer drug delivery through the EPR effect, prompting significant elevation of intratumoral drug concentrations and subsequent cellular death. In addition, sildenafil has demonstrated its implication in the modulation and potentiation of chemotherapeutic agents in a range of different types of cancer. This has been outlined in several in vitro and in vivo studies through the downregulation of Bcl-xL and FAP-1 expression, enhancing ROS generation, phosphorylating BAD and Bcl-2, upregulating caspase-3,8,9 activities, blocking cells at G0/G1 cell cycle phase, overcoming cancer cell resistance by inhibiting several ABC transporters through cGMP elevation, and increasing autophagosome and autolysosome levels; inducing tumor cell death.

Despite several clinical studies being underway, the need for further trials on patients remains of paramount importance to further understand the clinical impact they may perceive. These studies could possibly include the application of novel drug delivery formulations for combination therapies such as passively and actively targeting nanoparticles, external stimuli-responsive systems using light, focused ultrasound, and magnetic fields to release the drug therapy at the desired site of action, and controlled-release formulations where sildenafil may precede the chemotherapeutic agent, inducing its chemosensitizing action first and promoting higher cytotoxicity action of the latter. Such systems could certainly increase the efficacy and safety profiles of current oncological agents, enhancing the patient's quality of life and achieving a definite therapeutic outcome.

Author Contributions: Conceptualization, M.H. and K.G.; resources, M.H. and K.G.; writing—original draft preparation, M.H., A.E., V.P., A.N.F., M.A.A. and K.G.; writing—review and editing, M.H., A.E. and K.G.; supervision, M.H., V.P. and K.G.; project administration, M.H. and K.G.; funding acquisition, M.H. and K.G. All authors have read and agreed to the published version of the manuscript.

Funding: This research was funded by AGU Research Grant, E002-PI-04/18 to KG, and UOS targeted research project, 2101110345 to MH.

Institutional Review Board Statement: Not applicable.

Informed Consent Statement: Not applicable.

Conflicts of Interest: The authors declare no conflict of interest. The funders had no role in the design of the study; in the collection, analyses, or interpretation of data; in the writing of the manuscript, or in the decision to publish the results.

References

1. Utiger, R.D. A Pill for Impotence. *N. Engl. J. Med.* **1998**, *338*, 1458–1459. [CrossRef] [PubMed]
2. Terrett, N.K.; Bell, A.S.; Brown, D.; Ellis, P. Sildenafil (Viagra(TM)), a potent and selective inhibitor of type 5 CGMP phosphodiesterase with utility for the treatment of male erectile dysfunction. *Bioorg. Med. Chem. Lett.* **1996**, *6*, 1819–1824. [CrossRef]
3. Francis, S.H.; Blount, M.A.; Corbin, J.D. Mammalian cyclic nucleotide phosphodiesterases: Molecular mechanisms and physiological functions. *Physiol. Rev.* **2011**, *91*, 651–690. [CrossRef] [PubMed]
4. Rotella, D.P. Phosphodiesterase 5 inhibitors: Current status and potential applications. *Nat. Rev. Drug Discov.* **2002**, *1*, 674–682. [CrossRef] [PubMed]
5. Beavo, J.A. Cyclic nucleotide phosphodiesterases: Functional implications of multiple isoforms. *Physiol. Rev.* **1995**, *75*, 725–748. [CrossRef] [PubMed]
6. Andersson, K.E. PDE5 inhibitors—Pharmacology and clinical applications 20 years after sildenafil discovery. *Br. J. Pharmacol.* **2018**, *175*, 2554–2565. [CrossRef] [PubMed]
7. Blount, M.A.; Beasley, A.; Zoraghi, R.; Sekhar, K.R.; Bessay, E.P.; Francis, S.H.; Corbin, J.D. Binding of tritiated sildenafil, tadalafil, or vardenafil to the phosphodiesterase-5 catalytic site displays potency, specificity, heterogeneity, and cGMP stimulation. *Mol. Pharmacol.* **2004**, *66*, 144–152. [CrossRef]
8. Corbin, J.D.; Francis, S.H. Cyclic GMP phosphodiesterase-5: Target of sildenafil. *J. Biol. Chem.* **1999**, *274*, 13729–13732. [CrossRef]
9. Corbin, J.D.; Turko, I.V.; Beasley, A.; Francis, S.H. Phosphorylation of phosphodiesterase-5 by cyclic nucleotide-dependent protein kinase alters its catalytic and allosteric cGMP-binding activities. *Eur. J. Biochem.* **2000**, *267*, 2760–2767. [CrossRef]
10. Essayan, D.M. Cyclic nucleotide phosphodiesterases. *J. Allergy Clin. Immunol.* **2001**, *108*, 671–680. [CrossRef]
11. Goldstein, I.; Burnett, A.L.; Rosen, R.C.; Park, P.W.; Stecher, V.J. The Serendipitous Story of Sildenafil: An Unexpected Oral Therapy for Erectile Dysfunction. *Sex. Med. Rev.* **2019**, *7*, 115–128. [CrossRef]
12. Ghofrani, H.A.; Osterloh, I.H.; Grimminger, F. Sildenafil: From angina to erectile dysfunction to pulmonary hypertension and beyond. *Nat. Rev. Drug Discov.* **2006**, *5*, 689–702. [CrossRef]
13. Carson, C.C.; Lue, T.F. Phosphodiesterase type 5 inhibitors for erectile dysfunction. *BJU Int.* **2005**, *96*, 257–280. [CrossRef]
14. Barbaro, G.; Scozzafava, A.; Mastrolorenzo, A.; Supuran, C. Highly Active Antiretroviral Therapy: Current State of the Art, New Agents and Their Pharmacological Interactions Useful for Improving Therapeutic Outcome. *Curr. Pharm. Des.* **2005**, *11*, 1805–1843. [CrossRef]
15. Yafi, F.A.; Sharlip, I.D.; Becher, E.F. Update on the Safety of Phosphodiesterase Type 5 Inhibitors for the Treatment of Erectile Dysfunction. *Sex. Med. Rev.* **2018**, *6*, 242–252. [CrossRef]
16. Laties, A.M.; Fraunfelder, F.T.; Flach, A.J.; Tasman, W. Ocular safety of Viagra, (sildenafil citrate). *Trans. Am. Ophthalmol. Soc.* **1999**, *97*, 115–128.
17. Wang, H.; Liu, Y.; Huai, Q.; Cai, J.; Zoraghi, R.; Francis, S.H.; Corbin, J.D.; Robinson, H.; Xin, Z.; Lin, G.; et al. Multiple conformations of phosphodiesterase-5: Implications for enzyme function and drug development. *J. Biol. Chem.* **2006**, *281*, 21469–21479. [CrossRef]
18. Sung, B.J.; Hwang, K.Y.; Jeon, Y.H.; Lee, J.I.; Heo, Y.S.; Kim, J.H.; Moon, J.; Yoon, J.M.; Hyun, Y.L.; Kim, E.; et al. Structure of the catalytic domain of human phosphodiesterase 5 with bound drug molecules. *Nature* **2003**, *425*, 98–102. [CrossRef]
19. Supuran, C.; Mastrolorenzo, A.; Barbaro, G.; Scozzafava, A. Phosphodiesterase 5 Inhibitors—Drug Design and Differentiation Based on Selectivity, Pharmacokinetic and Efficacy Profiles. *Curr. Pharm. Des.* **2006**, *12*, 3459–3465. [CrossRef]
20. Salentin, S.; Schreiber, S.; Haupt, V.J.; Adasme, M.F.; Schroeder, M. PLIP: Fully automated protein-ligand interaction profiler. *Nucleic Acids Res.* **2015**, *43*, W443–W447. [CrossRef]
21. Ban, T.A. The role of serendipity in drug discovery. *Dialogues Clin. Neurosci.* **2006**, *8*, 335–344. [CrossRef]
22. Deckers, J.W. Classification of myocardial infarction and unstable angina: A re-assessment. *Int. J. Cardiol.* **2013**, *167*, 2387–2390. [CrossRef]
23. Jackson, G.; Benjamin, N.; Jackson, N.; Allen, M.J. Effects of sildenafil citrate on human hemodynamics. *Am. J. Cardiol.* **1999**, *83*, 13–20. [CrossRef]
24. Boolell, M.; Allen, M.J.; Ballard, S.A.; Gepi-Attee, S.; Muirhead, G.J.; Naylor, A.M.; Osterloh, I.H.; Gingell, C. Sildenafil: An orally active type 5 cyclic GMP-specific phosphodiesterase inhibitor for the treatment of penile erectile dysfunction. *Int. J. Impot. Res.* **1996**, *8*, 47–52.
25. Wallis, R.M.; Corbin, J.D.; Francis, S.H.; Ellis, P. Tissue distribution of phosphodiesterase families and the effects of sildenafil on tissue cyclic nucleotides, platelet function, and the contractile responses of trabeculae carneae and aortic rings in vitro. *Am. J. Cardiol.* **1999**, *83*, 3–12. [CrossRef]
26. Ignarro, L.J.; Bush, P.A.; Buga, G.M.; Wood, K.S.; Fukuto, J.M.; Rajfer, J. Nitric oxide and cyclic GMP formation upon electrical field stimulation cause relaxation of corpus cavernosum smooth muscle. *Biochem. Biophys. Res. Commun.* **1990**, *170*, 843–850. [CrossRef]

27. Perry, M.J.; Higgs, G.A. Chemotherapeutic potential of phosphodiesterase inhibitors. *Curr. Opin. Chem. Biol.* **1998**, *2*, 472–481. [CrossRef]
28. Hatzimouratidis, K.; Salonia, A.; Adaikan, G.; Buvat, J.; Carrier, S.; El-Meliegy, A.; McCullough, A.; Torres, L.O.; Khera, M. Pharmacotherapy for Erectile Dysfunction: Recommendations From the Fourth International Consultation for Sexual Medicine (ICSM 2015). *J. Sex. Med.* **2016**, *13*, 465–488. [CrossRef]
29. Bermejo, J.; Yotti, R.; García-Orta, R.; Sánchez-Fernández, P.L.; Castaño, M.; Segovia-Cubero, J.; Escribano-Subías, P.; San Román, J.A.; Borrás, X.; Alonso-Gómez, A.; et al. Sildenafil for improving outcomes in patients with corrected valvular heart disease and persistent pulmonary hypertension: A multicenter, double-blind, randomized clinical trial. *Eur. Heart J.* **2018**, *39*, 1255–1264. [CrossRef] [PubMed]
30. Galiè, N.; Ghofrani, H.A.; Torbicki, A.; Barst, R.J.; Rubin, L.J.; Badesch, D.; Fleming, T.; Parpia, T.; Burgess, G.; Branzi, A.; et al. Sildenafil Citrate Therapy for Pulmonary Arterial Hypertension. *N. Engl. J. Med.* **2005**, *353*, 2148–2157. [CrossRef] [PubMed]
31. Kolb, M.; Raghu, G.; Wells, A.U.; Behr, J.; Richeldi, L.; Schinzel, B.; Quaresma, M.; Stowasser, S.; Martinez, F.J. Nintedanib plus Sildenafil in Patients with Idiopathic Pulmonary Fibrosis. *N. Engl. J. Med.* **2018**, *379*, 1722–1731. [CrossRef] [PubMed]
32. Sastry, B.K.S.; Narasimhan, C.; Reddy, N.K.; Raju, B.S. Clinical efficacy of sildenafil in primary pulmonary hypertension: A randomized, placebo-controlled, double-blind, crossover study. *J. Am. Coll. Cardiol.* **2004**, *43*, 1149–1153. [CrossRef] [PubMed]
33. Pushpakom, S.; Iorio, F.; Eyers, P.A.; Escott, K.J.; Hopper, S.; Wells, A.; Doig, A.; Guilliams, T.; Latimer, J.; McNamee, C.; et al. Drug repurposing: Progress, challenges and recommendations. *Nat. Rev. Drug Discov.* **2018**, *18*, 41–58. [CrossRef] [PubMed]
34. Marwick, C. AZT (zidovudine) just a step away from FDA approval for AIDS therapy. *JAMA* **1987**, *257*, 1281–1282. [CrossRef]
35. Stewart, A.K. How thalidomide works against cancer. *Science* **2014**, *343*, 256–257. [CrossRef]
36. Rezaee, M.E.; Ward, C.E.; Brandes, E.R.; Munarriz, R.M.; Gross, M.S. A Review of Economic Evaluations of Erectile Dysfunction Therapies. *Sex. Med. Rev.* **2020**, *8*, 497–503. [CrossRef]
37. Sanchez, L.S.; De La Monte, S.M.; Filippov, G.; Jones, R.C.; Zapol, W.M.; Bloch, K.D. Cyclic-GMP-binding, cyclic-GMP-specific phosphodiesterase (PDE5) gene expression is regulated during rat pulmonary development. *Pediatr. Res.* **1998**, *43*, 163–168. [CrossRef]
38. Bhogal, S.; Khraisha, O.; Al Madani, M.; Treece, J.; Baumrucker, S.J.; Paul, T.K. Sildenafil for Pulmonary Arterial Hypertension. *Am. J. Ther.* **2019**, *26*, e520–e526. [CrossRef]
39. Mei, X.L.; Yang, Y.; Zhang, Y.J.; Li, Y.; Zhao, J.M.; Qiu, J.G.; Zhang, W.J.; Jiang, Q.W.; Xue, Y.Q.; Zheng, D.W.; et al. Sildenafil inhibits the growth of human colorectal cancer in vitro and in vivo. *Am. J. Cancer Res.* **2015**, *5*, 3311–3324.
40. Keats, T.; Rosengren, R.J.; Ashton, J.C. The Rationale for Repurposing Sildenafil for Lung Cancer Treatment. *Anticancer Agents Med. Chem.* **2018**, *18*, 367–374. [CrossRef]
41. Das, A.; Durrant, D.; Mitchell, C.; Mayton, E.; Hoke, N.N.; Salloum, F.N.; Park, M.A.; Qureshi, I.; Lee, R.; Dent, P.; et al. Sildenafil increases chemotherapeutic efficacy of doxorubicin in prostate cancer and ameliorates cardiac dysfunction. *Proc. Natl. Acad. Sci. USA* **2010**, *107*, 18202–18207. [CrossRef]
42. Das, A.; Durrant, D.; Mitchell, C.; Dent, P.; Batra, S.K.; Kukreja, R.C. Sildenafil (Viagra) sensitizes prostate cancer cells to doxorubicin-mediated apoptosis through CD95. *Oncotarget* **2016**, *7*, 4399–4413. [CrossRef]
43. Greish, K.; Fateel, M.; Abdelghany, S.; Rachel, N.; Alimoradi, H.; Bakhiet, M.; Alsaie, A. Sildenafil citrate improves the delivery and anticancer activity of doxorubicin formulations in a mouse model of breast cancer. *J. Drug Target.* **2018**, *26*, 610–615. [CrossRef]
44. El-Naa, M.M.; Othman, M.; Younes, S. Sildenafil potentiates the antitumor activity of cisplatin by induction of apoptosis and inhibition of proliferation and angiogenesis. *Drug Des. Dev. Ther.* **2016**, *10*, 3661–3672. [CrossRef]
45. Hassanvand, F.; Mohammadi, T.; Ayoubzadeh, N.; Tavakoli, A.; Hassanzadeh, N.; Sanikhani, N.S.; Azimi, A.I.; Mirzaei, H.R.; Khodamoradi, M.; Goudarzi, K.A.; et al. Sildenafil enhances cisplatin-induced apoptosis in human breast adenocarcinoma cells. *J. Cancer Res. Ther.* **2020**, *16*, 1412–1418. [CrossRef]
46. Hsu, J.-L.; Leu, W.-J.; Hsu, L.-C.; Ho, C.-H.; Liu, S.-P.; Guh, J.-H. Phosphodiesterase Type 5 Inhibitors Synergize Vincristine in Killing Castration-Resistant Prostate Cancer Through Amplifying Mitotic Arrest Signaling. *Front. Oncol.* **2020**, *10*, 1274. [CrossRef]
47. Roberts, J.L.; Poklepovic, A.; Booth, L. Curcumin interacts with sildenafil to kill GI tumor cells via endoplasmic reticulum stress and reactive oxygen/nitrogen species. *Oncotarget* **2017**, *8*, 99451–99469. [CrossRef]
48. Dent, P.; Booth, L.; Roberts, J.L.; Poklepovic, A.; Hancock, J.F. (Curcumin + sildenafil) enhances the efficacy of 5FU and anti-PD1 therapies in vivo. *J. Cell. Physiol.* **2020**, *235*, 6862–6874. [CrossRef]
49. Morales, J.C.; Li, L.; Fattah, F.J.; Dong, Y.; Bey, E.A.; Patel, M.; Gao, J.; Boothman, D.A. Review of poly (ADP-ribose) polymerase (PARP) mechanisms of action and rationale for targeting in cancer and other diseases. *Crit. Rev. Eukaryot. Gene Expr.* **2014**, *24*, 15–28. [CrossRef]
50. Muniyan, S.; Rachagani, S.; Parte, S.; Halder, S.; Seshacharyulu, P.; Kshirsagar, P.; Siddiqui, J.A.; Vengoji, R.; Rauth, S.; Islam, R.; et al. Sildenafil potentiates the therapeutic efficacy of docetaxel in advanced prostate cancer by stimulating NO-cGMP signaling. *Clin. Cancer Res.* **2020**, *26*. [CrossRef]
51. Chen, J.J.; Sun, Y.L.; Tiwari, A.K.; Xiao, Z.J.; Sodani, K.; Yang, D.H.; Vispute, S.G.; Jiang, W.Q.; Chen, S.D.; Chen, Z.S. PDE5 inhibitors, sildenafil and vardenafil, reverse multidrug resistance by inhibiting the efflux function of multidrug resistance protein 7 (ATP-binding Cassette C10) transporter. *Cancer Sci.* **2012**, *103*, 1531–1537. [CrossRef] [PubMed]

52. Marques, J.G.; Gaspar, V.M.; Markl, D.; Costa, E.C.; Gallardo, E.; Correia, I.J. Co-delivery of Sildenafil (Viagra(®)) and Crizotinib for synergistic and improved anti-tumoral therapy. *Pharm. Res.* **2014**, *31*, 2516–2528. [CrossRef] [PubMed]
53. Hajipour, H.; Ghorbani, M.; Kahroba, H.; Mahmoodzadeh, F.; Emameh, R.Z.; Taheri, R.A. Arginyl-glycyl-aspartic acid (RGD) containing nanostructured lipid carrier co-loaded with doxorubicin and sildenafil citrate enhanced anti-cancer effects and overcomes drug resistance. *Process. Biochem.* **2019**, *84*, 172–179. [CrossRef]
54. Ji, L.; Li, H.; Gao, P.; Shang, G.; Zhang, D.D.; Zhang, N.; Jiang, T. Nrf2 Pathway Regulates Multidrug-Resistance-Associated Protein 1 in Small Cell Lung Cancer. *PLoS ONE* **2013**, *8*, e63404. [CrossRef]
55. Mansoori, B.; Mohammadi, A.; Davudian, S.; Shirjang, S.; Baradaran, B. The Different Mechanisms of Cancer Drug Resistance: A Brief Review. *Adv. Pharm. Bull.* **2017**, *7*, 339–348. [CrossRef]
56. Di Nicolantonio, F.; Mercer, S.J.; Knight, L.A.; Gabriel, F.G.; Whitehouse, P.A.; Sharma, S.; Fernando, A.; Glaysher, S.; Di Palma, S.; Johnson, P.; et al. Cancer cell adaptation to chemotherapy. *BMC Cancer* **2005**, *5*, 78. [CrossRef]
57. Vasiliou, V.; Vasiliou, K.; Nebert, D.W. Human ATP-binding cassette (ABC) transporter family. *Hum. Genom.* **2009**, *3*, 281–290. [CrossRef]
58. Cree, I.A.; Knight, L.; di Nicolantonio, F.; Sharma, S.; Gulliford, T. Chemosensitization of solid tumor cells by alteration of their susceptibility to apoptosis. *Curr. Opin. Investig. Drugs* **2002**, *3*, 641–647.
59. Tewari, K.S.; Eskander, R.N.; Monk, B.J. Development of Olaparib for BRCA-Deficient Recurrent Epithelial Ovarian Cancer. *Clin. Cancer Res. Off. J. Am. Assoc. Cancer Res.* **2015**, *21*, 3829–3835. [CrossRef]
60. Gottesman, M.M.; Ambudkar, S. V Overview: ABC transporters and human disease. *J. Bioenerg. Biomembr.* **2001**, *33*, 453–458. [CrossRef]
61. Shi, Z.; Tiwari, A.K.; Shukla, S.; Robey, R.W.; Singh, S.; Kim, I.-W.; Bates, S.E.; Peng, X.; Abraham, I.; Ambudkar, S.V.; et al. Sildenafil reverses ABCB1- and ABCG2-mediated chemotherapeutic drug resistance. *Cancer Res.* **2011**, *71*, 3029–3041. [CrossRef]
62. Shi, Z.; Tiwari, A.K.; Patel, A.S.; Fu, L.W.; Chen, Z.S. Roles of sildenafil in enhancing drug sensitivity in cancer. *Cancer Res.* **2011**, *71*, 3735–3738. [CrossRef]
63. Preston, I.R.; Klinger, J.R.; Houtches, J.; Nelson, D.; Farber, H.W.; Hill, N.S. Acute and chronic effects of sildenafil in patients with pulmonary arterial hypertension. *Respir. Med.* **2005**, *99*, 1501–1510. [CrossRef]
64. Yuan, F.; Salehi, H.A.; Boucher, Y.; Vasthare, U.S.; Tuma, R.F.; Jain, R.K. Vascular permeability and microcirculation of gliomas and mammary carcinomas transplanted in rat and mouse cranial windows. *Cancer Res.* **1994**, *54*, 4564–4568.
65. Folkman, J. Angiogenesis in cancer, vascular, rheumatoid and other disease. *Nat. Med.* **1995**, *1*, 27–31. [CrossRef]
66. Hashizume, H.; Baluk, P.; Morikawa, S.; McLean, J.W.; Thurston, G.; Roberge, S.; Jain, R.K.; McDonald, D.M. Openings between defective endothelial cells explain tumor vessel leakiness. *Am. J. Pathol.* **2000**, *156*, 1363–1380. [CrossRef]
67. Matsumura, Y.; Maeda, H. A new concept for macromolecular therapeutics in cancer chemotherapy: Mechanism of tumoritropic accumulation of proteins and the antitumor agent smancs. *Cancer Res.* **1986**, *46*, 6387–6392.
68. Seymour, L.W.; Miyamoto, Y.; Maeda, H.; Brereton, M.; Strohalm, J.; Ulbrich, K.; Duncan, R. Influence of molecular weight on passive tumour accumulation of a soluble macromolecular drug carrier. *Eur. J. Cancer* **1995**, *31A*, 766–770. [CrossRef]
69. Greish, K.; Sawa, T.; Fang, J.; Akaike, T.; Maeda, H. SMA-doxorubicin, a new polymeric micellar drug for effective targeting to solid tumours. *J. Control. Release* **2004**, *97*, 219–230. [CrossRef]
70. Nagamitsu, A.; Inuzuka, T.; Greish, K.; Maeda, H. SMANCS dynamic therapy for various advanced solid tumors and promising clinical effects. *Drug Deliv. Syst.* **2007**, *22*, 510–521. [CrossRef]
71. Black, K.L.; Yin, D.; Ong, J.M.; Hu, J.; Konda, B.M.; Wang, X.; Ko, M.K.; Bayan, J.-A.; Sacapano, M.R.; Espinoza, A.; et al. PDE5 inhibitors enhance tumor permeability and efficacy of chemotherapy in a rat brain tumor model. *Brain Res.* **2008**, *1230*, 290–302. [CrossRef] [PubMed]
72. Zhang, P.; Zhang, Y.; Ding, X.; Xiao, C.; Chen, X. Enhanced nanoparticle accumulation by tumor-acidity-activatable release of sildenafil to induce vasodilation. *Biomater. Sci.* **2020**, *8*, 3052–3062. [CrossRef] [PubMed]
73. Sheffield-Moore, M.; Wiktorowicz, J.E.; Soman, K.V.; Danesi, C.P.; Kinsky, M.P.; Dillon, E.L.; Randolph, K.M.; Casperson, S.L.; Gore, D.; Horstman, A.M.; et al. Sildenafil increases muscle protein synthesis and reduces muscle fatigue. *Clin. Transl. Sci.* **2013**, *6*, 463–468. [CrossRef] [PubMed]
74. Treon, S.P.; Tournilhac, O.; Branagan, A.R.; Hunter, Z.; Xu, L.; Hatjiharissi, E.; Santos, D.D. Clinical Responses to Sildenafil in Waldenstrom's Macroglobulinemia. *Clin. Lymphoma* **2004**, *5*, 205–207. [CrossRef]
75. Danial, C.; Tichy, A.L.; Tariq, U.; Swetman, G.L.; Khuu, P.; Leung, T.H.; Benjamin, L.; Teng, J.; Vasanawala, S.S.; Lane, A.T. An open-label study to evaluate sildenafil for the treatment of lymphatic malformations. *J. Am. Acad. Dermatol.* **2014**, *70*, 1050–1057. [CrossRef]
76. Poklepovic, A.; Qu, Y.; Dickinson, M.; Kontos, M.C.; Kmieciak, M.; Schultz, E.; Bandopadhyay, D.; Deng, X.; Kukreja, R.C. Randomized study of doxorubicin-based chemotherapy regimens, with and without sildenafil, with analysis of intermediate cardiac markers. *CardioOncology* **2018**, *4*. [CrossRef]
77. Booth, L.; Roberts, J.L.; Rais, R.; Cutler, R.E.J.; Diala, I.; Lalani, A.S.; Hancock, J.F.; Poklepovic, A.; Dent, P. Neratinib augments the lethality of [regorafenib + sildenafil]. *J. Cell. Physiol.* **2019**, *234*, 4874–4887. [CrossRef]

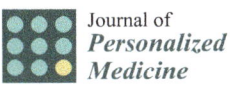

Review

Recent Advances in Tumor Targeting via EPR Effect for Cancer Treatment

Md Abdus Subhan [1,*], Satya Siva Kishan Yalamarty [2], Nina Filipczak [2], Farzana Parveen [2,3] and Vladimir P. Torchilin [2,4,*]

1. Department of Chemistry, Shah Jalal University of Science and Technology, Sylhet 3114, Bangladesh
2. CPBN, Department of Pharmaceutical Sciences, Northeastern University, Boston, MA 02115, USA; yalamarty.s@northeastern.edu (S.S.K.Y.); nina.filipczak@gmail.com (N.F.); farzanaparveenphd@gmail.com (F.P.)
3. Department of Pharmaceutics, Faculty of Pharmacy, The Islamia University of Bahawalpur, Punjab 63100, Pakistan
4. Department of Oncology, Radiotherapy and Plastic Surgery, I.M. Sechenov First Moscow State Medical University (Sechenov University), 119991 Moscow, Russia
* Correspondence: subhan-che@sust.edu (M.A.S.); v.torchilin@northeastern.edu (V.P.T.)

Abstract: Cancer causes the second-highest rate of death world-wide. A major shortcoming inherent in most of anticancer drugs is their lack of tumor selectivity. Nanodrugs for cancer therapy administered intravenously escape renal clearance, are unable to penetrate through tight endothelial junctions of normal blood vessels and remain at a high level in plasma. Over time, the concentration of nanodrugs builds up in tumors due to the EPR effect, reaching several times higher than that of plasma due to the lack of lymphatic drainage. This review will address in detail the progress and prospects of tumor-targeting via EPR effect for cancer therapy.

Keywords: EPR-based therapy; passive targeting; heterogeneity; solid-tumor; EPR-imaging techniques

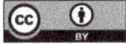

1. Introduction

The EPR effect was first discovered by Maeda and colleagues in solid murine tumors [1,2]. The polymer-drug conjugates were i.v. administered, and 10-to-100-fold higher concentrations were achieved relative to free drug administration [2–4]. Passively targeted cancer drugs at first reached the clinic about 30 years ago with the approval of an EPR-based drug, a PEGylated liposomal drug, DOXIL. Nanocarriers preferentially accumulate in the tumor through passive targeting due to a leaky vasculature and defective lymphatic drainage in solid tumors. The permeability of a chaotic vasculature and tumor microenvironment (TME) and retention can lead to the accumulation of macromolecules in TME by 70-fold. The leaky and defective vasculature created due to the rapid vascularization vital to the support of malignant tumors, coupled with imperfect lymphatic drainage, allows the EPR effect. The tumor vasculature is leaky and also irregular in diameter, shape, and density with discontinuous vessels. This results in several conditions, including heterogenous perfusion in the tumor, elevated interstitial fluid pressure from the extravasation of fluid, hypoxia, and an acidic environment [5]. EPR-based drug delivery depends on various factors, including circulation time, targeting, and the ability to overcome barriers, which are dependent on size, shape, and surface properties of the drug particles. Passive-targeting is mainly based on a diffusion mechanism. As a result, size is a crucial factor in the EPR-dependent delivery process. Studies have indicated that a nanoparticle size range of approximately 40 to 400 nm is suitable to ensure long circulation time, and enhanced accumulation in tumors with reduced renal clearance [6]. Shape and morphology also play important roles in passive targeting. Generally, rigid, spherical particles of size ranging from 50 to 200 nm have the highest tendency to long circulation, to avoid uptake by liver and spleen, but large enough to avoid kidney clearance [7,8]. Surface properties play a critical role in determining the internalization process of the drug particles into the target cell. To avoid opsonization and subsequent clearance by the RES, surface modification of polymers using PEG can be effective to a certain extent. Thus, the EPR-based drug delivery can be modulated by modifying the size, shape and sometimes by surface alteration of the nanoparticles.

Currently, a number of passively targeted nanoparticles are in clinical use including, Abraxene, Doxil, Marqibo, Myocet, and DuanoXome. Many other nanoparticles have shown promising therapeutic efficacy in clinical trials.

Major drawbacks of passive targeting include the inability to distinguish between healthy and diseased tissues, inadequate tumor accumulation, intra- and inter tumoral as well as inter-individual tumor heterogeneity. Different vascular and TME parameters contribute to the heterogeneity in EPR-mediated nanoparticle accumulation. These include vascular permeability, endothelial cell receptor expression, and vascular maturation at the vessel level. Several stromal parameters, including extracellular matrix (ECM), tumor cell density, hypoxia, and interstitial fluid pressure, contribute to heterogeneity in EPR-based tumor targeting responses. All of these pathophysiological parameters are factors necessary to be taken into consideration for the development of personalized and improved nanodrug treatments using the EPR effect. The extent of tumor accumulation always varies between tumor types, and in patients, making it necessary to determine the EPR effect. Thus, the application of direct and indirect imaging and other technologies is necessary to evaluate the degree of the EPR-effect. The presence of an EPR and non-EPR tumor in the EPR and non-EPR patients may help improve the EPR-based drug delivery systems for success in the clinic.

Dense cancer stroma is a critical component of the TME, where it has crucial roles in tumor initiation, progression, and metastasis. Most anticancer therapies target cancer cells specifically. However, tumor stromal factors can promote resistance of cancer cells to such therapies, ultimately resulting in deadly diseases such as PDAC (pancreatic ductal carcinoma). Therefore, novel anticancer therapies should be a combination of anticancer and anti-stroma therapeutic agents [9]. Approaches have been made to enhance the EPR-targeted drug accumulation to the tumor while considering cancer stromal barriers. For instance, in the use of the ADC (antibody-drug conjugate) drugs with a scaffold for cancer (CA) stromal (S) targeting (T) (CAST) [10]. In CAST therapy, stroma-targeting immunoconjugates bound to the stroma generate a scaffold, from which controlled release of cytotoxic drugs occurred and afterward diffused throughout the tumor tissue to damage both tumor cells and tumor vessels. The CAST therapy was thus reported as a new mode of cancer therapy, especially for refractory, stromal-rich cancers. Since the first CAST therapy was reported over 10 years ago, there have been several appreciated experimental studies and review works supporting and promoting CAST therapy [11–18].

Several strategies to overcome heterogeneity in EPR-based tumor accumulation can be employed to improve nanoparticle-based cancer treatments, including enhancing, combining, bypassing, and imaging. Enhancing pharmacological and physical means such as radiotherapy, hyperthermia, and sonoporation can be used to enhance the EPR effect. Combining active targeting with a pharmaceutically active ligand and the drug molecules encapsulated within a nanoparticle formulation can improve the EPR effect in a targeted tumor. Bypassing the EPR effect in cases of tumors with low or non-EPR, vascular targeting, or the use of triggerable nanocarriers to release the payload intra-vascularly can be used to enhance dr accumulation in spite of a low or non-EPR effect. To address the heterogeneity in EPR-mediated tumor targeting, direct or indirect imaging techniques, employing either nanotheranostics or companion nano-diagnostics to monitor the biodistribution and tumor accumulation or using standard imaging probes and protocols to visualize tumor blood vessels and the TME are required. Further, EPR-based tumor targeting can help to pre-select a patient for individualized therapies [19–22].

Thus, complementary active targeting with passive targeting, enhancing circulation, tumor accumulation, drug penetration in the target cell and finally release into the cytoplasm for action through circulation, accumulation, penetration, internalization, and release (CAPIR) cascade to improve the EPR effect is necessary for the development of effective cancer therapy and its translation to the clinic [23].

2. Passive Versus Active Tumor Targeting

Active targeting was at first employed to enhance the EPR-based drug delivery as a complementary approach with passively targeted drugs to improve tumor accumulation by nanoparticles to increase targeting efficiency and enhance their retention at targeted tumors [21]. Passively targeted drugs, which are dependent on the EPR effect, may not be sufficient to achieve effective targeting at target sites. However, a meta-analysis of preclinical data indicated that a median of only about 0.7% of injected dose (ID) of nanoparticles actually reaches the target tumor [21]. Several pre-clinical studies have also shown that only 0.1 to 0.2% of the ID are effective against cancer cells and show anticancer therapy with significant patient benefit [20,21].

Active targeting approaches are necessarily much more complex than a passive one. Several challenges associated with these active targeting strategies include physiological barriers and tumor heterogeneity and complex design and engineering needed for these drug delivery systems. The latter may pose major challenges and complicate pharmaceutical development and scale-up under GMP production and, significantly, to the overall cost of the therapy. In spite of several difficulties, one major advantage of active targeting is the ability to target sites disseminated throughout the body, including hematological malignancies and metastatic cancers in which the EPR is not effective [21].

Both passive and active targeting have their own limitations. To ensure clinical success of active targeting, pre-clinical tumor models need to be significantly improved to ensure effectiveness against diseases including solid tumors, hematological malignancies, and metastasis. There are significant barriers to passive targeting resulting in very low tumor accumulation leading to reduced therapeutic efficacy. Passive targeting may not distinguish between normal and diseased tissues. On the other hand, in cases of active targeting, increasing accumulation into tumor cells cannot guarantee the delivery of desired therapeutic agents to the target cells, as drug release may be hindered by the components within the cells. Moreover, endosomal escape of the drug and initiation of drug activating mechanisms is always challenging for targeted delivery. Conjugated nanoparticles may compromise the stealth capacity of the polymer because PEGylating may not be at a sufficient level. Encountering the tumor cell over-expressing receptors proteins without hurdles is a major limitation in targeted delivery. If the stealth properties of the nanoparticles are compromised, then the carriers may be rapidly uptaken/absorbed by the liver, spleen, and other RES organs, resulting in a very low accumulation of drugs in the target tumor.

For both passive and active targeting approaches, the development of companion diagnostic imaging technologies to evaluate the targeting efficiencies is very important. Selection of suitable patients and modifying treatments for specific patients may improve tumor accumulation, efficacy, and therapeutic outcome reducing the adverse effects, unnecessary treatments, and overall health expenses. Finally, active targeting can be used to complement passive targeting for better treatment results.

3. Factors Affecting the EPR Effect

The EPR effect has been observed by researchers working in cancer therapeutics for a long time. The preferential accumulation of these nanoparticles in the tumor region is a much more complex aspect than initially envisioned. This process includes several biological processes, including angiogenesis, hemodynamic regulation, vascular permeability, lymphangiogenesis, and heterogeneity of the tumor microenvironment. There is a lot of subject-to-subject variabilities related to these above-mentioned factors. The accumulation of the nanoparticles also depends on various factors, such as the physicochemical properties of each material. A rapidly growing tumor needs an enhanced blood supply as the blood vessels surrounding the tumor are enough to provide the oxygen required for cell growth. New blood vessels are formed to meet the nutritional demands of the tumor cells [24]. The process of angiogenesis surrounding the tumor is rapid, and due to this rapid growth, the blood vessels are irregular with discontinuous epithelium and lack of a basal membrane, constituting a leaky vasculature with fenestrations of 200 to 2000 nm [25–27]. This allows enhanced permeation of the blood components as it reduces resistance to extravasation into the tumor interstitium.

Unlike normal tissue, tumors have defective lymphatic drainage resulting in minimal uptake of their interstitial fluid [28]. Molecules smaller than 4 nm can be reabsorbed and diffuse back into the circulation, whereas the diffusion of larger nanoparticles is hindered by their hydrodynamic radii, which results in the accumulation of these nanoparticles in the tumor interstitium [29–31].

3.1. Extravasation

The concentration of colloids in the blood regulate extravasation with respect to the permeability of the vascular wall to nanoparticles and the nature of the extravascular environment as shown in Figure 1. The equation below describes the total flux of the material into the tumor, which is an additive function of diffusive and convective forces along with an unknown phenomenon denoted as *Black Box* [32].

$$J_{Total} = PA(C_v - C_i) + L_pA[(P_v - P_i) - \sigma(\pi_v - \pi_i)](1 - \sigma_F)C_v + Black\ Box$$

The browninan motion of the blood colloids creates a positive net flux towards the interstitium when a gradient occurs between vascular (C_v) and interstitial concentrations (C_i) [30]. The permeability (P) of the wall and the area (a) of the wall are measured by a modification of Fick's law. The diffusion coefficient of the colloid and restriction of passage by the vascular barrier is incorporated in permeability. The physicochemical properties of the colloid and the vessel wall equally affect the hindrance [26].

A convective force is generated due to the discharge of fluids from the vessel. The startling law describes the flux of the fluid, and the filtration coefficient of the fluid through the vessel is denoted by L_p. The hydrostatic pressures of vascular and interstitial parts are denoted by P_v and P_i. Vascular and interstitial oncotic pressures are denoted by π_v and π_i, respectively [30]. The σ is a capillary osmotic reflexion coefficient, which reflects the permeability of the capillary to large molecules such as proteins. It also describes how effective it is at pulling back fluid into the vascular space due to the oncotic pressure gradient. σ_F and C_v are the drag of the colloid by the fluid and colloid concentration in the vascular compartment, respectively.

The black box in the equation denotes the unknown phenomena by which colloids extravasate and reach the tumor. This lays the path to further exploration of the EPR effect. Some researchers believe that interactions with endothelial cells could cause increased permeability of the vessel. For example, cationic charges on the nanoparticles can cause more interactions and thus more permeability. Others consider these interactions a part of absorption and endocytosis by the endothelium [33–36]. Another important factor to consider for the black box is uncertain as a predictor of the concentration in the vasculature available for extravasation. The presence of phagocytic cells can cause an increase in the concentration of the nanoparticles in the vasculature of the tumor microenvironment due to the characteristic interaction of the nanoparticles to interact with phagocytic cells. [37]. Furthermore, the payload of these nanoparticles might have different properties compared to the nanoparticles. Thus, their release kinetics and their interactions within the tumor also have to be accounted for.

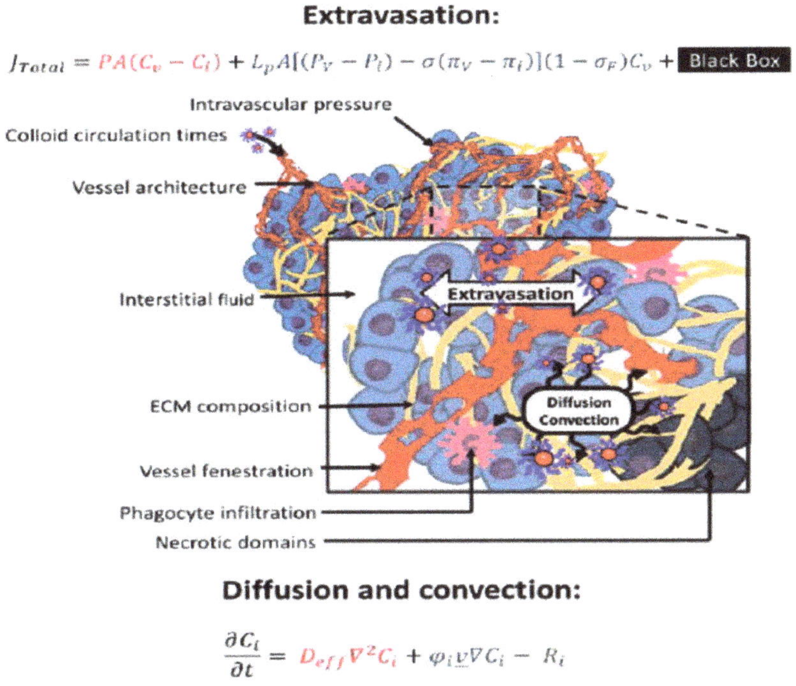

Extravasation:

$$J_{Total} = PA(C_v - C_i) + L_p A[(P_V - P_i) - \sigma(\pi_V - \pi_i)](1 - \sigma_F)C_v + \boxed{\text{Black Box}}$$

- Intravascular pressure
- Colloid circulation times
- Vessel architecture
- Interstitial fluid
- ECM composition
- Vessel fenestration
- Phagocyte infiltration
- Necrotic domains

Extravasation

Diffusion Convection

Diffusion and convection:

$$\frac{\partial C_i}{\partial t} = D_{eff} \nabla^2 C_i + \varphi_i \underline{v} \nabla C_i - R_i$$

Figure 1. The two phenomena of extravasation and later diffusion and convection of the colloid in the extracellular matrix both result in enhanced permeation and retention of the nanoparticles [32].

3.2. Diffusion and Convection in the Interstitium

The movement of the colloids once extravasated into interstitial fluid containing cancer, stromal cells, and extracellular matrix are guided by diffusive and convective forces. This is further described in the equation below:

$$\frac{\partial C_i}{\partial t} = D_{eff} \nabla^2 C_i + \varphi_i \underline{v} \nabla C_i - R_i$$

The change of the interstitial concentration over time results due to the diffusive component and convective component along with the effects of the tumor microenvironment on the colloid transport (R_i).

3.3. Tumor Vasculature and Biology

Untamed growth of the cells and angiogenic factors contribute to the disorganized vasculature and congested extravascular environments. These structural imperfections can promote the EPR effect and accumulation of nanoparticles in the tumor. The new blood vessels being formed are disordered and discontinuous with many fenestrations [38]. The cancer cells dictate the blood vessel architecture by releasing angiogenic factors [36]. Hence the type of cancer dictates the degree of leakiness of the endothelium and enhanced vascular permeability to macromolecules. They also depend on what stage the cancer is and the site it is located at [26,27,39]. These irregularities in the architecture of the vessels affect the flow and the pressure in the blood vessels, which can dictate the permeation and retention of the colloids. A highly proliferative tumor mass can also exert pressure on the blood vessels to hinder their perfusion. Thus, reduced pressure can lead to decreased convective forces and increased extravasation of both blood components and nanoparticles [26,28,38].

3.4. Tumor Extravascular Environment

The tumor extravascular environment is a haphazard, crowded entanglement of collagen fibers and glycosamine glycans (GAGs). Unlike normal tissues, the tumor microenvironment has solutes, proteins, and debris distributed unevenly [30,40]. Interstitial hydrodynamic and oncotic pressures play a key role in the convection of nanoparticles through the vascular wall, which are directly affected by the haphazard traffic of fluids [41]. The extracellular matrix will regulate the diffusive and convective forces that regulate the movement of nanoparticles once extravasated. The diffusive coefficient in the tumor interstitium is lower than in simple solutions for colloids and several in vivo and ex vivo studies have shown the same [42,43]. The viscosity of the environment and the diffusive paths can be altered by GAGs covalently linked to proteins such as collagen. The colloids of different sizes show high and low mobilities due to GAG chains that are organized in low and high viscosities, essentially making it a two-phase transfer process [43].

Resistance exerted on the interstitial transport correlated to the content and degree of organization of collagen in the ECM. The use of the collagenase enzyme may break the protein entanglement and restore mobility and help diffusion. Some research groups have shown that intratumoral injections of collagenase can enhance the mobility of viral vectors of 150 nm in size [43–45].

On the other hand, GAG-disrupting enzymes have not shown any significant effects. There were instances where injecting hyaluronidases decreased the diffusion of macromolecules and injecting heparinases that cleave heparin sulfate moieties restored the mobility of cationic macromolecules. The latter might be due to a decrease in the absorptive interactions of the colloids in the ECM [42–44].

Cells of the mononuclear phagocytic system have the tendency to extravasate to the tumor interstitium and inhibit the movement of the nanoparticles toward cancer cells. This happens due to the affinity of these macrophages to the colloids resulting in increased phagocytic activity [46]. Zamboni et al. showed that increased liposomal accumulation was seen in xenografts of ovarian cancer with increased CD11 positive cells in comparison to melanoma cells with lower dendritic cell expression [37]. The age of the individual also affects the clearance of nanoparticles such as liposomes. Older patients or patients with hepatic metastases have been shown to have higher exposure levels. Furthermore, older patients also tend to have lower hematological toxicities compared to patients below 60 years of age. This suggests that mononuclear phagocytes interact with nanoparticles, which could then affect the pharmacodynamics of the nanoparticles [47,48].

3.5. Changing Tumor Biology to Improve EPR

The tumor microenvironment can be optimized to enhance the distribution of nanoparticles in a tumor. As mentioned earlier, intratumoral injection of the enzymes to reorganize the extracellular matrix is an effective method. Similarly, reshaping the perivascular environment has been utilized in photo-immunotherapy or to deliver low molecular weight drugs. Preclinical models have shown increased accumulation and retention of the nanoparticles and oncolytic viruses with these approaches [45,49,50]. Increasing the perfusing pressure via improving transvascular convective movement is another approach. Administration of hypertensive drugs such as angiotensin II resulted in increased extravasation of the colloids with sufficient affinity to bind to the tumor and avoid being translocated back into the circulation. Moreover, the administration of angiotensin converting enzyme (ACE) inhibitors such as enalapril resulted in an increased accumulation of antibodies [2]. The ACE inhibitor blocked the degradation of bradykinin (a potent physiological vasodilatory peptide), which increased the permeability to large molecules [41,51]. Administration of both the ACE inhibitor and angiotensin II is a good approach to increase the EPR as angiotensin II will counteract the hypotensive effect of ACE inhibitor enalapril. EPR can be increased by employing other vasodilatory agents using nitric oxide, prostaglandins, and carbon monoxide [52–56].

3.6. Physicochemical Factors That Affect EPR

The physicochemical properties of the colloids play a key role in the EPR effect by altering their extravasation. The physicochemical properties of any external material for therapeutic or diagnostic purposes are important in drug delivery as they impact the way the host defense mechanisms clear them from the systemic circulation [57,58]. The size, charge, and shape of the nanoparticles are the important physicochemical properties that dictate the EPR effect. Table 1 lists the characteristic size, charge, and shape needed for increased enhanced permeation and retention.

Table 1. Properties of nanoparticles that affect the EPR.

	Properties of Nanoparticles		
	Size	Charge	Shape
Characteristics	<ul><li>It is evident from the mouse xenograft models that smaller molecules that are 3.3 to 10 kDa with 2 and 3 nm diffused deeper into the tumor compared to the large molecules [59].</li><li>Nanoparticles smaller than 70 nm tend to aggregate in the tumor if they are highly permeable [60].</li></ul>	<ul><li>Surface charge of the nanoparticles plays a key role in the clearance of the nanoparticles and thereby the residence time in the body. It also changes the opsonization profile of the nanoparticle [61].</li><li>An increased accumulation in the tumor site has been observed for nanoparticles that are cationic and sterically stabilized [62].</li><li>Both positively and negatively charged nanoparticles have an affinity to bind to the components in the extracellular matrix, thereby decreasing the diffusion in the interstitium [19].</li></ul>	<ul><li>Increased accumulation is observed in the nanoparticles that are elongated, such as carbon nanotubes with a high aspect ratio (100:1 to 500:1). Porous media can aid in the filtration process [63].</li><li>Nanorods 44 nm in length have been shown to extravasate more than 35 nm length rods by four-fold [64].</li></ul>

Furthermore, total blood exposure of these nanoparticles should be the key factor influencing the accumulation of the nanoparticles inside the tumor. The concentration of these colloids influences the diffusive and convective forces necessary in controlling the amount of extravasation into the interstitium. The efflux of the nanoparticles from the tumor can be hindered by maintaining higher concentrations in the bloodstream [32]. The above physicochemical properties can help the drug delivery scientists to design the nanoparticle in such a way as to increase the EPR effect and increase the drug concentration at the site of action.

4. Heterogeneity of EPR: A Clinically Relevant Phenomenon

In the last couple of years, research reports citing nanocarriers and EPR effect-based therapies have been increased markedly. The basic rationale for tumor targeting via EPR effect has been presented in thousands of research papers that claim improved therapeutic potentials and consider this phenomenon a royal gateway. However, at present, scientists and oncology specialists are of a view that these therapies are failing in the clinic and that the EPR effect is misinterpreted and overrated. This approach, "one size fits all," worked in lab animal tumor models but not in humans, possibly because they were transient in nature, thus limiting the bench to bedside translation of most targeted tumor therapies. The heterogenous outcomes of clinical trials have led to a new understanding that the EPR effect varies greatly between lab animals and humans as well as among different tumor types and metastases within the same individual. To address the complex nature of the EPR effect, the research is now moving towards a custom-fit approach to personalize the patient therapy for better outcomes and to identify the most responsive patients from clinical trials [20,65–68].

Human tumors differ greatly from animal tumors with respect to the rate of growth, size of the tumor, tumor-to-body weight ratio, and heterogeneity of the tumor microenvironment that collectively alters the pharmacokinetics of most drugs. The degree of tumor heterogeneity varies in different types of tumors as well as with the same types of tumors in different patients. Thus, complete control and performance monitoring throughout therapy might help develop successful clinical trials [69,70].

4.1. Heterogeneity of Tumor Blood Flow and Hypoxic Areas

The abnormal tumor growth requirements for nutrients and oxygen direct the neighboring tissues to proliferate and lead to the ingrowth of a vascular supply. The imbalance between oxygen supply and demand leads to hypoxia. The irregular branching order with enlarged vessels and chaotic blood flow within different parts of a tumor lead to the heterogenous distribution of drugs. The resulting hypoxic parts of tumors alter the EPR effect by activation of fibrinolysis, clotting, or bleeding in some tumor parts, result in poor delivery of drugs [65,71]. The activation of hypoxia-inducible factor (HIF) signaling is regulated by hypoxia through multiple mechanisms, including overexpression of Jagged 2 and Notch signaling, activation of CD24 expression, induction of integrin-like kinase, ILK and elevated levels of hypoxia induced genes such as B lymphocyte-induced maturation protein-1 (BLIMP1) that collectively promote metastatic stem cell phenotypes [72–77].

4.2. Heterogenous Vascular Permeability and Extravasation

The rapid tumor growth and improper development of blood vessels in murine tumors result in a much leakier vasculature as compared to human tumors that can lead to misinterpretation of the EPR effect [78]. This is generally not the case in humans, where not all tumors manifest a leaky vasculature and resultant enhanced permeability to macromolecules. However, there are certain human tumors that are very leaky, well-vascularized, and overexpress VEGF. Despite the above notion, some human tumors respond nearly as hypothesized, and the discovery of U.S. FDA approval of Doxil for AIDS-related Kaposi's sarcoma can be noted here. The liposomal doxorubicin extravasated and accumulated intact in tumors with a leaky vasculature [79].

4.3. Heterogenous Penetration

The clinical isolates from a variety of cancer patients support tumor related abnormal blood coagulation. This process starts when tumor cells erode the neighboring normal or tumor blood vessels resulting in microscopic hemorrhages. The insoluble fibrin (IF) clot formation and replacement with collagenous tissues start immediately to compensate for the tissue damage. This silent process called 'malignant cycle of blood coagulation' in cancer patients is similar to the normal wound healing process, however these fibrin clots survive with cancer cells. This fibrotic stroma provides a barrier to the penetration of chemotherapeutics and resultant treatment failure. This stromal barrier is more prominent in solid cancers that are invasive and hypercoagulable such as glioblastomas, pancreatic cancers, and stomach cancers [10–12].

When moving from the periphery to the center of tumors, drugs face heterogenous vessel stress and collapse due to proliferating cells as the density of tumor and interstitial fluid pressure increase that further hinders the transport of drug molecules [80]. The human tumors differ with respect to pericyte coverage (smooth muscle actin cells attached to endothelium) in that it is high and compact while low and loose in murine models. The tumors with a poor prognosis (brain tumors, renal carcinomas) have a fibrotic interstitium with more pericyte coverage (60–70%) as compared to tumors with better prognosis (ovarian carcinoma, colon cancers) with about a 10% coverage [81,82].

Adequate vascular pericyte coverage is crucial in normal cells' maintenance of the blood–brain barrier (BBB), where the loss of these cells leads to various brain disorders. The neoplastic pericytes derived after genetic modifications of glioma stem cells (GSC) develop a blood tumor barrier (BTB) that hampers the penetration of chemotherapeutics and results in treatment failure. The preferential overexpression of BMX-kinase in GSC-derived pericytes makes it a suitable target to disruption of the BTB and enhance the penetration of anticancer drugs. Zhou et al. identified ibrutinib as a potent tumor pericyte-disrupting drug. Their findings suggest that adequate synergism can be established by combining this treatment with some poorly penetrating anticancer drugs [83]. The pericytes serve as a gatekeeper against tumor progression and metastasis to other organs of the body. The clinical data also suggest that low pericyte coverage results in high mortality of cancer patients [84]. The basement membrane (BM) and extracellular matrix (ECM) also play an important role in determining the porosity and stiffness of human tumors that lead to heterogenous penetration, poor prognosis, and treatment failure [66]. Lee et al. reported non-invasive and cost-effective pulsed high intensity focused ultrasound technology as an ECM remodeling strategy as an alternative to intratumoral injection of collagenase and hyaluronidase for deep penetration of nanoparticles [85].

5. Strategies to Overcome Heterogeneity

Various treatment modalities based upon specific pathophysiology of tumor and EPR effect have been proposed with more than 7350 citations over the first report of EPR (as of June 2021 from Google Scholar). The CAST therapy received considerable attention from researchers after the successful development of new strategies to achieve highly localized concentration of topoisomerase-1 inhibitor, SN-38, conjugated with monoclonal antibody (mAb) targeted against collagen-4. This newly developed immunoconjugate was optimized to bound with stromal collagen creating a scaffold with sustained release of anticancer agent [13,14]. Gebleux and coworkers proposed non-internalizing antibody drug conjugates, ADC, that rely on extracellular release of drug thus preventing antigen barriers [15]. ADC might overcome heterogeneity of tumors by utilizing TME to facilitate cleavage of linkers and payload release [16]. Tumor endothelial marker-8 (TEM-8) is overexpressed in perivascular stromal cells and can be used as a useful stromal target for locally triggered drug release from anti TEM-8 ADC [17]. The heterogenous antigen distribution in malignant cells and the difference in targeted gene copy number among patients are serious challenges for researchers, and a single mAb may not be effective for all patients [14].

Many approaches have been proposed for mAb-based tumor targeting and mechanisms to overcome therapeutic resistance that is caused by the heterogeneity of tumor antigen and also the resistance executed by TME, including inefficient delivery to the tumor, alteration of effector functions in the TME, and Fc-γ receptor expression diversity and polymorphism. mAbs-based therapies are potential approaches to overcome these barriers using several diagnostic and prognostic biomarkers for envisaging response to mAb-based therapies [18].

EPR-effect has been proved by many preclinical animal models. However, results obtained from animal models are usually conflicting with clinical observations. Unlike hematological malignancies, in solid tumors, administered anticancer agents (ACA) must diffuse through the tumor mass, overcoming cancer stromal barriers and tumor mass itself. It has been demonstrated that hypercoagulability caused by cancer stroma, and the more aggressive cancer, the greater the deposition of insoluble fibrin (IF) in cancer tissue [14]. An ant-IF mAb was developed and conjugated with an ACA using V-L-K linker. The resultant ADC drug linker is degradable by plasmin. The plasmin is activated during the IF formation only. ACA is released from the ADC drug particularly when the conjugate binds to the IF. This novel approach was beneficial to deliver ACA to tumor cells through the stromal barrier due to the small size of the drug [14].

Numerous strategies have been used to modify the abnormal tumor microenvironment in humans by combination with nanomedicines. The direct permeability enhancement by various methods has been explored that take advantage of the EPR effect and facilitate the delivery of drugs/macromolecules inside tumors. Examples include the selective inhibition of angiotensin-converting enzymes [86,87], generation of NO or CO within tumors [56,87,88], blockage of VEGF and other angiogenic signaling factors [89–91], inhibition of pericyte recruitment and BM activation [92,93], and image guiding systems [94].

The recent advancements and technological innovations have allowed novel insights into the drastic differences between murine and human cancers that can hamper the clinical translation of tumor-targeted nanotherapeutics. The laboratory-established models are not true representatives of human cancer in many respects and require modifications to explain the heterogenous events responsible for compromised EPR effects in humans. To maximize the clinical outcomes of investigational cancer therapeutics, new strategies to mimic the individual tumors are required that closely recapitulate the patients' responses to preclinical drug testing [95,96]. This approach provides the potential for guided clinical decision-making in translational cancer research by individual performance metric calculation. Tailoring the cancer therapy to patient groups that are more prone to respond and benefit from the investigational treatment offer a potential solution to overcome the heterogeneity of the EPR effect. Patient-derived tumor xenografts (PDX) involve the engraftment of specific tumor tissues in immunocompromised mice. Izumchenko et al. integrated PDX models via implantation of 92 different solid cancers from a 237 cohort of patients into immunodeficient mice. They analyzed and compared the patient responses and PDX models after whole exome sequencing. Their findings suggested that these models accurately replicated the patient outcomes over a repetitive course of therapy, enabling an oncologist to assess the patient-specific cellular events [97]. The mouse models offered numerous benefits, such as their small size, ease of reproduction, transgenicity, and closely mimicked physiology. However, various limitations involving mice such as high cost, complex genetic manipulations, and prolonged duration of experimentation have forced researchers to utilize alternatives. Numerous current publications reported the use of chick chorioallantoic membrane (CAM) and Zebrafish for implantation as alternatives to mice. Hu and coworkers demonstrated that CAM is an efficient system to analyze pilot drug responses in patients with bladder tumors, accelerating the discovery of critical molecular mechanisms [98]. Mercatali et al. studied the metastatic potential of breast cancer after injecting primary culture of bone metastasis derived from a 67-year-old patient into zebrafish embryos. Their findings suggested zebrafish are a suitable substitute for mouse models and provide for a better understanding of chemotherapeutic sensitivity and prognostic marker identification [99]. Table 2 shows the status of some patient-derived tumor models.

Table 2. Recent progress and status of patient-derived tumor models.

Therapeutic Moiety/Combination	Target	Cancer Type	Animal Type	Reference
Erlotinib	EGFR	Glioblastoma	Athymic nude mice	[100]
Gefitinib and Enzalutamide	Androgen receptor and EGFR	non-small cell lung cancer and Prostate cancer	Chick chorioallantoic membrane (CAM)	[101]
Apatinib, Regorafenib, Cabozantinib, Ramucirumab	VEGFR2	Gastric cancers	Zebrafish	[102]
Ramucirumab	Her2, FGFR2, cMet	Gastric cancers	BALB/c nude mice	[103]
Bortezomib	CDK4 and MDM2	Liposarcoma	Mice	[104]
Pembrolizumab	PD-1/PD-L1	Soft Tissue Sarcoma	NSG mice	[105]
Erdafitinib	FGFR	Metastatic prostate cancer	Male mice	[106]
β-elemene and cisplatin-coloaded liposomes	Codelivery to reverse MDR	Lung cancer	$C_{57}BL/6$ mice	[107]

6. Targeting Tumor Tissues via an EPR Effect

Since the discovery of the EPR concept, it has been utilized widely for many applications (Figure 2), especially for the delivery of anticancer drugs. The EPR effect helps promote a favorable biodistribution of nanoparticles in blood and a high level of nanoparticle accumulation in solid tumors. However, for the optimal development of nanoparticles for enhanced drug delivery by EPR effect, multiple factors should be considered, including blood half-life of nanoparticles, minimal nonspecific delivery, and effective elimination from the body [108].

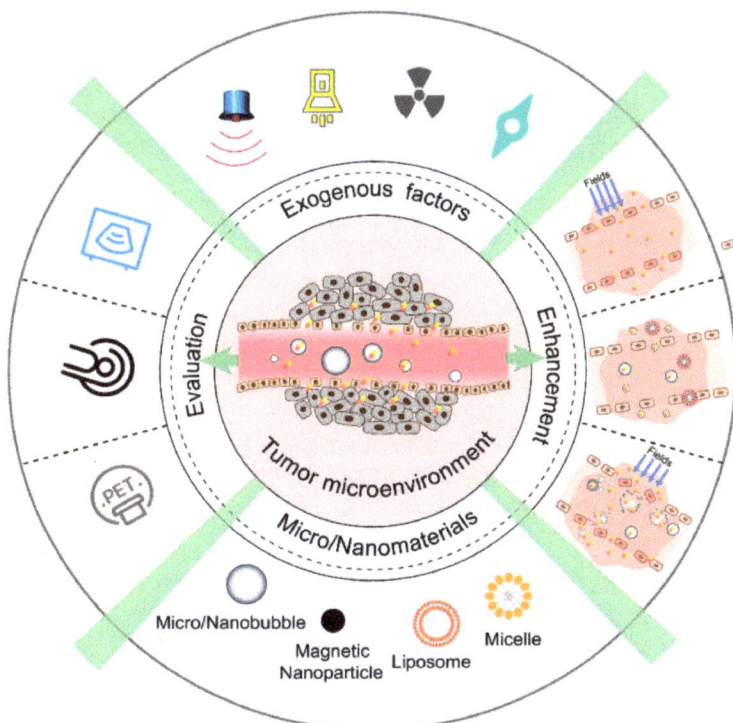

Figure 2. Common strategies utilizing the EPR effect [109].

The EPR effect discovery was a milestone in drug delivery systems, and expectations for utilizing this effect in a selective anticancer drug delivery were high. However, the transition of nano-drug delivery medicine from benchtop to clinic has been very difficult. An EPR effect-mediated drug accumulation has been proved with various natural and synthetic molecules with molecular sizes greater than 40 kDa or 7 to 8 nm in diameter. Encapsulation of small molecules inside macromolecular vehicles, including liposomes, nanospheres, or polymeric micelles, led to full utilization of the EPR effect and made it a universal method for targeting the tumor side known as passive targeting. The characteristics of the EPR effect are at disposal for this method of targeting, including (i) defective architecture of blood vessels, known as a "leaky vasculature," with large gaps (around 400 nm) between capillary endothelial cell linings; (ii) overproduction of vascular mediators including bradykinin and nitric oxide [NO]); and (iii) improved retention of the macromolecules in tumor tissue due to impaired lymphatic recovery [110,111].

6.1. Chemotherapeutics Targeted through EPR Effect

Taken together, it can be said that successful drug delivery via EPR effect is based on the properties of the molecule/carrier, including (i) biocompatibility; (ii) molecular size greater than renal clearance threshold (40 kDa); (iii) neutral or slightly negative charge; (iv) drug retention time greater than a few hours (v) circulation time longer than a few hours [65,110]. Among these factors influencing the EPR effect, the most important are molecular size and biocompatibility. To prevent renal clearance, low molecular weight drugs are conjugated to polymers or to natural blood components that circulate long in the plasma, such as serum albumin or lipoproteins. The best-known example of such a polymer is poly (styrene-maleic anhydride) (SMA). It has been proven that the conjugation of peptides and proteins with a polymer of this type (1.5 kDa) allows extending the circulation time of anti-cancer proteins and peptides by binding the conjugates to plasma albumin. It has also been shown that conjugation with SMA protects proteins from enzymatic degradation and reduces the immunogenicity of modified proteins. An example of such a conjugate is neocarzinostatin and SMA (SMANCs) used for the treatment of hepatoma, which accumulates in solid tumors through the EPR effect and which was the basis for other conjugates based on the same mechanism of action [112–114]

The copolymer to which a wide variety of anti-cancer drugs including doxorubicin, has been attached is based on N-(2-hydroxypropyl)methacrylamide (HPMA) for delivery to tumors via the EPR effect [115–117]. Conjugates of HPMA copolymer with an anticancer drug are active in many models and have low immunogenicity, which makes it possible to improve such a conjugate to target and control its subcellular localization of the drug based on its mechanism of action [116,118,119].

Another method for drug delivery through the EPR effect is to entrap the drugs into nanoparticles. The disadvantage of this solution is that large-sized nanoparticles will be absorbed by organs of the reticuloendothelial system (RES), such as the liver and spleen, resulting in slower elimination from the body and a potential for toxicity [120]. For this purpose, the concept of stealth liposome was developed. Conjugation of phospholipids with polyethylene glycol (PEG) leads to the formation of a protective, hydrophilic layer on the liposome surface. This layer prevents recognition of the liposomes by opsonin and other complement components, thereby preventing clearance through the RES system and increasing the half-life of the liposomes. As stealth liposomes, the appropriate size of the liposomes prevents loss due to renal filtration, while pegylation, in turn, ensures that the RES system does not recognize the nanoparticles, which leads to the preferential accumulation of liposomes in tumor tissues through the EPR effect [121,122]. The first liposomal formulation that met these guidelines and was approved by the FDA was Doxil®, a formulation containing doxorubicin hydrochloride used in the treatment of AIDS-related Kaposi's sarcoma, multiple myeloma, and ovarian cancer using the EPR effect. To date, the FDA has approved many other liposomal formulations such as DaunoXome®, which contains daunorubicin, and Marquibo®, which contains vincristine sulfate for cancer therapy [123] as well as other types of nanoparticle including polymeric micelles containing paclitaxel (Genexol® PM), micelles built with PEG and a poly(γ-benzyl L-glutamate, containing cisplatin [124] and albumin nanoparticles with paclitaxel (Abraxane®) [125]. A new strategy to overcome the dilemma between the EPR effect and renal clearance was the development of multifunctional particles such as FeTNPs. These molecules were designed based on the coordinated interaction of phenolic groups and iron, composed of ferric iron, tannic acid (TA), and poly (glutamic acid) -graft-methoxy poly (ethylene glycol) (PLG-g-mPEG). FeTNPs are characterized by their effective accumulation in tumor tissue based on the EPR effect and the possibility of being disassembled dynamically by deferoxamine mesylate (DFO) to accelerate the elimination of nanoparticles, thus reducing the potential for toxicity [126].

Another extremely important physicochemical parameter that affects the time of systemic circulation and intratumoral processes is the presence of a surface charge, which can control the opsonization profile of the material, its recognition by the MPS cell, and its overall plasma circulation profile. The desired parameter has a neutral or slightly negative surface charge, while a positive charge was believed to lower the circulation time. However, the non-pegylated, positively charged liposomes containing 1,2-diacyl-trimethylammonium propane (DOTAP) lipid have been shown to have higher tumor-to-surrounding tissue ratios than their negative or neutral counterparts. The positive charges are believed to promote NP interactions with tumor blood vessels and compromise their predisposition to deeper diffusion in the tumor while preventing their redistribution in the systemic circulation. This phenomenon has been exploited for therapeutic purposes by targeting an endothelial tumor vessel with anti-angiogenic and antitumor drugs in preclinical and clinical models [33,127].

6.2. Targeting DNA, siRNA, and Other Nucleotides

The main strategy to target nucleic acids via the EPR effect is to encapsulate/conjugate them with nanoparticles. Similar to anticancer drugs, for specific tumor delivery of siRNA, sufficient longevity of loaded siRNA carriers is required [128]. Currently, polyethyleneimine (PEI) is one of the most studied and successful cationic polymers for nucleic acid delivery, including siRNA. Unfortunately, PEI of high molecular weight did not show high transfection efficiency and also showed significant systemic toxicity. To reduce the toxicity of a PEI-based delivery system, polyethyleneimine is most often combined with other polymers such as PEG [129] or dendrimers [130]. These have led to the successful clinical use of PEI to deliver sensitive genetic biomaterials [129].

To improve the PEI-based genetic material delivery system, a conjugate of a lipid, PEI, and polyethylene glycol (PEG) with a hypoxia-sensitive linker (azobenzene; a derivative of nitroimidazole) was developed. The advantage of this approach is that under hypoxic conditions, the azobenzene linker is degraded, thus releasing the protective PEG layer, exposing the siRNA to allow hypoxia-dependent cellular uptake. This method uses the enhancement of the EPR effect by targeting the carrier to a specific tumor environment. This strategy may allow for an effective supply of genetic material and can be used as a therapy for drug-resistant tumors [131,132].

6.3. Targeting Imaging Agents

The EPR effect is an important tool for specific nanoparticle targeting in cancer therapy as well as for diagnostic purposes. Diagnostic techniques such as fluorescence imaging, positron emission tomography (PET), magnetic resonance imaging (MRI), computed tomography (CT), or single-photon emission computed tomography (SPECT) require delivery of small molecules to a tumor site, which is a challenging task [133,134]. Nowadays, imaging plays an important role in clinical oncology by serving as the main tool to identify solid tumors and determine therapeutic responses. Unfortunately, imaging techniques including CT and MRI have limited sensitivity and thus, cannot provide specific and functional information on the disease due to usage of non-targeted contrast agents. Therefore, there is a definite need for new contrast agents or modified existing ones. Significant progress was seen with recently developed biodegradable nanostructures of iron oxide for MRI and luminescent quantum dots (QDs), a new class of light-emitting particles. The nanoparticles were built of PLGA-mPEG polymer and showed prolonged circulation half-life and improved imaging effects [135,136].

Recently, liposomes containing 89Zr have also been formulated for photodynamic therapy and PET imaging. Liposomes with a multicompartment-membrane were developed containing tween-80, where 89Zr was conjugated with a deferoxamine chelator with tetrakis (4-carboxyphenyl) porphyrin. These radiolabeled liposomes showed enhanced EPR effects, improved photodynamics, and in vivo stability [137]. Copper-64 containing PEGylated liposomes were also developed to clearly observe the EPR effect through PET imaging [138].

Similarly, for fluorescent imaging, various strategies have been developed. Fluorescent dyes have been conjugated to macromolecules to enhance the EPR effect, including tetramethylrhodamine isothiocyanate (TRITC)-conjugated, with high-molecular-weight [MW 67,000] bovine serum albumin (BSA). Another polymer, N-(2-hydroxypropyl)methacrylamide (HPMA) (13 kDa), was also conjugated with zinc protoporphyrin (ZnPP). Formed micelles were about 80 nm in diameter and produced a clear tumor image similar to BSA-TRIC conjugate [139].

Nowadays, superparamagnetic iron oxide nanoparticles (SPION) are being used as an MRI contrast agent for tumor imaging. SPION are usually built of magnetite (Fe_3O_4) or maghemite (Fe_2O_3), encapsulated within an aqueous core. The marketed SPION contrast agent that has been used for tumor imaging is known as Endorem®. Modification of SPION with the ultrasmall size is USPION, known as Sinerem®. These nanoparticles with a size below 50 nm are mostly used for the detection of brain tumors [140].

Although we understand more about the EPR effect and many approaches have been taken to utilize this phenomenon in cancer treatment and diagnosis, there are still many challenges left. Thus, significant research has been focused on the enhancement of the EPR effect.

7. Approaches for Promoting EPR of Nanodrugs in Cancer

There is a large intra- and inter-personal heterogeneity in EPR-based tumor targeting, which is reflected in the outcome of clinical trials showing unexpected lower success rates. Based on the nature, heterogeneity, and complexity of the EPR effect, the development of systems and approaches for enhancing, combining, bypassing, and imaging the EPR tumor-targeting are crucial.

In healthy tissues, low MW drugs easily extravasate out of blood vessels, whereas nanodrugs are often unable to do so because of size. On the other hand, in tumors, abnormally wide fenestrations in the blood vessels allow the extravasation of nanoparticles with sizes of up to several hundreds of nm. Additionally, the relative absence of lymphatic drainage leads to an effective and selective accumulation of nanodrugs in tumors.

Multiple vascular and TME parameters contribute to heterogeneity in EPR-mediated tumor accumulation. Biological barriers that contribute to heterogeneity in EPR-based tumor targeting include high cellularity, dense ECM, hypoxia, interstitial fluid pressure (IFP), vascular permeability, endothelial cell receptor expression, and vascular maturation at the vessel level.

Many pharmaceutical and physical approaches can be used to enhance tumor accumulation and efficiency of the EPR-based drug delivery. Important pharmacological approaches include modulating VEGF signaling with angiotensin agonists and antagonists, TNFα, vessel-promoting treatments, and nitric oxide-producing agents. Physical approaches include hyperthermia, ultrasound, radiotherapy.

Regulation of particle size and encapsulation in micelles can improve circulation time and enhance accumulation via the EPR effect. Encapsulation of doxorubicin in liposomes, Doxil, enhances plasma half-life by up to 2–3 days compared to free drug. In many liposomal and micellar nanodrug formulations, surface modification with the stealthy polymer, PEG, decreased aggregation, opsonization with plasma protein and enhanced the circulation half-life [20].

Anti-angiogenic drugs can be used to deprive tumors of nutrients and oxygen. For instance, at an intermediate dose of anti-angiogenic drug, bevacizumab was employed to normalize the disorganized tumor vasculature into a highly vascularized one to enhance drug delivery. The use of intermediate doses of Doxil or Abraxane enhanced the accumulation of paclitaxel in tumors by restoring convective drug delivery with reduced IFP, and without decreasing the concentration of doxorubicin in a size-dependent manner. Bevacizumab-mediated vascular normalization enhances the antitumor response of Doxil-based chemotherapy of ovarian cancer in a clinical setting [141].

TNFα is a potential inflammatory molecule. It led to a 10-fold higher EPR-induced accumulation of radio-labeled liposomes in mouse tumors compared to non-TNFα treated ones. Fibromuna, an antibody fused to TNFα used in melanoma treatment, has been used in combination with doxorubicin for sarcoma treatment and in combination with melphalan used for isolated limb perfusion to avoid amputation of a cancerous limb [142,143]. Although clinical trials with several TNFα-based drugs are promising, their use has been limited to local delivery due to their systemic toxicity [20].

Accumulation by EPR in tumors can be enhanced with Angiotensin II receptor blockers (ARB) that promote vessel permeability and dilation through the loosening of the endothelial cadherin-mediated intracellular connections [53]. The ARBs can modulate the expression of ECM, leading to vessel decompression and an enhanced EPR [144]. For example, losartan can decompress tumor blood vessels, increase vascular perfusion and EPR-targeted drug delivery [145]. Instead of increasing vessel permeability and dilation of vessels using ARBs, vasoconstriction using angiotensin II can also be used to enhance the EPR-mediated drug delivery. Angiotensin II can induce systemic vasoconstriction in healthy blood vessels. However, since tumor blood vessels are immature and lack a uniformly differentiated and structured smooth muscle cell layer, they do not contract in response to AT-II. As a result, the AT-II drugs can enhance the EPR drug accumulation through an increased blood flow into the tumor blood vessels compared to healthy blood vessels. Thus, AT-II can lead to better perfusion of tumor tissues and enhanced EPR-based drug accumulation in tumors. However, this treatment option may be limited to patients with normal BP levels.

Approaches to vessel promotion of increased angiogenesis instead of inhibiting the angiogenesis can result in more vessels and a higher delivery of drugs. Cligentide can bind to $\alpha v \beta 3$ integrins to prompt anti-angiogenesis [146]. Verapamil, a calcium channel blocker, induced higher blood flow and enhanced blood vessel perfusion. The combination therapy using cligentide, verapamil, and gemcitabine enhanced survival in a mouse model of pancreatic cancer due to a reduced tumor burden. This combination therapy significantly increased vessel density and reduced hypoxia, exhibiting possible benefits of vessel promotion in combination with chemotherapy. Similarly, erythropoietin in NSCLC models, increased vessel density by 50%, doubled the relative tissue blood volume, through the vessel promotion, which resulted in up to a 100% increased cisplatin delivery [147].

Radiation therapy can increase vascular leakiness through upregulation of fibroblast growth factor [148]. The combination of nanodrug therapy and radiotherapy can enhance the EPR-based drug delivery. Combination therapy using Doxil with radiotherapy in osteosarcoma xenograft mice delayed tumor growth compared to the control [9]. However, un-encapsulated nanodrugs, when combined with radiotherapy, may have severe side effects [149]. In fact, ionizing radiation has an effect on different cell types in TME. Besides increasing vascular leakiness, radiotherapy can prompt MDR and metastasis [150]. Thus, applying radiotherapy in combination with nanodrug therapy required precautionary steps.

Hyperthermia can be used in combination with chemo- and radiotherapy for locally well-defined solid tumors. This can be applied through radiofrequency, microwave-focused ultrasound, and intracavity perfusion. Hyperthermia increases tumor blood flow and enhances vascular permeability and promotes drug and oxygen supply to tumors. Thus, hyperthermia can be used to enhance EPR-mediated drug delivery, especially in non-leaky tumors with a very low level of baseline nanodrug accumulation [151]. Extravasation of 100 nm liposomes was enhanced significantly upon increasing temperature [152]. The combination of hyperthermia with temperature-sensitive nanodrugs can be an effective EPR-based drug delivery system.

In low EPR tumors upon sonoporation, liposome accumulation was enhanced up to 100% [20]. Sonoporation in combination with gemcitabine-based therapy in pancreatic cancer demonstrated positive impact [153]. Usually, CNS drug therapies are not effective due to the BBB. However, sonoporation prompted a spatially and temporally controlled BBB opening facilitating enhanced drug delivery [154]. Ultrasound (US)-mediated brain vascular opening demonstrated that MRI-focused US treatment in combination with Doxil enhanced drug accumulation in a gliosarcoma model [155]. Clinical trials to evaluate minimal US required for safely open the BBB are currently ongoing [156].

Photodynamic therapy (PDT), based on a photosensitizing agent and ROS formation, can damage nucleic acids and proteins, leading to cell death. A mAb-photosensitizer conjugate, panitumumab-IR700, against the EGFR in combination with laser light and liposomal daunorubicin was used to treat tumors [157]. Treatment of tumors with EGFR targeted photosensitizer, prior to daunorubicin treatment led to super-enhanced permeability and retention (SUPR), enhanced tumor accumulation, and therapeutic efficacy. However, clinical limitations of PDT, including penetration depth of laser light and short migration distance by ROS, render the treatment options for wide-spread tumors and metastasis located deep in the body almost impossible.

The pretreatment with intralipid increased accumulation of nanomedicine in tumors due to induced reduction in liver uptake. This increased accumulation, therefore, led to significantly improved therapeutic effects, which were validated by using the Doxil drug. As a fascinating result, intralipid pretreatment prolonged the plasma half-life of nanomedicines in normal healthy mice but not in tumor-bearing mice, which suggests that tumors may be an alternative route of nanodrug delivery when liver delivery is suppressed [158].

The combination of two different drugs within a formulation can be beneficial for EPR targeting. CPX-1 is a liposome containing irinotecan and fluoxuridine in a 1:1 molar ratio enhanced EPR-accumulation of CPX-1 in colorectal cancer [159]. Combination of Abraxane with gemcitabine for the treatment of metastatic PDAC, and a combination of abraxane with carboplatin for the treatment of NSCLC have shown promise in the clinic [160]. Trastuzumab, together with different chemotherapeutics, are used for the treatment of HER2-positive metastatic breast cancer [161]. An EGFR-targeted nanobody linked to a polymeric micelle (PM), nanobody modified DOX-PM, inhibited tumor growth and prolonged survival [162].

The combination of an anti-PD-L1 with an immunogenic cell death-inducing nanoscale coordination polymer (NCP), loaded with oxaliplatin, as well as photosensitizer for PDT showed success in cancer therapy [157]. Combination therapy using nanoformulations suitable for combined PDT and immune checkpoint blockade was also successful against TNBC [163].

Combination of several drugs in a nanocarrier and application ADCs accumulated drugs through an EPR effect and enhanced delivery of all drugs with different mechanisms to the tumor cell, without cross-resistance. This combination therapeutic approach enhances the impact of individual drug components, aids synergistic effects, reduces side effects due to the encapsulation of drugs into a nanocarrier resulting in an enhanced nano-immunotherapeutic outcome [164].

Patients with a low EPR tumor with a non-leaky vasculature need either active delivery or a bypassing of the EPR effect to trigger drug release into the tumor. Several approaches have been developed to deliver nanoparticles without reliance on an EPR effect [5]. Fluorescent peptides that form nanoparticles in situ in tumors, and treatment responses that can be detected by imaging, have been developed [165]. Similarly, an assembly of GNPs and fluorescent contrast agents has been used for the detection of drug delivery in tumors [166].

For low EPR tumors, an injectable nanoparticle generator (iNPG) has been developed to enhance drug delivery to tumors. The iNPG releases the drug-polymer conjugate due to natural tropism and enhanced vascular dynamics and forms self-assembled nanoparticles in situ, which are transported to the perinuclear region to bypass the drug efflux pump. The iNPG system was effective in TNBC, MDA-MB-231, and 4T1 mouse models of metastasis [21,167].

Another EPR-independent approach to improve tumor targeting in low EPR tumors and metastatic cancer sites that are unreachable by EPR targeting is by cell-mediated delivery of nanoparticles. Conjugating nanocapsules encapsulating the topoisomerase I drug SN-38 to the T cell surface, used to traffic through the lymphatic system, resulted in a 90-fold increase of SN-38 drugs in lymph nodes relative to free drug [168]. Immune cell-induced delivery of nanoparticles can improve drug accumulation in disseminated tumors and metastasis. Such a safer targeted delivery of IFN-γ can promote the differentiation of tumor-enhancing M2 macrophages to antitumor M1 [21].

To better clinical results, patients showing a sufficient level of EPR may be pre-selected. Suitable, efficient probes and protocols are necessary for patient pre-selection for clinical trials in considering factors, including vascular leakiness and perfusion, macrophage content, and density of ECM. To quantify the EPR effect in tumor targeting, direct and indirect imaging techniques have been promising. MRI scanning was used to characterize and correlate parameters including RBV and vessel permeability with the accumulation of fluorophore-labeled nanoparticles in several tumor models to detect biomarkers of EPR-mediated drug accumulation that have been studied [169]. The accumulation of polystyrene nanoparticles in different tumor models has been evaluated using multi-modal imaging techniques [170].

The PET nano-reporter, can serve as a companion nano-diagnostic for Doxil, loaded with chelators allowing for ^{89}Zr-labeling and PET imaging to evaluate the therapeutic outcome by predicting the drug accumulation. Nano-reporter and doxorubicin concentrations in tumors correlated well with therapeutic efficiency, indicating a good therapeutic response [171]. A paramagnetic, ferumoxytol, was studied as a companion nano-diagnostic with polymeric nanoparticles encapsulating docataxel, to differentiate tumors with high, medium and low accumulation of docetaxel and ferumoxytol. The highest docetaxel accumulation and tumor response was observed for high ferumoxytol accumulated tumors [20].

^{64}Cu-labelled, HER2-targeted PEGylated liposomes containing doxorubicin were used to study the EPR effect in primary and metastatic breast cancers by quantitative PET imaging and biopsies to determine the doxorubicin accumulation in the tumor and therapeutic efficacy [172].

The various direct and indirect imaging strategies discussed above for EPR determination have their own advantages and difficulties. However, the use of indirect imaging is promising for EPR measurement and patient pre-selection for therapy. The clinically approved and imageable companion diagnostic, ferumoxytol, has shown potential in patient pre-selection, evaluation of EPR effect, and improvement of EPR-based tumor targeting [20].

The typical xenograft mouse model uses inoculation of simple human cell lines and immuno-compromised mice. Nanodrug accumulation is lower in immuno-deficient mice compared to immuno-competent mice. These mouse models are highly homogeneous compared to the patient tumor with a typically low degree of heterogeneity. Tumors in mice usually have a relatively large size. However, compared to the size of the tumor in patients, they are usually relatively small. The murine tumors also lack the patient's TME and stromal factors due to their very different growth kinetics, usually days and weeks in mice, when contrasted with months and even years in patients. Metastasis is often ignored in xenograft models. With EPR-mediated drug delivery, tumor location plays a crucial role, with a tendency for higher accumulation in orthotopic tumors. Age differences between human and mouse may further affect the EPR, as mice at a very young age are usually selected for tumor inoculation and tumors grow rapidly However, human tumors, at old age, may grow slowly and progress only over several years [5,20].

Organoids and PDX models are very attractive for preclinical research because of the regrowth of human tumors. The tumor cells are harvested through biopsy or surgery. Upon growth in PDX model or organoids, most of the tumor stroma and TME features, and structure are retained. PDX models facilitate the study of several parameters, including TME and vascularization of the tumor and accumulation of drugs indicating the extent of EPR. However, there still exist limitations for translating PDX and organoids study benefits to clinic, since PDX models depend on immuno-compromised mice and organoids and PDX models require time and labor-intensive workflow with low engraftment rates.

8. The EPR Effect and Beyond: Enhancement of Therapeutic Efficacy of Cancer Nanomedicine

EPR-mediated drug systems have prodigious therapeutic potential. However, intra- and inter-tumoral, inter-patient heterogeneity in EPR effect, and physiological barriers associated with it pose a big challenge in drug delivery. Actively targeted drug delivery systems are greatly beneficial for the treatment of hematological malignancies. For solid tumors, active targeting must rely on EPR-mediated accumulation in tumors. To assess the EPR effect, the development of fast, quantitative EPR-imaging technologies is necessary. Several strategies have also been proposed that bypass the EPR effect, including cell-mediated delivery of nanoparticles and immune-modulating payload release in tumors. Such approaches should be useful for the treatment of low-EPR tumors, hematological malignancies, and metastatic cancers. Besides, local delivery of drugs using nanoparticles, hydrogels, implants, etc., can bypass physiological barriers of EPR-targeted delivery [5,20,21]. Moreover, the CAST therapy might be another approach to compensate for the inadequate effect of the EPR targeting [14]. Recently, mAb-based therapies for solid tumors has been proposed to overcome tumor heterogeneity, efficient delivery to tumor, durable therapeutic and clinical outcome in a large subset of patients, and enhanced prognosis [18]. Table 3 shows some selected EPR-based drug delivery systems [173].

Table 3. Selected EPR-based therapeutic systems.

Carrier	Ligand	Imaging/Therapeutic Agent	Applications
Nanoemulsion	PEGylated hydrophilic molecules (Killiphore ELP)	Iodinated monoglyceride and iodinated castor oil contrast agent	Blood pool imaging agents, accumulated particularly in liver and spleen and imaged by X-ray, CT.
Albumin nps	-	Tacrolimus (TAC)	TAC-loaded HAS nps, target inflamed joints of rheumatoid arthritis tissues
Polymeric nps	C18PMH-PEG	Fe_3O_4 contarst agents and doxorubicin drug	Magnetically controlled drug delivery and for T2-weighted MRI imaging
Lipid nanocapsules	Polysaccharide lipochitosan and liopdextran	DiD fluorescent dye	Selective to HEK293 (β3) cells bearing mice, detected by imaging

Development of more predictive animal models, including PDX and organoids, and EPR-imaging techniques and adoption of GLP, standardization guidelines, are necessary for translation of ERP-based therapies to the clinic. Development of PDX and organoid libraries to share information of the EPR patients, EPR tumors, and outcome of EPR-mediated drug delivery research will be helpful to predict appropriate therapy for the patients more rapidly and accurately. Scheme 1 shows the proposed workflow in the development of EPR-based drug delivery systems.

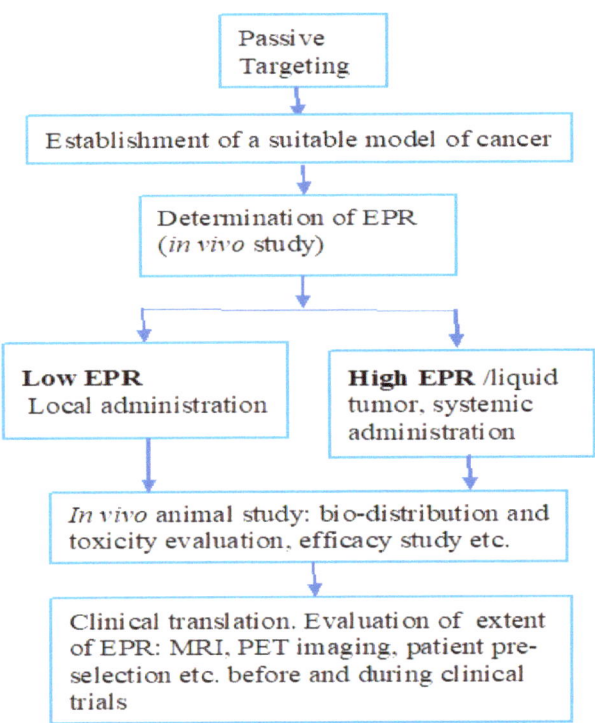

Scheme 1. Proposed workflow in the development of an EPR-based drug delivery system.

Active targeting can also be used as a complementary approach to EPR-mediated tumor targeting to enhance drug delivery, accumulation, and retention in tumors [174]. Finally, pharmacological and physical co-treatments, nanoparticle-based combination therapies, bio-inspired design of nanoparticles allowing tumor-selective drug release, advanced imaging techniques coupled with HTP computing technologies, and development of 3D-models of cells, better animal models, and organoids are necessary to improve the application and efficacy of EPR-targeted drug delivery for cancer therapy in both clinical and pre-clinical settings.

9. Conclusions and Future Perspective

EPR-targeted drug delivery was first discovered by Maeda and colleagues in solid murine tumors and reached the clinic about 30 years ago with the approval of the first EPR-based drug. Interpersonal and intra-, as well as inter-tumoral heterogeneity, is a major difficulty in EPR drug delivery studies. Since drug accumulation through EPR effect in the tumor may not be enough to obtain therapeutic effect, penetration, internalization, effective drug delivery, and cytoplasmic release are crucial for improvements with anticancer therapy. Actively targeted drug delivery systems have been highly useful for the treatment of hematological malignancies, whereas, for solid tumors, active targeting must rely on EPR-mediated accumulation in tumors. Quantification of the EPR-effect is thus necessary. To assess the EPR effect, the development of fast, quantitative EPR-imaging technologies is essential. Combination therapeutic approaches using nanoparticles, complementary use of passive and active targeting, and pharmaceutical as well physical co-treatments are crucial for enhancing EPR-based drug delivery systems. Humanized advanced animal models, 3D-models and organoids development, and patient pre-selection may improve EPR-based tumor targeting and clinical translation.

Author Contributions: Conceptualization, M.A.S.; manuscript preparation and revisions, M.A.S., S.S.K.Y.; N.F.; F.P. and V.P.T., coordination and supervision of the project V.P.T. All authors have read and agreed to the published version of the manuscript.

Funding: This research received no external funding.

Institutional Review Board Statement: Not applicable.

Informed Consent Statement: Not applicable.

Acknowledgments: The authors dedicated this article to Hiroshi Maeda. The authors thank William C. Hartner for helpful comments and preparation of the manuscript.

Conflicts of Interest: The authors declare that they have no known competing financial interests or personal relationships that could have appeared to influence the work reported in this paper.

References

1. Matsumura, Y.; Maeda, H. A new concept for macromolecular therapeutics in cancer chemotherapy: Mechanism of tumor-itropic accumulation of proteins and the antitumor agent smancs. *Cancer Res.* **1986**, *46*, 6387–6392.
2. Matsumura, Y.; Kimura, M.; Yamamoto, T.; Maeda, H. Involvement of the Kinin-generating Cascade in Enhanced Vascular Per-meability in Tumor Tissue. *Jpn. J. Cancer Res.* **1988**, *79*, 1327–1334. [CrossRef] [PubMed]
3. Wu, J.; Akaike, T.; Maeda, H. Modulation of enhanced vascular permeability in tumors by a bradykinin antagonist, a cyclooxygenase inhibitor, and a nitric oxide scavenger. *Cancer Res.* **1998**, *58*, 159–165. [PubMed]
4. Van Vlerken, L.E.; Duan, Z.; Seiden, M.V.; Amiji, M.M. Modulation of intracellular ceramide using polymeric nanoparticles to over come multidrug resistance in cancer. *Cancer Res.* **2007**, *67*, 4843–4850. [CrossRef] [PubMed]
5. Huynh, E.; Zheng, G. Cancer nanomedicine: Addressing the dark side of the enhanced permeability and retention effect. *Nanomedicine* **2015**, *10*, 1993–1995. [CrossRef]
6. Liechty, W.B.; Peppas, N.A. Expert opinion: Responsive polymer nanoparticles in cancer therapy. *Eur. J. Pharm. Biopharm.* **2012**, *80*, 241–246. [CrossRef]
7. Hillaireau, H.; Couvreur, P. Nanocarriers' entry into the cell: Relevance to drug delivery. *Cell. Mol. Life Sci.* **2009**, *66*, 2873–2896. [CrossRef]
8. Rejman, J.; Oberle, V.; Zuhorn, I.; Hoekstra, D. Size-dependent internalization of particles via the pathways of clathrin- and caveolae-mediated endocytosis. *Biochem. J.* **2004**, *377*, 159–169. [CrossRef] [PubMed]
9. Valkenburg, K.C.; De Groot, A.E.; Pienta, K.J. Targeting the tumour stroma to improve cancer therapy. *Nat. Rev. Clin. Oncol.* **2018**, *15*, 366–381. [CrossRef]
10. Matsumura, Y. Cancer stromal targeting (CAST) therapy. *Adv. Drug Deliv. Rev.* **2012**, *64*, 710–719. [CrossRef]
11. Matsumura, Y. Principle of CAST strategy. In *Cancer Drug Delivery Systems Based on the Tumor Microenvironment*; Matsumura, Y., Tarin, D., Eds.; Springer: Tokyo, Japan, 2020; pp. 255–268.
12. Yasunaga, M.; Manabe, S.; Tarin, D.; Matsumura, Y. Cancer-Stroma Targeting Therapy by Cytotoxic Immunoconjugate Bound to the Collagen 4 Network in the Tumor Tissue. *Bioconjug. Chem.* **2011**, *22*, 1776–1783. [CrossRef]
13. Yasunaga, M.; Manabe, S.; Matsumura, Y. New Concept of Cytotoxic Immunoconjugate Therapy Targeting Cancer-Induced Fibrin Clots. *Cancer Sci.* **2011**, *102*, 1396–1402. [CrossRef] [PubMed]
14. Matsumura, Y. Cancer stromal targeting therapy to overcome the pitfall of EPR effect. *Adv. Drug Deliv. Rev.* **2020**, *154–155*, 142–150. [CrossRef] [PubMed]
15. Gebleux, R.; Stringhini, M.; Casanova, R.; Soltermann, A.; Neri, D. Non-internalizing antibody-drug conjugates display potent anticancer activity upon proteolytic release of mono Methyl auristatin E in the sub-endothelial extracellular matrix. *Int. J. Cancer* **2018**, *140*, 1670–1679. [CrossRef] [PubMed]
16. Szot, C.; Saha, S.; Zhang, X.M.; Zhu, Z.; Hilton, M.B.; Morris, K.; Seaman, S.; Dunleavey, J.M.; Hsu, K.-S.; Yu, G.-J.; et al. Tumor strom-targeting antibody-drug conjugate triggers local-ized anticancer drug release. *J. Clin. Investig.* **2018**, *128*, 2927–2943. [CrossRef] [PubMed]
17. Drago, J.Z.; Modi, S.; Chandarlapaty, S. Unlocking the potential of antibody-drug conjugates for cancer therapy. *Nat. Rev. Clin. Oncol.* **2021**, *18*, 327–344. [CrossRef]
18. Shah, A.; Rauth, S.; Aithal, A.; Kaur, K.; Ganguly, K.; Orzechowski, C.; Varshney, G.C.; Jain, M.; Batra, S.K. The current landscape of antibody-based therapies in solid malignancies. *Theranostics* **2021**, *11*, 1493–1512. [CrossRef]
19. Wakaskar, R.R. Passive and Active Targeting in Tumor Microenvironment. *Int. J. Drug Dev. Res.* **2017**, *9*, 37–41.
20. Susanne, K.G.; Jan-Niklas MBenjamin, T. Tumor targeting vis EPR: Strategies to enhance patient responses. *Adv. Drug Deliv. Rev.* **2018**, *130*, 17–38.
21. Daniel, R.; Nitin, J.; Wei, T.; Jeffrey, M.K.; Dan, P. Progress and challenges towards targeted delivery of cancer therapeutics. *Nat. Commun.* **2018**, *9*, 1410.
22. Torchilin, V.P. Passive and active drug targeting: Drug delivery to tumors as an example. In *Drug Delivery, Handbook of Experimental Pharmacology*; Schafer-Korting, M., Ed.; Springer: Berlin/Heidelberg, Germany, 2010; Volume 197, pp. 4–36.

23. He, B.; Sui, X.; Yu, B.; Wang, S.; Shen, Y.; Cong, H. Recent advances in drug delivery systems for enhancing drug penetration into tumors. *Drug Deliv.* **2020**, *27*, 1474–1490. [CrossRef]
24. Bates, D.O.; Hillman, N.J.; Williams, B.; Neal, C.R.; Pocock, T.M. Regulation of microvascular permeability by vascular endothelial growth factors. *J. Anat.* **2002**, *200*, 581–597. [CrossRef]
25. Jain, R.K. The next frontier of molecular medicine: Delivery of therapeutics. *Nat. Med.* **1998**, *4*, 655–657. [CrossRef]
26. Jain, R.K.; Stylianopoulos, T. Delivering nanomedicine to solid tumors. *Nat. Rev. Clin. Oncol.* **2010**, *7*, 653–664. [CrossRef]
27. Hobbs, S.K.; Monsky, W.L.; Yuan, F.; Roberts, W.G.; Griffith, L.; Torchilin, V.P.; Jain, R.K. Regulation of transport pathways in tumor vessels: Role of tumor type and microenvironment. *Proc. Natl. Acad. Sci. USA* **1998**, *95*, 4607–4612. [CrossRef]
28. Padera, T.P.; Stoll, B.R.; Tooredman, J.B.; Capen, D.; di Tomaso, E.; Jain, R.K. Pathology: Cancer cells compress intratumour vessels. *Nature* **2004**, *427*, 695. [CrossRef] [PubMed]
29. Jain, R.K. Transport of molecules across tumor vasculature. *Cancer Metastasis Rev.* **1987**, *6*, 559–593. [CrossRef]
30. Swartz, M.A. The physiology of the lymphatic system. *Adv. Drug Deliv. Rev.* **2001**, *50*, 3–20. [CrossRef]
31. Noguchi, Y.; Wu, J.; Duncan, R.; Strohalm, J.; Ulbrich, K.; Akaike, T.; Maeda, H. Early Phase Tumor Accumulation of Macromolecules: A Great Difference in Clearance Rate between Tumor and Normal Tissues. *Jpn. J. Cancer Res.* **1998**, *89*, 307–314. [CrossRef] [PubMed]
32. Bertrand, N.; Wu, J.; Xu, X.; Kamaly, N.; Farokhzad, O.C. Cancer nanotechnology: The impact of passive and active targeting in the era of modern cancer biology. *Adv. Drug Deliv. Rev.* **2014**, *66*, 2–25. [CrossRef]
33. Stylianopoulos, T.; Soteriou, K.; Fukumura, D.; Jain, R.K. Cationic nanoparticles have superior transvascular flux into solid tumors: Insights from a mathe-matical model. *Ann. Biomed. Eng.* **2013**, *41*, 68–77. [CrossRef] [PubMed]
34. Dellian, M.; Yuan, F.; Trubetskoy, V.S.; Torchilin, V.P.; Jain, R.K. Vascular permeability in a human tumour xenograft: Molecular charge dependence. *Br. J. Cancer* **2000**, *82*, 1513–1518. [PubMed]
35. Schmitt-Sody, M.; Strieth, S.; Krasnici, S.; Sauer, B.; Schulze, B.; Teifel, M.; Michaelis, U.; Naujoks, K.; Dellian, M. Neovascular targeting therapy: Paclitaxel encapsulated in cationic liposomes improves antitumoral efficacy. *Clin. Cancer Res.* **2003**, *9*, 2335–2341. [PubMed]
36. Krasnici, S.; Werner, A.; Eichhorn, M.E.; Schmitt-Sody, M.; Pahernik, S.A.; Sauer, B.; Schulze, B.; Teifel, M.; Michaelis, U.; Naujoks, K.; et al. Effect of the surface charge of liposomes on their uptake by angiogenic tumor vessels. *Int. J. Cancer* **2003**, *105*, 561–567. [CrossRef]
37. Zamboni, W.C.; Eiseman, J.L.; Strychor, S.; Rice, P.M.; Joseph, E.; Zamboni, B.A.; Donnelly, M.K.; Shurer, J.; Parise, R.A.; Tonda, M.E.; et al. Tumor disposition of pegylated liposomal CKD-602 and the reticuloendothelial system in preclinical tumor models. *J. Liposome Res.* **2010**, *21*, 70–80. [CrossRef]
38. Carmeliet, P.; Jain, R.K. Principles and mechanisms of vessel normalization for cancer and other angiogenic diseases. *Nat. Rev. Drug Discov.* **2011**, *10*, 417–427. [CrossRef]
39. Hashizume, H.; Baluk, P.; Morikawa, S.; McLean, J.W.; Thurston, G.; Roberge, S.; Jain, R.K.; McDonald, D.M. Openings between Defective Endothelial Cells Explain Tumor Vessel Leakiness. *Am. J. Pathol.* **2000**, *156*, 1363–1380. [CrossRef]
40. Swartz, M.A.; Fleury, M. Interstitial Flow and Its Effects in Soft Tissues. *Annu. Rev. Biomed. Eng.* **2007**, *9*, 229–256. [CrossRef] [PubMed]
41. Netti, P.; Hamberg, L.M.; Babich, J.W.; Kierstead, D.; Graham, W.; Hunter, G.J.; Wolf, G.L.; Fischman, A.; Boucher, Y.; Jain, R.K. Enhancement of fluid filtration across tumor vessels: Implication for delivery of macromolecules. *Proc. Natl. Acad. Sci. USA* **1999**, *96*, 3137–3142. [CrossRef] [PubMed]
42. Lieleg, O.; Baumgärtel, R.M.; Bausch, A.R. Selective filtering of particles by the extracellular matrix: An electrostatic bandpass. *Biophys. J.* **2009**, *97*, 1569–1577. [CrossRef]
43. Alexandrakis, G.; Brown, E.B.; Tong, R.T.; McKee, T.D.; Campbell, R.B.; Boucher, Y.; Jain, R.K. Two-photon fluorescence correlation microscopy reveals the two-phase nature of transport in tumors. *Nat. Med.* **2004**, *10*, 203–207. [CrossRef]
44. Netti, P.A.; Berk, D.A.; Swartz, M.A.; Grodzinsky, A.J.; Jain, R.K. Role of extracellular matrix assembly in interstitial transport in solid tumors. *Cancer Res.* **2000**, *60*, 2497–2503.
45. McKee, T.; Grandi, P.; Mok, W.; Alexandrakis, G.; Insin, N.; Zimmer, J.P.; Bawendi, M.G.; Boucher, Y.; Breakefield, X.O.; Jain, R.K. Degradation of Fibrillar Collagen in a Human Melanoma Xenograft Improves the Efficacy of an Oncolytic Herpes Simplex Virus Vector. *Cancer Res.* **2006**, *66*, 2509–2513. [CrossRef] [PubMed]
46. Prabhakar, U.; Maeda, H.; Jain, R.K.; Sevick-Muraca, E.M.; Zamboni, W.; Farokhzad, O.C.; Barry, S.T.; Gabizon, A.; Grodzinski, P.; Blakey, D.C. Challenges and Key Considerations of the Enhanced Permeability and Retention Effect for Nanomedicine Drug Delivery in Oncology. *Cancer Res.* **2013**, *73*, 2412–2417. [CrossRef] [PubMed]
47. Caron, W.P.; Song, G.; Kumar, P.; Rawal, S.; Zamboni, W.C. Interpatient Pharmacokinetic and Pharmacodynamic Variability of Carrier-Mediated Anticancer Agents. *Clin. Pharmacol. Ther.* **2012**, *91*, 802–812. [CrossRef] [PubMed]
48. Zamboni, W.C.; Maruca, L.J.; Strychor, S.; Zamboni, B.A.; Ramalingam, S.; Edwards, R.P.; Kim, J.; Bang, Y.; Lee, H.; Friedland, D.M.; et al. Bidirectional pharmacodynamic interaction between pegylated liposomal CKD-602 (S-CKD602) and monocytes in patients with refractory solid tumors. *J. Liposome Res.* **2010**, *21*, 158–165. [CrossRef] [PubMed]
49. Sano, K.; Nakajima, T.; Choyke, P.L.; Kobayashi, H. Markedly Enhanced Permeability and Retention Effects Induced by Photo-immunotherapy of Tumors. *ACS Nano* **2012**, *7*, 717–724. [CrossRef]

50. Diop-Frimpong, B.; Chauhan, V.P.; Krane, S.; Boucher, Y.; Jain, R.K. Losartan inhibits collagen I synthesis and improves the distribution and efficacy of nanotherapeu-tics in tumors. *Proc. Natl. Acad. Sci. USA* **2011**, *108*, 2909–2914. [CrossRef]
51. Noguchi, A.; Takahashi, T.; Yamaguchi, T.; Kitamura, K.; Noguchi, A.; Tsurumi, H.; Takashina, K.; Maeda, H. Enhanced tumor localization of monoclonal antibody by treatment with kininase II inhibitor and angio-tensin II. *Jpn. J. Cancer Res.* **1992**, *83*, 240–243. [CrossRef]
52. Maeda, H. Nitroglycerin enhances vascular blood flow and drug delivery in hypoxic tumor tissues: Analogy between angina pectoris and solid tumors and enhancement of the EPR effect. *J. Control. Release* **2010**, *142*, 296–298. [CrossRef]
53. Maeda, H. Macromolecular therapeutics in cancer treatment: The EPR effect and beyond. *J. Control. Release* **2012**, *164*, 138–144. [CrossRef] [PubMed]
54. Fang, J.; Qin, H.; Nakamura, H.; Tsukigawa, K.; Shin, T.; Maeda, H. Carbon monoxide, generated by heme oxygenase-1, mediates the enhanced permeability and retention effect in solid tumors. *Cancer Sci.* **2012**, *103*, 535–541. [CrossRef] [PubMed]
55. Islam, W.; Fang, J.; Imamura, T.; Etrych, T.; Subr, V.; Ulbrich, K.; Maeda, H. Augmentation of the Enhanced Permeabil-ity and Retention Effect with Nitric Oxide–Generating Agents Improves the Therapeutic Effects of Nanomedicines. *Mol. Cancer Ther.* **2018**, *17*, 2643–2653. [CrossRef] [PubMed]
56. Fang, J.; Islam, R.; Islam, W.; Yin, H.; Subr, V.; Etrych, T.; Ulbrich, K.; Maeda, H. Augmentation of EPR Effect and Efficacy of Anticancer Nanomedicine by Carbon Monoxide Generating Agents. *Pharmaceutics* **2019**, *11*, 343. [CrossRef] [PubMed]
57. Alexis, F.; Pridgen, E.; Molnar, L.K.; Farokhzad, O.C. Factors Affecting the Clearance and Biodistribution of Polymeric Nanoparti-cles. *Mol. Pharm.* **2008**, *5*, 505–515. [CrossRef] [PubMed]
58. Bertrand, N.; Leroux, J.-C. The journey of a drug-carrier in the body: An anatomo-physiological perspective. *J. Control. Release* **2012**, *161*, 152–163. [CrossRef]
59. Dreher, M.R.; Liu, W.; Michelich, C.R.; Dewhirst, M.W.; Yuan, F.; Chilkoti, A. Tumor Vascular Permeability, Accumulation, and Penetration of Macromolecular Drug Carriers. *J. Natl. Cancer Inst.* **2006**, *98*, 335–344. [CrossRef]
60. Cabral, H.; Matsumoto, Y.; Mizuno, K.; Chen, Q.; Murakami, M.; Kimura, M.; Terada, Y.; Kano, M.R.; Miyazono, K.; Uesaka, M.; et al. Accumulation of sub-100 nm polymeric micelles in poorly permeable tumours depends on size. *Nat. Nanotechnol.* **2011**, *6*, 815–823. [CrossRef]
61. Salvador-Morales, C.; Zhang, L.; Langer, R.; Farokhzad, O.C. Immunocompatibility properties of lipid-polymer hybrid nanoparti-cles with heterogeneous sur-face functional groups. *Biomaterials* **2009**, *30*, 2231–2240. [CrossRef]
62. Meng, H.; Xue, M.; Xia, T.; Ji, Z.; Tarn, D.Y.; Zink, J.I.; Nel, A.E. Use of Size and a Copolymer Design Feature to Improve the Biodistribution and the Enhanced Permeability and Retention Effect of Doxorubicin-Loaded Mesoporous Silica Nanoparticles in a Murine Xenograft Tumor Model. *ACS Nano* **2011**, *5*, 4131–4144. [CrossRef]
63. Ruggiero, A.; Villa, C.H.; Bander, E.; Rey, D.A.; Bergkvist, M.; Batt, C.A.; Manova-Todorova, K.; Deen, W.M.; Scheinberg, D.A.; McDevitt, M.R. Paradoxical glomerular filtration of carbon nanotubes. *Proc. Natl. Acad. Sci. USA* **2010**, *107*, 12369–12374. [CrossRef]
64. Chauhan, V.; Popović, Z.; Chen, O.; Cui, J.; Fukumura, D.; Bawendi, M.G.; Jain, R.K. Fluorescent Nanorods and Nanospheres for Real-Time In Vivo Probing of Nanoparticle Shape-Dependent Tumor Penetration. *Angew. Chem. Int. Ed.* **2011**, *50*, 11417–11420. [CrossRef]
65. Maeda, H. Toward a full understanding of the EPR effect in primary and metastatic tumors as well as issues related to its heterogeneity. *Adv. Drug Deliv. Rev.* **2015**, *91*, 3–6. [CrossRef]
66. Danhier, F. To exploit the tumor microenvironment: Since the EPR effect fails in the clinic, what is the future of nanomedicine? *J. Control. Release* **2016**, *244*, 108–121. [CrossRef] [PubMed]
67. Nichols, J.W.; Bae, Y.H. EPR: Evidence and fallacy. *J. Control. Release* **2014**, *190*, 451–464. [CrossRef] [PubMed]
68. Lammers, T.; Kiessling, F.; Hennink, W.E.; Storm, G. Drug targeting to tumors: Principles, pitfalls and (pre-) clinical progress. *J. Control. Release* **2012**, *161*, 175–187. [CrossRef] [PubMed]
69. Natfji, A.A.; Ravishankar, D.; Osborn, H.; Greco, F. Parameters Affecting the Enhanced Permeability and Retention Effect: The Need for Patient Selection. *J. Pharm. Sci.* **2017**, *106*, 3179–3187. [CrossRef]
70. Maeda, H.; Khatami, M. Analyses of repeated failures in cancer therapy for solid tumors: Poor tumor-selective drug delivery, low therapeutic efficacy and unsustainable costs. *Clin. Transl. Med.* **2018**, *7*, 11. [CrossRef] [PubMed]
71. Michiels, C.; Tellier, C.; Feron, O. Cycling hypoxia: A key feature of the tumor microenvironment. *Biochim. Biophys. Acta (BBA) Bioenergy* **2016**, *1866*, 76–86. [CrossRef]
72. Xing, F.; Okuda, H.; Watabe, M.; Kobayashi, A.; Pai, S.K.; Liu, W.; Pandey, P.R.; Fukuda, K.; Hirota, S.; Sugai, T. Hypox-ia-induced Jagged2 promotes breast cancer metastasis and self-renewal of cancer stem-like cells. *Oncogene* **2011**, *30*, 4075–4086. [CrossRef]
73. Lee, K.W.; Castilho, A.; Cheung, V.C.H.; Tang, K.H.; Ma, S.; Ng, I.O.-L. CD24+ Liver Tumor-Initiating Cells Drive Self-Renewal and Tumor Initiation through STAT3-Mediated NANOG Regulation. *Cell Stem Cell* **2011**, *9*, 50–63. [CrossRef]
74. Thomas, S.; Harding, M.A.; Smith, S.C.; Overdevest, J.B.; Nitz, M.D.; Frierson, H.F.; Tomlins, S.A.; Kristiansen, G.; Theodorescu, D. CD24 Is an Effector of HIF-1–Driven Primary Tumor Growth and Metastasis. *Cancer Res.* **2012**, *72*, 5600–5612. [CrossRef]
75. Hannigan, G.E.; Troussard, A.A.; Dedhar, S. Integrin-linked kinase: A cancer therapeutic target unique among its ILK. *Nat. Rev. Cancer* **2005**, *5*, 51–63. [CrossRef]
76. Pang, M.-F.; Siedlik, M.J.; Han, S.; Stallings-Mann, M.; Radisky, D.C.; Nelson, C.M. Tissue Stiffness and Hypoxia Modulate the Integrin-Linked Kinase ILK to Control Breast Cancer Stem-like Cells. *Cancer Res.* **2016**, *76*, 5277–5287. [CrossRef] [PubMed]

77. Chiou, S.-H.; Risca, V.I.; Wang, G.; Yang, D.; Grüner, B.M.; Kathiria, A.S.; Margaret, K.; Vaka, D.; Chu, P.; Kozak, M.; et al. BLIMP1 Induces Transient Metastatic Heterogeneity in Pancreatic Cancer. *Cancer Discov.* **2017**, *7*, 1184–1199. [CrossRef] [PubMed]
78. Shi, J.; Kantoff, P.W.; Wooster, R.; Farokhzad, J.S.O.C. Cancer nanomedicine: Progress, challenges and opportunities. *Nat. Rev. Cancer* **2017**, *17*, 20–37. [CrossRef]
79. Barenholz, Y.C. Doxil®—The first FDA-approved nano-drug: Lessons learned. *J. Control. Release* **2012**, *160*, 117–134. [CrossRef] [PubMed]
80. Matsumoto, Y.; Nichols, J.W.; Toh, K.; Nomoto, T.; Cabral, H.; Miura, Y.; Christie, R.J.; Yamada, N.; Ogura, T.; Kano, M.R.; et al. Vascular bursts enhance permeability of tumour blood vessels and improve nanoparticle delivery. *Nat. Nanotechnol.* **2016**, *11*, 533–538. [CrossRef]
81. Casazza, A.; Di Conza, G.; Wenes, M.; Finisguerra, V.; Deschoemaeker, S.; Mazzone, M. Tumor stroma: A complexity dictat-ed by the hypoxic tumor microenvironment. *Oncogene* **2014**, *33*, 1743–1754. [CrossRef]
82. Miao, L.; Huang, L. Exploring the Tumor Microenvironment with Nanoparticles. *Cancer Treat. Res.* **2015**, *166*, 193–226. [CrossRef]
83. Zhou, W.; Chen, C.; Shi, Y.; Wu, Q.; Gimple, R.C.; Fang, X.; Huang, Z.; Zhai, K.; Ke, S.Q.; Ping, Y.-F.; et al. Targeting Glioma Stem Cell-Derived Pericytes Disrupts the Blood-Tumor Barrier and Improves Chemotherapeutic Efficacy. *Cell Stem Cell* **2017**, *21*, 591–603.e4. [CrossRef]
84. Cooke, V.G.; LeBleu, V.S.; Keskin, D.; Khan, Z.; O'Connell, J.T.; Teng, Y.; Duncan, M.B.; Xie, L.; Maeda, G.; Vong, S. Pericyte depletion results in hypoxia-associated epithelial-to-mesenchymal transition and metastasis mediated by met signaling path-way. *Cancer Cell* **2012**, *21*, 66–81. [CrossRef]
85. Lee, S.; Han, H.; Koo, H.; Na, J.H.; Yoon, H.Y.; Lee, K.E.; Lee, H.; Kim, H.; Kwon, I.C.; Kim, K. Extracellular matrix remod-eling in vivo for enhancing tumor-targeting efficiency of nanoparticle drug carriers using the pulsed high intensity focused ultrasound. *J. Control. Release* **2017**, *263*, 68–78. [CrossRef]
86. Nassiri, M.; Babina, M.; Dölle, S.; Edenharter, G.; Ruëff, F.; Worm, M. Ramipril and metoprolol intake aggravate human and murine anaphylaxis: Evidence for direct mast cell priming. *J. Allergy Clin. Immunol.* **2015**, *135*, 491–499. [CrossRef] [PubMed]
87. Fang, J.; Liao, L.; Yin, H.; Nakamura, H.; Shin, T.; Maeda, H. Enhanced bacterial tumor delivery by modulating the EPR ef-fect and therapeutic potential of Lactobacillus casei. *J. Pharm. Sci.* **2014**, *103*, 3235–3243. [CrossRef] [PubMed]
88. Studenovsky, M.; Sivak, L.; Sedlacek, O.; Konefal, R.; Horkova, V.; Etrych, T.; Kovar, M.; Rihova, B.; Sirova, M. Polymer ni-tric oxide donors potentiate the treatment of experimental solid tumours by increasing drug accumulation in the tumour tissue. *J. Control. Release* **2018**, *269*, 214–224. [CrossRef] [PubMed]
89. Li, F.; Wang, Y.; Chen, W.-L.; Wang, D.-D.; Zhou, Y.-J.; You, B.-G.; Liu, Y.; Qu, C.-X.; Yang, S.-D.; Chen, M.-T.; et al. Co-delivery of VEGF siRNA and Etoposide for Enhanced Anti-angiogenesis and Anti-proliferation Effect via Multi-functional Nanoparticles for Orthotopic Non-Small Cell Lung Cancer Treatment. *Theranostics* **2019**, *9*, 5886–5898. [CrossRef] [PubMed]
90. Hori, Y.; Ito, K.; Hamamichi, S.; Ozawa, Y.; Matsui, J.; Umeda, I.O.; Fujii, H. Functional Characterization of VEGF- and FGF-induced Tumor Blood Vessel Models in Human Cancer Xenografts. *Anticancer Res.* **2017**, *37*, 6629–6638. [CrossRef]
91. Yao, Y.; Wang, T.; Liu, Y.; Zhang, N. Co-delivery of sorafenib and VEGF-siRNA via pH-sensitive liposomes for the synergistic treatment of hepatocellular carcinoma. *Artif. Cells Nanomed. Biotechnol.* **2019**, *47*, 1374–1383. [CrossRef] [PubMed]
92. Theek, B.; Baues, M.; Gremse, F.; Pola, R.; Pechar, M.; Negwer, I.; Koynov, K.; Weber, B.; Barz, M.; Jahnen-Dechent, W. His-tidine-rich glycoprotein-induced vascular normalization improves EPR-mediated drug targeting to and into tumors. *J. Control. Release* **2018**, *282*, 25–34. [CrossRef]
93. Wu, Q.; Yuan, X.; Bai, J.; Han, R.; Li, Z.; Zhang, H.; Xiu, R. MicroRNA-181a protects against pericyte apoptosis via directly targeting FOXO1: Implication for ameliorated cognitive deficits in APP/PS1 mice. *Aging* **2019**, *11*, 6120–6133. [CrossRef] [PubMed]
94. Ergen, C.; Niemietz, P.M.; Heymann, F.; Baues, M.; Gremse, F.; Pola, R.; van Bloois, L.; Storm, G.; Kiessling, F.; Trautwein, C.; et al. Liver fibrosis affects the targeting properties of drug delivery systems to macrophage subsets in vivo. *Biomaterials* **2019**, *206*, 49–60. [CrossRef] [PubMed]
95. Jung, J. Human Tumor Xenograft Models for Preclinical Assessment of Anticancer Drug Development. *Toxicol. Res.* **2014**, *30*, 1–5. [CrossRef]
96. Lai, Y.; Wei, X.; Lin, S.; Qin, L.; Cheng, L.; Li, P. Current status and perspectives of patient-derived xenograft models in cancer research. *J. Hematol. Oncol.* **2017**, *10*, 106. [CrossRef] [PubMed]
97. Izumchenko, E.; Paz, K.; Ciznadija, D.; Sloma, I.; Katz, A.; Vasquez-Dunddel, D.; Ben-Zvi, I.; Stebbing, J.; McGuire, W.; Harris, W.; et al. Patient-derived xenografts effectively capture responses to oncology therapy in a heterogeneous cohort of patients with solid tumors. *Ann. Oncol.* **2017**, *28*, 2595–2605. [CrossRef]
98. Hu, J.; Ishihara, M.; Chin, A.I.; Wu, L. Establishment of xenografts of urological cancers on chicken chorioallantoic mem-brane (CAM) to study metastasis. *Precis. Clin. Med.* **2019**, *2*, 140–151. [CrossRef] [PubMed]
99. Mercatali, L.; La Manna, F.; Groenewoud, A.; Casadei, R.; Recine, F.; Miserocchi, G.; Pieri, F.; Liverani, C.; Bongiovanni, A.; Spadazzi, C.; et al. Development of a Patient-Derived Xenograft (PDX) of Breast Cancer Bone Metastasis in a Zebrafish Model. *Int. J. Mol. Sci.* **2016**, *17*, 1375. [CrossRef]
100. Randall, E.C.; Emdal, K.B.; Laramy, J.K.; Kim, M.; Roos, A.; Calligaris, D.; Regan, M.S.; Gupta, S.K.; Mladek, A.C.; Carlson, B.L.; et al. Integrated mapping of pharmacokinetics and pharmacodynamics in a patient-derived xenograft model of glioblastoma. *Nat. Commun.* **2018**, *9*, 4904. [CrossRef]

101. Pawlikowska, P.; Tayoun, T.; Oulhen, M.; Faugeroux, V.; Rouffiac, V.; Aberlenc, A.; Pommier, A.L.; Honore, A.; Marty, V.; Bawa, O.; et al. Exploitation of the chick embryo chorioallantoic membrane (CAM) as a platform for anti-metastatic drug testing. *Sci. Rep.* **2020**, *10*, 16876. [CrossRef] [PubMed]
102. Wu, J.-Q.; Fan, R.-Y.; Zhang, S.-R.; Li, C.-Y.; Shen, L.-Z.; Wei, P.; He, Z.-H.; He, M.-F. A systematical comparison of anti-angiogenesis and anti-cancer efficacy of ramucirumab, apatinib, regorafenib and cabozantinib in zebrafish model. *Life Sci.* **2020**, *247*, 117402. [CrossRef]
103. Wang, H.; Lu, J.; Tang, J.; Chen, S.; He, K.; Jiang, X.; Jiang, W.; Teng, L. Establishment of patient-derived gastric cancer xen-ografts: A useful tool for preclinical evaluation of targeted therapies involving alterations in HER-2, MET and FGFR2 signal-ing pathways. *BMC Cancer* **2017**, *17*, 191. [CrossRef] [PubMed]
104. Jo, E.B.; Hong, D.; Lee, Y.S.; Lee, H.; Park, J.B.; Kim, S.J. Establishment of a Novel PDX Mouse Model and Evaluation of the Tumor Suppression Efficacy of Bortezomib Against Liposarcoma. *Transl. Oncol.* **2019**, *12*, 269–281. [CrossRef]
105. Choi, B.; Lee, J.S.; Kim, S.J.; Hong, D.; Park, J.B.; Lee, K.-Y. Anti-tumor effects of anti-PD-1 antibody, pembrolizumab, in hu-manized NSG PDX mice xenografted with dedifferentiated liposarcoma. *Cancer Lett.* **2020**, *478*, 56–69. [CrossRef]
106. Palanisamy, N.; Yang, J.; Shepherd, P.D.A.; Li-Ning-Tapia, E.M.; Labanca, E.; Manyam, G.C.; Ravoori, M.K.; Kundra, V.; Araujo, J.C.; Efstathiou, E.; et al. The MD Anderson Prostate Cancer Patient-derived Xenograft Series (MDA PCa PDX) Captures the Molecular Landscape of Prostate Cancer and Facilitates Marker-driven Therapy Development. *Clin. Cancer Res.* **2020**, *26*, 4933–4946. [CrossRef]
107. Cao, M.; Long, M.; Chen, Q.; Lu, Y.; Luo, Q.; Zhao, Y.; Lu, A.; Ge, C.; Zhu, L.; Chen, Z. Development of β-elemene and cis-platin co-loaded liposomes for effective lung cancer therapy and evaluation in patient-derived tumor xenografts. *Pharm. Res.* **2019**, *36*, 121. [CrossRef]
108. Choi, H.S.; Frangioni, J.V. Nanoparticles for Biomedical Imaging: Fundamentals of Clinical Translation. *Mol. Imaging* **2010**, *9*, 291–310. [CrossRef] [PubMed]
109. Duan, L.; Yang, L.; Jin, J.; Yang, F.; Liu, D.; Hu, K.; Wang, Q.; Yue, Y.; Gu, N. Micro/nano-bubble-assisted ultrasound to enhance the EPR effect and potential theranostic applications. *Theranostics* **2020**, *10*, 462–483. [CrossRef]
110. Maeda, H.; Tsukigawa, K.; Fang, J. A Retrospective 30 Years after Discovery of the Enhanced Permeability and Reten-tion Effect of Solid Tumors: Next-Generation Chemotherapeutics and Photodynamic Therapy—Problems, Solutions, and Pro-spects. *Microcirculation* **2016**, *23*, 173–182. [CrossRef]
111. Nakamura, H.; Jun, F.; Maeda, H. Development of next-generation macromolecular drugs based on the EPR effect: Challenges and pitfalls. *Expert Opin. Drug Deliv.* **2014**, *12*, 53–64. [CrossRef] [PubMed]
112. Maeda, H. SMANCS and polymer-conjugated macromolecular drugs: Advantages in cancer chemotherapy. *Adv. Drug Deliv. Rev.* **2001**, *46*, 169–185. [CrossRef]
113. Maeda, H.; Sawa, T.; Konno, T. Mechanism of tumor-targeted delivery of macromolecular drugs, including the EPR effect in solid tumor and clinical overview of the prototype polymeric drug SMANCS. *J. Control. Release* **2001**, *74*, 47–61. [CrossRef]
114. Fang, J.; Sawa, T.; Maeda, H. Factors and mechanism of "EPR" effect and the enhanced antitumor effects of macromolec-ular drugs including SMANCS. *Adv. Exp. Med. Biol.* **2003**, *519*, 29–49. [PubMed]
115. Peterson, C.M.; Shiah, J.-G.; Sun, Y.; Kopečková, P.; Minko, T.; Straight, R.C.; Kopeček, J. HPMA Copolymer Delivery of Chemotherapy and Photodynamic Therapy in Ovarian Cancer. *Chem. Biol. Pteridines Folates* **2005**, *519*, 101–123. [CrossRef]
116. Kopeček, J. HPMA copolymer–anticancer drug conjugates: Design, activity, and mechanism of action. *Eur. J. Pharm. Biopharm.* **2000**, *50*, 61–81. [CrossRef]
117. Ulbrich, K.; Hola, K.; Šubr, V.; Bakandritsos, A.; Tuček, J.; Zbořil, R. Targeted Drug Delivery with Polymers and Magnetic Nanoparticles: Covalent and Noncovalent Approaches, Release Control, and Clinical Studies. *Chem. Rev.* **2016**, *116*, 5338–5431. [CrossRef]
118. Chytil, P.; Kostka, L.; Etrych, T. HPMA Copolymer-Based Nanomedicines in Controlled Drug Delivery. *J. Pers. Med.* **2021**, *11*, 115. [CrossRef]
119. Nakamura, H.; Liao, L.; Hitaka, Y.; Tsukigawa, K.; Subr, V.; Fang, J.; Ulbrich, K.; Maeda, H. Micelles of zinc protoporphyrin conjugated to N-(2-hydroxypropyl)methacrylamide (HPMA) copolymer for imaging and light-induced antitumor effects in vivo. *J. Control. Release* **2013**, *165*, 191–198. [CrossRef]
120. Tan, L.; Wan, J.; Guo, W.; Ou, C.; Liu, T.; Fu, C.; Zhang, Q.; Ren, X.; Liang, X.-J.; Ren, J.; et al. Renal-clearable quaternary chalcogenide nanocrystal for photoacoustic/magnetic resonance imaging guided tumor photothermal therapy. *Biomaterials* **2018**, *159*, 108–118. [CrossRef] [PubMed]
121. Akbarzadeh, A.; Rezaei-Sadabady, R.; Davaran, S.; Joo, S.W.; Zarghami, N.; Hanifehpour, Y.; Samiei, M.; Kouhi, M.; Nejati-Koshki, K. Liposome: Classification, preparation, and applications. *Nanoscale Res. Lett.* **2013**, *8*, 102. [CrossRef]
122. Li, J.; Wang, X.; Zhang, T.; Wang, C.; Huang, Z.; Luo, X.; Deng, Y. A review on phospholipids and their main applications in drug delivery systems. *Asian J. Pharm. Sci.* **2015**, *10*, 81–98. [CrossRef]
123. Bulbake, U.; Doppalapudi, S.; Kommineni, N.; Khan, W. Liposomal Formulations in Clinical Use: An Updated Review. *Pharmaceutics* **2017**, *9*, 12. [CrossRef]
124. Oerlemans, C.; Bult, W.; Bos, M.; Storm, G.; Nijsen, J.F.W.; Hennink, W.E. Polymeric Micelles in Anticancer Therapy: Targeting, Imaging and Triggered Release. *Pharm. Res.* **2010**, *27*, 2569–2589. [CrossRef] [PubMed]

125. Davis, M.E.; Chen, Z.G.; Shin, D.M. Nanoparticle therapeutics: An emerging treatment modality for cancer. *Nat. Rev. Drug Discov.* **2008**, *7*, 771–782. [CrossRef] [PubMed]
126. Wang, Y.; Wang, Z.; Xu, C.; Tian, H.; Chen, X. A disassembling strategy overcomes the EPR effect and renal clearance dilemma of the multifunctional theranostic nanoparticles for cancer therapy. *Biomaterials* **2019**, *197*, 284–293. [CrossRef] [PubMed]
127. Löhr, J.M.; Haas, S.L.; Bechstein, W.; Bodoky, G.; Cwiertka, K.; Fischbach, W.; Fölsch, U.R.; Jäger, D.; Osinsky, D.; Prausova, J.; et al. Cationic liposomal paclitaxel plus gemcitabine or gemcitabine alone in patients with advanced pancreatic cancer: A randomized controlled phase II trial. *Ann. Oncol.* **2012**, *23*, 1214–1222. [CrossRef] [PubMed]
128. Wagner, E.; Ogris, M.; Günther, M. Specific Targets in Tumor Tissue for the Delivery of Therapeutic Genes. *Curr. Med. Chem. Agents* **2005**, *5*, 157–171. [CrossRef]
129. Wang, J.; Meng, F.; Kim, B.-K.; Ke, X.; Yeo, Y. In-vitro and in-vivo difference in gene delivery by lithocholic acid-polyethyleneimine conjugate. *Biomaterials* **2019**, *217*, 119296. [CrossRef]
130. Pan, J.; Mendes, L.P.; Yao, M.; Filipczak, N.; Garai, S.; Thakur, G.A.; Sarisozen, C.; Torchilin, V.P. Polyamidoamine dendrimers-based nanomedicine for combination therapy with siRNA and chemotherapeutics to overcome multidrug resistance. *Eur. J. Pharm. Biopharm.* **2019**, *136*, 18–28. [CrossRef]
131. Perche, F.; Biswas, S.; Patel, N.R.; Torchilin, V.P. Hypoxia-Responsive Copolymer for siRNA Delivery. *Adv. Struct. Saf. Stud.* **2016**, *1372*, 139–162. [CrossRef]
132. Joshi, U.; Filipczak, N.; Khan, M.M.; Attia, S.A.; Torchilin, V. Hypoxia-sensitive micellar nanoparticles for co-delivery of siRNA and chemotherapeutics to overcome multi-drug resistance in tumor cells. *Int. J. Pharm.* **2020**, *590*, 119915. [CrossRef]
133. Rosenkrantz, A.; Friedman, K.; Chandarana, H.; Melsaether, A.; Moy, L.; Ding, Y.-S.; Jhaveri, K.; Beltran, L.S.; Jain, R. Current Status of Hybrid PET/MRI in Oncologic Imaging. *Am. J. Roentgenol.* **2016**, *206*, 162–172. [CrossRef] [PubMed]
134. Herzog, E.; Taruttis, A.; Beziere, N.; Lutich, A.A.; Razansky, D.; Ntziachristos, V. Optical Imaging of Cancer Heterogeneity with Multispectral Optoacoustic Tomography. *Radiology* **2012**, *263*, 461–468. [CrossRef]
135. Dilnawaz, F.; Singh, A.; Mohanty, C.; Sahoo, S.K. Dual drug loaded superparamagnetic iron oxide nanoparticles for targeted cancer therapy. *Biomaterials* **2010**, *31*, 3694–3706. [CrossRef]
136. Wang, Y.; Ng, Y.W.; Chen, Y.; Shuter, B.; Yi, J.; Ding, J.; Wang, S.-C.; Feng, S.S. Formulation of Superparamagnetic Iron Oxides by Nanoparticles of Biodegradable Polymers for Magnetic Resonance Imaging. *Adv. Funct. Mater.* **2008**, *18*, 308–318. [CrossRef]
137. Yu, B.; Goel, S.; Ni, D.; Ellison, P.A.; Siamof, C.M.; Jiang, D.; Cheng, L.; Kang, L.; Yu, F.; Liu, Z.; et al. Reassembly of (89) Zr-Labeled Cancer Cell Membranes into Multicompartment Membrane-Derived Liposomes for PET-Trackable Tumor-Targeted Theranostics. *Adv. Mater.* **2018**, *30*, e1704934. [CrossRef] [PubMed]
138. Hansen, A.E.; Petersen, A.L.; Henriksen, J.R.; Børresen, B.; Rasmussen, P.; Elema, D.R.; Rosenschöld, P.M.A.; Kristensen, A.T.; Kjær, A.; Andresen, T.L. Positron Emission Tomography Based Elucidation of the Enhanced Permeability and Retention Effect in Dogs with Cancer Using Copper-64 Liposomes. *ACS Nano* **2015**, *9*, 6985–6995. [CrossRef]
139. Maeda, H.; Nakamura, H.; Fang, J. The EPR effect for macromolecular drug delivery to solid tumors: Improvement of tumor uptake, lowering of systemic toxicity, and distinct tumor imaging in vivo. *Adv. Drug Deliv. Rev.* **2013**, *65*, 71–79. [CrossRef]
140. Brigger, I.; Dubernet, C.; Couvreur, P. Nanoparticles in cancer therapy and diagnosis. *Adv. Drug Deliv. Rev.* **2002**, *54*, 631–651. [CrossRef]
141. Chauhan, V.P.; Stylianopoulos, T.; Martin, J.D.; Popović, Z.; Chen, O.; Kamoun, W.S.; Bawendi, M.G.; Fukumura, D.; Jain, R.K. Normalization of tumour blood vessels improves the delivery of nanomedicines in a size-dependent manner. *Nat. Nanotechnol.* **2012**, *7*, 383–388. [CrossRef]
142. Philogen, S.A. *Intratumoral Administration of L19IL2/L19TNF*; US National Library of Medicine: Bethesda, MD, USA, 2016.
143. Eggermont, A.A.; Koops, H.S.H.; Klausner, J.J.; Kroon, B.B.; Schlag, P.M.; Liénard, D.; Van Geel, A.A.; Hoekstra, H.H.; Meller, I.I.; Nieweg, O.O.; et al. Isolated Limb Perfusion with Tumor Necrosis Factor and Melphalan for Limb Salvage in 186 Patients with Locally Advanced Soft Tissue Extremity Sarcomas. *Ann. Surg.* **1996**, *224*, 756–765. [CrossRef]
144. Binnemars-Postma, K.A.; Hoopen, H.W.T.; Storm, G.; Prakash, J. Differential uptake of nanoparticles by human M1 and M2 polarized macrophages: Protein corona as a critical determinant. *Nanomedicine* **2016**, *11*, 2889–2902. [CrossRef] [PubMed]
145. Chauhan, V.P.; Martin, J.D.; Liu, H.; Lacorre, D.A.; Jain, S.R.; Kozin, S.V.; Stylianopoulos, T.; Mousa, A.S.; Han, X.; Adstamongkonkul, P.; et al. Angiotensin inhibition enhances drug delivery and potentiates chemotherapy by decompressing tumour blood vessels. *Nat. Commun.* **2013**, *4*, 2516. [CrossRef]
146. Mas-Moruno, C.; Rechenmacher, F.; Kessler, H. Cilengitide: The first anti-angiogenic small molecule drug candidate design, syn-thesis and clinical evaluation. *Anticancer Agents Med. Chem.* **2010**, *10*, 753–768. [CrossRef] [PubMed]
147. Doleschel, D.; Rix, A.; Arns, S.; Palmowski, K.; Gremse, F.; Merkle, R.; Salopiata, F.; Klingmüller, U.; Jarsch, M.; Kiessling, F.; et al. Erythropoietin Improves the Accumulation and Therapeutic Effects of Carboplatin by Enhancing Tumor Vascularization and Perfusion. *Theranostics* **2015**, *5*, 905–918. [CrossRef]
148. Park, J.S.; Qiao, L.; Su, Z.Z.; Hinman, D.; Willoughby, K.; McKinstry, R.; Yacoub, A.; Duigou, G.J.; Young, C.S.; Grant, S.; et al. Ionizing radiation modulates vascular endothelial growth factor (VEGF) expression through multiple mitogen activated pro-tein kinase dependent pathways. *Oncogene* **2001**, *20*, 3266–3280. [CrossRef]
149. Machtay, M.; Moughan, J.; Trotti, A.; Garden, A.S.; Weber, R.S.; Cooper, J.S.; Forastiere, A.A.; Ang, K.K. Factors Associated with Severe Late Toxicity after Concurrent Chemoradiation for Locally Advanced Head and Neck Cancer: An RTOG Analysis. *J. Clin. Oncol.* **2008**, *26*, 3582–3589. [CrossRef]

150. Barker, H.E.; Paget, J.T.E.; Khan, A.A.; Harrington, K.J. The Tumour Microenvironment after Radiotherapy: Mechanisms of Re-sistance and Recurrence. *Nat. Rev. Cancer* **2015**, *15*, 409–425. [CrossRef]
151. Lammers, T.; Peschke, P.; Kühnlein, R.; Subr, V.; Ulbrich, K.; Debus, J.; Huber, P.; Hennink, W.; Storm, G. Effect of radiotherapy and hyperthermia on the tumor accumulation of HPMA copolymer-based drug delivery systems. *J. Control. Release* **2007**, *117*, 333–341. [CrossRef]
152. Kong, G.; Braun, R.D.; Dewhirst, M.W. Characterization of the Effect of Hyperthermia on Nanoparticle Extravasation from Tumor Vasculature. *Cancer Res.* **2001**, *61*, 3027–3032.
153. Dimcevski, G.; Kotopoulis, S.; Bjånes, T.; Hoem, D.; Schjøtt, J.; Gjertsen, B.T.; Biermann, M.; Molven, A.; Sorbye, H.; McCormack, E.; et al. A human clinical trial using ultrasound and microbubbles to enhance gemcitabine treatment of inoperable pancreatic cancer. *J. Control. Release* **2016**, *243*, 172–181. [CrossRef]
154. Lammers, T.; Koczera, P.; Fokong, S.; Gremse, F.; Ehling, J.; Vogt, M.; Pich, A.; Storm, G.; Van Zandvoort, M.; Kiessling, F. Theranostic USPIO-Loaded Microbubbles for Mediating and Monitoring Blood-Brain Barrier Permeation. *Adv. Funct. Mater.* **2015**, *25*, 36–43. [CrossRef]
155. Treat, L.H.; McDannold, N.; Zhang, Y.; Vykhodtseva, N.; Hynynen, K. Improved Anti-Tumor Effect of Liposomal Doxorubicin after Targeted Blood-Brain Barrier Disruption by MRI-Guided Focused Ultrasound in Rat Glioma. *Ultrasound Med. Biol.* **2012**, *38*, 1716–1725. [CrossRef]
156. Blood-Brain-Barrier Opening Using Focused Ultrasound with IV Contrast Agents in Patients with Early Alzheimer's Disease—ClinicalTrials.gov. (n.d.). Available online: https://clinicaltrials.gov/ct2/show/NCT02986932 (accessed on 5 June 2021).
157. Sano, K.; Nakajima, T.; Choyke, P.L.; Kobayashi, H. The Effect of Photoimmunotherapy Followed by Liposomal Daunorubicin in a Mixed Tumor Model: A Demonstration of the Super-Enhanced Permeability and Retention Effect after Photoimmunother-apy. *Mol Cancer Ther.* **2014**, *13*, 426–432. [CrossRef]
158. Islam, R.; Gao, S.; Islam, W.; Šubr, V.; Zhou, J.-R.; Yokomizo, K.; Etrych, T.; Maeda, H.; Fang, J. Unraveling the role of Intralipid in suppressing off-target delivery and augmenting the therapeutic effects of anticancer nanomedicines. *Acta Biomater.* **2021**, *126*, 372–383. [CrossRef]
159. Goel, S.; Duda, D.G.; Xu, L.; Munn, L.L.; Boucher, Y.; Fukumura, D.; Jain, R.K. Normalization of the vasculature for treatment of cancer and other diseases. *Physiol. Rev.* **2011**, *91*, 1071–1121. [CrossRef] [PubMed]
160. Cobleigh, M.A.; Vogel, C.L.; Tripathy, D.; Robert, N.J.; Scholl, S.; Fehrenbacher, L.; Wolter, J.M.; Paton, V.; Shak, S.; Lieberman, G.; et al. Multinational Study of the Efficacy and Safety of Humanized Anti-HER2 Monoclonal Antibody in Women Who Have HER2-Overexpressing Metastatic Breast Cancer That Has Progressed after Chemotherapy for Metastatic Disease. *J. Clin. Oncol.* **1999**, *17*, 2639. [CrossRef]
161. Talelli, M.; Oliveira, S.; Rijcken, C.J.; Pieters, E.H.; Etrych, T.; Ulbrich, K.; van Nostrum, R.C.; Storm, G.; Hennink, W.E.; Lammers, T. Intrinsically active nanobody-modified polymeric micelles for tumor-targeted combination therapy. *Biomaterials* **2013**, *34*, 1255–1260. [CrossRef]
162. Duan, X.; Chan, C.; Guo, N.; Han, W.; Weichselbaum, R.R.; Lin, W. Photodynamic Therapy Mediated by Nontoxic Core-Shell Nano particles Synergizes with Immune Checkpoint Blockade to Elicit Antitumor Immunity and Antimetastatic Effect on Breast Cancer. *J. Am. Chem. Soc.* **2016**, *138*, 16686–16695. [CrossRef] [PubMed]
163. Jiang, W.; Yuan, H.; Chan, C.K.; Von Roemeling, C.A.; Yan, Z.; Weissman, I.L.; Kim, B.Y.S. Lessons from immuno-oncology: A new era for cancer nanomedicine? *Nat. Rev. Drug Discov.* **2017**, *16*, 369–370. [CrossRef]
164. Ye, D.; Shuhendler, A.J.; Cui, L.; Tong, L.; Tee, S.S.; Tikhomirov, G.; Felsher, D.W.; Rao, J. Bioorthogonal cyclizationmediated in situ self-assembly of small-molecule probes for imag-ing caspase activity in vivo. *Nat. Chem.* **2014**, *6*, 519–526. [CrossRef] [PubMed]
165. Perrault, S.D.; Chan, W.C.W. In vivo assembly of nanoparticle components to improve targeted cancer imaging. *Proc. Natl. Acad. Sci. USA* **2010**, *107*, 11194–11199. [CrossRef]
166. Xu, R.; Zhang, G.; Mai, J.; Deng, X.; Segura-Ibarra, V.; Wu, S.; Shen, J.; Liu, H.; Hu, Z.; Chen, L.; et al. An injectable nanoparticle generator enhances delivery of cancer therapeutics. *Nat. Biotechnol.* **2016**, *34*, 414–418. [CrossRef]
167. Huang, B.; Abraham, W.D.; Zheng, Y.; López, S.C.B.; Luo, S.S.; Irvine, D.J. Active targeting of chemotherapy to disseminated tumors using nanoparticle-carrying T cells. *Sci. Transl. Med.* **2015**, *7*, 291ra94. [CrossRef]
168. Karageorgis, A.; Dufort, S.; Sancey, L.; Henry, M.; Hirsjärvi, S.; Passirani-Malleret, C.; Benoit, J.-P.; Gravier, J.; Texier, I.; Montigon, O.; et al. An MRI-based classification scheme to predict passive access of 5 to 50-nm large nanoparticles to tumors. *Sci. Rep.* **2016**, *6*, 21417. [CrossRef]
169. Sulheim, E.; Kim, J.; van Wamel, A.; Kim, E.; Snipstad, S.; Vidic, I.; Grimstad, I.H.; Widerøe, M.; Torp, S.H.; Lundgren, S.; et al. Multi-modal characterization of vasculature and nanoparticle accumulation in five tumor xenograft models. *J. Control. Release* **2018**, *279*, 292–305. [CrossRef] [PubMed]
170. Pérez-Medina, C.; Abdel-Atti, D.; Tang, J.; Zhao, Y.; Fayad, Z.A.; Lewis, J.S.; Mulder, W.J.M.; Reiner, T. Nanoreporter PET predicts the efficacy of anti-cancer nanotherapy. *Nat. Commun.* **2016**, *7*, 11838. [CrossRef] [PubMed]
171. Miller, M.A.; Gadde, S.; Pfirschke, C.; Engblom, C.; Sprachman, M.M.; Kohler, R.H.; Yang, K.S.; Laughney, A.M.; Wojtkiewicz, G.; Kamaly, N.; et al. Predicting therapeutic nanomedicine efficacy using a companion magnetic resonance imaging nano particle. *Sci. Transl. Med.* **2015**, *7*, 314ra183. [CrossRef]

172. Lee, H.; Shields, A.F.; Siegel, B.A.; Miller, K.D.; Krop, I.; Ma, C.X.; Lorusso, P.M.; Munster, P.N.; Campbell, K.; Gaddy, D.F.; et al. 64Cu-MM-302 Positron Emission Tomography Quantifies Variability of Enhanced Permeability and Retention of Nanoparticles in Relation to Treatment Response in Patients with Metastatic Breast Cancer. *Clin. Cancer Res.* **2017**, *23*, 4190–4202. [CrossRef] [PubMed]
173. Attia, M.F.; Antona, N.; Wallyn, J.; Omrand, Z.; Vandamme, T.F. An overview of active and passive targeting strategies to improve the nanocarriers efficiency to tumour sites. *J. Pharm. Pharmacol.* **2019**, *71*, 1185–1198. [CrossRef] [PubMed]
174. Shi, Y.; Van der Meel, R.; Chen, X.; Lammers, T. The EPR effect and beyond: Strategies to improve tumor targeting and cancer nanomedicine treatment efficacy. *Theranostics* **2020**, *10*, 7921–7924. [CrossRef]

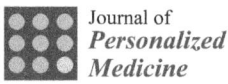 Journal of
Personalized
Medicine

Review

In Situ Delivery and Production System (*i*DPS) of Anti-Cancer Molecules with Gene-Engineered *Bifidobacterium*

Shun'ichiro Taniguchi

Department of Hematology and Medical Oncology, Shinshu University School of Medicine, Matsumoto City 390-8621, Japan; stangch@shinshu-u.ac.jp

Abstract: To selectively and continuously produce anti-cancer molecules specifically in malignant tumors, we have established an in situ delivery and production system (*i*DPS) with *Bifidobacterium* as a micro-factory of various anti-cancer agents. By focusing on the characteristic hypoxia in cancer tissue for a tumor-specific target, we employed a gene-engineered obligate anaerobic and non-pathogenic bacterium, *Bifidobacterium*, as a tool for systemic drug administration. This review presents and discusses the anti-tumor effects and safety of the *i*DPS production of numerous anti-cancer molecules and addresses the problems to be improved by directing attention mainly to the hallmark vasculature and so-called enhanced permeability and retention effect of tumors.

Keywords: solid cancer; microenvironment; hypoxia; cancer therapy; DDS; anaerobic bacteria; *Bifidobacterium*; bacterial therapy; *i*DPS; EPR

Citation: Taniguchi, S. In Situ Delivery and Production System (*i*DPS) of Anti-Cancer Molecules with Gene-Engineered *Bifidobacterium*. *J. Pers. Med.* **2021**, *11*, 566. https://doi.org/10.3390/jpm11060566

Academic Editor: Jun Fang

Received: 19 May 2021
Accepted: 15 June 2021
Published: 17 June 2021

Publisher's Note: MDPI stays neutral with regard to jurisdictional claims in published maps and institutional affiliations.

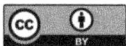

Copyright: © 2021 by the author. Licensee MDPI, Basel, Switzerland. This article is an open access article distributed under the terms and conditions of the Creative Commons Attribution (CC BY) license (https://creativecommons.org/licenses/by/4.0/).

1. Introduction

1.1. Molecular Target Cancer Therapy and its Limitations

One of the greatest advances in recent cancer research is the identification of driving genes, which are specific to cancer type and critically responsible for cellular growth. Many molecular targeting drugs have now been developed, leading to increased specificity to cancers and fewer side effects on bone marrow and digestive organs, the most common areas harmed by classic chemotherapeutic anti-cancer drugs [1]. However, there remain obstacles in cancer treatment, such as the appearance of drug-resistant cells from heterogeneous cancer cell populations, which leads to recurrence. There are also new types of side effects differing qualitatively from those of conventional cytotoxic anti-cancer drugs [2]. In the case of solid cancers, simple but troublesome problems exist in that the exposed dose of drugs is often insufficient to kill cancer cells as compared with hematopoietic cancers, which are more readily exposed to anti-cancer drugs. Accordingly, it is essential to develop a selective drug administration system to deliver large amounts of anti-cancer drugs to solid tumors and overcome the situation.

In their review on the hallmarks of recent cancer research leading to the identification of driving genes and development of molecular targeting drugs and antibody drugs, Hanahan and Weinberg pointed out the importance of the characteristic microenvironment of cancer, including low oxygen pressure (pO_2) and immune avoidance conditions [3], as targets for emerging therapies [4]. Thus, it may be desirable to focus on the tumor microenvironment rather than attack individual cancers, which contain heterogenous populations of cells [5] that can produce drug resistance.

1.2. The Enhanced Permeability and Retention (EPR) Effect

To overcome the above difficulties, it was suggested that anti-cancer drugs of a high molecular weight should be employed to make use of the characteristic vasculature of tumor tissues [6]. In malignant tumors, leaky vasculature with 100–1000 nm pores is generally formed due to the rapid but immature formation of vessels in association with cancer growth. In addition to fragile blood vessels [7,8], there is usually poor lymphatic drainage, resulting in the retention of large molecules in tumor tissue. This phenomenon was discovered by Maeda, who named it the EPR effect. By focusing on EPR, many trials have managed to successfully target tumor tissues [9].

1.3. Our Approach Targeting the Low pO_2 in Solid Cancers with Bifidobacterium

We have been working to establish a system for the selective and continuous production of anti-cancer molecules in tumors [10,11]. For this purpose, we directed our attention to the hypoxic conditions in solid cancers for a therapeutic target. As a tool for the local production of anti-cancer drugs, we adopted the obligate anaerobic and non-pathogenic bacterium, *Bifidobacterium*. Our first paper in 1980 showed the selective growth of *Bifidobacterium* in the cancer tissues of tumor-bearing mice where the bacilli were intravenously injected [12]. Currently, several gene-engineered *Bifidobacterium* lines have been established to produce numerous anti-cancer molecules in a process we have termed the in situ delivery and production system (*i*DPS). A new anti-tumor drug made with the *i*DPS is now undergoing clinical testing.

1.4. Hypoxia and Immature Blood Vasculature in Malignant Tumors

Tumor hypoxia is a well-known phenomenon [13–15]. The median pO_2 in tumor tissues is lower than that in normal tissues, which is never below 10 mm Hg. Hypoxia is generally observed in tumor tissues in spite of active angiogenesis. This paradoxical phenomenon has been attributed to impaired vascular communication and networks leading to functional, but chaotic, shunting and dysfunctional microcirculation [16]. Thus, even in the presence of blood vessels carrying fresh oxygen and nutrients, shunts to other blood vessels form easily, such that the downstream vessel will be not supplied, leading to hypoxia and/or necrosis [16].

Our project idea of the *i*DPS originally derived from Malmgren's work of injecting anaerobic *Clostridium tetani* spores into animals [17]. In his experiments, tumor-bearing mice died of tetanus due to the strongly toxic neuro-active substances produced by germinated *Clostridium tetani*, while normal mice survived. This was a strong piece of biological evidence for hypoxia existing in tumors; the spores of the anaerobic bacteria had germinated and produced strong toxins in the hypoxic conditions of the tumors, and the highly toxic poison leaked from the tumor tissues to kill the host despite very small amounts. This led us to the idea of non-pathogenic anaerobic bacteria as a tool for safely and selectively targeting solid cancers while sparing the host.

1.5. Bacterial Therapy for Cancer

Bacterial cancer therapy has a long history. The accidental tumor regression by clostridial infection clinically observed by Vautier in 1813 [18] launched a number of bacterial therapy experiments. Later, the recovery of a patient with inoperable lymphosarcoma by erysipelas prompted Coley to begin treating cancer patients with live erysipelas agents and/or bacterial toxins [19]. However, ensuing trials were limited, likely due to the difficulty in controlling toxicity and a shift to chemotherapy and radiation treatment. Recently, however, bacterial therapy has been revived with the use of genetic manipulation and is a promising method for cancer therapy [20–23].

Nowadays, several clinical studies on bacterial cancer therapies, including our own, are underway in the United States. In most cases, *Salmonella* or *Clostridium* is used. The earliest clinical trials approved by the American Food and Drug Administration (FDA) were carried out by Rosenberg's group at the National Institutes of Health (NIH) using *Salmonella* [24] and by a group at Johns Hopkins University with *Clostridium* [25]. Other trials have produced anti-tumor responses in both animals and human clinical studies [26–28]. In the above cases, the bacteria are attenuated due to their highly virulent nature. Despite concerns on the appearance of revertants and whether facultative anaerobic bacteria can be completely removed from normal aerobic tissues and cells, recent clinical trials have largely managed to maintain host safety [23].

The EPR Effect's Importance in Bacterial Therapy

Maeda's group noted that though EPR effect is applicable to particles of μm size (i.e., bacteria) or macromolecules of ~1000 kDa, nanocarriers with diameters of ~100 nm are known to achieve better or optimal EPR-based tumor accumulation [29]. Thus, the accumulation of even aerobic bacteria in tumors may be explained by the EPR effect [30]. Importantly, this effect can be augmented by vascular dynamic modifiers, such as nitroglycerin, from which nitric oxide is produced in the hypoxic conditions of tumors. In his attempts to target tumors with lactobacillus, Maeda's group showed that the number of bacteria localized in tumors increased by ten-fold as compared with controls [30].

2. Our Trials for Bacterial Therapy

2.1. Selective Localization of i.v. Injected Bifidobacterium in Tumors

Figure 1 shows our first data reported in 1980 [12] on the growth of i.v. injected *Bifidobacterium* in tumors (Figure 1a) along with the results of our genetically engineered *Bifidobacterium* (Figure 1b) (Farumashia,15, (5), 438–440, 2015 [in Japanese]). In both cases, *Bifidobacterium* selectively grew in tumor tissues and became rapidly diminished in the blood and normal tissues, including the relatively hypoxic bone marrow known as a niche for hematopoietic stem cells. No acute toxicity was observed, and the survival of mice i.v. injected with *Bifidobacterium* was comparable with that of control animals, demonstrating the absence of chronic toxicity [12].

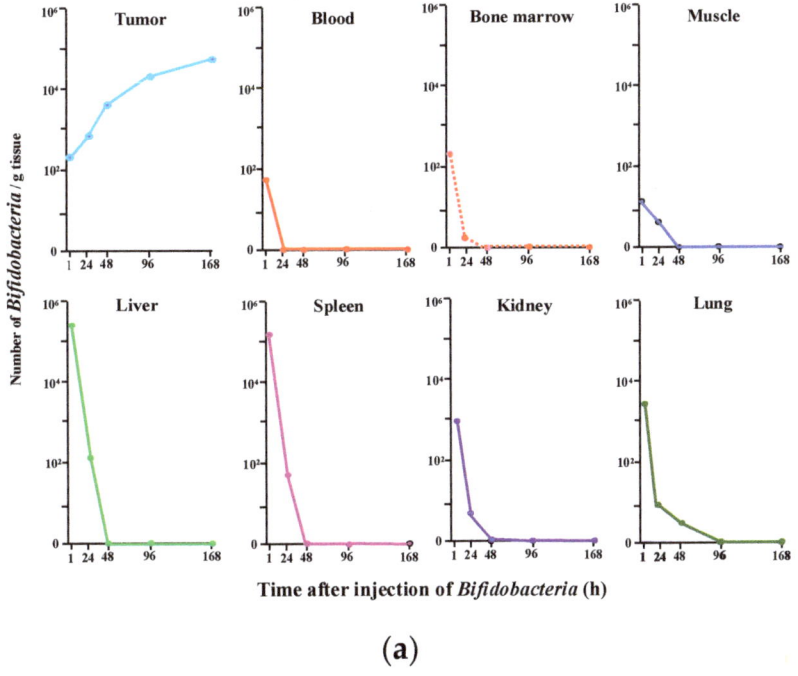

(a)

Figure 1. Cont.

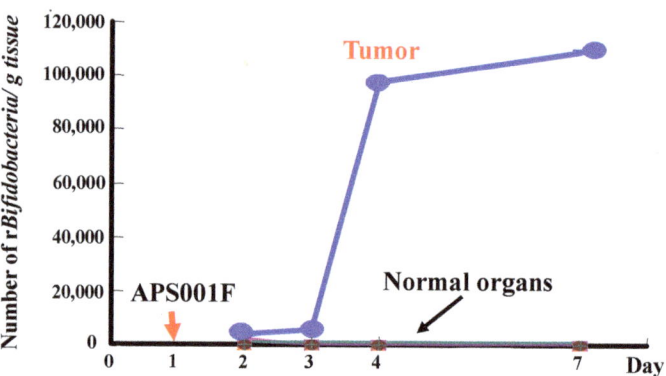

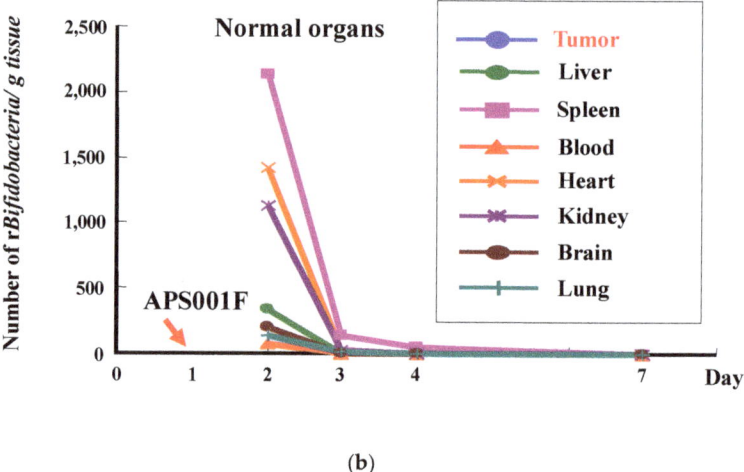

(b)

Figure 1. (**a**) Specific distribution of *Bifidobacterium (bifidum)* in tumor tissues following a single *i.v.* injection of 5×10^6 c.f.u./mouse into Ehlich solid tumor-bearing mice. Each point represents the mean c.f.u./g tissue (*n* = 8). This figure was adopted from a previous study [12]. (**b**) Recombinant *Bifidobacterium (longum)* (6.9×10^8 c.f.u./mouse) was injected *i.v.* on day 1. Bacterial cells in each tissue were counted on day 2, 3, 4, and 7 by plating assays. * Mean c.f.u./g tissue (*n* = 5). This figure was adopted from Farumashia,15, (5), 438–440 (in Japanese).

It was noteworthy that the survival of the normal animals in Malmgren's experiments [17] indicated that the *Clostridium* spores did not geminate in the bone marrow, thus demonstrating that bone marrow pO_2 was insufficiently low for obligate anaerobic bacteria germination and/or an inadequate EPR effect to trap the spores or bacteria. This phenomenon also likely occurred in our experiments.

2.2. *Transformation of Bifidobacterium with an Expression Vector for Cytosine Deaminase (CD)*

Although we initially sought to transform the bacteria to produce anti-cancer molecules, no plasmid was available for *Bifidobacterium* in the 1980s. In 1997, however, an expression vector developed by Kano's group [31] launched a series of collaborative trials for the creation of anti-cancer drugs by *Bifidobacterium*. We first inserted the CD gene of *E. coli* into the vector. The CD enzyme can convert the low-toxic 5FC, a prodrug of 5FU, to the toxic anti-cancer drug 5FU. 5FC is a well-known drug for mycosis, with almost no systemic toxicity by oral administration. We transformed *Bifidobacterium* with the CD expression vector and began experiments on solid cancers using genetically engineered *Bifidobacterium* in combination with 5FC [32–35]. This was the first step towards our *i*DPS.

2.3. Therapy Experiments on Solid Cancers Using Transformed Bifidobacterium with 5FC

The procedure for our cancer treatment with *Bifidobacterium* carrying the CD gene is as follows [11,36]. First, we *i.v.* injected the transformed *Bifidobacterium* into tumor-bearing animals. Several days later when the specific localization of the bacteria inside the tumor tissues was expected, we commenced oral 5FC administration to the animals. Although the prodrug spread throughout the body, it was converted to 5FU only in tumor tissues by *Bifidobacterium* expressing CD. We then checked for tumor growth suppression and systemic toxicity by 5FU. In the first experiment, we used an autochthonous DMBA-induced rat breast cancer system, and comparable results were obtained in various tumor-bearing animals. The selective localization of *Bifidobacterium* in tumors was confirmed by tissue homogenate cultures in vitro and Gram-positive staining of *Bifidobacterium* in the tumor tissues. CD expression in *Bifidobacterium* was ascertained by immunostaining with anti-CD antibodies.

The success of our therapy system, i.e., the suppression of tumor growth in chemically induced autochthonous rat breast cancer, can be seen in Figure 2a. When we treated human breast carcinoma transplanted into immunodeficient nude mice, tumor suppression was again witnessed without systemic toxicity (Figure 2b). Indeed, relatively large 5FU production was detected exclusively in tumors and not in normal tissues (Figure 2c). An important point was that no apparent adverse effects were observed, which was also the case in dogs, monkeys, and other large animal tests.

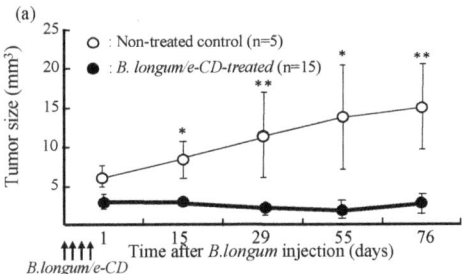

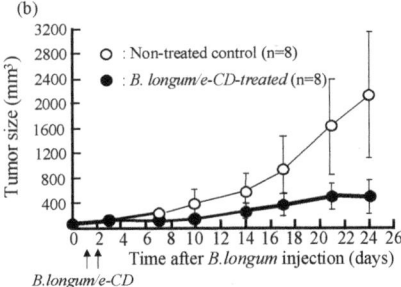

Figure 2. *Cont.*

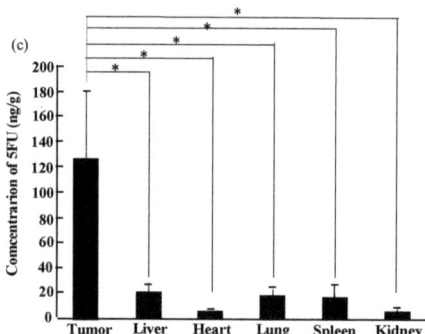

Figure 2. Anti-tumor effects of i.v. injected cytosine deaminase of *Escherichia coli* (e-CD)-transformed *Bifidobacterium longum* (*B. longum/e-CD*) combined with oral 5-fluorocytosine (5FC). (**a**) Comparison of tumor volumes of non-injected rats ($n = 5$) with those of *B. longum/e-CD* i.v. injected rats ($n = 15$). Rats bearing 7,12-dimethylbenz(a)anthracene-induced mammary tumors received i.v. *B. longum/e-CD* and 500 mg/kg/day 5FC. * $p < 0.05$; ** $p < 0.01$. (**b**) Anti-tumor assessment of *B. longum/e-CD* in nude mice transplanted with KPL-1 human mammary tumor cells. Tumor-bearing nude mice ($n = 8$) were given a dose of transformed bacteria cells i.v. (5.9×10^9 c.f.u./mouse), followed by oral 5FC for 21 days. (**c**) Measurement of 5-fluorouracil (5FU) concentration in various tissues in rats bearing MRMT-1 mammary gland carcinoma. Rats were given *B. longum/e-CD* at 1.1×10^{10} c.f.u./rat i.v. and 5FC by intragastric gavage for 4 days starting on day 4 after bacterium injection. The concentration of 5FU in normal tissues and tumor tissues was measured. Rats given 5FC without injection of *B. longum/e-CD* were used as controls. * $p < 0.05$. These figures were adopted from a previous study [11,36].

We later sought to increase enzyme activity by modifying the active site of CD according to Mahan's method [37]. Since the original substrate for CD is not 5FC, but rather cytosine, the enzymatic activity and affinity to 5FC was relatively low as compared with that to cytosine. When we changed the amino acid at position 314 of the active center of the enzyme from aspartic acid to alanine, the conversion rate of 5FC to 5FU was increased by approximately ten-fold. In clinical trials, the modified expression vector was further tailored by removing the resistance gene to an antibiotic, spectinomycin, to protect against horizontal transmission.

2.4. Immunological Safety

To test for immunological toxicity and possible severe anaphylaxis from repeated injection of the bacteria into animals, we evaluated for active systemic anaphylaxis (ASA) reactions and passive cutaneous anaphylaxis (PCA) caused by IgG with a sensitive guinea pig system (Table 1). In terms of ASA reactions, the positive control ovalbumin induced severe shock, whereas little, if any, reactions were seen for *Bifidobacterium*. Regarding PCA, although IgG antibody formation against *Bifidobacterium* had been suggested, experiments using animals immunized with *Bifidobacterium* confirmed the safety and therapeutic efficiency of the system.

We further examined for the induction of inflammatory cytokines related to *Bifidobacterium* in collaboration with an expert of infectious immunity, Tsutsui, Hyogo College of Medicine in Japan. As shown in Figure 3, the *E. coli* control predictably induced the cytokines seen in sepsis, while *Bifidobacterium* did little [12]. Since cytokine production occurs through Toll-like receptors, which are the main players in innate immunity, those results suggested that *Bifidobacterium* was recognized neither by Toll-like receptors in vivo [38], nor by other innate immunity systems activating IL-1β through inflammasomes in the cytosol [39]. It is well known that inflammasomes are activated by the flagella of *Salmonella* to induce IL-1β.

Table 1. Antigenic tests to estimate the toxicity of B. longum/S-eCD.

(a) ASA Reaction								
Group	Sensitized Antigen	Cause Antigen	No. of Animals	Antigen Challenge Outcome				
				(−)	(+/−)	(+)	(++)	(+++)
A	B.longum/S-eCD	B.longum/S-eCD	5	4	1	0	0	0
B	B.longum/S-eCD + FCA	B.longum/S-eCD	5	5	0	0	0	0
C	OVA + FCA	OVA	5	0	0	5	5	4
D	Saline + FCA	B.longum/S-eCD	5	5	0	0	0	0
(b) PCA Reaction								
Group	Sensitized Antigen	Cause Antigen	No. of Animals	PCA Titer				
				(×1)	(×4)	(×16)	(×64)	(×256)
A	B.longum/S-eCD	B.longum/S-eCD	5	0	0	0	0	0
B	B.longum/S-eCD + FCA	B.longum/S-eCD	5	3	2	2	2	2
C	OVA + FCA	OVA	5	5	5	5	5	4
D	Saline + FCA	B.longum/S-eCD	5	0	0	0	0	0

Note: (a) Actively immunized guinea pigs were injected intravenously with B. longum/S-eCD or OVA 14 days after the final sensitization. Anaphylaxis symptoms were quantified by the following criteria: −, no symptoms; ±, scrub of face or ear and/or scratch of nose; +, coughing or locomotion ataxia; ++, convulsion or roll, but no death observed within 1 h; and +++, death observed within 1 h. (b) In the PCA reaction, immunized guinea pigs were killed and blood samples were collected 14 days after final sensitization to obtain each antiserum. Normal guinea pigs were shaved, and 0.05 mL of each serum dilution was injected intradermally into the dorsal skin. After 4 h, the animals were injected i.v. with 1 mL of antigen (B. longum/S-eCD or OVA) and 0.5 mL of 1% Evans blue solution. After 30 min, the animals were killed, the dorsal skin was peeled off, and blue spots within the intradermal sites were measured. A PCA reaction was judged to be positive when the blue spot measured more than 5 mm^2 in dimension. This table was adopted from a previous study [36].

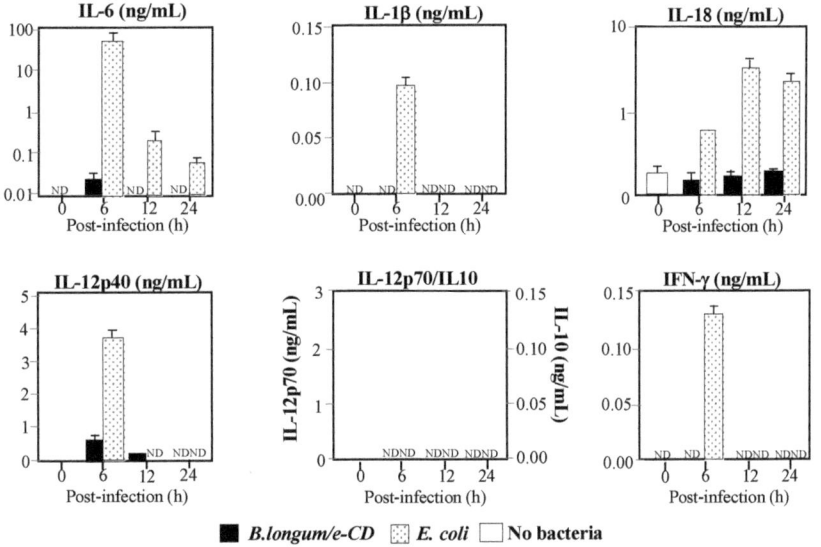

Figure 3. Production of inflammatory cytokines in C57BL/6 mice injected i.v. with cytosine deaminase of *Escherichia coli* (e-CD)-transformed *Bifidobacterium longum* (B. longum/e-CD) or non-pathogenic E. coli (control). Cytokines were assessed by ELISA at 6 h after injection. Closed bars, blood of mice injected with B. longum/e-CD; dotted bars, blood of mice injected with non-pathogenic E. coli; open bars, normal blood. IFN, interferon; IL, interleukin; ND, not detected. This figure was adopted from a previous study [10,11].

Concerning the above findings, an interesting report found that extracellular vesicles in the blood inhibited the induction of NFκB expression by *Bifidobacterium* [40]. NFκB is a well-known master gene for inflammatory cytokines. When *Bifidobacterium* was allowed to act on cultured human embryonic kidney cells, NFκB was induced in the absence of serum. However, serum addition to the medium suppressed NFκB expression in a concentration-dependent manner. It was also shown that extracellular vesicles in the serum played a key role in suppressing NFκB. Those results suggested that the lack, if any, little of inflammatory cytokine induction in mice by *Bifidobacterium* was partially attributed to extracellular vesicles in the blood.

In the field of probiotic research, human intestinal flora changes have been examined for relationships between flora variety and health conditions. Shortly after birth, *Bifidobacterium* becomes the main gut flora and coexists with the organism throughout life at gradually decreasing amounts [41,42]. It is likely that humans and other mammals have some immune tolerance against *Bifidobacterium*. These facts strengthen our notion that *Bifidobacterium* can be safely used for an *i*DPS to produce anti-cancer molecules in humans. Moreover, *Bifidobacterium* has been included in commensal microbiome work to enhance the cancer therapy efficiency of anti-PD-1 antibodies [43].

2.5. Translational Research

For the purpose of applying *i*DPS/5FC for clinical cancer treatment in humans, rigorous testing was performed according to Chemistry, Manufacturing and Control (CMC) and Good Manufacturing Practice (GMP) guidelines. CMC requires showing the physicochemical properties of the product in detail, while GMP necessitates the provision of quality assurance that products are consistently produced and controlled to quality standards. Since CMC and GMP are generally difficult processes even with simple chemical compounds, certification for living bacteria has been much more challenging.

We have performed the precise characterization of various aspects of *Bifidobacterium*, including its membrane composition, stability of the expression vector in which the antibiotic resistance gene for selective pressure and other sequences were removed for safety, and bacterial survival measurement methods. Every attempt has been made to establish virus-free and sterile preparations for GMP. Finally, through investigational new drug discussion, our proposed first-in-man clinical trial was approved by the American FDA, with NIH Recombinant DNA Advisory Committee approval of our protocol on biosafety. The first-in-man phase 1 and 2 tests were approved in 2013 and carried out sponsored by a bio-venture company, Anaeropharma Science Inc., Tokyo, Japan. Whereas the phase 1 test is almost completed, phase 2 has regrettably been postponed by the current COVID-19 pandemic.

The concept for applying the *i*DPS using genetically modified *Bifidobacterium* on human cancer therapy is much the same as that with animals. Since the line of CD-expressing *Bifidobacterium* for application on humans is named APS001F, the clinical trial has been entitled "A Phase I/II Safety, Pharmacokinetic, and Pharmacodynamic Study of APS001F with Flucytosine (5FC) and Maltose for the Treatment of Advanced and/or Metastatic Solid Tumors" [44].

2.6. Combination Therapy of APS001F Plus 5FC (APS001F/5FC) in Combination with the Immune Checkpoint Inhibitor (ICPI) Anti-PD-1

With recent developments in cancer treatment, the prominent anti-tumor effects of ICPIs, such as anti-CTLA4 and anti-PD-1 antibodies, have been demonstrated worldwide [45–47]. To augment the effects of ICPIs, combination treatments with chemotherapy, molecular targeting anti-cancer agents, and/or radiation therapy have been tested. However, the associated side effects often increased in tandem with anti-tumor action. We expected our *i*DPS using *Bifidobacterium* to enhance ICPI treatment by 5FU in tumors without raising side effects by enhancing immune reactions through innate immunity locally stimulated by *Bifidobacterium*.

Combination therapy experiments of the *i*DPS with APS001F/5FC and anti-mPD-1 antibodies have already yielded promising results [48]. The almost completed clinical phase 1 test of APS001F/5FC also serves for prechecking whether the combination of anti-PD-1 antibodies, which are already available for clinical use, with APS001F/5FC can be a potential treatment candidate. The rationality for this next step was made through investigation of the literature [49–52] as follows: (1) combining ICPIs and anti-cancer drugs, including 5FU, reportedly enhances anti-tumor effects, (2) 5FU has the potential to suppress myeloid-derived suppressor cell inhibition of anti-tumor immune reactions, and (3) the systemic administration of 5FU at a high dose rather impairs anti-tumor immunity. The third consideration may be attributed to the systemic toxicity of 5FU, which is improved by the *i*DPS with APS001F/5FC.

Combining APS001F/5FC with anti-PD-1 antibodies in therapeutic experiments enhanced treatment effects (Figure 4a) without increasing side effects. We first observed that the tumor growth in animals treated with anti-PD-1 antibodies was slightly suppressed. When combined with APS001F/5FC, however, this effect was significantly augmented. Animal survival was also prolonged, including a complete remission case [48].

By analyzing the immune cells in tumors during combination therapy, we witnessed a remarkable decrease in regulatory T (Treg) cells, which inhibit anti-tumor immune activity, and consequently the ratio of CD8 cells to Treg cells was greatly increased (Figure 4b) through a yet unspecified mechanism. In this therapy system, 5FU was produced in situ in tumor tissues and Treg cells were suppressed without a change in CD8 activity, likely raising the anti-tumor effect of combination therapy. We strongly believe that APS001F/5FC in future clinical trials will exert promising effects in combination with anti-PD-1 antibodies and other ICPIs. Furthermore, combined treatment with anti-tumor drugs and ICPIs may be possible with a single gene-engineered *Bifidobacterium* clone. Although technically challenging, we have already succeeded in establishing such a co-expression system with *Bifidobacterium*.

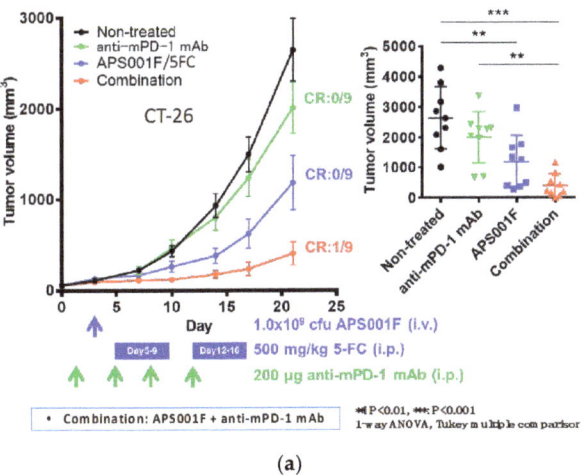

(a)

Figure 4. *Cont.*

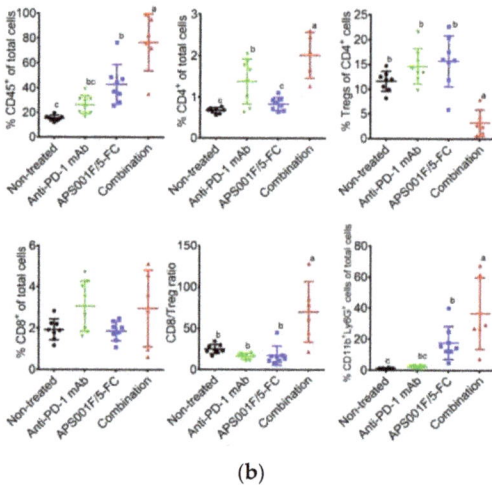

(b)

Figure 4. Anti-tumor effects of APS001F/5FC, anti-PD-1 mAb, and their combination were evaluated in a syngeneic CT26 mouse model. Experiment schedule. Mice were *s.c.* inoculated with 1×10^5 CT26 cells (day -13), and stratification was done on day 0. APS001F was administered *i.v.* at 1.0×10^9 c.f.u./mouse via the tail vein on day 3 with 200 mg maltose supplementation (days 3 through 16). 5-FC was administered *i.p.* at 250 mg/kg twice a day (500 mg/kg/day) on days 5 through 9 and days 12 through 16. Anti-PD-1 mAb was administered *i.p.* at 200 μg/mouse on days 1, 4, 8, and 11. Tumor volume was measured twice a week. (**a**) Change in tumor volume after treatment with APS001F/5-FC, anti-PD-1 mAb, and their combination. Results are the mean ± standard error of the mean of 9 mice. Analyses of 4 groups on day 21 were conducted using Tukey's method of multiple comparisons. Means sharing a letter are not significantly different. Tumor Growth Inhibition was calculated on day 21. (**b**) Flow cytometric analysis of tumor cells in mice engrafted with CT26 cells. Results are the mean ± standard deviation of 8 mice. %CD45$^+$ of total cells, %CD4$^+$ of total cells, %Tregs (CD45$^+$ CD4$^+$ CD25$^+$ Foxp3$^+$ cells) of CD4$^+$ cells, %CD8$^+$ of total cells, CD8/Treg ratio, and %neutrophils (CD45$^+$ CD11b$^+$ Ly-6G$^+$ cells) of total cells, and %TAMs (CD45$^+$ CD11b$^+$ Ly-6G$^-$Ly-6C^{low} cells) of total cells were analyzed. Analyses of 4 groups were conducted using Tukey's method of multiple comparisons. Means sharing a letter are not significantly different. This figure was adopted from a previous study [48].

2.7. Establishment of a Protein-Secreting System

We are underway to engineer *Bifidobacterium* that not only express, but also secrete, proteins such as anti-tumor antibodies and cytokines (Scheme 1). In spite of the prominent effects of ICPIs, there remain problems including autoimmune diseases and other severe side effects. Immune checkpoint molecules, such as CTLA4 and PD-1, inactivate T-cell killing to terminate excessive inflammatory reactions in the body. It is physiologically important to halt unnecessary immunoreactions, and blocking those molecules tends to induce immune toxicities in the host [53–55].

To improve this situation, it will be useful to establish an *i*DPS for immune checkpoint-modifying antibodies, including anti-CTLA4 and anti-PD-1 antibodies, and immune modifiers, such as anti-tumor cytokines, with *Bifidobacterium*. We have therefore been attempting to establish *Bifidobacterium* that both express and secrete immunological anti-cancer molecules (Scheme 1), such as anti-CTLA4 and/or anti-PD-1 antibodies, in addition to such immune-stimulating anti-tumor cytokines as TNFα and INFγ.

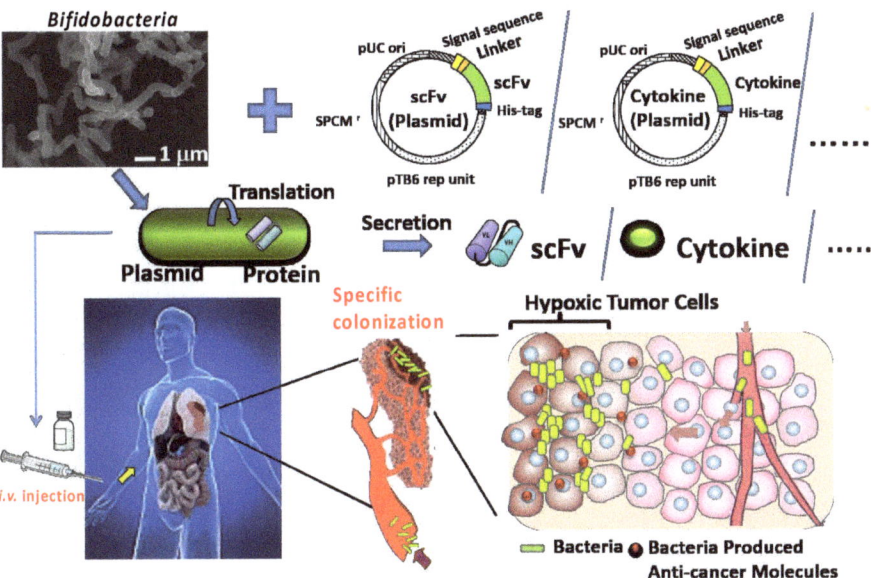

Scheme 1. The in situ delivery and production system (*i*DPS) as a platform technology for producing various anti-tumor scFvs and cytokines.

2.7.1. Anti-HER2 scFv

As it is generally difficult to produce the original structure of antibodies with bacteria, we firstly tried to create single-chain variable fragments (scFvs), which were fusion proteins of variable light and heavy chains connected with a linker for each antibody, such that the scFv could be called a single-chain antibody.

In our attempts to produce scFvs for immune checkpoint molecules, we started by expressing and secreting a biologically active scFv already made and confirmed by another system. For this purpose, we turned to an anti-HER2 antibody, trastuzumab, since a biologically active scFv for trastuzumab had been developed by Akiyama at the Shizuoka Cancer Center in Japan. Trastuzumab is well known and widely used as a molecular targeting antibody for human breast cancer, but occasionally induces cardiotoxicities [56,57]. Thus, we sought to establish *Bifidobacterium* secretion of the biologically active scFv for anti-HER2 antibodies.

We succeeded in making not only an expression, but also a secretion, system for a biologically active scFv derived from the anti-HER2 trastuzumab with *Bifidobacterium* (Figure 5) [58]. Production of the scFv to human HER2 was confirmed by Western blot analysis. We also verified biochemical activity by FACS and immunological staining [58]. The genetically modified bacteria were injected into nude mice bearing the human HER2-positive breast cancer, NCI-N87. We witnessed selective localization of the bacteria inside the tumor, secretion of anti-HER2 single-chain antibodies, and ultimately a suppressive effect on tumor growth (Figure 5) [58]. This success in creating *Bifidobacterium* to express and secrete the biologically active trastuzumab scFv prompted us to establish *i*DPS with *Bifidobacterium* for ICPIs.

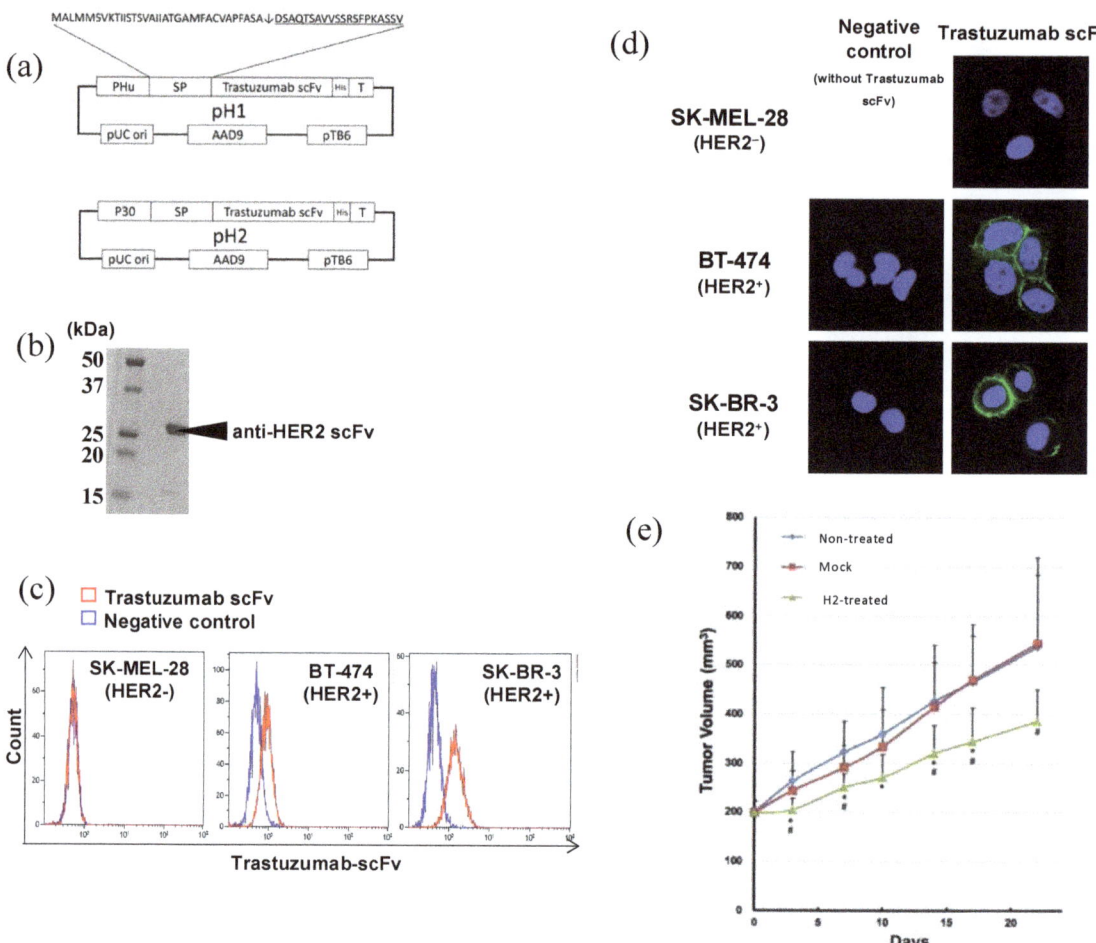

Figure 5. (**a**) Structure of the pH1 and pH2 plasmids. (**b**) Molecular size of the trastuzumab scFV produced by *Bifidobacterium*. Results for H1 scFv are shown. Regarding H2, identically sized scFv was confirmed at a markedly higher expression amount. (**c**) FACS analysis. SK-MEL-28 (HER2−), BT-474 (HER2 +/−), and SK-BR-3 (HER2+) cells were stained with His-tag-purified trastuzumab scFv. Blue line: control (buffer alone). Red line: stained with trastuzumab scFv from H2. (**d**) Immunostaining of cultured cells by His-tag-purified trastuzumab scFv from *B. longum* H2. Immunofluorescent staining. Blue: nucleus. Green: stained with trastuzumab scFv from H2. Right panels: stained with trastuzumab scFv. Left panels: negative control (without trastuzumab scFv). Original magnification of all images was ×400. (**e**) Growth suppression of a human HER2(+) carcinoma transplanted into nude mice by recombinant *Bifidobacterium* H2. *B. longum* mock and H2 were i.v. administered to NCI-N87 human gastric cancer tumor-bearing mice twice a week. Mean ± standard deviation values of 8 mice. *: $p < 0.05$ versus non-treated group, #: $p < 0.05$ versus mock-treated group. This figure was adopted from a previous study [58].

2.7.2. scFvs for ICP Antagonistic or Agonistic Antibodies, including Anti-PD-1, Anti-CTLA4, Anti-41BB, and Anti-Tumor Cytokines

We next established *Bifidobacterium* to secrete scFvs of anti-PD-1 [59], anti-CTLA4 [60], and anti-41BB (an immune checkpoint agonist) [61] antibodies. All scFvs produced by the *i*DPS were detected exclusively in tumor tissues and exhibited immunological activity and anti-tumor effects without remarkable side effects.

In addition to scFvs, we have also established *Bifidobacterium* expressing and secreting INFγ and/or TNFα, which displayed notable anti-tumor effects [62,63]. It is well known that the clinical application of INFγ and TNFα is difficult due to their severe systemic toxicity in spite of strong anti-tumor effects [64]. However, this was not the case in our *i*DPS using *Bifidobacterium*. When we systemically *i.v.* injected *Bifidobacterium* that could secrete INFγ and/or TNFα into tumor-bearing animals, high amounts of cytokines were detected in tumors, with little in the blood and thus no systemic toxicity. In addition to the anti-tumor properties of *Bifidobacterium* expressing and secreting the cytokines, the enhancement of anti-tumor effects by combination with ICPI antibodies or a popular anti-cancer drug, Adriamycin, was observed as well. Taken together, drugs that have been unsuitable for clinical use due to strong systemic toxicity despite formidable anti-cancer properties may be revisited through the use of our *i*DPS. Most recently, a *Bifidobacterium* clone, APS002, has been established to secrete diabodies against EGFR/HER3 and CD3 and redirect T cells to EGFR/HER3-positive cancer cells. This clone inhibited the growth of human EGFR-positive cancer cells transplanted into humanized immunodeficient mice [65], indicating a possible clinical application of this engineered *Bifidobacterium*.

3. For Further Improvement of the *i*DPS

3.1. Notes for the Presnt iDPS

3.1.1. Animal Experiments

The established methods for *i*DPS so far are detailed in our previous papers, especially in [11] and patent information [63]. In animal experiments with *Bifidobacteria*, we used chemically induced autochthonous tumor system, mouse tumor model, and allogenic transplanted human tumors in immunodeficient mice (Figures 1 and 2). Generally, autochthonous cancer is relatively difficult to cure compared with a transplanted tumor, because the tumor is comprised of cells which have escaped from host immune surveillance. In this sense, it is thought to mimic the human cancer system. In transplantation of cancer cells, the number of cells should be as small as possible to mimic a human tumor system where one nodule is produced from single or a few cancer cells. In such systems, we have experienced that *Bifidobacteria* tended to be localized even in small tumors. While *Bifidobacterium* could be safely administered to immunodeficient mice, immunodeficient mice are always infected with various bacteria as compared with normal mice because they are immunodeficient. Thus, during the assay of the number of *Bifidobacteria* in various tissues, it was required to remove intrinsically contaminated germs in in vitro bacterial culture system. Our genetically engineered *Bifidobacteria* have 5FU resistance in addition to spectinomycin, so that we were able to eliminate such germs and to identify the colony of *Bifidobacterium* by using both drugs in vitro bacterial culture.

In the assay for inflammatory cytokines, there was little or no induction of such cytokines in our mouse system (Figure 3), however, it probably depends on the type of animal, including human. More detailed analysis is needed from the viewpoint of molecular immunology.

In our present chemotherapy system (Figure 2), 5FC have been used as the prodrug. Since a *Bifidobacterium* clone expressing β-glucuronidase has also been established to activate prodrugs inactivated by glucuronic acid conjugation. Such clone will be useful to reuse drugs that have strong anti-tumor properties but severe systemic side effects.

In the protein secretory system (Figure 5), the optimum secretory signal peptide depended on the secretory protein. We have searched various secretory signals of the *Bifidobacterium*'s own secretory proteins and adequate promoter for the gene as well. In order to improve combination therapy, we have established various vectors to co-express/secrete anti-tumor cytokines and/or scFvs for various antitumor antibodies, which will be useful for combination therapies of cancer in the future.

At the preclinical level, there are some studies using *Bifidobacteria*, though there seems to be only our group that has advanced to clinical trials. One of the preclinical studies similar to ours demonstrated the successful delivery and efficient expression of

Tumstatin, a powerful angiostatin, with genetically engineered *Bifidobacterium*, leading to antitumor effects through inducing apoptosis of tumorous vascular endothelial cells [66]. They observed that *Bifidobacterium longum*, selectively localizes to and proliferates in the hypoxia location within solid tumor. The other investigated the therapeutic effect of new recombinant *Bifidobacterium breve* strain expressing interleukin (IL)-24 gene on head and neck tumor xenograft in mice and reported that new recombinant bacterium has the capability of targeting tumor tissue *in vivo* [67]. These reports are consistent with our results in terms of selective localization of *Bifidobacterium* in tumors.

3.1.2. As for Safety of *i*DPS with *Bifidobacterium*

For the clinical trial, bacteria dosage was initiated at less than a NOAEL (no observed adverse effect level) in the most sensitive dogs, and the dose was gradually increased with the minimum homing dose for rat transplanted cancer as a guide [44].

Since the *Bifidobacterium* we use is derived from enterobacteria in human, which is also used as intestinal regulators and yogurt as a probiotics, and thus it has been considered to be a priori non-toxic from experience. However, to evaluate the toxicity of genetically modified *B. longum*, a number of preclinical studies have been also carried out in several animal species, including normal mice, nude mice, normal rats, nude rats, dogs and monkeys. Both pharmacological and preliminary general toxicity studies were done, none of which revealed serious unfavorable toxicities [10]. Various antibiotics were examined to eliminate excess *Bifidobacteria* after treatment, and many antibiotics were found to be effective. In particular, we have confirmed that it can be easily removed with commonly used penicillin antibiotics (data, not shown).

3.1.3. The Specific Advantages of Using Bifidobacterium for Our *i*DPS

The specific advantages of using *Bifidobacterium* and the reason why we have been using *Bifidobacterium longum* for our *i*DPS are as follows: (1) It is an obligate anaerobic bacterium, so that it can discriminate hypoxic malignant tumor tissues for the colony formation from normal tissues. (2) It does neither produce toxic substances, nor has flagella which activate inflammasome to induce IL-1β. (3) It has been generally regarded as a good bacterium derived from human intestinal bacteria, so that it is easy to think about safety a priori even if it is administered into the blood, thus leading to a sense of security for the recipient. In addition, (4) it has also been shown to work positively in treatment with antitumor immune check point inhibitor, anti-PD-1 antibody.

Since an expression vector has become available firstly for *Bifidobacterium longum*, this *Bifidobacterium longum* has been used as a tool for *i*DPS and we came to apply for IND with *longum*. However, if safety is ensured by other probiotic species and the use of expression vectors becomes possible for them, they could become a better tool, so that it seems important to continue to search such species in the future.

3.2. Seeking an Ideal Micro-Factory with Guaranteed Safety

Nowadays, bacteria can be modified to endow new phenotypes using gene engineering [18,23]. It will be important to improve the efficiency of *i*DPSs by modifying *Bifidobacterium* to develop ideal delivery and in situ production systems. The success and safety of *i.v.* administration of APS001F with living *Bifidobacterium* in our clinical phase 1 trial was an encouraging first step. Based on the clinically confirmed safety of systemic *Bifidobacterium* injection, we will next modify *i*DPS setups to produce an ideal micro-factory of various anti-cancer molecules for selectively and continuously treating all types of solid cancer.

To strengthen the concept of *i*DPS tolerance in clinical applications, its molecular safety mechanism needs deeper understanding from the viewpoint of the innate and acquired immunological reactions to *i.v.* injected *Bifidobacterium*. We believe that we can ameliorate our system towards completely and safely eradicating cancer.

There are several issues to consider when improving and strengthening *i*DPS microfactories in tumors. First, it will be necessary to increase the number of bacteria in tumors to provide clear therapeutic effects. One way is the simple quantitative approach of increasing the inoculation size as we have not yet determined the tolerable maximal dose. Concerning qualitative modifications, it will be critical to consider two main factors: (1) The dynamics of tumoral blood flow preventing bacteria entrance into the tumor, and (2) The capture of bacteria by reticuloendothelial cells and neutrophils that rapidly reduces bacterial density in the blood.

3.2.1. Modification of Tumor Hemodynamics with Vasodilators to Enhance the EPR Effect

In our research, the number of bacteria detected in each tumor-bearing animal varied and depended on the tumor type. In order to consistently obtain a large number of bacteria in any type of tumor, we will need to consider modifying the hemodynamics of lesions by directing attention to the EPR effect [9].

Inside the tumor, it is well known that blood vessels occasionally become blocked by poor blood flow dynamics, which may hinder the entrance of *Bifidobacterium* and other macromolecules. In future clinical trials, transiently exposing tumor blood vessels to vasodilators, such as nitroglycerin, may contribute to improved *i*DPSs. Since nitroglycerin reportedly augments the anti-tumor effects of chemotherapies [68–71], it seems logical to use this agent to enhance the accumulation of *Bifidobacterium* in tumors by increasing the EPR effect. Maeda's group targeted cancers with lactobacillus in animal experiments in combination with nitroglycerin and showed that the number of bacteria localized in tumors increased by ten-fold versus controls [30].

As an additional factor related to poor blood flow in tumors, we may have to consider thrombus inhibition of the intra-tumoral accessibility of anti-cancer drugs. Thrombosis can occur in cancer patients [72–74], in whom blood clots may form easily in tumor tissues [75]. The local administration of recombinant plasminogen activators may be effective to dissolve such clots [76]. If bacteria are equipped with such an enzyme by gene-engineering, their accumulation in tumors will likely become enhanced.

Another factor to potentially improve the bacterial accumulation is to make the bacteria smaller. In a liposome study of pancreatic cancer, smaller liposomes could deliver greater amounts of anti-cancer drugs to the lesion and augment therapeutic effects [77]. Tunability of bacterial size has been investigated [78]. Interestingly, it was reported that deletion of the *Bacillus subtilis ponA* gene encoding for PBP1 (a class A penicillin-binding protein), a bifunctional peptidoglycan synthase, led to thinner cells [79], indicating that it may be possible to change the size of the bacteria by gene engineering.

3.2.2. Transient Evasion from Bacteria Trapping by the Reticuloendothelial System (RES) and/or Neutrophils

Clinical trials using bacteria for cancer treatment have found that the amount of bacteria accumulation in tumors appears to be less than expected based on the results of animal experiments [23].

One reason may be a more rapid capture of injected bacteria by the RES and/or neutrophils than in animal trials. A similar phenomenon is seen for liposome-type drugs. The RES in the human liver and spleen is a major obstacle to the tumor delivery of macromolecular drugs and liposomes [80,81], the effect of which seems to be stronger than in animal systems. Therefore, higher doses may be needed to achieve satisfactory therapeutic effects in humans along with a method to temporarily avoid trapping by the RES.

In one study, covering liposomes with polyethylene glycol (PEG) by so-called PEGylation enabled a breakthrough in the field of liposomes to avoid RES trapping. PEGylation has been also attempted at the cellular level with promising results [82,83]. Additional trials may bring about the same and/or improved effects as PEGylation. In that way, the removal of membrane molecules on bacteria responsible for phagocytosis by the RES and/or neutrophils by gene-targeting [84] will help avoid trapping by the RES. Furthermore, the genes encoding the antigens recognized by reticulocyte-endothelial cells and neutrophils can be replaced with ones produce anti-cancer molecules. As a result, the bacteria will evade detection by the RES and neutrophils, leading not only to an increase in bacterial number entering the tumor microcirculation, but also enabling the bacteria to more stably express anti-cancer molecules.

In addition to genome editing, a sophisticated method to control plasmid copy number has been reported [85], which will be a powerful tool for enhancing bacterial cancer therapy in the future.

3.2.3. Other Factors for Improving the iDPS

Regarding other factors contributing to the improvement of iDPSs, bacterial proteolytic activity [86] might be able to widen the localization area of bacteria, thus also being effective to spread anti-cancer substances produced by bacterial micro-factories to the whole tumor region from the central necrosis and/or periphery of the necrotic region where the anaerobic bacteria are colonized. For better distribution of anti-cancer substances in tumor tissue, there may be other ways to conjugate anti-tumor substances with oligopeptides to penetrate tumor masses and consequently widen the diffusion area of therapeutic agents [87].

It is also possible that specific and effective energy sources or nutrients that selectively stimulate the growth of bacteria in solid cancers can increase the number of intra-tumoral bacteria, even if the initial localization number is small. In the case of *Bifidobacterium*, lactulose was firstly used to enhance bacterial number in animal experiments. Lactulose is a disaccharide made up of galactose and fructose that cannot be used by mammalian cells as an energy source. Although considered an ideal bacterial energy source, the i.v. administration of lactulose is not permitted in the clinical setting. Therefore, maltose has been used in phase 1 testing as an alternative energy source. The search for an ideal nutrient in clinical trials continues for *Bifidobacterium* [88]. If lactic acid can be used as an energy source, it will be abundantly supplied by the tumor as a metabolite of cancer cell glycolysis. Other bacteria, such as *Veillonella*, consume lactic acid as reported in a meta-omics analysis of elite athletes as a performance-enhancing microbe that functions via lactate metabolism [89]. Transferring this metabolic phenotype to *Bifidobacterium* through gene transfer techniques may create a better micro-factory for anti-cancer drug production.

4. Conclusions

The present review of our novel iDPS with *Bifidobacterium* demonstrates its strong potential to safely improve the current problems of solid cancer treatment. Further advances will lower medical expenses through the continuous production of anti-cancer agents and cost-effectively reintroduce discontinued drugs that have strong anti-tumor properties but severe systemic side effects.

With a concerted global effort, it will be possible to pursue and realize an ideal bacterial-based system, no matter what difficulties await; all that is needed is to remove the unnecessary and undesirable genes and replace them with beneficial ones. Our novel iDPS with *Bifidobacterium* represents a promising therapeutic candidate for solid tumors as an in situ self-propagating micro-factory.

Funding: These works were supported by grants from the Japan Science and Technology Agency and the New Energy and Industrial Technology Development Organization, Collaborative Research Funds from Anaeropharma Science Inc. to Shinshu University, a Grant-in-Aid for Scientific Research from the Japan Society for the Promotion of Science, and an award from the Kobayashi Foundation for Cancer Research.

Institutional Review Board Statement: Not applicable.

Informed Consent Statement: Not applicable.

Data Availability Statement: Not applicable.

Acknowledgments: These works were done by graduate students and colleagues at Shinshu University School of Medicine and Anaeropharma Science Inc. I thank all of them for their technical support and useful discussions, and N. Kimura and the late T. Baba for their guidance when I was a graduate student at Kyushu University. Since autumn 2020, research concerning the *i*DPS has been transferred to Azusapharma Science Inc.

Conflicts of Interest: As a disclosure statement for conflicts of interest, S. Taniguchi is a former Science Advisor of Anaeropharma Science Inc.

References

1. Kumar, B.; Singh, S.; Skvortsova, I.; Kumar, V. Promising Targets in Anti-cancer Drug Development: Recent Updates. *Curr. Med. Chem.* **2017**, *24*, 4729–4752. [CrossRef] [PubMed]
2. Olgen, S. Overview on Anticancer Drug Design and Development. *Curr. Med. Chem.* **2018**, *25*, 1704–1719. [CrossRef] [PubMed]
3. Hanahan, D.; Weinberg, R.A. Hallmarks of cancer: The next generation. *Cell* **2011**, *144*, 646–674. [CrossRef]
4. Wang, J.J.; Lei, K.F.; Han, F. Tumor microenvironment: Recent advances in various cancer treatments. *Eur. Rev. Med. Pharmacol. Sci.* **2018**, *22*, 3855–3864.
5. McGranahan, N.; Swanton, C. Biological and therapeutic impact of intratumor heterogeneity in cancer evolution. *Cancer Cell* **2015**, *27*, 15–26. [CrossRef]
6. Maeda, H.; Nakamura, H.; Fang, J. The EPR effect for macromolecular drug delivery to solid tumors: Improvement of tumor uptake, lowering of systemic toxicity, and distinct tumor imaging in vivo. *Adv. Drug Deliv. Rev.* **2013**, *65*, 71–79. [CrossRef]
7. Stylianopoulos, T.; Martin, J.D.; Snuderl, M.; Mpekris, F.; Jain, S.R.; Jain, R.K. Coevolution of solid stress and interstitial fluid pressure in tumors during progression: Implications for vascular collapse. *Cancer Res.* **2013**, *73*, 3833–3841. [CrossRef]
8. Taniguchi, S.; Takeoka, M.; Ehara, T.; Hashimoto, S.; Shibuki, H.; Yoshimura, N.; Shigematsu, H.; Takahashi, K.; Katsuki, M. Structural fragility of blood vessels and peritoneum in calponin h1-deficient mice, resulting in an increase in hematogenous metastasis and peritoneal dissemination of malignant tumor cells. *Cancer Res.* **2001**, *61*, 7627–7634. [PubMed]
9. Fang, J.; Islam, W.; Maeda, H. Exploiting the dynamics of the EPR effect and strategies to improve the therapeutic effects of nanomedicines by using EPR effect enhancers. *Adv. Drug Deliv. Rev.* **2020**, *157*, 142–160. [CrossRef]
10. Taniguchi, S.; Fujimori, M.; Sasaki, T.; Tsutsui, H.; Shimatani, Y.; Seki, K.; Amano, J. Targeting solid tumors with non-pathogenic obligate anaerobic bacteria. *Cancer Sci.* **2010**, *101*, 1925–1932. [CrossRef]
11. Taniguchi, S.; Shimatani, Y.; Fujimori, M. Tumor-Targeting Therapy Using Gene-Engineered Anaerobic-Nonpathogenic Bifidobacterium longum. *Methods Mol. Biol.* **2016**, *1409*, 49–60. [PubMed]
12. Kimura, N.T.; Taniguchi, S.; Aoki, K.; Baba, T. Selective localization and growth of Bifidobacterium bifidum in mouse tumors following intravenous administration. *Cancer Res.* **1980**, *40*, 2061–2068. [PubMed]
13. Brown, J.M. The hypoxic cell: A target for selective cancer therapy—Eighteenth Bruce F. Cain Memorial Award lecture. *Cancer Res.* **1999**, *59*, 5863–5870.
14. Vaupel, P.; Höckel, M.; Mayer, A. Detection and characterization of tumor hypoxia using pO2 histography. *Antioxid Redox Signal* **2007**, *122*, 1–35. [CrossRef] [PubMed]
15. O'Connor, J.P.B.; Robinson, S.P.; Waterton, J.C. Imaging tumor hypoxia with oxygen-enhanced MRI and BOLD MRI. *Br. J. Radiol.* **2019**, *92*, 20180642. [CrossRef] [PubMed]
16. Pries, A.R.; Höpfner, M.; le Noble, F.; Dewhirst, M.W.; Secomb, T.W. The shunt problem: Control of functional shunting in normal and tumor vasculature. *Nat. Rev. Cancer* **2010**, *10*, 587–593. [CrossRef] [PubMed]
17. Malmgren, R.A.; Flanigan, C.C. Localization of the vegetative form of Clostridium tetani in mouse tumors following intravenous spore administration. *Cancer Res.* **1955**, *15*, 473–478.
18. Mowday, A.M.; Guise, C.P.; Ackerley, D.F.; Minton, N.P.; Lambin, P.; Dubois, L.J.; Theys, J.; Smaill, J.B.; Patterson, A.V. Advancing Clostridia to Clinical Trial: Past Lessons and Recent Progress. *Cancers* **2016**, *8*, 63. [CrossRef]
19. Nauts, H.C.; Swift, W.E.; Coley, B.L. The treatment of malignant tumors by bacterial toxins as developed by the late William B. Coley, M.D., reviewed in the light of modern research. *Cancer Res.* **1946**, *6*, 205–216.
20. Forbes, N.S. Engineering the perfect (bacterial) cancer therapy. *Nat. Rev. Cancer* **2010**, *10*, 785–794. [CrossRef]
21. Sarotra, P.; Medhi, B. Use of Bacteria in Cancer Therapy. *Recent Results Cancer Res.* **2016**, *209*, 111–121.
22. Hoffman, R.M. Future of Bacterial Therapy of Cancer. *Methods Mol. Biol.* **2016**, *1409*, 177–184.
23. Zhou, S.; Gravekamp, C.; Bermudes, D.; Liu, K. Tumour-targeting bacteria engineered to fight cancer. *Nat. Rev. Cancer* **2018**, *18*, 727–743. [CrossRef]
24. Toso, J.F.; Sznol, M.; Rosenberg, S.A. Phase I study of the intravenous administration of attenuated Salmonella typhimurium to patients with metastatic melanoma. *J. Clin. Oncol.* **2002**, *20*, 142–152. [CrossRef] [PubMed]
25. Roberts, N.J.; Zhang, L.; Janku, F.; Collins, A.; Bai, R.Y.; Staedtke, V.; Rusk, A.W.; Tung, D.; Miller, M.; Roix, J.; et al. Intratumoral injection of Clostridium novyi-NT spores induces antitumor responses. *Sci. Transl. Med.* **2014**, *6*, 249ra111. [CrossRef] [PubMed]
26. Nemunaitis, J.; Sznol, M. Pilot trial of genetically modified, attenuated Salmonella expressing the E. coli cytosine deaminase gene in refractory cancer patients. *Cancer Gene Ther.* **2003**, *10*, 737–744. [CrossRef]

27. Thamm, D.H.; Kurzman, I.D.; King, I.; Li, Z.; Sznol, M.; Dubielzig, R.R.; Vail, D.M.; MacEwen, E.G. Systemic administration of an attenuated, tumor-targeting Salmonella typhimurium to dogs with spontaneous neoplasia: Phase I evaluation. *Clin. Cancer Res.* **2005**, *11*, 4827–4834. [CrossRef] [PubMed]
28. Fritz, S.E.; Henson, M.S.; Greengard, E.; Winter, A.L.; Stuebner, K.M.; Yoon, U.; Wilk, V.L.; Borgatti, A.; Augustin, L.B.; Modiano, J.F.; et al. A phase I clinical study to evaluate safety of orally administered, genetically engineered *Salmonella enterica serovar Typhimurium* for canine osteosarcoma. *Vet. Med. Sci.* **2016**, *2*, 179–190. [CrossRef]
29. Fang, J.; Long, L.; Maeda, H. Enhancement of Tumor-Targeted Delivery of Bacteria with Nitroglycerin Involving Augmentation of the EPR Effect. *Methods Mol. Biol.* **2016**, *1409*, 9–23. [PubMed]
30. Fang, J.; Liao, L.; Yin, H.; Nakamura, H.; Shin, T.; Maeda, H. Enhanced bacterial tumor delivery by modulating the EPR effect and therapeutic potential of Lactobacillus casei. *J. Pharm. Sci.* **2014**, *103*, 3235–3243. [CrossRef]
31. Matsumura, H.; Takeuchi, A.; Kano, Y. Construction of *Escherichia coli-Bifidobacterium longum* shuttle vector transforming *B. longum* 105-A and 108-A. *Biosci. Biotechnol. Biochem.* **1997**, *61*, 1211–1212. [CrossRef] [PubMed]
32. Yazawa, K.; Fujimori, M.; Amano, J.; Kano, Y.; Taniguchi, S. Bifidobacterium longum as a delivery system for cancer gene therapy: Selective localization and growth in hypoxic tumors. *Cancer Gene Ther.* **2000**, *7*, 269–274. [CrossRef]
33. Yazawa, K.; Fujimori, M.; Nakamura, T.; Sasaki, T.; Amano, J.; Kano, Y.; Taniguchi, S. Bifidobacterium longum as a delivery system for gene therapy of chemically induced rat mammary tumors. *Breast Cancer Res. Treat.* **2001**, *66*, 165–170. [CrossRef] [PubMed]
34. Nakamura, T.; Sasaki, T.; Fujimori, M.; Yazawa, K.; Kano, Y.; Amano, J.; Taniguchi, S. Cloned cytosine deaminase gene expression of Bifidobacterium longum and application to enzyme/pro-drug therapy of hypoxic solid tumors. *Biosci. Biotechnol. Biochem.* **2002**, *66*, 2362–2366. [CrossRef]
35. Hidaka, A.; Hamaji, Y.; Sasaki, T.; Taniguchi, S.; Fujimori, M. Exogenous cytosine deaminase gene expression in Bifidobacterium breve I-53-8w for tumor-targeting enzyme/prodrug therapy. *Biosci. Biotechnol. Biochem.* **2007**, *71*, 2921–2926. [CrossRef]
36. Sasaki, T.; Fujimori, M.; Hamaji, Y.; Hama, Y.; Ito, K.; Amano, J.; Taniguchi, S. Genetically engineered Bifidobacterium longum for tumor-targeting enzyme-prodrug therapy of autochthonous mammary tumors in rats. *Cancer Sci.* **2006**, *97*, 649–657. [CrossRef] [PubMed]
37. Mahan, S.D.; Ireton, G.C.; Knoeber, C.; Stoddard, B.L.; Black, M.E. Random mutagenesis and selection of Escherichia coli cytosine deaminase for cancer gene therapy. *Protein. Eng. Des. Sel.* **2004**, *17*, 625–633. [CrossRef] [PubMed]
38. Kawai, T.; Akira, S. TLR signaling. *Semin. Immunol.* **2007**, *19*, 24–32. [CrossRef]
39. Taniguchi, S.; Sagara, J. Regulatory molecules involved in inflammasome formation with special reference to a key mediator protein, ASC. *Semin. Immunopathol.* **2007**, *29*, 231–238. [CrossRef]
40. Van Bergenhenegouwen, J.; Kraneveld, A.D.; Rutten, L.; Kettelarij, N.; Garssen, J.; Vos, A.P. Extracellular vesicles modulate host-microbe responses by altering TLR2 activity and phagocytosis. *PLoS ONE* **2014**, *9*, e89121.
41. Kato, K.; Odamaki, T.; Mitsuyama, E.; Sugahara, H.; Xiao, J.Z.; Osawa, R. Age-Related Changes in the Composition of Gut Bifidobacterium Species. *Curr. Microbiol.* **2017**, *74*, 987–995. [CrossRef]
42. Azad, M.B.; Konya, T.; Maughan, H.; Guttman, D.S.; Field, C.J.; Chari, R.S.; Sears, M.R.; Becker, A.B.; Scott, J.A.; Kozyrskyj, A.L. CHILD Study Investigators. Gut microbiota of healthy Canadian infants: Profiles by mode of delivery and infant diet at 4 months. *CMAJ* **2013**, *185*, 385–394. [CrossRef]
43. Matson, V.; Fessler, J.; Bao, R.; Chongsuwat, T.; Zha, Y.; Alegre, M.L.; Luke, J.J.; Gajewski, T.F. The commensal microbiome is associated with anti-PD-1 efficacy in metastatic melanoma patients. *Science* **2018**, *359*, 104–108. [CrossRef]
44. Phase I/II Study of APS001F With Flucytosine and Maltose in Solid Tumors, US National Library of Medicine, ClinicalTrials.gov. Available online: https://clinicaltrials.gov/ct2/show/NCT01562626 (accessed on 26 March 2012).
45. Gotwals, P.; Cameron, S.; Cipolletta, D.; Cremasco, V.; Crystal, A.; Hewes, B.; Mueller, B.; Quaratino, S.; Sabatos-Peyton, C.; Petruzzelli, L.; et al. Prospects for combining targeted and conventional cancer therapy with immunotherapy. *Nat. Rev. Cancer* **2017**, *17*, 286–301. [CrossRef]
46. Pardoll, D.M. The blockade of immune checkpoints in cancer immunotherapy. *Nat. Rev. Cancer* **2012**, *12*, 252–264. [CrossRef] [PubMed]
47. Vanneman, M.; Dranoff, G. Combining immunotherapy and targeted therapies in cancer treatment. *Nat. Rev. Cancer* **2012**, *12*, 237–251. [CrossRef]
48. Shioya, K.; Matsumura, T.; Seki, Y.; Shimizu, H.; Nakamura, T.; Taniguchi, S. Potentiated antitumor effects of APS001F/5-FC combined with anti-PD-1 antibody in a CT26 syngeneic mouse model. *Biosci. Biotechnol. Biochem.* **2021**, *85*, 324–331. [CrossRef]
49. Vincent, J.; Mignot, G.; Chalmin, F.; Ladoire, S.; Bruchard, M.; Chevriaux, A.; Martin, F.; Apetoh, L.; Rébé, C.; Ghiringhelli, F. 5-Fluorouracil selectively kills tumor-associated myeloid-derived suppressor cells resulting in enhanced T cell-dependent antitumor immunity. *Cancer Res.* **2010**, *70*, 3052–3061. [CrossRef] [PubMed]
50. Zitvogel, L.; Galluzzi, L.; Smyth, M.J.; Kroemer, G. Mechanisms of action conventional and targeted anticancer therapies: Reinstating immunosurveillance. *Immunity* **2013**, *39*, 74–88. [CrossRef]
51. Kadoyama, K.; Miki, I.; Tamura, T.; Brown, J.B.; Sakaeda, T.; Okuno, Y. Adverse event profiles of 5- fluorouracil and capecitabine: Data mining of the public version of the FDA adverse event reporting system, AERS, and reproducibility of clinical observations. *Int. J. Med. Sci.* **2012**, *9*, 33–39. [CrossRef] [PubMed]

52. Wu, Y.; Deng, Z.; Wang, H.; Ma, W.; Zhou, C.; Zhang, S. Repeated cycles of 5-fluorouracil chemotherapy impaired anti-tumor functions of cytotoxic T cells in a CT26 tumor-bearing mouse model. *BMC Immunol.* **2016**, *17*, 29. [CrossRef] [PubMed]
53. Bajwa, R.; Cheema, A.; Khan, T.; Amirpour, A.; Paul, A.; Chaughtai, S.; Patel, S.; Patel, T.; Bramson, J.; Gupta, V.; et al. Adverse Effects of Immune Checkpoint Inhibitors (Programmed Death-1 Inhibitors and Cytotoxic T-Lymphocyte-Associated Protein-4 Inhibitors): Results of a Retrospective Study. *J. Clin. Med. Res.* **2019**, *11*, 225–236. [CrossRef]
54. Johncilla, M.; Grover, S.; Zhang, X.; Jain, D.; Srivastava, A. Morphological spectrum of immune check-point inhibitor therapy-associated gastritis. *Histopathology* **2020**, *76*, 531–539. [CrossRef] [PubMed]
55. George, J.; Bajaj, D.; Sankaramangalam, K.; Yoo, J.W.; Joshi, N.S.; Gettinger, S.; Price, C.; Farrell, J.J. Incidence of pancreatitis with the use of immune checkpoint inhibitors (ICI) in advanced cancers: A systematic review and meta-analysis. *Pancreatology* **2019**, *19*, 587–594. [CrossRef]
56. Nemeth, B.T.; Varga, Z.V.; Wu, W.J.; Pacher, P. Trastuzumab cardiotoxicity: From clinical trials to experimental studies. *Br. J. Pharmacol.* **2017**, *174*, 3727–3748. [CrossRef]
57. Cameron, D.; Piccart-Gebhart, M.J.; Gelber, R.D.; Procter, M.; Goldhirsch, A.; de Azambuja, E.; Castro, G., Jr.; Untch, M.; Smith, I.; Gianni, L.; et al. Herceptin Adjuvant (HERA) Trial Study Team. 11 years' follow-up of trastuzumab after adjuvant chemotherapy in HER2-positive early breast cancer: Final analysis of the HERceptin Adjuvant (HERA) trial. *Lancet* **2017**, *389*, 1195–1205. [CrossRef]
58. Kikuchi, T.; Shimizu, H.; Akiyama, Y.; Taniguchi, S. In situ delivery and production system of trastuzumab scFv with Bifidobacterium. *Biochem. Biophys. Res. Commun.* **2017**, *493*, 306–312. [CrossRef]
59. Shioya, K.; Wang, L.; Matsumura, T.; Shimizu, H.; Kanari, Y.; Seki, Y.; Shimatani, Y.; Taniguchi, S. Anti-PD-1 antibody scFV producing recombinant Bifidobacterium exerts antitumor effect in a large fraction of the treated mice compared to full-length anti-PD-1 antibody. AACR Special Conference; 1–4 October 2017, Boston, USA. *Cancer Immunol. Res.* **2018**, *6*, A23.
60. Shioya, K.; Kataoka, S.; Wang, L.; Matsumura, T.; Shimizu, H.; Kanari, Y.; Seki, Y.; Shimatani, Y.; Fujimori, M.; Taniguchi, S. anti-CTLA-4 antibody scFv producing recombinant Bifidobacterium secretes CTLA-4 blocker specifically inside hypoxic tumor and suppresses tumor growth in syngeneic mice model., AACR Special Conference on Tumor Immunology and Immunotherapy; 20–23 October 2016, Boston, USA. *Cancer Immunol. Res.* **2017**, *5*, A29.
61. Matsumura, T.; Shioya, K.; Kanari, Y.; Shimatani, Y.; Kataoka, S.; Taniguchi, S.; Nakamura, T. Cancer immunotherapy with agonistic anti-4-1BB scFv producing and secreting Bifidobacterium in syngeneic mouse model., AACR Annual Meeting; 14–18 April 2018, Chicago, IL, USA. *Cancer Res.* **2018**, *78*, A2735.
62. Seki, Y.; Shioya, K.; Kobayashi, S.; Shimatani, Y.; Fujimori, M.; Taniguchi, S. Enhanced anti-tumor effects by a combination approach of interferon-producing recombinant Bifidobacterium and anti-mPD-1 antibody in syngeneic mouse model. AACR Annual Meeting, 1–5 April 2017, Washington, DC, USA. *Cancer Res.* **2017**, *77*, A2631.
63. Patent Information. Available online: https://patents.google.com/patent/WO2011093465A1/ja (accessed on 17 June 2021).
64. Van Horssen, R.; Ten Hagen, T.L.; Eggermont, A.M. TNF-alpha in cancer treatment: Molecular insights, antitumor effects, and clinical utility. *Oncologist* **2006**, *11*, 397–408. [CrossRef] [PubMed]
65. Kobayashi, S.; Shioya, K.; Yuji Seki, Y.; Matsumura, T.; Kanari, Y.; Shimatani, Y.; Nakazawa, H.; Umetsu, M.; Kataoka, S.; Nakamura, T. Anti-tumor activity of Bifidobacterium secreting dual specific T cell redirecting antibody against EGFR/HER3-expressing cancer. AACR Annual Meeting; 22–24 June 2020, Philadelphia, PA, USA. *Cancer Res.* **2020**, *80*, AS689.
66. Wei, C.; Xun, A.Y.; Wei, X.X.; Yao, J.; Wang, J.Y.; Shi, R.Y.; Yang, G.H.; Li, Y.X.; Xu, Z.L.; Lai, M.G.; et al. Bifidobacteria expressing tumstatin protein for antitumor therapy in tumor-bearing mice. *Technol. Cancer Res. Treat.* **2015**, *15*, 498–508. [CrossRef]
67. Wang, L.; Vuletic, I.; Deng, D.; Crielaard, W.; Xie, Z.; Zhou, K.; Zhang, J.; Sun, H.; Ren, Q.; Gu, C. *Bifidobacterium breve* as a delivery vector of IL-24 gene therapy for bead and neck squamous cell carcinoma in vivo. *Gene Ther.* **2017**, *24*, 699–705. [CrossRef]
68. Yasuda, H.; Yamaya, M.; Nakayama, K.; Sasaki, T.; Ebihara, S.; Kanda, A.; Asada, M.; Inoue, D.; Suzuki, T.; Okazaki, T.; et al. Randomized phase II trial comparing nitroglycerin plus vinorelbine and cisplatin with vinorelbine and cisplatin alone in previously untreated stage IIIB/IV non-small-cell lung cancer. *J. Clin. Oncol.* **2006**, *24*, 688–694. [CrossRef] [PubMed]
69. Yasuda, H.; Nakayama, K.; Watanabe, M.; Suzuki, S.; Fuji, H.; Okinaga, S.; Kanda, A.; Zayasu, K.; Sasaki, T.; Asada, M.; et al. Nitroglycerin treatment may enhance chemosensitivity to docetaxel and carboplatin in patients with lung adenocarcinoma. *Clin. Cancer Res.* **2006**, *12*, 6748–6757. [CrossRef]
70. Yasuda, H.; Yanagihara, K.; Nakayama, K.; Mio, T.; Sasaki, T.; Asada, M.; Yamaya, M.; Fukushima, M. Therapeutic applications of nitric oxide for malignant tumor in animal models and human studies. In *Nitric Oxide and Cancer*; Bonavida, B., Ed.; Springer Science: New York, NY, USA, 2009.
71. Siemens, D.R.; Heaton, J.P.; Adams, M.A.; Kawakami, J.; Graham, C.H. Phase II study of nitric oxide donor for men with increasing prostate-specific antigen level after surgery or radiotherapy for prostate cancer. *Urology* **2009**, *74*, 878–883. [CrossRef] [PubMed]
72. Tieken, C.; Versteeg, H.H. Anticoagulants versus cancer. *Thromb Res.* **2016**, *140* (Suppl. 1), S148–S153. [CrossRef]
73. Gadomska, G.; Ziołkowska, K.; Boinska, J.; Filipiak, J.; Rość, D. Activation of TF-Dependent Blood Coagulation Pathway and VEGF-A in Patients with Essential Thrombocythemia. *Medicina* **2019**, *55*, 54. [CrossRef]
74. Dvorak, H.F. Tumors: Wounds that do not heal-redux. *Cancer Immunol. Res.* **2015**, *3*, 1–11. [CrossRef]
75. Samoszuk, M.; Deng, T.; Hamamura, M.J.; Su, M.Y.; Asbrock, N.; Nalcioglu, O. Increased blood clotting, microvascular density, and inflammation in eotaxin-secreting tumors implanted into mice. *Am. J. Pathol.* **2004**, *165*, 449–456. [CrossRef]

76. Islam, M.S. Thrombolytic Therapy by Tissue Plasminogen Activator for Pulmonary Embolism. *Adv. Exp. Med. Biol.* **2017**, *906*, 67–74.
77. Cabral, H.; Matsumoto, Y.; Mizuno, K.; Chen, Q.; Murakami, M.; Kimura, M.; Terada, Y.; Kano, M.R.; Miyazono, K.; Uesaka, M.; et al. Accumulation of sub-100 nm polymeric micelles in poorly permeable tumours depends on size. *Nat. Nanotechnol.* **2011**, *6*, 815–823. [CrossRef]
78. Cesar, S.; Huang, K.C. Thinking big: The tunability of bacterial cell size. *FEMS Microbiol. Rev.* **2017**, *41*, 672–678. [CrossRef] [PubMed]
79. Tocheva, E.I.; López-Garrido, J.; Hughes, H.V.; Fredlund, J.; Kuru, E.; Vannieuwenhze, M.S.; Brun, Y.V.; Pogliano, K.; Jensen, G.J. Peptidoglycan transformations during Bacillus subtilis sporulation. *Mol. Microbiol.* **2013**, *88*, 673–686. [CrossRef]
80. Zahednezhad, F.; Saadat, M.; Valizadeh, H.; Zakeri-Milani, P.; Baradaran, B. Liposome and immune system interplay: Challenges and potentials. *J. Control. Release* **2019**, *305*, 194–209. [CrossRef]
81. Suk, J.S.; Xu, Q.; Kim, N.; Hanes, J.; Ensign, L.M. PEGylation as a strategy for improving nanoparticle-based drug and gene delivery. *Adv. Drug Deliv. Rev.* **2016**, *99*, 28–51. [CrossRef] [PubMed]
82. Scott, M.D.; Chen, A.M. Beyond the red cell: Pegylation of other blood cells and tissues. *Transfus. Clin. Biol.* **2004**, *11*, 40–46. [CrossRef] [PubMed]
83. Chen, A.M.; Scott, M.D. Current and future applications of immunological attenuation via pegylation of cells and tissue. *BioDrugs* **2001**, *15*, 833–847. [CrossRef]
84. Zuo, F.; Zeng, Z.; Hammarström, L.; Marcotte, H. Inducible Plasmid Self-Destruction (IPSD) Assisted Genome Engineering in Lactobacilli and Bifidobacteria. *ACS Synth. Biol.* **2019**, *8*, 1723–1729. [CrossRef]
85. Mruk, I.; Kobayashi, I. To be or not to be: Regulation of restriction-modification systems and other toxin-antitoxin systems. *Nucleic Acids Res.* **2014**, *42*, 70–86. [CrossRef] [PubMed]
86. Shirai, H.; Tsukada, K. Bacterial proteolytic activity improves drug delivery in tumors in a size, pharmacokinetic, and binding affinity dependent manner—A mechanistic understanding. *J. Control. Release* **2020**, *321*, 348–362. [CrossRef] [PubMed]
87. Hamley, I.W. Small Bioactive Peptides for Biomaterials Design and Therapeutics. *Chem. Rev.* **2017**, *117*, 14015–14041. [CrossRef] [PubMed]
88. Hidalgo-Cantabrana, C.; Delgado, S.; Ruiz, L.; Ruas-Madiedo, P.; Sánchez, B.; Margolles, A. Bifidobacteria and Their Health-Promoting Effects. *Microbiol. Spectr.* **2017**, *5*. [CrossRef]
89. Scheiman, J.; Luber, J.M.; Chavkin, T.A.; MacDonald, T.; Tung, A.; Pham, L.D.; Wibowo, M.C.; Wurth, R.C.; Punthambaker, S.; Tierney, B.T.; et al. Meta-omics analysis of elite athletes identifies a performance-enhancing microbe that functions via lactate metabolism. *Nat. Med.* **2019**, *25*, 1104–1109. [CrossRef]

Article

Enhanced Anticancer Activity of Nanoformulation of Dasatinib against Triple-Negative Breast Cancer

Fatemah Bahman [1], Valeria Pittalà [2,*], Mohamed Haider [3,4] and Khaled Greish [5,*]

1. Department of Molecular Genetics, Kuwait Ministry of Health, Kuwait City 50000, Kuwait; fato88.fb@gmail.com
2. Department of Drug and Health Science, University of Catania, 95125 Catania, Italy
3. Department of Pharmaceutics and Pharmaceutical Technology, College of Pharmacy, University of Sharjah, Sharjah 27272, United Arab Emirates; mhaider@sharjah.ac.ae
4. Department of Pharmaceutics and Industrial Pharmacy, Faculty of Pharmacy, Cairo University, Cairo 71526, Egypt
5. Department of Molecular Medicine and Nanomedicine Unit, Princess Al-Jawhara Center for Molecular Medicine, College of Medicine and Medical Sciences, Arabian Gulf University, Manama 329, Bahrain
* Correspondence: valeria.pittala@unict.it (V.P.); khaledfg@agu.edu.bh (K.G.); Tel.: +39-0957-738-4269 (V.P.); +973-1723-7393 (K.G.); Fax: +973-1724-6022 (K.G.)

Abstract: Triple negative breast cancer (TNBC) is the most aggressive breast cancer accounting for around 15% of identified breast cancer cases. TNBC lacks human epidermal growth factor receptor 2 (HER2) amplification, is hormone independent estrogen (ER) and progesterone receptors (PR) negative, and is not reactive to current targeted therapies. Existing treatment relies on chemotherapeutic treatment, but in spite of an initial response to chemotherapy, the inception of resistance and relapse is unfortunately common. Dasatinib is an approved second-generation inhibitor of multiple tyrosine kinases, and literature data strongly support its use in the management of TNBC. However, dasatinib binds to plasma proteins and undergoes extensive metabolism through oxidation and conjugation. To protect dasatinib from fast pharmacokinetic degradation and to prolong its activity, it was encapsulated on poly(styrene-co-maleic acid) (SMA) micelles. The obtained SMA–dasatinib nanoparticles (NPs) were evaluated for their physicochemical properties, in vitro antiproliferative activity in different TNBC cell lines, and in vivo anticancer activity in a syngeneic model of breast cancer. Obtained results showed that SMA–dasatinib is more potent against 4T1 TNBC tumor growth in vivo compared to free drug. This enhanced effect was ascribed to the encapsulation of the drug protecting it from a rapid metabolism. Our finding highlights the often-overlooked value of nanoformulations in protecting its cargo from degradation. Overall, results may provide an alternative therapeutic strategy for TNBC management.

Keywords: TNBC; dasatinib; poly(styrene-co-maleic acid) micelles; nanoformulation; metabolism; EPR; nanomedicine; targeted therapy

1. Introduction

Breast cancers are the top widespread type of tumor among females in the U.S., and in 2021, it is predicted that 280,000 new breast cancers will be diagnosed [1,2]. The disease is globally affecting about 1 in 8 women in the U.S. during their lifetime. Breast cancer mortality could be attributed to metastasis by 80–90% [3].

Triple negative breast cancer (TNBC) is a long-lasting orphan disease and among the most clinically challenging breast cancer subtype. TNBC is the most aggressive and heterogeneous breast tumor that lacks all of three therapeutically relevant biomarkers including estrogen receptor (ER), progesterone receptor (PR), and human epidermal growth factor receptor 2 (HER2) [4]. The conventional treatment for TNBC involves surgical excision and radiotherapy with a combination of adjuvant chemotherapies [5,6]. Despite current therapeutic regimens, patients affected by TNBC show frequently fatal prognosis and are exposed to early relapse and metastatic spread, as a result of resistance to chemotherapies [5]. Despite initially TNBC exhibiting more chemo-sensitivity than other groups of breast cancer, it shows high propensity to spread and metastasize to vital organs, for instance the lungs and brain, rendering the survival rate still significantly lower than patients with non TNBC across any phase of diagnosis [7–9]. These aggressive phenotypes can be at least to some extent ascribed to the incidence of breast cancer stem cells (BCSCs). In addition, the lack of targeted therapies increases the use of traditional chemotherapy often accompanied by severe side effects. The subclassification of TNBC based on gene expression profiling analysis includes basal like 1 (BL1) and basal like 2 (BL2), immunomodulatory (IM), mesenchymal (M), mesenchymal stem like (MSL), and luminal androgen receptor positive (LAR) [10–12]. This classification is paving the way to the identification of more specific molecular targets for TNBC treatment. In fact, these subtypes show different drug sensitivity profiles to anticancer treatments such as cisplatin for BL1 and BL2, PI3K, and proto-oncogene tyrosine-protein kinase (Src) inhibitors [13].

Src is a protein tyrosine kinase that regulates various cancerous events at an intracellular level, such as cellular adhesion, invasion, growth, survival, and vascular endothelial growth factor (VEGF) expression [14,15]. In addition, Src regulates an osteoclast function in normal bone and bone metastases [16]. A number of literature reports have evidenced in TNBC an abnormal activation and amplification of Src or Src-family kinases (SFK) and an involvement in metastasis regulation [17]. Not surprisingly, TNBC shows increased sensitivity to Src inhibitors compared to other cancer subgroups [18–20]. In addition, it has been demonstrated that ER and HER2 expression levels affect the beneficial effects of Src inhibitors in TNBC [21]. Therefore, Src can be considered as a new molecular target for TNBC therapy, and Src inhibitors have long been proposed as new antitumoral treatments, since they are able to prevent cell growth in liver, colon, breast, and ovarian cancers.

Dasatinib (Figure 1) is a Src, BCR-ABL, c-KIT, PDGFR-α and PDGFR-β, and ephrin receptor kinase blockers accepted by the Food and Drug Administration (FDA) for treating cases of Philadelphia chromosome positive leukemias (chronic myeloid leukemia; CML) [22,23]. Preclinical studies demonstrated significant inhibition of malignant breast cells growth through reducing the percentage of aldehyde dehydrogenase-positive (ALDH+) BCSCs within the BL-2 subtype of breast cancer [13,24]. Considering that BCSCs are often responsible for the onset of chemotherapy resistance, dasatinib has been considered for the treatment of TNBC [24,25]. Similarly, preclinical studies evidenced synergistic or additive dasatinib activity with chemotherapy, implying that this Src inhibitor can offer clinical benefit in TNBC [26]. Regrettably, patients suffering from TNBC have inadequate benefit from Src inhibitors treatment [27–29]. In fact, despite promising preclinical results, a phase II clinical trial by administering dasatinib as a single agent highlighted only a 9% clinical benefit rate, and other clinical trials terminated due to futility (e.g., NCT00817531, NCT00780676, etc.) [29]. Moreover, dasatinib suffers from some limitations related to its pharmacokinetic profile. Oral absorption of dasatinib is quick and produces around 80% of bioavailability; however, it is rapidly eliminated through CYP3A4-mediated metabolism, with a $T_{1/2}$ of 3–4 h. In addition, dasatinib bioavailability has reduced the its ability to modify gastric pH value (antacids, H_2-receptor blockers, proton pump inhibitors) and is modified according to the concomitant treatment with CYP3A4 inducers or inhibitors [30].

In recent years, considerable attention has been devoted to strategic application of nanoscience to pharmaceutical development with the aim of improving efficacy, delivery at the site of action, safety, physicochemical properties, and the absorption, distribution, metabolism, and excretion (ADME) profile of bioactive compounds [31]. In particular, nanoparticle formulations (NPs) can guarantee increased bioavailability of drugs administered orally, enhanced half-life of intravenous drugs (by reducing both metabolism and elimination), and augmented drug concentration in specific tissues [32]. Taking in account the dasatinib ADME profile, encapsulation of the drug into NPs may improve the drug efficacy, minimize side effects, and permit the active principle to assemble at the malignant tumor site by means of the enhanced permeability and retention (EPR) effect [33,34]. In addition, using the SMA micellar system to generate dasatinib NPs has multiple advantages over other nanoformulations. It produces a micelle with a nearly neutral or slightly negative charge reducing opsonization of the micelles, recognition by the reticuloendothelial system, and elimination from the blood circulation [35]. In our previous work utilizing dasatinib micelles compared to free drug, we had shown enhanced anticancer activity both in vitro and in vivo against various glioblastoma cell lines and in animal model of the disease [36]. In this study, we encapsulated dasatinib into polystyrene co-melic acid (SMA) micelles to generate micellar dasatinib system (SMA–dasatinib) that has been characterized for physicochemical properties including size, loading, charge, and release rate. In addition, SMA–dasatinib has been assessed for their anticancer effect in vitro using 4T1, MDA-MB-231, and MCF-7 cell lines and in vivo in a syngenic model of TNBC. The cell lines chosen represents a spectrum of commonly used breast cancer cell lines of both hormonal responsive and TNBC of human and murine origin. Our choice of cell lines will allow the comparison of dasatinib formulation in different biological environments and further allows the comparison of our results to earlier and subsequent research in the field. Encouraging obtained results will pave the way for further study in the management of TNBC.

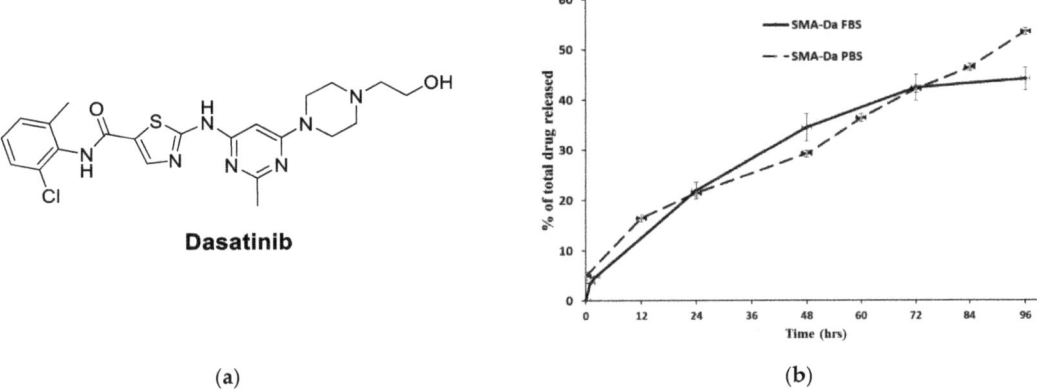

Figure 1. (a) Chemical structure of dasatinib; (b) SMA–dasatinib drug release studies. Cumulative release of the free drug from SMA–dasatinib micelles at pH 7.4 in PBS and FBS.

2. Materials and Methods

Dasatinib were retained from LC Laboratories (Woburn, MA, USA). Polystyrene co-maleic anhydride (molecular weight~1600), Roswell Park Memorial Institute (RPMI) 1640 medium, Hank's balanced salt solution, fetal bovine serum (FBS), bovine serum albumin (BSA), and TrypLE express were bought from ThermoFisher Scientific (Dubai, United Arab Emirates). N-(3-dimethylaminopropyl)-N-ethylcarbodiimide hydrochloride (EDAC), L-glutamine, antibiotic solution of penicillin/streptomycin were acquired from (Merck Hertfordshire, UK). All consumable materials including petri dishes, conical tubes (15 mL and 50 mL), cell culture flasks (25 and 75 cm^2), and dialysis tubing were purchased from (Merck Hertfordshire, UK).

2.1. SMA–Dasatinib Micelles Synthesis

SMA–micelles were synthesized as previously reported [36]. Briefly, SMA was hydrolyzed by adding the SMA powder to 1 M NaOH solution at 70 °C to reach a concentration of 10 mg/mL. After this time, the pH of the obtained solution of SMA was adjusted to pH 5.0. This was followed by adding EDAC (1:1 weight ratio with SMA). Dasatinib was dissolved in dimethyl sulfoxide (DMSO) at 25% weigh ratio to SMA. Dasatinib was added to the solution, and pH was kept at 5 by adding 0.1 HCL until pH remained stable at 5.0. Then, the pH was raised up to reach 11.0 and kept until it become stable. The pH was then dropped to 7.4, and the solution was filtered 4 times by meand of a Millipore Labscale TFF system with a Pellicon XL 10 KDa cutoff membrane. Finally, the concentrated SMA–dasatinib micelles were frozen at −80 °C and the following day lyophilized (5 mTorr and −52 °C) to achieve a stable SMA–dasatinib powder.

2.2. SMA–Dasatinib Micelles Characterization

The SMA micelles loading was determined by using three different samples of 1.0 mg/mL of SMA–dasatinib micelles dissolved in DMSO for measuring absorbance at 320 nm of dasatinib to a previously prepared standard curve of the drug intending to determine the ratio between the micelle and the loaded dasatinib.

For size distribution and zeta potential determination of SMA–dasatinib micelles, a Malvern ZEN3600 Zetasizer Nano series was used (Malvern Instruments Inc., Westborough, MA, USA) by using 1 mg/mL of the SMA–dasatinib nanomicelles dissolved in both double DW as a solvent for size measurement or for charge measurement. Then, to measure the release rate of free drug (dasatinib) from SMA micellar system, two separate experiments have been performed by measuring the release in PBS and in FBS. A 2 mg of the SMA–dasatinib were dissolved in 2 mL of PBS or FBS, respectively, and inserted into a 10 kDa cutoff dialysis membrane that was flooded in 20 mL of PBS or FBS for 72 h. At specified time points, the surrounding water was collected from outside the dialysis bag and replaced with PBS or FBS, and the absorbance was measured at 320 nm.

2.3. Cell Culture

The cell lines 4T1, MDA-MB-231, and MCF-7 were obtained from American Type Culture Collection (ATCC) (Manassas, VA, USA). RPMI medium supplemented with 5% fetal bovine serum (FBS) was used to culture the cell lines while being maintained in a humidified atmosphere at 37 °C, 5% CO_2.

In Vitro Anti-Proliferative Effect of Dasatinib and SMA–Dasatinib Micelles

Cells were seeded in 96-well plates (density: 4T1 5×10^3, MDA-MB-231 5×10^3, MCF-7 5×10^3 cells/well, respectively) and incubated for 24 h at 37 °C in 5% CO_2 and then treated with a different of concentrations of dasatinib 0 to 10 µM) or SMA–dasatinib (0 to 10 µM). The cytotoxicity was assessed after 48 h incubation using a sulforhodamine B (SRB) assay, as described previously [37]. Free SMA and DMSO at concentrations equivalent to that used for testing dasatinib were used as controls. Cells were fixed using 10% trichloroacetic acid and stained with SRB. The cytotoxicity experiments were performed in triplicate ($n = 3$). Then, the 50% growth inhibition (IC_{50}) was assessed by using SRB assay after 48 h incubation. HepG-2 cells also were seeded at a density of 50,000 cells/cm^2 onto a 25 cm^2 flask. Then, cells were treated by various concentration of dasatinib and SMA–dasatinib. Twenty-four hours after incubation, the supernatants were collected and diluted accordingly to retreat 4T1 cells. Data were represented as mean ± SD of three independent experiments of each cell lines.

2.4. Effect of Dasatinib and DMA-Dasatinib Treatment in In Vivo Syngeneic Model

The Laboratory Animal Care Facility of the Arabian Gulf University (AGU), Bahrain, supplied the Female Balb/c mice (6–12 weeks old, mean weight 20–25 gm). Animals were maintained under standard conditions such as controlled temperature (25 °C), a 12 h photoperiod, and had access to food and drinking water ad libitum. All animal experiments were performed based on the rules and regulations of AGU Animal Care Policy and approved by the Research and Ethics Committee, REC approval No: G- E003-PI-04/17.

To propagate the tumor, female Balb/c mice ($n = 3$) were treated subcutaneously with 1 million 4T1 mammary carcinoma cells in both sides (right and left side) of the mice back. The tumor then was collected and cut down into small pieces of average size 1–3 mm^3 in sterile PBS to sustain tumor viability. Following this, 5 mice of each group were cleanshaven, anesthetized, and injected with one small piece of the 4T1 tumor tissue subcutaneously. When the tumors reached 100 mm^3 in size, mice were casually divided into three groups $n = 5$ in each group (negative control, dasatinib, and SMA–dasatinib) subjected to drug treatment. Dasatinib was given once at a dose of 5 mg/kg via the tail vein, whereas SMA–dasatinib at a dose of 5 mg/kg (dasatinib equivalent dose) dissolved in PBS was given by IV injection. The first day of drug treatment was established as day 0. Tumor volume was measured by manual caliper; the size was assessed by using this formula:

$$V (mm^3) = ((\text{transverse section (W)})^2 \times \text{longitudinal cross section (L)})/ 2).$$

Tumor sizes were normalized by using the original tumor measure and represented as mean ± standard error of the mean (SEM). Additionally, the body weight of mice was estimated every day and normalized daily for 10 days.

2.5. In Vivo Biodistribution of Dasatinib and SMA–Dasatinib

Cells of 4T1 were injected into female Balb/c mice, bilaterally on the flanks to obtain 1–3 mm^3 tumor size. When cancer volume reached 100 mm^3, mice were casually divided into 2 groups (4 mice per group). Mice were injected with both dasatinib or the equivalent in SMA–dasatinib at 50 mg/kg via the tail vein. Mice were sacrificed 24 h after drugs injection and different organs were collected. Organs such as heart, lungs, liver, spleen, kidneys, and tumor tissue were examined for dasatinib content. SMA–dasatinib was taken out using the method reported earlier [38]. In brief, organs were crushed, weighed, and snap-frozen before pulverization. Obtained frozen tissue powder (1 mg) was treated with 67% ethanol and 1 mL of HCl 4M. The suspension was incubated at 70 °C for 30 min, sonicated, and centrifuged to take out dasatinib from tissue samples. Dasatinib amount was measured by absorbance at 332 nm and compared to a dasatinib calibration curve. The amount of dasatinib was standardized to the weight of tissue and to the whole weight of the organs from which it was extracted.

2.6. Statistical Analysis

The data from both experiments in vitro and in vivo were evaluated using GraphPad prism software. Tumor size measurements are expressed as group means ± SEM in the treatment groups. Cytotoxicity experiments with dasatinib and SMA–dasatinib are reported as means ± SD. The statistical significance of difference between groups were performed using a two-tailed t-test. Statistical differences were considered significant if the *p*-value was <0.05.

3. Results

3.1. Synthesis and Characterization of SMA–Dasatinib

SMA–dasatinib was synthesized and characterized by a low critical micelle concentration (CMC), as previously described [36]. Furthermore, the structural variation of hydrophobic styrene and hydrophilic maleic groups stimulates the quick construction of SMA micelles and facilitates the encapsulation of dasatinib. The loading of SMA–dasatinib was 11.5%, calculated as the weight ratio of the dasatinib over the total amount of SMA micelle weight. Micelles average size measuring showed that SMA–dasatinib micelles were 198 nm and had a polydispersity index (PDI) of 0.17, which was determined by dynamic light scattering (DLS). As shown in Table 1, the zeta potential of SMA–dasatinib is near neutral with a value of 0.0035 mV, which can sustain the micelle in the blood circulation for a long time by lowering the clearance by the reticuloendothelial system and allows accumulation in the tumor [39].

Table 1. Characterization of SMA–dasatinib [1].

Micelle	Recovery	Loading (wt./wt.)	Size (nm)	PDI [2]	Zeta Potential (mV)
SMA–dasatinib	65%	11.5%	198	0.17	−0.0035

[1] Data are shown as mean values ± standard deviation (SD). Values are the mean of triplicate experiments; [2] PDI = polydispersity index.

Thus, the average size of SMA–dasatinib is within the size range to facilitate its accumulation in tumor tissue by the effect of enhanced permeability and retention (EPR) [40]. Moreover, the release rate of the drug from the micelles was more efficient in an environment mimicking extracellular pH than in the blood (53 vs. 44%) following 96 h incubation).

The release of dasatinib from SMA micelles was assessed at physiological pH 7.4 in PBS and FBS, respectively, for 96 h (Figure 1). The SMA–dasatinib micelles were stable in solution with about half of the formulation released after 96 h. Moreover, in the first 2 h, the cumulative release was around 5%, as shown in Figure 1. The stability of the micellar system depends on the slow release in the blood circulation, which promotes the SMA–dasatinib accumulation at the tumor site through the EPR effect. A previous study has demonstrated the endocytosis of SMA micelle through caveolin-1 [41]. Therefore, SMA–dasatinib will be internalized by endocytosis and the release of dasatinib into the TNBC tumor cells.

3.2. Cytotoxicity of Dasatinib and SMA–Dasatinib versus Breast Cancer Cell Lines

The assessment of the cytotoxic effect of SMA–dasatinib and dasatinib on cell viability was achieved using different breast cancer cell lines, such as human MDA-MB-231, 4T1, and MCF-7 cells. A cell's cytotoxicity of dasatinib and SMA–dasatinib was determined by means of the SRB assay. Equivalent concentrations of free SMA and DMSO were used to dissolve the dasatinib and yielded no cytotoxic effect.

The treatment of MCF-7 cells (Figure 2A and Table 2) evidenced that either dasatinib and SMA–dasatinib showed no noteworthy difference in their cytotoxic activity after 48 h incubation and both displayed an $IC_{50} > 10$ µM. An IC_{50} value of 6.1 ± 2.2 µM was obtained for the dasatinib treatment of MDA-MB-231 cells, while SMA–dasatinib exhibited an IC_{50} value of 8.16 ± 3.1 µM (Figure 2B and Table 2). An enhanced effect could be partially attributed to greater internalization capability of MDA-MB-231 cells compared to MCF-7 cells [26].

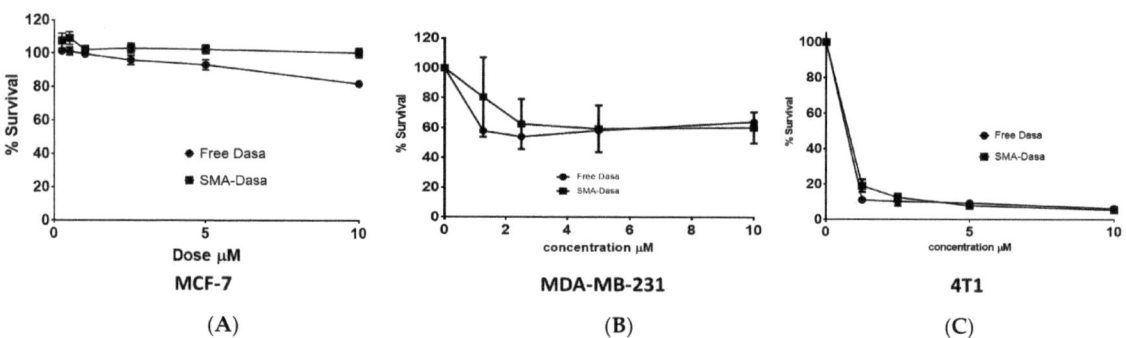

Figure 2. Cytotoxicity of dasatinib and SMA–dasatinib (**A**) against MCF-7, (**B**) MDA-MB-231, (**C**) and 4T1 cells. The cells were treated for 72 h with specific concentrations of dasatinib and SMA–dasatinib micelles. The cell number was determined using the SRB assay. Data are expressed as mean ± SEM ($n = 3$).

Table 2. Experimental IC_{50} values (μM) of free dasatinib and SMA–dasatinib towards human MDA-MB-231, 4T1, and MCF-7 cells.

Cell Line	IC_{50} (μM) [1,2]	
	Dasatinib	SMA–Dasatinib
MCF7	>10	>10
MDA-MB-231	6.1 ± 2.2	8.16 ± 3.1
4T1	0.014 ± 0.003	0.083 ± 0.01
Hep-G2	>10	>10
4T1 after Hep-G2	0.21 ± 0.04	0.09 ± 0.012

[1] IC_{50} value determination was performed using GraphPad Prism. Data are reported as IC_3 values in μM ± standard deviation (SD). Values are the mean of triplicate experiments. [2] The IC_{50} value calculations were calculated according to GraphPad prism algorithm and were included to have a numerical reference value of comparison, although it is clear that a plateau is reached after certain concentrations in MCF-7 and MDA-MB 231 cell lines.

Both MDA-MB-231 and MCF-7 reached a plateau, which can be explained by the inherent dependence of the breast cancer cell lines on tyrosine kinases signaling for growth and division. Cells of 4T1 treated with free dasatinib and SMA–dasatinib showed a significant cytotoxic effect when compared to MCF-7 and MDA-MB-231 cells with IC_{50} of 0.014 ± 0.003 and 0.083 ± 0.01 μM, respectively (Figure 2C and Table 2).

3.3. Effect of Dasatinib and SMA–Dasatinib on the Development of 4T1 Tumors

The anticancer activity of dasatinib and SMA–dasatinib was evaluated using Balb/c mice harboring 4T1 tumor over a treatment period of 10 days. Figure 3A shows that during the first days' treatment with free dasatinib (5 mg/kg) tumor growth seems to be delayed, while overall tumor size did not change significantly after 10 days in comparison to control-treated mice. Very differently, treatment with SMA–dasatinib almost entirely stopped the tumor growth for the duration of the study.

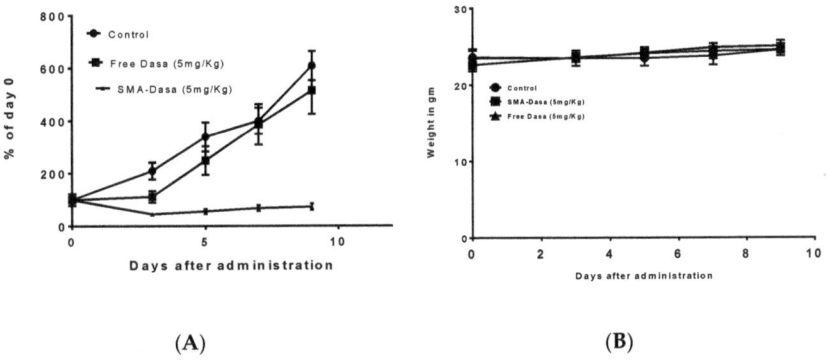

(A)   (B)

Figure 3. In vivo antitumor activity of dasatinib and SMA–dasatinib on 4T1 tumor bearing Balb/c mice. Mice were treated for 10 days with single dose of either dasatinib 5 mg/kg and SMA–dasatinib 5 mg/kg. Control group was injected with PBS (pH 7.4). Tumor volume changes (**A**) and body weight changes (**B**) were monitored over the treatment period. Data are presented as the mean of triplicate experiments ± standard error.

The therapeutic efficacy of dasatinib and SMA–dasatinib treatments were not associated with any statistically significant weight loss during the treatment period, as shown in Figure 3B and Table 3.

Table 3. Body weight changes upon treatment with dasatinib and SMA–dasatinib were monitored over the treatment period [1].

Day	Control	Dasatinib	SMA–Dasatinib
0	23.5	23.5	22.6
9	24.6	25.1	24.6
Mean weight	23.8	24.2	23.9
Std. deviation	0.4637	0.7537	0.7987

[1] Data are presented as the mean of triplicate experiments ± standard error.

3.4. In Vivo Biodistribution of Dasatinib and SMA–Dasatinib

The biodistribution of dasatinib and SMA–dasatinib were measured in vivo; to this extent, immunocompetent Balb/c mice harboring 4 T1 tumors were intravenously injected with equivalent doses of dasatinib or SMA–dasatinib, and the concentration of dasatinib in various organs and tumor has been measured. As reported in Figure 4, dasatinib and SMA–dasatinib are distributed to the heart, liver, lung, kidney, and spleen. There was an increased accumulation of dasatinib following SMA–dasatinib injection in the spleen, kidney, and lung when compared to the free dasatinib injection (Figure 4A). No significant statistical difference was observed in the heart and liver. Additionally, in the tumor when comparing SMA–dasatinib to the free dasatinib injection (Figure 4B), no statistically significant difference was observed.

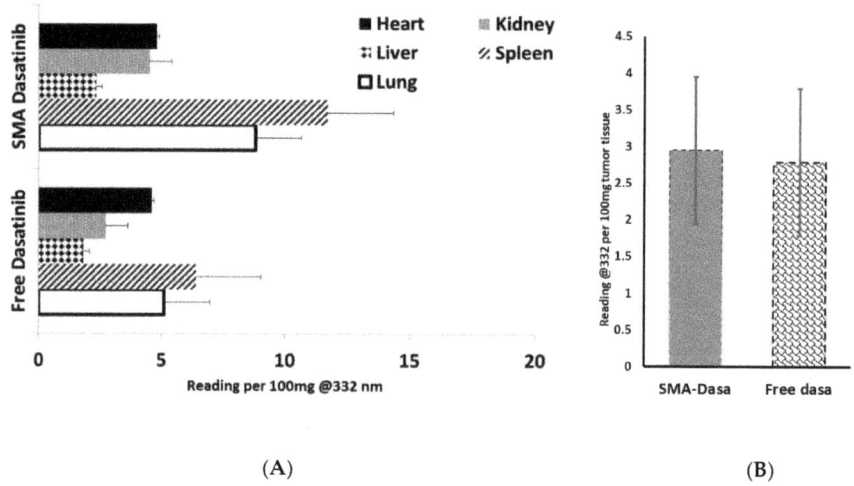

Figure 4. (**A**) Tissue and (**B**) tumor distribution of free dasatinib and SMA–dasatinib at 24 h after intravenous injection of dasatinib or SMA–dasatinib (50 mg/kg) to Balb/c mice bearing 4T1 tumors (n = 5). Representation of the relative content of dasatinib per 100 mg tissue expressed in free and micellar dasatinib.

3.5. Cytotoxicity of Dasatinib and SMA–Dasatinib Versus HepG2 Cell Line and 4T1 after Passage in HepG2

The effect of SMA–dasatinib and dasatinib on HepG2 cell viability was assessed by using SRB assay. HepG2 cells upon treatment with dasatinib and SMA–dasatinib micelles did not show any significant toxicity (Figure 5A) after 48 h incubation and both displayed an IC_{50} > 10 µM (Table 2). However, when the supernatants obtained from HepG2 treatment with dasatinib and SMA–dasatinib, respectively, were added to 4T1 cells the correspondent IC_{50s} varied noticeably. While the SMA–dasatinib cytotoxicity did not change (IC_{50} = 0.09 vs. 0.083 µM, respectively, Table 2); dasatinib cytotoxicity resulted in a 15-fold decrease in cytotoxicity (IC_{50} = 0.21 vs. 0.014 µM, respectively, Table 2).

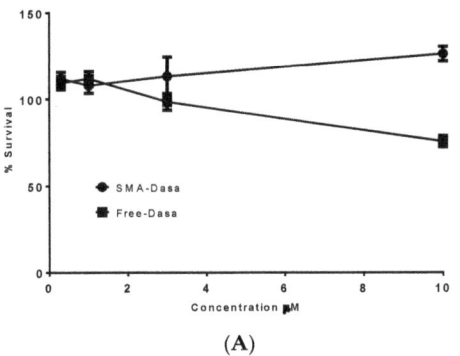 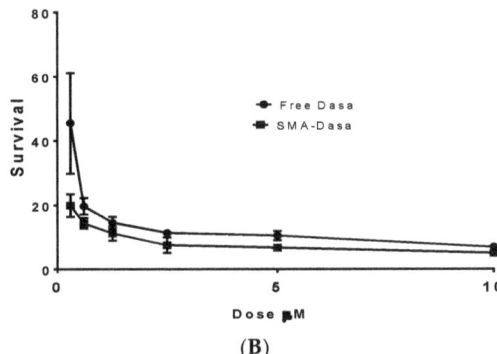

(A)   (B)

Figure 5. Cytotoxicity of dasatinib and SMA–dasatinib (**A**) against HepG2 cells, (**B**) 4T1 cells after treatment with HepG2. The cells were treated for 48 h with specific concentrations of dasatinib and SMA–dasatinib micelles. The cell number was determined using the SRB assay. Data are expressed as mean ± SEM (n = 8).

4. Discussion

Dasatinib is a multi-target kinase inhibitor, including BCR/ABL kinases and Src family kinases (SFK) that are closely linked to multiple signal pathways that regulate proliferation, invasion, survival, metastasis, and angiogenesis [42]. Dasatinib showed promising results in the treatment of TNBC as a single agent or as a neoadjuvant; nevertheless, its use is limited by its poor aqueous solubility (6.49×10^{-4} mg/mL). Moreover, after oral administration, dasatinib is subjected to extensive first pass metabolism, where multiple CYP enzymes appear to have the potential to metabolize the drug [43]. Our current work aims at encapsulating dasatinib into SMA micelles to generate an SMA–dasatinib micellar system that can improve its solubility in water, protect the drug against enzymatic degradation, potentiate its chemotherapeutic effect, and minimize the rate of drug resistance.

The characterization of SMA–dasatinib micelles showed successful encapsulation of the drug with a loading capacity of 11.5%. Given that effective molecular size for EPR is 20–200 nm, the micellar size of 198 nm favors the accumulation of the nanoparticles in the tumor cells. In addition, the particle size of the prepared drug-loaded micelles should improve their circulation time and extend their plasma half-life by avoiding their rapid elimination from the kidney. The surface charge of the obtained prepared SMA–dasatinib micelles was almost neutrall, which is desirable to limit their interaction with active plasma constituents such as complement system and coagulation factors. Further, a near neutral charge will ensure selective EPR-based extravasation through tumor vasculature with minimal interaction with normal endothelial cell membrane. The micellar formulations showed a sustained slow-release rate of the drug for 96 h in both PBS and FBS (Figure 2), which shows that they can function as a reservoir for delivering a consistent level of dasatinib once concentrated extracellularly at tumor tissues and, hence, prolong the exposure of tumor cells to effective doses of the drug.

The examination of dasatinib-induced inhibition of metabolic activity on three commonly studied TNBC cell lines showed different responses. The MCF7 cell line was the least sensitive to treatment with SMA–dasatinib and free drug ($IC_{50} > 10$ μM) compared to MDA-MB-231 (IC_{50} 8.16 and 6.1 μM, respectively). This correlates with previous studies, which suggested that MDA-MB-231 are more sensitive due to the presence of active ABL kinase and their greater drug internalization capacity [26,44]. The 4T1 cell line exhibited a significantly high sensitivity to dasatinib and SMA–dasatinib (IC_{50} = 0.014 and 0.083 μM, respectively) compared to MDA-MB-231 and MCF7, which may be due to their sensitivity to Src (Kin-2) receptor tyrosine kinase blockade [45]. Interestingly, there was no significant difference in the cytotoxic effect of the SMA–dasatinib and the free drug on the different types of TNBC cell lines in vitro. Nevertheless, Figure 4 showed that treatment with SMA–dasatinib significantly inhibited the tumor growth in vivo compared to animals treated with the free drug. Both treatments resulted in no significant weight loss in treated animals, indicating that it is relatively safe to use dasatinib and SMA–dasatinib micelles in this animal model.

The biodistribution after IV administration showed a significantly high accumulation of SMA–dasatinib in the spleen compared to the free drug. This could possibly be due to the fact the size of SMA–dasatinib micelles is larger than the fenestration of the liver vasculature, which can reduce the hepatic uptake of the micelles and may decrease the metabolism of the drug. On the other hand, there was no significant difference between the tumor distribution of dasatinib and SMA–dasatinib. Dasatinib is characterized by a large volume of distribution and human plasma protein binding. In vitro studies showed that plasma protein binding of dasatinib can reach 96%, creating a depot from which the drug slowly releases its free form. It may also increase the molecular size of the drug and enhance its accumulation at the tumor site by EPR effect similar to SMA–dasatinib [46].

Treatment of HepG2 cells with dasatinib and SMA–dasatinib micelles did not show significant toxicity ($IC_{50} > 10$ µM). This is probably due to low expression levels of Src kinase, which reduced the sensitivity of the cell line to the drug [42]. The passage of dasatinib and SMA–dasatinib through HepG2 before treatment of 4T1 cells was carried out to check the effect of metabolism on the cytotoxic ability of the treatments. Dasatinib is significantly metabolized by CYP3A4 in the liver generating an active metabolite with similar potency to the drug; however, it represents only 5% of dasatinib in plasma. The co-administration of potent CYP3A4 inducer results in a considerable reduction on Cmax and AUC of the drug [43]. Treatment of 4T1 cells with supernatants obtained from HepG2 treatment showed a significant decrease in cytotoxicity of the free dasatinib, while the cytotoxic effect of SMA–dasatinib remained unchanged. The encapsulation of dasatinib offered protection for the drug against enzymatic degradation. The size of the produced micelles enhanced its accumulation at the tumor site by EPR effect and reduced its liver uptake. Our work is an emphasis of the overlooked advantage of nano-delivery systems in terms of cargo protection against degradation. This potential advantage was first described by Maeda back in 1991 [47]. Neocarzinostatin (NCS) is a very potent anticancer pretentious agent; however, NCS half-life is almost 1.9 min in tested mice. Using the nanoformulation of SMANCS protected the drug from the proteolytic activities in the plasma as well as extending its half-life by one order of magnitude. Further, this early work proved the safety of clinical use of SMA as a polymeric carrier for various biological payloads. Overall, our work further emphasizes the metabolic advantages of SMA–dasatinib nanosystems with a potential application for treating TNBC.

5. Conclusions

In this work, we have successfully synthesized and characterized an SMA nanomicellar system encapsulating the TKI dasatinib. Both the free drug and its nanoformulation have shown comparable cytotoxic activity in vitro against an array of breast cancer cell lines. The TKI and its nanoformulation proved to be more effective against TNBC cell lines compared to a hormone-sensitive cell line. In an animal model of 4T1 TNBC, the nanoformulations was about seven-fold more effective in controlling 4T1 implanted tumors. This pronounced in vivo activity was attributed to the protection of an SMA micellar system of TKI from the enzymatic degradation. Overall, our work can renew the interest in dasatinib as an effective treatment modality against TNBC.

Author Contributions: Conceptualization, funding acquisition, project administration, supervision, writing—review and editing, K.G.; methodology, validation, F.B.; software, formal analysis, data curation, writing—original draft preparation, supervision, writing—review and editing, M.H. and V.P. All authors have read and agreed to the published version of the manuscript.

Funding: This research was funded by Arabian Gulf University Research grant to KG, grant No: G003-PI-04/17.

Institutional Review Board Statement: The study was conducted according to the guidelines of the Declaration of Helsinki and approved by the Research and Ethics Committee of Arabian Gulf university, approval No E003-PI-04/17 approved on 11 December 2017 and extended to November 2022.

Data Availability Statement: The data presented in this study are available on request from the corresponding authors.

Acknowledgments: We sincerely acknowledge the technical support of Reem Al Zahrani and Sebastian Taurin.

Conflicts of Interest: The authors declare no conflict of interest.

References

1. Siegel, R.L.; Miller, K.D.; Fuchs, H.E.; Jemal, A. Cancer Statistics, 2021. *CA A Cancer J. Clin.* **2021**, *71*, 7–33. [CrossRef]
2. Bray, F.; Ferlay, J.; Soerjomataram, I.; Siegel, R.L.; Torre, L.A.; Jemal, A. Global cancer statistics 2018: GLOBOCAN estimates of incidence and mortality worldwide for 36 cancers in 185 countries. *CA A Cancer J. Clin.* **2018**, *68*, 394–424. [CrossRef]
3. Chaffer, C.L.; Weinberg, R.A. A Perspective on Cancer Cell Metastasis. *Science* **2011**, *331*, 1559. [CrossRef]
4. Hubalek, M.; Czech, T.; Müller, H. Biological Subtypes of Triple-Negative Breast Cancer. *Breast Care* **2017**, *12*, 8–14. [CrossRef]
5. Waks, A.G.; Winer, E.P. Breast Cancer Treatment: A Review. *JAMA* **2019**, *321*, 288–300. [CrossRef] [PubMed]
6. Yagata, H.; Kajiura, Y.; Yamauchi, H. Current strategy for triple-negative breast cancer: Appropriate combination of surgery, radiation, and chemotherapy. *Breast Cancer* **2011**, *18*, 165–173. [CrossRef] [PubMed]
7. Anders, C.; Carey, L.A. Understanding and treating triple-negative breast cancer. *Oncology (Williston Park)* **2008**, *22*, 1233–1239, discussion 1239–1240, 1243. [PubMed]
8. Yin, L.; Duan, J.-J.; Bian, X.-W.; Yu, S.-c. Triple-negative breast cancer molecular subtyping and treatment progress. *Breast Cancer Res.* **2020**, *22*, 61. [CrossRef] [PubMed]
9. Yao, Y.; Chu, Y.; Xu, B.; Hu, Q.; Song, Q. Risk factors for distant metastasis of patients with primary triple-negative breast cancer. *Biosci. Rep.* **2019**, *39*. [CrossRef] [PubMed]
10. McLaughlin, R.P.; He, J.; van der Noord, V.E.; Redel, J.; Foekens, J.A.; Martens, J.W.M.; Smid, M.; Zhang, Y.; van de Water, B. A kinase inhibitor screen identifies a dual cdc7/CDK9 inhibitor to sensitise triple-negative breast cancer to EGFR-targeted therapy. *Breast Cancer Res.* **2019**, *21*, 77. [CrossRef]
11. Wang, D.-Y.; Jiang, Z.; Ben-David, Y.; Woodgett, J.R.; Zacksenhaus, E. Molecular stratification within triple-negative breast cancer subtypes. *Sci. Rep.* **2019**, *9*, 19107. [CrossRef]
12. Perou, C.M. Molecular stratification of triple-negative breast cancers. *Oncologist* **2010**, *15* (Suppl. 5), 39–48. [CrossRef]
13. Lehmann, B.D.; Bauer, J.A.; Chen, X.; Sanders, M.E.; Chakravarthy, A.B.; Shyr, Y.; Pietenpol, J.A. Identification of human triple-negative breast cancer subtypes and preclinical models for selection of targeted therapies. *J. Clin. Investig.* **2011**, *121*, 2750–2767. [CrossRef]
14. Yeatman, T.J. A renaissance for SRC. *Nat. Rev. Cancer* **2004**, *4*, 470–480. [CrossRef]
15. Finn, R.S. Targeting Src in breast cancer. *Ann. Oncol.* **2008**, *19*, 1379–1386. [CrossRef]
16. Araujo, J.; Logothetis, C. Targeting Src signaling in metastatic bone disease. *Int. J. Cancer* **2009**, *124*, 1–6. [CrossRef] [PubMed]
17. Thakur, R.; Trivedi, R.; Rastogi, N.; Singh, M.; Mishra, D.P. Inhibition of STAT3, FAK and Src mediated signaling reduces cancer stem cell load, tumorigenic potential and metastasis in breast cancer. *Sci. Rep.* **2015**, *5*, 10194. [CrossRef] [PubMed]
18. Wheeler, D.L.; Iida, M.; Dunn, E.F. The role of Src in solid tumors. *Oncologist* **2009**, *14*, 667–678. [CrossRef] [PubMed]
19. Ahluwalia, M.S.; de Groot, J.; Liu, W.M.; Gladson, C.L. Targeting SRC in glioblastoma tumors and brain metastases: Rationale and preclinical studies. *Cancer Lett.* **2010**, *298*, 139–149. [CrossRef]
20. Summy, J.M.; Gallick, G.E. Src family kinases in tumor progression and metastasis. *Cancer Metastasis Rev.* **2003**, *22*, 337–358. [CrossRef]
21. Fan, P.; McDaniel, R.E.; Kim, H.R.; Clagett, D.; Haddad, B.; Jordan, V.C. Modulating therapeutic effects of the c-Src inhibitor via oestrogen receptor and human epidermal growth factor receptor 2 in breast cancer cell lines. *Eur. J. Cancer* **2012**, *48*, 3488–3498. [CrossRef]
22. Steinberg, M. Dasatinib: A tyrosine kinase inhibitor for the treatment of chronic myelogenous leukemia and philadelphia chromosome-positive acute lymphoblastic leukemia. *Clin. Ther.* **2007**, *29*, 2289–2308. [CrossRef]
23. Brave, M.; Goodman, V.; Kaminskas, E.; Farrell, A.; Timmer, W.; Pope, S.; Harapanhalli, R.; Saber, H.; Morse, D.; Bullock, J.; et al. Sprycel for chronic myeloid leukemia and Philadelphia chromosome-positive acute lymphoblastic leukemia resistant to or intolerant of imatinib mesylate. *Clin. Cancer Res.* **2008**, *14*, 352–359. [CrossRef]
24. Kurebayashi, J.; Kanomata, N.; Moriya, T.; Kozuka, Y.; Watanabe, M.; Sonoo, H. Preferential antitumor effect of the Src inhibitor dasatinib associated with a decreased proportion of aldehyde dehydrogenase 1-positive cells in breast cancer cells of the basal B subtype. *BMC Cancer* **2010**, *10*, 568. [CrossRef]
25. Tian, J.; Raffa, F.A.; Dai, M.; Moamer, A.; Khadang, B.; Hachim, I.Y.; Bakdounes, K.; Ali, S.; Jean-Claude, B.; Lebrun, J.-J. Dasatinib sensitises triple negative breast cancer cells to chemotherapy by targeting breast cancer stem cells. *Br. J. Cancer* **2018**, *119*, 1495–1507. [CrossRef]

26. Pichot, C.S.; Hartig, S.M.; Xia, L.; Arvanitis, C.; Monisvais, D.; Lee, F.Y.; Frost, J.A.; Corey, S.J. Dasatinib synergizes with doxorubicin to block growth, migration, and invasion of breast cancer cells. *Br. J. Cancer* **2009**, *101*, 38–47. [CrossRef]
27. Gucalp, A.; Sparano, J.A.; Caravelli, J.; Santamauro, J.; Patil, S.; Abbruzzi, A.; Pellegrino, C.; Bromberg, J.; Dang, C.; Theodoulou, M.; et al. Phase II trial of saracatinib (AZD0530), an oral SRC-inhibitor for the treatment of patients with hormone receptor-negative metastatic breast cancer. *Clin. Breast Cancer* **2011**, *11*, 306–311. [CrossRef] [PubMed]
28. Campone, M.; Bondarenko, I.; Brincat, S.; Hotko, Y.; Munster, P.N.; Chmielowska, E.; Fumoleau, P.; Ward, R.; Bardy-Bouxin, N.; Leip, E.; et al. Phase II study of single-agent bosutinib, a Src/Abl tyrosine kinase inhibitor, in patients with locally advanced or metastatic breast cancer pretreated with chemotherapy. *Ann. Oncol.* **2012**, *23*, 610–617. [CrossRef]
29. Finn, R.S.; Bengala, C.; Ibrahim, N.; Roché, H.; Sparano, J.; Strauss, L.C.; Fairchild, J.; Sy, O.; Goldstein, L.J. Dasatinib as a single agent in triple-negative breast cancer: Results of an open-label phase 2 study. *Clin. Cancer Res.* **2011**, *17*, 6905–6913. [CrossRef] [PubMed]
30. Levêque, D.; Becker, G.; Bilger, K.; Natarajan-Amé, S. Clinical Pharmacokinetics and Pharmacodynamics of Dasatinib. *Clin. Pharmacokinet.* **2020**, *59*, 849–856. [CrossRef] [PubMed]
31. Bahman, F.; Taurin, S.; Altayeb, D.; Taha, S.; Bakhiet, M.; Greish, K. Oral Insulin Delivery Using Poly (Styrene Co-Maleic Acid) Micelles in a Diabetic Mouse Model. *Pharmaceutics* **2020**, *12*, 1026. [CrossRef]
32. Greish, K.; Sawa, T.; Fang, J.; Akaike, T.; Maeda, H. SMA-doxorubicin, a new polymeric micellar drug for effective targeting to solid tumours. *J. Control. Release* **2004**, *97*, 219–230. [CrossRef] [PubMed]
33. Qian, X.-L.; Zhang, J.; Li, P.-Z.; Lang, R.-G.; Li, W.-D.; Sun, H.; Liu, F.-F.; Guo, X.-J.; Gu, F.; Fu, L. Dasatinib inhibits c-src phosphorylation and prevents the proliferation of Triple-Negative Breast Cancer (TNBC) cells which overexpress Syndecan-Binding Protein (SDCBP). *PLoS ONE* **2017**, *12*, e0171169. [CrossRef]
34. Maeda, H.; Nakamura, H.; Fang, J. The EPR effect for macromolecular drug delivery to solid tumors: Improvement of tumor uptake, lowering of systemic toxicity, and distinct tumor imaging in vivo. *Adv. Drug Deliv. Rev.* **2013**, *65*, 71–79. [CrossRef] [PubMed]
35. Greish, K.; Fang, J.; Inutsuka, T.; Nagamitsu, A.; Maeda, H. Macromolecular therapeutics: Advantages and prospects with special emphasis on solid tumour targeting. *Clin. Pharm.* **2003**, *42*, 1089–1105. [CrossRef] [PubMed]
36. Greish, K.; Jasim, A.; Parayath, N.; Abdelghany, S.; Alkhateeb, A.; Taurin, S.; Nehoff, H. Micellar formulations of Crizotinib and Dasatinib in the management of glioblastoma multiforme. *J. Drug Target.* **2018**, *26*, 692–708. [CrossRef]
37. Vichai, V.; Kirtikara, K. Sulforhodamine B colorimetric assay for cytotoxicity screening. *Nat. Protoc.* **2006**, *1*, 1112–1116. [CrossRef]
38. Greish, K.; Fateel, M.; Abdelghany, S.; Rachel, N.; Alimoradi, H.; Bakhiet, M.; Alsaie, A. Sildenafil citrate improves the delivery and anticancer activity of doxorubicin formulations in a mouse model of breast cancer. *J. Drug Target.* **2018**, *26*, 610–615. [CrossRef]
39. Davis, M.E.; Chen, Z.; Shin, D.M. Nanoparticle therapeutics: An emerging treatment modality for cancer. *Nat. Rev. Drug Discov.* **2008**, *7*, 771–782. [CrossRef]
40. He, C.; Hu, Y.; Yin, L.; Tang, C.; Yin, C. Effects of particle size and surface charge on cellular uptake and biodistribution of polymeric nanoparticles. *Biomaterials* **2010**, *31*, 3657–3666. [CrossRef]
41. Nehoff, H.; Parayath, N.N.; Domanovitch, L.; Taurin, S.; Greish, K. Nanomedicine for drug targeting: Strategies beyond the enhanced permeability and retention effect. *Int. J. Nanomed.* **2014**, *9*, 2539–2555. [CrossRef]
42. Chang, A.Y.; Wang, M. Molecular mechanisms of action and potential biomarkers of growth inhibition of dasatinib (BMS-354825) on hepatocellular carcinoma cells. *BMC Cancer* **2013**, *13*, 267. [CrossRef]
43. Duckett, D.R.; Cameron, M.D. Metabolism considerations for kinase inhibitors in cancer treatment. *Expert Opin. Drug Metab. Toxicol.* **2010**, *6*, 1175–1193. [CrossRef]
44. Huang, F.; Reeves, K.; Han, X.; Fairchild, C.; Platero, S.; Wong, T.W.; Lee, F.; Shaw, P.; Clark, E. Identification of candidate molecular markers predicting sensitivity in solid tumors to dasatinib: Rationale for patient selection. *Cancer Res.* **2007**, *67*, 2226–2238. [CrossRef] [PubMed]
45. Rao, S.; Larroque-Lombard, A.L.; Peyrard, L.; Thauvin, C.; Rachid, Z.; Williams, C.; Jean-Claude, B.J. Target modulation by a kinase inhibitor engineered to induce a tandem blockade of the epidermal growth factor receptor (EGFR) and c-Src: The concept of type III combi-targeting. *PLoS ONE* **2015**, *10*, e0117215. [CrossRef] [PubMed]
46. Kamath, A.V.; Wang, J.; Lee, F.Y.; Marathe, P.H. Preclinical pharmacokinetics and in vitro metabolism of dasatinib (BMS-354825): A potent oral multi-targeted kinase inhibitor against SRC and BCR-ABL. *Cancer Chemother. Pharm.* **2008**, *61*, 365–376. [CrossRef]
47. Maeda, H. SMANCS and polymer-conjugated macromolecular drugs: Advantages in cancer chemotherapy. *Adv. Drug Deliv. Rev.* **1991**, *6*, 181–202. [CrossRef]

Article

EPR-Effect Enhancers Strongly Potentiate Tumor-Targeted Delivery of Nanomedicines to Advanced Cancers: Further Extension to Enhancement of the Therapeutic Effect

Waliul Islam [1,2], Shintaro Kimura [1,3], Rayhanul Islam [4], Ayaka Harada [5], Katsuhiko Ono [1], Jun Fang [4,*], Takuro Niidome [5], Tomohiro Sawa [1] and Hiroshi Maeda [1,2,6,†]

1. Department of Microbiology, Graduate School of Medical Sciences, Kumamoto University, Kumamoto 860-8556, Japan; bcmb.waliul@gmail.com (W.I.); s.kimura@stateart.co.jp (S.K.); onokat@kumamoto-u.ac.jp (K.O.); sawat@kumamoto-u.ac.jp (T.S.)
2. BioDynamics Research Foundation, Kumamoto 862-0954, Japan
3. StateArt Inc., Tokyo 103-0012, Japan
4. Faculty of Pharmaceutical Sciences, Sojo University, Kumamoto 860-0082, Japan; rayhanulislam88@gmail.com
5. Faculty of Advanced Science and Technology, Kumamoto University, Kumamoto 860-8555, Japan; 144t1817@gmail.com (A.H.); niidome@kumamoto-u.ac.jp (T.N.)
6. Tohoku University, Sendai 980-8572, Japan
* Correspondence: fangjun@ph.sojo-u.ac.jp
† The author passed away during article revision.

Abstract: For more than three decades, enhanced permeability and retention (EPR)-effect-based nanomedicines have received considerable attention for tumor-selective treatment of solid tumors. However, treatment of advanced cancers remains a huge challenge in clinical situations because of occluded or embolized tumor blood vessels, which lead to so-called heterogeneity of the EPR effect. We previously developed a method to restore impaired blood flow in blood vessels by using nitric oxide donors and other agents called EPR-effect enhancers. Here, we show that two novel EPR-effect enhancers—isosorbide dinitrate (ISDN, Nitrol®) and sildenafil citrate—strongly potentiated delivery of three macromolecular drugs to tumors: a complex of poly(styrene-co-maleic acid) (SMA) and cisplatin, named Smaplatin® (chemotherapy); poly(N-(2-hydroxypropyl)methacrylamide) polymer-conjugated zinc protoporphyrin (photodynamic therapy and imaging); and SMA glucosamine-conjugated boric acid complex (boron neutron capture therapy). We tested these nanodrugs in mice with advanced C26 tumors. When these nanomedicines were administered together with ISDN or sildenafil, tumor delivery and thus positive therapeutic results increased two- to four-fold in tumors with diameters of 15 mm or more. These results confirmed the rationale for using EPR-effect enhancers to restore tumor blood flow. In conclusion, all EPR-effect enhancers tested showed great potential for application in cancer therapy.

Keywords: isosorbide dinitrate; sildenafil citrate; EPR effect; EPR-effect enhancers; heterogeneity of the EPR effect; nitric oxide donors; tumor blood flow

1. Introduction

The enhanced permeability and retention (EPR) effect is believed to be a universal mechanism occurring in most solid tumors and a key issue for selective delivery of nanomedicines to tumors [1–6]. Suppressed blood flow or obstructed blood vessels in advanced cancers lead to heterogeneity of the EPR effect [7–12]. Criticisms of the EPR effect were recently raised [13,14], probably because of inaccurate understanding of the EPR effect together with the use of inappropriate nanomedicines, particularly those lacking good stability in vivo and those with an inadequate or poor experimental design [7–9]. For instance, if the release of active pharmaceutical ingredients from liposomes is too slow because the complexes are very stable, even though they accumulates in tumors by EPR effect, the therapeutic outcome is poor [7–12,15].

The EPR effect was first demonstrated in mouse tumor models in which the tumor size was usually smaller than 10 mm and the tumors were highly vasculated; nanomedicines thus had high permeability. In contrast, human tumors diagnosed in clinical situations are frequently larger than 3 mm and up to 10 cm or more. In such large tumors, blood flow is often suppressed or blood vessels are occluded because of the formation of vascular clots or thrombi [9–12,15–18]. This blood-flow suppression thus results in little or no drug delivery and, therefore, a highly limited EPR effect [9,12,15–18]. However, Ding et al. observed that more than 87% of human renal tumors manifested a considerable EPR effect with significant diversity and heterogeneity in different patients [19]. Also, Lee et al. reported that nanoparticles conjugated with positron-emitting radionuclei such as ^{64}Cu resulted the EPR effect in breast cancer, including metastatic cancer [20]. We demonstrated similar results by using arterial angiography of the polymer-conjugate drug SMANCS, i.e., neocarzinostatin (NCS) conjugated to poly(styrene-co-maleic acid) (SMA), in lipiodol [21–24]. In these situations, restoration of tumor blood flow led to successful treatments with nanomedicines [1,23,24]. The review article by Maeda covers these issues [24].

In our studies to overcome the problem of occluded blood flow in advanced tumors, we achieved a breakthrough by using the nitric oxide (NO) donors nitroglycerin (NG), L-arginine (L-Arg), hydroxyurea (HU), and an ACE (angiotensin-converting enzyme) inhibitor as well as other agents including carbon monoxide (CO)-releasing micelles, such as SMA-encapsulated CO-releasing molecule-2 (SMA/CORM2) and polyethylene glycol-hemin (PEG-hemin) [7–12,25–27]. Some of these NO-releasing agents are routinely used in clinical situations. They generate NO in tumors in a selective manner so that tumor blood vessels open mostly through the effect of vasodilation. NO thereby facilitates the EPR effect and delivery of drugs to tumors [7,9–12,25]. These enhancers increased drug delivery to different implanted tumors (S180, C26, and B16) two- to three-fold in mice. They also improved the therapeutic effect two- to three-fold in autochthonous colon tumors induced chemically with azoxymethane and 2% dextran sodium sulfate in mice and 7,12-dimethylbenz[a]anthracene-induced advanced breast tumors in rats [9,12,25]. These two tumor models are similar to naturally occurring tumors and tumors seen in clinical conditions.

In this study, we investigated three EPR-effect enhancers—isosorbide dinitrate (ISDN), sildenafil citrate, and L-Arg—in C26 tumor models in mice, which exhibit less tumor blood flow and are not easy to cure compared to S180 tumor model. ISDN is an organic nitrate compound used to treat angina pectoris, heart failure, and esophageal spasms; to treat and prevent cardiac infarction; and to restore blood flow to the heart [28–30]. ISDN is absorbed at several sites, including the gastrointestinal tract, mucous membranes, and skin, depending on the formulation [31], after which the nitroxyl (-O-NO$_2$) moiety releases the nitrite ion [32]. Nitrite (NO$_2$) is converted to NO by nitrite reductase [32,33]. A patient with lung adenocarcinoma with multiple tumor masses was treated with Nitrol® (ISDN) by means of arterial infusion of SMANCS/lipiodol (0.5 mg/0.5 mL total), the outcome being marked tumor suppression even after only one infusion of SMANCS/lipiodol. This patient remained in good health and free of tumors, as judged by computed tomography (CT), after at least one year and six months [11]. However, a positive effect of the intravenous infusion of Nitrol® and polymer-drug conjugate in an aqueous formulation was not fully demonstrated in this clinical setting. In contrast, sildenafil citrate, another EPR enhancer recently described to have a positive effect in tumor delivery [34], is widely used for male erectile dysfunction. It is a selective inhibitor of phosphodiesterase type 5 that enhances extravasation in target tissues by inhibiting cGMP degradation [35], with results similar to those of NO; however, it does not contain a nitro group.

We report here our utilization of these vascular mediators in combination with three macromolecular drugs to increase delivery of the drugs to tumors and thereby improve therapeutic efficacy in advanced C26 tumors in mice. These three drugs tested are the following: a complex of SMA encapsulated cisplatin (registered name Smaplatin®), in which cisplatin is used in cancer chemotherapy [36]; SMA glucosamine-conjugated boric acid complex (SGB-complex) that was designed for boron neutron capture therapy (BNCT) [37]; and poly(N-(2-hydroxypropyl methacrylamide) (P-HPMA) copolymer-conjugated zinc protoporphyrin (PZP), used for photodynamic therapy (PDT) [38]. Our data showed about two- to four-fold enhancement of therapeutic outcome for all these drugs. These findings again indicate the importance of EPR-effect enhancers to restore tumor blood flow for successful treatment of solid tumors.

2. Materials and Methods

2.1. Chemicals

ISDN was purchased from Eisai Co. Ltd., Tokyo, Japan. Sildenafil citrate was purchased from Yoshindo Co. Ltd., Toyama, Japan. *cis*-Diamminedichloroplatinum(II) (CDDP, cisplatin®) was purchased from Sigma-Aldrich, Tokyo, Japan. SMA (molecular size 5500–6500 Da) was obtained from KJ Chemicals, Tokyo, Japan. Smaplatin®, with a particle size of 100.2 nm as described previously [36]; SGB-complex, with a diameter of 12–15 nm, containing about 16–18% (w/w) glucosamine; and 7–8% (w/w) boric acid was synthesized by Maeda's group [37]. P-HPMA-conjugated zinc protoporphyrin (PZP) [38] was developed previously for PDT. All other reagents and solvents of reagent grade were from commercial sources and were used without additional purification.

2.2. Animals, Cells, and Tumor Models

All animals used in in vivo studies were maintained at 22 ± 1 °C and 55 ± 5% relative humidity with a 12-h light/dark cycle. Each cage contained 4 mice in this study. All experiments were approved by the Animal Ethics Committee of Kumamoto University and carried out according to the Laboratory Protocol of Animal Handling, Kumamoto University, Kumamoto, Japan. Mice were randomly assigned to study groups, and endpoints of experiments were governed by tumor volume (up to ~4000 mm^3). Male BALB/c mice, all 6 weeks old, were purchased from SLC, Shizuoka, Japan.

For solid tumor model experiments, mouse colon cancer C26 cells were maintained and cultured in vitro by using Dulbecco's Modified Eagle's Medium (Wako Pure Chemical Industry, Osaka, Japan) and supplemented with 10% fetal bovine serum (Biosera, Kansas City, MO, USA) and antibiotics (100 U/mL penicillin and 100 μg/mL streptomycin) (Nacalai Tesque, Kyoto, Japan) in 5% CO_2/air at 37 °C. Cultured C26 cells were collected and suspended in physiological saline to a concentration of 2×10^7 cells/mL. We implanted 0.1 mL of cell suspension in the dorsal skin of BALB/c mice to obtain C26 solid tumors.

2.3. Enhancement of Drug Delivery by Using ISDN and Sildenafil Citrate in Advanced C26 Tumors

For this study, we utilized BALB/c mice, 6 weeks old, that had relatively large-sized (diameter of >15 mm) or advanced tumors. Tumor diameters measured about 15 mm at 15–18 days after injection of C26 cells into the dorsal skin. Those mice bearing tumors without wound, collapse, and necrosis were included in this study. PZP (10 mg/kg) was then infused intravenously (iv) or was infused as part of the combination treatment with EPR-effect enhancers, which were injected after the PZP infusion: ISDN at 30 mg/kg intraperitoneally (ip) or sildenafil citrate at 30 mg/kg subcutaneously (sc). At 24 h after the PZP infusion, mice were killed, and blood samples were withdrawn; other tissues, including the heart, lung, liver, spleen, kidney, intestine, and tumor, were collected after perfusion with 20 mL of phosphate-buffered saline to remove blood from the tissues. Each tissue sample was added to 100 mg/mL dimethyl sulfoxide and homogenized very well. Samples were then centrifuged at 12,000× g for 30 min, and supernatants were collected. Finally, the amounts of PZP in the plasma and each tissue were measured in supernatants by means of fluorescence spectroscopy (excitation wavelength 422 nm, emission wavelength 590 nm).

2.4. Improvement in Drug Delivery to Tumors by ISDN as Evaluated by Inductively Coupled Plasma Mass Spectroscopy (ICP-MS)

We used two drugs, SGB-complex and Smaplatin®, to quantify the increased drug delivery induced by ISDN. When tumor diameters were 15–16 mm, we injected 15 mg/kg SGB-complex (boric acid equivalent) or 10 mg/kg Smaplatin® (cisplatin equivalent) into mice via the tail vein. The EPR-effect enhancer ISDN, at 30 mg/kg, was administered ip immediately after the drug injection. After 24 h, mice were killed, and blood samples and other tissues were collected as described above. For elemental quantification by ICP-MS, specimens of about 100 mg of tumor and normal tissues, including the liver, spleen, kidney, intestine, heart, lung, and skin, were excised and placed into test tubes, followed by the addition of a 1:1 mixture of concentrated nitric acid and sulfuric acid (0.25 mL), and samples were digested at 80 °C for 2 h. Samples were then cooled, 10 mL of deionized water was added to each tube, followed by vortexing, and then samples (about 1 mL) were analyzed by using ICP-MS. The amounts (parts per billion, ppb) of ^{10}B and platinum in each tissue were measured and compared.

2.5. Ex Vivo Imaging of PZP with ISDN and Sildenafil Citrate in Advanced Mouse C26 Tumors

When tumor diameters were about 18 mm, we infused 5 mg/kg PZP (ZnPP equivalent) iv. We administered the EPR enhancer ISDN or sildenafil citrate immediately after the PZP infusion. After 24 h, mice were killed, and tumor tissues were removed and subjected to fluorescence imaging by IVIS (IVIS XR; Caliper Life Sciences, Hopkinton, MA, USA). As a positive control, we used L-Arg at 50 mg/mouse in combination with PZP in similar experimental settings.

2.6. Augmentation of the Therapeutic Effects of Micellar Anticancer Agents Used in Combination with EPR-Effect Enhancers

To evaluate the therapeutic results of using two EPR-effect enhancers (ISDN and sildenafil citrate) with Smaplatin® or SGB-complex, we administered Smaplatin® iv at 6 mg/kg as the high dose or 3 mg/kg as the low dose to mice with C26 tumors when the tumors had diameters of 10–12 mm. For the combination therapy with the low Smaplatin® dose, we added ISDN at 30 mg/kg ip or sildenafil citrate at 10 or 30 mg/kg sc. For the combination therapy with the SGB-complex, 10 mg/kg or 5 mg/kg (boric acid equivalent) was infused iv, and immediately after the infusion, the enhancers were injected. In a control experiment, we investigated another EPR-effect enhancer, L-Arg, together with Smaplatin®, with 50 mg/mouse L-Arg being injected ip.

Tumor volumes and body weights were determined throughout the experimental period. After we measured the length (L) and width (W) of the tumors, we calculated tumor volume (mm^3) as $(W^2 \times L)/2$.

2.7. Cytotoxicity of ISDN and Sildenafil Citrate in HeLa and C26 Cells

In vitro cytotoxicity of ISDN and sildenafil was determined by using the MTT method with HeLa and colon carcinoma C26 cells. Both types of cells (1×10^4 cells/well) were plated in 96-well culture plates and cultured overnight in D-MEM with 10% FBS and antibiotics (100U penicillin/mL and 100 μg/mL of streptomycin) at 37 °C under 5% CO$_2$ and 95% air atmosphere. The medium was then replaced with fresh medium, and treatment proceeded with various concentrations of ISDN and sildenafil. After treatment, cells were incubated at 37 °C for 24 h. The MTT assay was then performed, and the toxicity was quantified as the fraction of surviving cells compared with that without drug treatment (control).

2.8. Statistical Analyses

In all experiments, error bars represent the standard deviation (SD) unless otherwise noted. Data were analyzed by using analysis of variance followed by the Bonferroni t-test.

A difference was considered to be statistically significant when $p < 0.05$; $n \geq 5$ samples for each group unless noted.

3. Results

3.1. Augmentation of Delivery of Nanomedicines to C26 Tumors in Mice by Using ISDN or Sildenafil Citrate

We investigated the use of ISDN and sildenafil citrate to increase delivery of different nanomedicines to advanced tumors that were 15–18 mm in diameter (about 2000–3000 mm^3), in C26 tumors-model mice. The three nanomedicines used were PZP, SGB-complex, and Smaplatin®. Table S1 summarizes their characteristics [36–38]. We first determined tumor delivery of PZP by means of fluorescence spectroscopy. Data showed high accumulation of PZP in tumors except in the liver and spleen. When PZP was used in combination with ISDN or sildenafil citrate, tumor accumulation increased about two-fold at 24 h after iv administration of PZP compared with use of PZP alone but no EPR enhancers (Figure 1). As an interesting finding, drug delivery increased significantly only in tumor tissue; in other normal tissues, no significant drug accumulation was seen (Figure 1). Therefore, restoration of blood flow by using EPR-effect enhancers improved EPR effect-based drug delivery to this tumor. This finding (Figure 1) is consistent with our previous data: when P-HPMA-conjugated pirarubicin (P-THP) [39] or P-HPMA-conjugated pyropheophorbide [40] was administered in combination with an NO donor, NG, L-Arg, or HU, drug accumulation in tumors increased two- to three-fold in S180 and C26 tumor-bearing mice [12,25]. As a notable result, ISDN enhanced drug accumulation about 20% more than did sildenafil citrate (Figure 1). The reason for this result with ISDN is not clear, but one possibility may be that direct NO production by ISDN occurred selectively in tumor tissue.

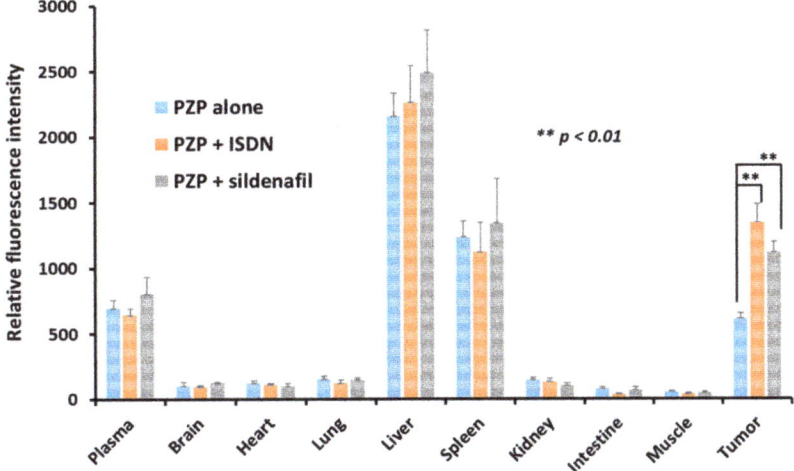

Figure 1. Enhancement of delivery of PZP to tumors by using EPR-effect enhancers. Male, 6-week-old, BALB/c mice bearing Colon 26 tumor were given 10 mg/kg PZP iv; ISDN at 30 mg/kg intraperitoneally or sildenafil citrate at 30 mg/kg subcutaneously immediately after PZP. The amount of drug in each tissue was quantified by using fluorescence spectroscopy, with the excitation wavelength of 422 nm (corresponding to ZnPP). Data are expressed as means ± SD. See text for details.

We also studied delivery of SGB-complex and Smaplatin® given with ISDN in the same tumor model and observed increased delivery of the boron in the SGB-complex and the platinum in Smaplatin® to the tumor tissues, as determined by ICP-MS. We found that 15 mg/kg SGB-complex given iv in combination with 30 mg/kg ISDN given ip led to significantly enhanced delivery of ^{10}B to tumor tissues by about two-fold at 24 h after drug administration; no other tissue demonstrated similar results (Figure 2A). Also, 10 mg/kg

Smaplatin® given with ISDN demonstrated increased accumulation in tumor tissues 1.5- to 2-fold at 24 h after iv infusion (Figure 2B). Again, these data indicate the importance of EPR-effect enhancers to increase delivery of drugs to late-stage tumors.

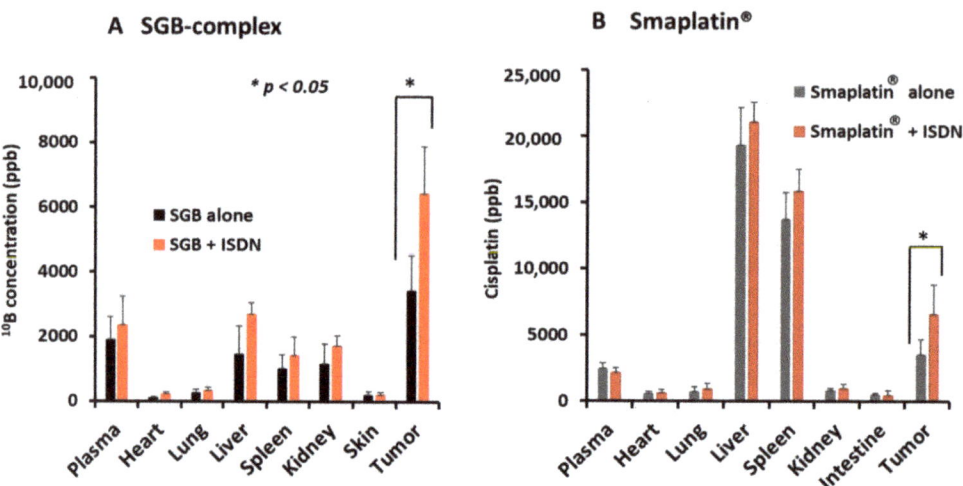

Figure 2. ISDN-enhanced accumulation of SGB-complex (**A**) and Smaplatin® (**B**) in C26 tumor tissues. SGB-complex at 15 mg/kg (boric acid equivalent) or Smaplatin at 10 mg/kg (Cisplatin equivalent) was administered iv; 30 mg/kg ISDN was administered ip as an EPR-effect enhancer. At 24 h after drug treatment, the amounts of ^{10}B and platinum in tissues were quantified by means of ICP-MS according to the manufacturer's procedure. Data are expressed as means ± SD. (n = 5) See text for details.

3.2. Enhanced Drug Delivery to Advanced Tumors by Using ISDN or Sildenafil Citrate as Revealed by Ex Vivo Fluorescence Imaging

We continued to investigate the enhancement of delivery of PZP nanoparticles given alone or with ISDN or sildenafil citrate by using ex vivo fluorescence imaging by IVIS to study cut surfaces of tumor tissues. In this study, we utilized large-size tumors about 18 mm in diameter (3000 mm^3), i.e., advanced C26 tumors in which tumor blood flow may be suppressed or blood vessels may be embolized by clots. Fluorescence intensity data showed that, again, ISDN enhanced drug delivery about three-fold at 24 h after PZP infusion compared with PZP alone (Figure 3A,B). Sildenafil citrate also improved PZP delivery about two-fold compared with PZP alone (Figure 3A,B). In addition, by using this ex vivo tumor-imaging method, we confirmed enhanced drug delivery with L-Arg, 50 mg/mouse: PZP accumulation increased about three- to four-fold after 24 h of iv infusion compared with PZP without L-Arg (Supplementary Figure S1).

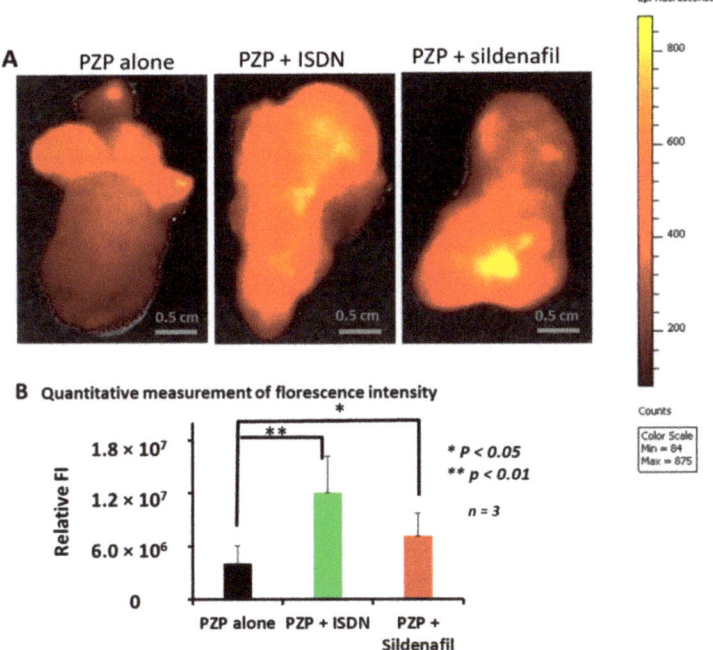

Figure 3. Ex vivo imaging of advanced mouse tumors after treatment with PZP plus ISDN or sildenafil. To study EPR-effect enhancers, we used late-stage C26 tumors (about 18 mm in diameter). PZP, 5 mg/kg, was injected iv, after which ISDN or sildenafil was administered. After 24 h of iv infusion, tumors were removed from mice, and fluorescence images were obtained by IVIS. Both enhancers augmented drug delivery to tumors about two- to three-fold (**A**). (**B**) shows the comparison quantitative measurement of PZP drug accumulation with/without EPR-effect enhancers based on the fluorescence intensity. Data are expressed as means ± SD (n = 3).

3.3. Improvement in the Antitumor Effects of Nanomedicines by Using EPR-Effect Enhancers

We studied two EPR-effect enhancers—ISDN and sildenafil citrate—given in combination with different concentrations of the two micellar nanomedicines, Smaplatin® and SGB-complex (Table S1), in C26 tumors. We found that 3 mg/kg Smaplatin® given with 30 mg/kg ip ISDN resulted in a better therapeutic effect at day 30 than that for 6 mg/kg Smaplatin® given alone (no ISDN) (Figure 4A). In contrast, 3 mg/kg Smaplatin® given alone showed very little antitumor effect at day 12 or later (Figure 4A). These data suggest that ISDN enhanced the therapeutic effect of Smaplatin® about three- to four-fold in C26 tumor-bearing mice, a result that was consistent with our previous findings for P-THP given in combination with NO-generating agents (NG, L-Arg, and HU) [7,10,25], all of which selectively generated NO in tumor tissues. These agents produced two- to three-fold greater antitumor effects in various tumor models [7,10,25].

Smaplatin®, 3 mg/kg, given with 10 mg/kg sildenafil citrate sc suppressed tumor growth about 1.5-fold at day 7 after treatment (Figure 4B). To study whether the therapeutic effect would be enhanced by using a different sildenafil citrate concentration, we used 30 mg/kg sildenafil citrate at day 8 and found that the combination treatment enhanced the antitumor effect about two-fold at day 30 (Figure 4B).

We also found that the combination treatment of Smaplatin® with L-Arg in the C26 tumor model improved the therapeutic efficacy of Smaplatin® two-fold (Supplementary Figure S2).

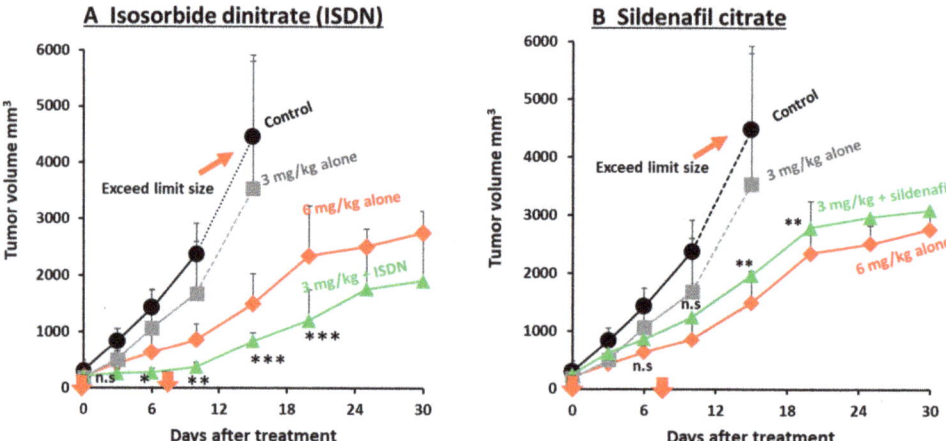

Figure 4. Improvement in the therapeutic effect of different concentrations of Smaplatin® by using ISDN (**A**) and sildenafil (**B**) in C26 tumors. When tumor diameters measured about 12 mm, 6 mg/kg or 3 mg/kg Smaplatin® was injected iv; ISDN (30 mg/kg, ip) or sildenafil (30 mg/kg sc) was given with 3 mg/kg Smaplatin®. The 3 mg/kg Smaplatin® given with ISDN showed improved therapeutic efficacy compared with 6 mg/kg Smaplatin® given alone (**A**); the result for 3 mg/kg Smaplatin® plus sildenafil was similar to that for 6 mg/kg Smaplatin® given alone (**B**). Arrows indicate times of drug administration. * $p < 0.05$, ** $p < 0.01$, *** $p < 0.001$, combination group vs Smaplatin® 3 mg/kg group. Data are expressed as means ± SD. ($n = 5$).

In addition, we confirmed an enhanced therapeutic effect by using another micellar drug, SGB-complex, which was developed for BNCT. We previously reported that SGB-complex itself suppressed tumor growth in vivo and in vitro by inhibiting glycolysis and by damaging functions of mitochondrial membranes in cancer cells [37]. To increase the antitumor effect of the SGB-complex, in our study here, we used ISDN or sildenafil citrate as an EPR-effect enhancer. We observed almost no therapeutic effect when 5 mg/kg SGB-complex alone was infused iv, whereas 5 mg/kg SGB-complex given iv in combination with 30 mg/kg ISDN produced an enhanced antitumor effect compared with that for 10 mg/kg SGB-complex given alone (Figure 5A). These data suggest that combination therapy with ISDN can enhance the therapeutic effect of nanomedicines about two- to three-fold. Sildenafil citrate was also given twice, at day zero (10 mg/kg sc) and day eight (30 mg/kg sc), and we found an improved antitumor effect of about two-fold (Figure 5B).

To see the cytotoxicity of ISDN and sildenafil, we examined two cancer cells, e.g., HeLa and C26, and we found both EPR-effect enhancers did not show any significant cytotoxicity in both cells after 24 h incubation based on MTT assay (Supplementary Figure S3). Furthermore, we evaluated the in vivo toxicity of Smaplatin® (Supplementary Figure S4A) and SGB-complex (Supplementary Figure S4B) with or without EPR-effect enhancer (ISDN or sildenafil) by monitoring the mouse body-weight changes. We observed that the combination treatment did not exhibit any notable body-weight changes up to 30 days after treatment (Supplementary Figure S4).

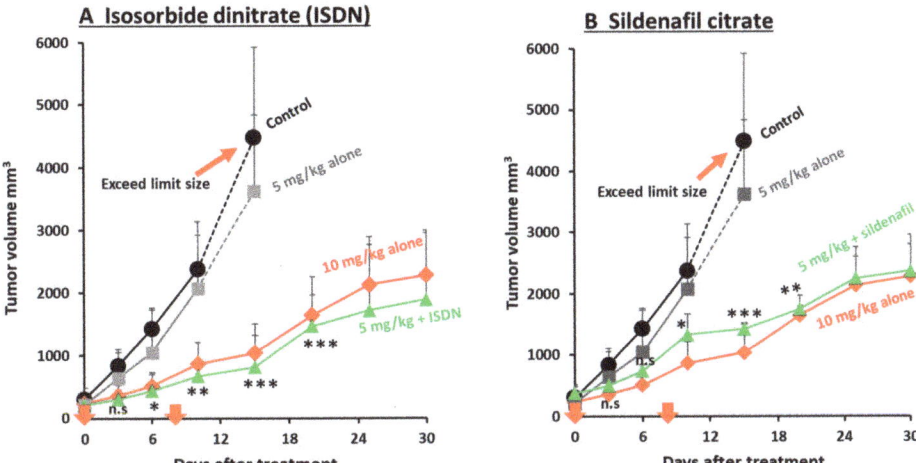

Figure 5. Improvement in the antitumor effect of SGB-complex by using EPR-effect enhancers in the C26 tumor model. (**A**) Antitumor effect of the SGB-complex given with ISDN. (**B**) Antitumor efficacy of the SGB-complex given with sildenafil. ISDN increased the antitumor effect of the SGB-complex about 3-fold; sildenafil, 1.5- to 2-fold. Arrows indicate times of drug administration. Data are expressed as means ± SD. * $p < 0.05$, ** $p < 0.01$, *** $p < 0.001$, combination group vs. SGB 5 mg/kg group. See text for details.

4. Discussion

Commonly used cancer chemotherapeutic agents, including immunotherapy drugs, have shown failure rates of 90% (±5%) for solid tumors [15]. One reason for this low success rate is that most drugs currently used in clinics to treat solid tumors are low-molecular-weight compounds. As a consequence, these drugs travel throughout the body and diffuse indiscriminately when administered iv. They thus cause severe adverse effects in normal tissues and organs and result in a lower therapeutic effect [7,9,12,15,24,41,42]. In contrast, when biocompatible nanodrugs are administered iv, they remain in circulating blood for a long time, and they gradually penetrate tumor tissue and selectively accumulate there because of the EPR effect [7,15,24]. One criticism raised about the EPR effect was that this effect was not observed in human cancers. However, Lee et al. recently demonstrated the presence of the EPR effect in breast cancer, including metastatic tumors [20], and Ding et al. reported a positive EPR effect in about 87% of patients with renal cancer [19]. These data are consistent with the clinical findings of Maeda's group with SMANCS/lipiodol infused into tumor-feeding arteries, with this method showing remarkable results. Their method of using an arterial infusion of SMANCS/lipiodol (drug) selectively delivered the drug to tumors by virtue of the EPR effect, and the selective delivery was clearly visualized by using CT [3,5,11,12,22–24]. Also demonstrated in radio scintigraphy imaging of a tumor using γ-emitting gallium-67 citrate, when it was infused iv, it formed a complex with transferrin (90 kDa) in the plasma. This complex behaves as a nanomedicine. After 48–72 h, this complex accumulated selectively in solid tumors, as visualized by a γ-scintillation camera [43], which provides clear evidence of the EPR effect.

The heterogeneity of the EPR effect presents another problem in that tumor blood vessels are frequently embolized or occluded, and blood flow is suppressed, as discussed above. When tumor blood flow is obstructed, no typical EPR effect is observed even when nanomedicines are administered [7,8,18,24]. We had previously reported restoration of obstructed tumor blood flow by using NO donors, L-Arg, NG, and HU [7,10–12,25], and micellar forms of CO donors such as SMA/CORM2 and PEG-hemin or an inducer of heme oxygenase-1 (HO-1), which also generates CO [26,27]. These vascular mediators remarkably increased the tumor delivery of nanomedicine by augmenting tumor blood flow and vascular permeability, consequently improving the therapeutic efficacy of nanomedicines two- to three-fold in various tumor models in mice and rats and also in humans [23,44].

In this report, we confirmed that the two EPR-effect enhancers ISDN and sildenafil citrate, in addition to L-Arg, improved delivery of three different micellar drugs—Smaplatin®, SGB-complex, and PZP—to tumors, and we also confirmed the therapeutic effect of these three nanomedicines on C26 tumors in mice. Table S1 summarizes the physicochemical properties of these three nanomedicines.

We first investigated the delivery of PZP to mouse tumors by using ISDN and sildenafil citrate, which enhanced delivery about two-fold (Figure 1). We previously showed that PZP produced an excellent anticancer effect in various tumor models when used with light irradiation in PDT. In addition, even without light irradiation, PZP also suppressed HO-1 in cancer cells [38,45], inhibited HSP-32 (tumor survival factor), and downregulated oncogene expression so that it ultimately suppressed tumor growth [46,47]. PZP showed relative high liver and spleen accumulation, which is commonly seen for many nanomedicines because liver and spleen are rich in reticuloendothelial systems to capture macromolecules. However, NO donors did not significantly increase the drug accumulation in liver and spleen but only remarkably increased tumor accumulation, suggesting these EPR enhancers will not increase the side effects of nanomedicine. Furthermore, for PZP that is used for PDT upon light irradiation, the side effects or toxicities to the liver and spleen are not significant because light irradiation is applied to the tumor but not to the liver or spleen. Smaplatin® is a pH-sensitive micellar drug (cisplatin complexed with SMA polymer [36]) that releases free cisplatin in an acidic milieu after tumor-selective accumulation, and the released cisplatin inhibits DNA synthesis of cancer cells [36]. We showed that ISDN improved delivery of these nanomedicines to tumors, thereby increasing anticancer efficacy more than 3-fold; sildenafil improved delivery 1.5- to 2-fold (Figures 2B and 4A). We also confirmed that the use of SGB-complex with ISDN resulted in an improved therapeutic effect, by two- to three-fold, in the same tumor model and by the same mechanisms (Figures 2A and 5A).

In Figures 1 and 2, high uptake is seen for PZP and Smaplatin® in the liver and spleen, so called by reticuloendothelial system (RES). To suppress this uptake, we are now investigating how to avoid this issue by pretreating lipid microparticles of Intralipid® or lipiodol by blocking scavenger receptor of RES. This strategy seems effective to prevent RES uptake [48]

SGB-complex was initially designed for use in BNCT. We discovered by chance that this complex can inhibit hypoxia-adapted tumor-cell growth under mildly hypoxic conditions (pO_2, 6–10%) by inhibiting glycolysis and by damaging functions of mitochondrial membranes in cancer cells [37] without neutron irradiation. SGB-complex also significantly suppressed tumor growth two- to three-fold when used with ISDN in vivo compared with SGB-complex alone (Figure 5A). We later confirmed a much improved therapeutic effect after utilization of neutron irradiation [37]. Therefore, we expect that the use of EPR-effect enhancers plus neutron irradiation will enhance the therapeutic effects of this method even more. Experiments investigating this possibility are under way and should usher in a new era in BNCT.

We also confirmed the EPR-enhancing effect of sildenafil citrate. The mode of action of sildenafil citrate is not by generation of NO, but the ultimate result of using it was similar to that related to NO generation. Das and Fisher and their colleagues showed that sildenafil citrate enhanced apoptosis and the antitumor efficacy of doxorubicin in a xenograft model of prostate-tumor-bearing mice [49,50]. This finding may be attributed to the EPR-enhancing effect. We report here that sildenafil citrate enhanced the delivery of PZP to advanced tumors by two- to three-fold, as judged by fluorescence imaging (Figures 1 and 3); it also improved the anticancer efficacy of both SGB-complex and Smaplatin® by about 1.5- to 2-fold (Figures 4B and 5B). Moreover, we confirmed that ISDN or sildenafil citrate itself did not show any toxicity in vitro (Supplementary Figure S3), and in the combination treatment with nanomedicine, we did not find significant body-weight loss in mice (Supplementary Figure S4A,B). These data suggest that EPR enhancers play a critical role for the improvement of tumor drug delivery of nanomedicines and thus enhancement of the therapeutic effect.

5. Conclusions

We present here examples of the effective influence of the EPR enhancers ISDN and sildenafil citrate, which we evaluated with three micellar polymer drugs—SGB complex, Smaplatin®, and PZP—in a mouse model with relatively advanced C26 tumors. Smaplatin® releases free cisplatin in tumor tissues and damages cancer cells by inhibiting their DNA synthesis [36]. SGB-complex, in contrast, generates free boric acid in tumors which exhibit microenvironmental acidic pH, and boric acid thus generated competes with phosphate in phosphorylation reaction of glucose by hexokinase in glycolysis. As a result, it inhibits glycolysis in cancer cells; the glucosamine moiety of this complex seems to damage functions of mitochondrial membranes in cancer cells [37]. We also showed that the delivery to tumors and antitumor effects of Smaplatin® and SGB-complex were enhanced by using ISDN and sildenafil citrate by about 2- to 4-fold and 1.5- to 2-fold, respectively (Figures 2, 4 and 5). A similar EPR effect-enhancing result was observed with another fluorescent macromolecular drug PZP, with two-fold enhancement (Figures 1 and 3). Previous studies of the NO donors L-Arg, NG, and HU and the ACE inhibitor (ACE-1) showed about two-fold enhancement of therapeutic effects in the same C26 and S180 tumors in mice. These data further confirm the efficacy of EPR-effect enhancers in the treatment of advanced cancer.

Supplementary Materials: The following are available online at https://www.mdpi.com/article/10.3390/jpm11060487/s1, Figure S1: Enhancement of tumor drug delivery of PZP using L-arginine evaluated by fluorescence imaging (IVIS), Figure S2: Improvement of therapeutic effect of Smaplatin® by using L-arginine in C26 tumor, Figure S3: Cytotoxicity of ISDN and sildenafil citrate in HeLa and C26 cells, Figure S4: In vivo toxicity of Smaplatin® and SGB-complex with EPR effect enhancers revealed by body weight change, Table S1: Characteristics of micellar drugs used in this study.

Author Contributions: H.M. designed this study. W.I. performed most of the in vitro and in vivo experiments. A.H. and T.N. performed the transmission electron microscopy. W.I., S.K., and K.O. completed the ICP-MS analysis. R.I., W.I., and J.F. conducted the fluorescence imaging by IVIS. H.M. and W.I. wrote the manuscript. H.M., T.S., T.N., and W.I. discussed the content and refinements of the manuscript. All authors have read and agreed to the published version of the manuscript.

Funding: This work was supported in part by a Bilateral Joint Research Project between the Japan Society for the Promotion of Science (JSPS) and the Czech Academy of Sciences (CAS) to H. Maeda and J. Fang (29400001). This work was also supported by Grants-in-Aid for Scientific Research category (C) to J. Fang (25430162 and 16K08217); categories (A) and Priority Areas to H. Maeda (17016076 and 18H04059) from the JSPS; A-STEP from JST to H. Maeda (AS242Z01542Q); and No. 3 Anticancer Research-General 001 from the Ministry of Health, Labor, and Welfare (MLHW), Japan, to H. Maeda. This work was also supported by research funds from the BioDynamics Research Foundation to H. Maeda.

Institutional Review Board Statement: All animal experiments were approved by the Animal Ethics Committee of Kumamoto University and carried out according to the Laboratory Protocol of Animal Handling, Kumamoto University, Kumamoto, Japan. Mice were randomly assigned to study groups, and endpoints of experiments were governed by tumor volume (up to ~4000 mm^3).

Informed Consent Statement: Not applicable.

Data Availability Statement: The data presented in this study are available on request from the corresponding author or first author of this article.

Acknowledgments: W. Islam is the recipient of a fellowship from the BioDynamics Research Foundation (2017–2021), awarded from The Ichiro Kanehara Foundation for the Promotion of Medical Sciences and Medical Care (2018), and a Mitsubishi Corporation International Scholarship (JEES Sponsor-Crowned Scholarship) (2020–2021). We would like to acknowledge the important effort of Judith B. Gandy in AZ, USA, for her excellent English editing and Asami Yamashiro for the preparation of the manuscript.

Conflicts of Interest: The authors declare no conflict of interest.

References

1. Fang, J.; Nakamura, H.; Maeda, H. The EPR Effect: Unique Features of Tumor Blood Vessels for Drug Delivery, Factors Involved, and Limitations and Augmentation of the Effect. *Adv. Drug Deliv. Rev.* **2011**, *63*, 136–151. [CrossRef] [PubMed]
2. Maeda, H. Polymer Therapeutics and the EPR Effect. *J. Drug Target.* **2017**, *25*, 781–785. [CrossRef] [PubMed]
3. Maeda, H. Vascular Permeability in Cancer and Infection as Related to Macromolecular Drug Delivery, with Emphasis on the EPR Effect for Tumor-Selective Drug Targeting. *Proc. Jpn. Acad. Ser. B* **2012**, *88*, 53–71. [CrossRef] [PubMed]
4. Matsumura, Y.; Maeda, H. A New Concept for Macromolecular Therapeutics in Cancer Chemotherapy: Mechanism of Tumoritropic Accumulation of Proteins and the Antitumor Agent Smancs. *Cancer Res.* **1986**, *46*, 6387–6392. [PubMed]
5. Maeda, H. Tumor-Selective Delivery of Macromolecular Drugs via the EPR Effect: Background and Future Prospects. *Bioconjug. Chem.* **2010**, *21*, 797–802. [CrossRef]
6. Maeda, H. The Link between Infection and Cancer: Tumor Vasculature, Free Radicals, and Drug Delivery to Tumors via the EPR Effect. *Cancer Sci.* **2013**, *104*, 779–789. [CrossRef]
7. Fang, J.; Islam, W.; Maeda, H. Exploiting the Dynamics of the EPR Effect and Strategies to Improve the Therapeutic Effects of Nanomedicines by Using EPR Effect Enhancers. *Adv. Drug Deliv. Rev.* **2020**. [CrossRef]
8. Maeda, H.; Islam, W. Overcoming barriers for tumor-targeted drug delivery: The power of macromolecular anticancer drugs with the EPR effect and the modulation of vascular physiology. In *Polymer-Protein Conjugates*; Pasut, G., Zalipsky, S., Eds.; Elsevier: Amsterdam, the Netherlands, 2020; pp. 41–58, ISBN 978-0-444-64081-9.
9. Maeda, H.; Tsukigawa, K.; Fang, J. A Retrospective 30 Years After Discovery of the Enhanced Permeability and Retention Effect of Solid Tumors: Next-Generation Chemotherapeutics and Photodynamic Therapy—Problems, Solutions, and Prospects. *Microcirculation* **2016**, *23*, 173–182. [CrossRef]
10. Seki, T.; Fang, J.; Maeda, H. Enhanced Delivery of Macromolecular Antitumor Drugs to Tumors by Nitroglycerin Application. *Cancer Sci.* **2009**, *100*, 2426–2430. [CrossRef]
11. Maeda, H. Macromolecular Therapeutics in Cancer Treatment: The EPR Effect and Beyond. *J. Control. Release* **2012**, *164*, 138–144. [CrossRef]
12. Maeda, H. Nitroglycerin Enhances Vascular Blood Flow and Drug Delivery in Hypoxic Tumor Tissues: Analogy between Angina Pectoris and Solid Tumors and Enhancement of the EPR Effect. *J. Control. Release* **2010**, *142*, 296–298. [CrossRef]
13. Sindhwani, S.; Syed, A.M.; Ngai, J.; Kingston, B.R.; Maiorino, L.; Rothschild, J.; MacMillan, P.; Zhang, Y.; Rajesh, N.U.; Hoang, T.; et al. The Entry of Nanoparticles into Solid Tumours. *Nat. Mater.* **2020**, *19*, 566–575. [CrossRef]
14. Park, K. Questions on the Role of the EPR Effect in Tumor Targeting. *J. Control. Release* **2013**, *172*, 391. [CrossRef]
15. Maeda, H.; Khatami, M. Analyses of Repeated Failures in Cancer Therapy for Solid Tumors: Poor Tumor-Selective Drug Delivery, Low Therapeutic Efficacy and Unsustainable Costs. *Clin. Transl. Med.* **2018**, *7*, 11. [CrossRef]
16. Strongman, H.; Gadd, S.; Matthews, A.; Mansfield, K.E.; Stanway, S.; Lyon, A.R.; Dos-Santos-Silva, I.; Smeeth, L.; Bhaskaran, K. Medium and Long-Term Risks of Specific Cardiovascular Diseases in Survivors of 20 Adult Cancers: A Population-Based Cohort Study Using Multiple Linked UK Electronic Health Records Databases. *Lancet* **2019**, *394*, 1041–1054. [CrossRef]
17. Young, A.; Chapman, O.; Connor, C.; Poole, C.; Rose, P.; Kakkar, A.K. Thrombosis and Cancer. *Nat. Rev. Clin. Oncol.* **2012**, *9*, 437–449. [CrossRef]
18. Navi, B.B.; Reiner, A.S.; Kamel, H.; Iadecola, C.; Okin, P.M.; Tagawa, S.T.; Panageas, K.S.; DeAngelis, L.M. Arterial Thromboembolic Events Preceding the Diagnosis of Cancer in Older Persons. *Blood* **2019**, *133*, 781–789. [CrossRef]
19. Ding, Y.; Xu, Y.; Yang, W.; Niu, P.; Li, X.; Chen, Y.; Li, Z.; Liu, Y.; An, Y.; Liu, Y.; et al. Investigating the EPR Effect of Nanomedicines in Human Renal Tumors via Ex Vivo Perfusion Strategy. *Nano Today* **2020**, *35*, 100970. [CrossRef]
20. Lee, H.; Shields, A.F.; Siegel, B.A.; Miller, K.D.; Krop, I.; Ma, C.X.; LoRusso, P.M.; Munster, P.N.; Campbell, K.; Gaddy, D.F.; et al. 64Cu-MM-302 Positron Emission Tomography Quantifies Variability of Enhanced Permeability and Retention of Nanoparticles in Relation to Treatment Response in Patients with Metastatic Breast Cancer. *Clin. Cancer Res.* **2017**, *23*, 4190–4202. [CrossRef]
21. Maeda, H.; Matsumoto, T.; Konno, T.; Iwai, K.; Ueda, M. Tailor-Making of Protein Drugs by Polymer Conjugation for Tumor Targeting: A Brief Review on Smancs. *J. Protein Chem.* **1984**, *3*, 181–193. [CrossRef]
22. Maeda, H. SMANCS and Polymer-Conjugated Macromolecular Drugs: Advantages in Cancer Chemotherapy. *Adv. Drug Deliv. Rev.* **2001**, *46*, 169–185. [CrossRef]
23. Nagamitsu, A.; Greish, K.; Maeda, H. Elevating Blood Pressure as a Strategy to Increase Tumor-Targeted Delivery of Macromolecular Drug SMANCS: Cases of Advanced Solid Tumors. *Jpn. J. Clin. Oncol.* **2009**, *39*, 756–766. [CrossRef]
24. Maeda, H. The 35th Anniversary of the Discovery of EPR Effect: A New Wave of Nanomedicines for Tumor-Targeted Drug Delivery—Personal Remarks and Future Prospects. *J. Pers. Med.* **2021**, *11*, 229. [CrossRef]
25. Islam, W.; Fang, J.; Imamura, T.; Etrych, T.; Subr, V.; Ulbrich, K.; Maeda, H. Augmentation of the Enhanced Permeability and Retention Effect with Nitric Oxide-Generating Agents Improves the Therapeutic Effects of Nanomedicines. *Mol. Cancer Ther.* **2018**, *17*, 2643–2653. [CrossRef]
26. Fang, J.; Qin, H.; Seki, T.; Nakamura, H.; Tsukigawa, K.; Shin, T.; Maeda, H. Therapeutic Potential of Pegylated Hemin for Reactive Oxygen Species-Related Diseases via Induction of Heme Oxygenase-1: Results from a Rat Hepatic Ischemia/Reperfusion Injury Model. *J. Pharmacol. Exp. Ther.* **2011**, *339*, 779–789. [CrossRef]
27. Fang, J.; Islam, R.; Islam, W.; Yin, H.; Subr, V.; Etrych, T.; Ulbrich, K.; Maeda, H. Augmentation of EPR Effect and Efficacy of Anticancer Nanomedicine by Carbon Monoxide Generating Agents. *Pharmaceutics* **2019**, *11*, 343. [CrossRef]

28. Chavey, W.E.; Bleske, B.E.; Harrison, R.V.; Hogikyan, R.V.; Kesteron, S.; Nicklas, J.M. Pharmacologic Management of Heart Failure Caused by Systolic Dysfunction. *Am. Fam. Physician* **2008**, *77*, 957–964.
29. Zoller, D.; Lüttgenau, J.; Steffen, S.; Bollwein, H. The Effect of Isosorbide Dinitrate on Uterine and Ovarian Blood Flow in Cycling and Early Pregnant Mares: A Pilot Study. *Theriogenology* **2016**, *85*, 1562–1567. [CrossRef]
30. Sciorati, C.; Staszewsky, L.; Zambelli, V.; Russo, I.; Salio, M.; Novelli, D.; Di Grigoli, G.; Moresco, R.M.; Clementi, E.; Latini, R. Ibuprofen plus Isosorbide Dinitrate Treatment in the Mdx Mice Ameliorates Dystrophic Heart Structure. *Pharmacol. Res.* **2013**, *73*, 35–43. [CrossRef]
31. Bogaert, M.G. Pharmacokinetics of Organic Nitrates in Man: An Overview. *Eur. Heart J.* **1988**, *9* (Suppl. A), 33–37. [CrossRef]
32. Divakaran, S.; Loscalzo, J. The Role of Nitroglycerin and Other Nitrogen Oxides in Cardiovascular Therapeutics. *J. Am. Coll. Cardiol.* **2017**, *70*, 2393–2410. [CrossRef] [PubMed]
33. Fung, H.L.; Chung, S.J.; Bauer, J.A.; Chong, S.; Kowaluk, E.A. Biochemical Mechanism of Organic Nitrate Action. *Am. J. Cardiol.* **1992**, *70*, 4B–10B. [CrossRef]
34. Greish, K.; Fateel, M.; Abdelghany, S.; Rachel, N.; Alimoradi, H.; Bakhiet, M.; Alsaie, A. Sildenafil Citrate Improves the Delivery and Anticancer Activity of Doxorubicin Formulations in a Mouse Model of Breast Cancer. *J. Drug Target.* **2018**, *26*, 610–615. [CrossRef] [PubMed]
35. Riazi, K.; Roshanpour, M.; Rafiei-Tabatabaei, N.; Homayoun, H.; Ebrahimi, F.; Dehpour, A.R. The Proconvulsant Effect of Sildenafil in Mice: Role of Nitric Oxide–CGMP Pathway. *Br. J. Pharmacol.* **2006**, *147*, 935–943. [CrossRef]
36. Saisyo, A.; Nakamura, H.; Fang, J.; Tsukigawa, K.; Greish, K.; Furukawa, H.; Maeda, H. PH-Sensitive Polymeric Cisplatin-Ion Complex with Styrene-Maleic Acid Copolymer Exhibits Tumor-Selective Drug Delivery and Antitumor Activity as a Result of the Enhanced Permeability and Retention Effect. *Colloids Surf. B Biointerfaces* **2016**, *138*, 128–137. [CrossRef]
37. Islam, W.; Matsumoto, Y.; Fang, J.; Harada, A.; Niidome, T.; Ono, K.; Tsutsuki, H.; Sawa, T.; Imamura, T.; Sakurai, K.; et al. Polymer-Conjugated Glucosamine Complexed with Boric Acid Shows Tumor-Selective Accumulation and Simultaneous Inhibition of Glycolysis. *Biomaterials* **2021**, *269*, 120631. [CrossRef]
38. Nakamura, H.; Liao, L.; Hitaka, Y.; Tsukigawa, K.; Subr, V.; Fang, J.; Ulbrich, K.; Maeda, H. Micelles of Zinc Protoporphyrin Conjugated to N-(2-Hydroxypropyl)Methacrylamide (HPMA) Copolymer for Imaging and Light-Induced Antitumor Effects in Vivo. *J. Control. Release* **2013**, *165*, 191–198. [CrossRef]
39. Nakamura, H.; Etrych, T.; Chytil, P.; Ohkubo, M.; Fang, J.; Ulbrich, K.; Maeda, H. Two Step Mechanisms of Tumor Selective Delivery of N-(2-Hydroxypropyl)Methacrylamide Copolymer Conjugated with Pirarubicin via an Acid-Cleavable Linkage. *J. Control. Release* **2014**, *174*, 81–87. [CrossRef]
40. Fang, J.; Šubr, V.; Islam, W.; Hackbarth, S.; Islam, R.; Etrych, T.; Ulbrich, K.; Maeda, H. N-(2-Hydroxypropyl)Methacrylamide Polymer Conjugated Pyropheophorbide-a, a Promising Tumor-Targeted Theranostic Probe for Photodynamic Therapy and Imaging. *Eur. J. Pharm. Biopharm.* **2018**, *130*, 165–176. [CrossRef]
41. Islam, W.; Fang, J.; Etrych, T.; Chytil, P.; Ulbrich, K.; Sakoguchi, A.; Kusakabe, K.; Maeda, H. HPMA Copolymer Conjugate with Pirarubicin: In Vitro and Ex Vivo Stability and Drug Release Study. *Int. J. Pharm.* **2018**, *536*, 108–115. [CrossRef]
42. Maeda, H. Toward a Full Understanding of the EPR Effect in Primary and Metastatic Tumors as Well as Issues Related to Its Heterogeneity. *Adv. Drug Deliv. Rev.* **2015**, *91*, 3–6. [CrossRef]
43. Barth, R.F. Boron Neutron Capture Therapy at the Crossroads: Challenges and Opportunities. *Appl. Radiat. Isot. Data Instrum. Methods Use Agric. Ind. Med.* **2009**, *67*, S3–S6. [CrossRef]
44. Dozono, H.; Yanazume, S.; Nakamura, H.; Etrych, T.; Chytil, P.; Ulbrich, K.; Fang, J.; Arimura, T.; Douchi, T.; Kobayashi, H.; et al. HPMA Copolymer-Conjugated Pirarubicin in Multimodal Treatment of a Patient with Stage IV Prostate Cancer and Extensive Lung and Bone Metastases. *Target. Oncol.* **2016**, *11*, 101–106. [CrossRef]
45. Nakamura, H.; Fang, J.; Gahininath, B.; Tsukigawa, K.; Maeda, H. Intracellular Uptake and Behavior of Two Types Zinc Protoporphyrin (ZnPP) Micelles, SMA-ZnPP and PEG-ZnPP as Anticancer Agents; Unique Intracellular Disintegration of SMA Micelles. *J. Control. Release* **2011**, *155*, 367–375. [CrossRef]
46. Fang, J.; Greish, K.; Qin, H.; Liao, L.; Nakamura, H.; Takeya, M.; Maeda, H. HSP32 (HO-1) Inhibitor, Copoly(Styrene-Maleic Acid)-Zinc Protoporphyrin IX, a Water-Soluble Micelle as Anticancer Agent: In Vitro and in Vivo Anticancer Effect. *Eur. J. Pharm. Biopharm.* **2012**, *81*, 540–547. [CrossRef]
47. Herrmann, H.; Kneidinger, M.; Cerny-Reiterer, S.; Rülicke, T.; Willmann, M.; Gleixner, K.V.; Blatt, K.; Hörmann, G.; Peter, B.; Samorapoompichit, P.; et al. The Hsp32 Inhibitors SMA-ZnPP and PEG-ZnPP Exert Major Growth-Inhibitory Effects on D34+/CD38+ and CD34+/CD38- AML Progenitor Cells. *Curr. Cancer Drug Targets* **2012**, *12*, 51–63. [CrossRef]
48. Islam, R.; Gao, S.; Islam, W.; Šubr, V.; Zhou, J.-R.; Yokomizo, K.; Etrych, T.; Maeda, H.; Fang, J. Unraveling the Role of Intralipid in Suppressing Off-Target Delivery and Augmenting the Therapeutic Effects of Anticancer Nanomedicines. *Acta Biomater.* **2021**. [CrossRef]
49. Das, A.; Durrant, D.; Mitchell, C.; Dent, P.; Batra, S.K.; Kukreja, R.C. Sildenafil (Viagra) Sensitizes Prostate Cancer Cells to Doxorubicin-Mediated Apoptosis through CD95. *Oncotarget* **2016**, *7*, 4399–4413. [CrossRef]
50. Fisher, P.W.; Salloum, F.; Das, A.; Hyder, H.; Kukreja, R.C. Phosphodiesterase-5 Inhibition with Sildenafil Attenuates Cardiomyocyte Apoptosis and Left Ventricular Dysfunction in a Chronic Model of Doxorubicin Cardiotoxicity. *Circulation* **2005**, *111*, 1601–1610. [CrossRef]

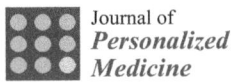

Review

The 35th Anniversary of the Discovery of EPR Effect: A New Wave of Nanomedicines for Tumor-Targeted Drug Delivery—Personal Remarks and Future Prospects

Hiroshi Maeda [1,2,3,4]

1 BioDynamics Research Foundation, Kumamoto 862-0954, Japan; maedabdr@sweet.ocn.ne.jp
2 Department of Microbiology, Kumamoto University School of Medicine, Kumamoto 862-0954, Japan
3 Tohoku University, Sendai 980-8572, Japan
4 Osaka University Medical School, Osaka 565-0871, Japan

Abstract: This Special Issue on the enhanced permeability and retention (EPR) effect commemorates the 35th anniversary of its discovery, the original 1986 Matsumura and Maeda finding being published in *Cancer Research* as a new concept in cancer chemotherapy. My review here describes the history and heterogeneity of the EPR effect, which involves defective tumor blood vessels and blood flow. We reported that restoring obstructed tumor blood flow overcomes impaired drug delivery, leading to improved EPR effects. I also discuss gaps between small animal cancers used in experimental models and large clinical cancers in humans, which usually involve heterogeneous EPR effects, vascular abnormalities in multiple necrotic foci, and tumor emboli. Here, I emphasize arterial infusion of oily formulations of nanodrugs into tumor-feeding arteries, which is the most tumor-selective drug delivery method, with tumor/blood ratios of 100-fold. This method is literally the most personalized medicine because arterial infusions differ for each patient, and drug doses infused depend on tumor size and anatomy in each patient. Future developments in EPR effect-based treatment will range from chemotherapy to photodynamic therapy, boron neutron capture therapy, and therapies for free radical diseases. This review focuses on our own work, which stimulated numerous scientists to perform research in nanotechnology and drug delivery systems, thereby spawning a new cancer treatment era.

Keywords: EPR effect; enhanced permeability and retention effect; nanomedicines; cancer therapy; drug delivery; nanotechnology; tumor-selective drug delivery; photodynamic therapy; boron neutron capture therapy

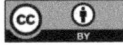

1. Background: Discovery of the Enhanced Permeability and Retention (EPR) Effect, Criticism, and Reality

1.1. Status Quo of Enhanced Permeability and Retention (EPR) Effect and Tumor Targeting

Thirty-five years of investigation into the EPR effect [1–4] have led to the true value of this discovery being increasingly recognized [5–8]. A recent report by the multinational European Technology Platform on Nanomedicine, set up with the European Commission, stated *"the nanomedicine field is concretely able to design products that overcome critical barriers in conventional medicine in a unique manner"* [9]. This view agrees with the opinions of Lammers et al. [10], Martins et al. [11], and our own [4–7,12,13]. These viewpoints, however, disagreed with those of Prof. Park [14] and Wilhelm and Tavares [15].

In my opinion, these negative opinions of the EPR effect are based on experimental data for poorly designed nanomedicines. Most of the examples of failed cases reflect the use of so-called nanomedicines with very poor plasma half-lives ($t_{1/2}$) in vivo, or active pharmaceutical ingredients (APIs) in nanomedicines that rapidly became free low-molecular-weight (LMW) drugs. Therefore, similar to the parental LMW APIs, they lacked an essential requirement for nanomedicines of reasonably long $t_{1/2}$ values (i.e., several hours or longer in circulation in vivo). Failures include examples of block copolymer micelle carriers containing doxorubicin such as NK911 (code No. of the drug by Nippon Kayaku Co., Ltd.) or drug-polymer conjugates of inadequate size (less than 30 kDa). Their plasma $t_{1/2}$ values were too short in humans (<3 h). Cases reported by Wilhelm and Tavares [15] demonstrated the same problems. The size of macromolecular drugs that exhibit the EPR effect should be larger than 40 KDa to above 250 KDa, or above a molecular size larger than renal clearance (>5 nm to 100 nm). When the enhancers of the EPR effect are used, it is observed that a limit of this endothelial cell gaps will be increased as discussed later [1–7]. Furthermore, these findings suggest that the biocompatibility of these conjugates or nanomedicines must not be sufficient to demonstrate good stability during circulation. In contrast, if micellar or liposomal drugs are too stable, they may not release APIs from complexes or nanomedicines, even if they are delivered to tumors via the EPR effect, as is the case with Doxil (doxorubicin [DOX]-containing liposomes), which has a surface coating of polyethylene glycol (PEG) [16].

One should also realize that the milieu into which such drugs are infused is 100% blood, meaning a physiologically acceptable nature is required, and that the drugs are not subject to clearance by reticuloendothelial or phagocytic cells. Blood is quite different from physiological saline or deionized water because it contains many dye-binding proteins; dense negative charges also exist on vascular surfaces and will interact with APIs; and APIs may be abstracted from the micellar complex with APIs (drugs) before getting to tumor. Our previous reviews documented these problems related to failed cases [4–7,12,13].

1.2. Issue Concerns Passive Targeting to Tumor vs. the EPR Effect Driven Tumor Targeting

I want to emphasize, in this occasion, a critical difference between "passive targeting" and "EPR-effect based tumor targeted drug delivery". During the arterial angiography, a LMW x-ray contrast agent such as Angioconray® is infused intraarterially (i.a.), then this x-ray contrast agent of a LMW nature is taken up more selectively into the tumor tissues than normal tissues. This is indeed passive targeting. However, this LMW contrast agent administered will be rapidly washed out within a minute or so, as seen by x-ray imaging. In contrast, when macromolecular agents of >40 KDa or albumin binding dye Evans blue is injected i.v., they will be more selectively accumulated in the tumor tissue than normal tissues, and retained in the tumor for a prolonged period, more than several hours to weeks. This does not happen for LMW agents as they will be washed out rapidly. Similar to macromolecular drugs, when the lipidic contrast agent Lipiodol®, which is iodinated and ethylated poppy seed oil, is injected into the tumor feeding artery, Lipiodol becomes microparticles as it is broken up during its passing through the branched capillaries. Consequently, Lipiodol behaves like nanoparticles, and it will be retained in tumor tissue selectively more than several hours to months as easily seen by x-ray CAT scan, but this does not happen in normal tissues. This account is discussed in detail later.

Arterial infusion of LMW anticancer agents was tried extensively in the past as well as bolus intratumor injection, but both modalities were not so effective. Then, slow continuous arterial infusion using a infusion pump was conducted, though the drugs being infused will diffuse back quickly to the circulating blood, and result is more or less similar to i.v. infusion.

In conclusion, passive targeting only showed a short period of tumor retention, which is almost insignificant compared to the prolonged time of drug retention seen in EPR driven tumor delivery of macromolecular anti-cancer agents. The key issue here is that the passive targeting of drug does not implicate prolonged tumor retention of the drugs. This is the rationale of the EPR effect driven cancer therapy with longer retention time in tumors, but it needs to use nanomedicines, but not by LMW drugs.

In addition, the initial finding of the EPR effect was based primarily on experiments with tumor models in mice, whereas many large advanced tumors that are frequently seen in clinical situations differ from the small tumors in mice [12,13]. Nevertheless, we have ample evidence of the EPR effect occurring in human cancers. For example, neocarzinostatin (NCS) conjugated to poly(styrene-co-maleic acid) (SMA)—the conjugate named SMANCS—dissolved in Lipiodol® and given intra-arterially accumulated selectively in human solid tumors, as described below. Traditional radioscintigraphy with radioactive ^{67}Ga, which binds to the plasma protein transferrin (90 kDa), showed selective accumulation of ^{67}Ga in tumors by virtue of the EPR effect. More recently, intravenously injected nanomedicines demonstrated a tumor-selective EPR effect in breast cancer [17] and renal cancer [18].

1.3. Inflammation and EPR Effect Observed in Bacterial Infection Protease and Permeability Inducing Factors; Bradykinin and Other Mediators

As a historical aside, before I describe the vascular permeability of solid tumors, I should mention that we first studied bacterial infection and inflammation with a focus on the role of proteases produced by bacteria [19–22]. We then found that the bradykinin-generating cascade of endogenous proteases was activated by exogenous proteases produced by bacterial infection. That is, the sequence of the cascade was Hageman factor or factor XII → kallikrein → kininogen → bradykinin (kinin) (Figure 1). Kinin is a nonapeptide (RPPGFSPFR) cleaved off from kininogen in the plasma, and it induces vascular permeability, severe pain, and various signaling molecules. All microbial proteases including fungi trigger the cascade system, of which multiple steps are affected (Supplementary Figure S1) [21,22]. Activated endogenous proteases function in two important pathways: (i) thrombin activation and then fibrin formation, and (ii) kinin generation (Supplementary Figure S1), which is a key factor in vascular permeability in tumors, bacterial infections, and inflammation [23–27]. Ascitic and pleural effusions in carcinomatosis also largely depend on kinin generation in vivo [23–30].

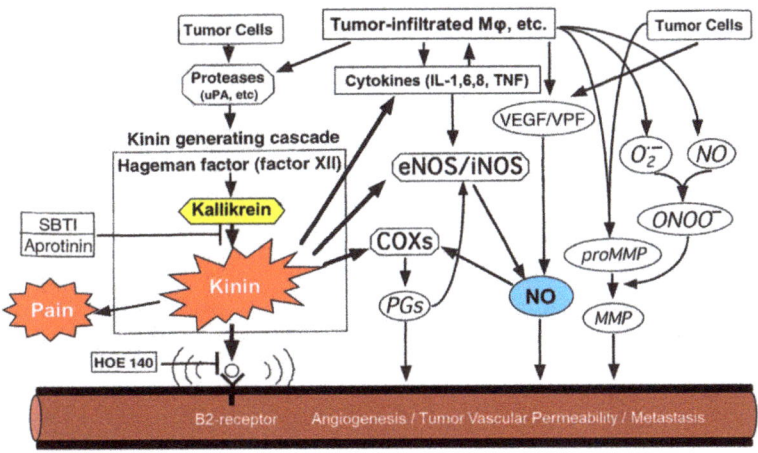

Figure 1. The enhanced permeability and retention (EPR) effect in tumor vasculature. The mechanism of this tumor-selective macromolecular drug targeting depends on various effectors affecting vascular tone, as shown here. Aprotinin is an inhibitor of kallikrein; HOE-140 is a peptide antagonist of kinin. SBTI, soybean trypsin inhibitor; NO, nitric oxide; eNOS, endothelial nitric oxide synthase; iNOS, inducible form of nitric oxide synthase; COXs, cyclooxygenases; PGs, prostaglandins; MMP, metalloproteinase; ONOO$^-$, peroxynitrite; O$_2^-$, superoxide anion radical; MΦ, macrophage; VEGF, vascular endothelial growth factor; VPF, vascular permeability factor; uPA, urokinase plasminogen activator; IL, interleukin; TNF, tumor necrosis factor; B2 receptor, bradykinin B2 receptor (see also Supplementary Figure S1, adapted from ref [23]).

In large advanced tumors, blood vessels are often occluded or embolized, although individual tumor pathology varies. For example, some liver metastases, pancreatic tumors, and prostate cancers have avascular areas with less vascular density, whereas primary liver and kidney cancers have extremely high vascular densities and therefore a correspondingly significant EPR effect (see also the discussion below). However, animal research ethics committees at most institutions restrict the use of large tumors, more than 5000 mm^3, in experimental settings. Such large tumors have occluded or embolized tumor blood vessels, as above-mentioned, and the degree of vascular density can be demonstrated by means of arterial angiography with a contrast agent such as Lipiodol®.

Since 1983, we have been studying blood vessels and their characteristics [6–8,31–36] in human cancers of the liver, kidney, lung, and other solid tumors. Contrast-enhanced arterial angiography showed highly stained areas that indeed corresponded to the EPR effect. We also demonstrated the effect of EPR effect enhancers in the above tumors including angiotensin II induced high blood pressure [34–36]. In contrast, pancreatic, prostate, and metastatic liver cancers showed low-density staining, thus indicating poor blood flow or avascular nature of tumors. These tumors have either occluded blood flow, or a weak or heterogeneous EPR effect.

2. Nanomedicines: Proceeding from Tissue EPR Effects to Tumor Cellular Uptake to Molecular Targets in Tumor Cells

After a nanomedicine has reached a tumor, the drug (the API) must enter the tumor cells and then affect target molecules in the cells. Doxil is delivered to tumor tissues because of its high stability in vivo and does have an EPR effect [16,37], but it has a low rate of API (DOX) release from the liposomes. DOX, liberated from Doxil, also has a low rate of internalization by tumor cells, which is a crucial issue. Although once DOX is internalized into cells, then to the nucleus, it forms an intercalated complex with target DNA. In this case, DOX is retained in the nucleus for a long time [38]. However, slow cell uptake of DOX is more critical before bending to the target. For instance, we found great different rates of internalization of DOX vs. pirarubicin, which is a derivative of DOX in which one mole of extra tetrahydropyranyl group is added. Pirarubicin showed a 10- to 100-fold higher rate of internalization, even though both DOX and pirarubicin possess the same anthracycline structure as their biologically active component [12,39,40] (see Figure 2). This rapid intracellular uptake of free pirarubicin continued even after the conjugation of pirarubicin with the N-(2-hydroxypropyl) methacrylamide (HPMA) polymer (Figure 2A). In contrast, the same DOX-polymer conjugate showed an extremely poor cellular uptake, and its biological activity was also poor (Figure 2B). The superior cellular uptake of pirarubicin may be attributed to the pyranyl group (i.e., its structure), which is similar to that of glucose (pyranose). Pyranose can be utilized in the cell uptake step by the glucose transporter system of tumor cells, which is highly upregulated in tumor cells.

With regard to the physicofchemical properties of macromolecular drugs (nanomedicines), we have described the importance of hydrophobicity and pH in the tumor microenvironment, which affects protonation and deionization of the carboxyl group in SMANCS, for instance [41–43]. That is, in addition to the styrene group's hydrophobicity, which results in an affinity to cell membranes; the maleyl carboxyl group becomes a pH sensor in the tumor environment. When the pH becomes lower than neutral, that is, the COO$^-$ is fully ionized to the protonated form (–COOH), hydrophobicity increases [41–43]. The result is a 100- to 200-fold increase in uptake by tumor cells in culture. As an additional advantage of this amphiphilic polymer conjugate, SMANCS and its parental proteinaceous antitumor agent (NCS) are active against drug (DOX)-resistant cell lines [44].

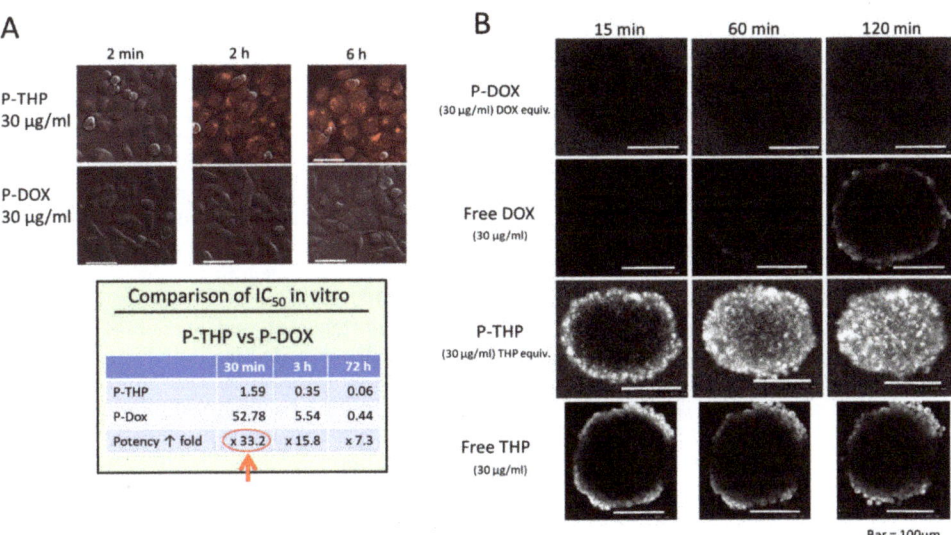

Figure 2. Comparison of the cellular uptake of P-THP—the poly(hydroxypropylmethaacrylamide [HPMA]) conjugate of pirarubicin (THP)—and P-DOX (HPMA polymer-DOX conjugate) by human pancreatic cancer cells (SUIT-2) in vitro. (**A**) Polymeric P-THP shows a far greater uptake by tumor cells compared with P-DOX: at 30 min, P-THP had a 33.2-fold higher uptake, and its cytotoxicity had greatly increased (see Table at lower left). (**B**) Penetration of P-DOX, DOX, P-THP, and THP into spheroidal tumor colon cancer (Adapted with permission from ref. [39,40]. 2016 American Chemical Society, 2019 American Chemical Society). Far greater penetration of P-THP into the tumor spheroid (similar to Figure 2, Table) is seen.

3. Future Prospects for the EPR Effect: Toward Clinical Application

3.1. Restoration of Tumor Blood Flow and Augmentation of the EPR Effect

The discussion above on the EPR effect for cancer-selective drug delivery is based on the assumption that tumor blood flow is normal—without vascular embolization, semi-necrotic areas that have poor blood flow, or necrotic tissue with blocked blood flow. However, the EPR effect, as just discussed, is often reduced in clinical settings, which is a most critical issue for proper tumor drug delivery [12,44–46]. The success of cancer chemotherapy with nanomedicines as based on the EPR effect thus requires normal tumor blood flow. For this purpose, we have worked on vasodilators or EPR effect enhancers including nitroglycerin [4–8,13,34–36], isosorbide dinitrate, L-arginine, and angiotensin I-converting enzyme inhibitors such as enalapril, among others. Our earlier and recent publications have emphasized this topic [8,9,12,13,34–36,45–47]. In this Special Issue, readers will find other tactics to enhance the EPR effect such as using bubble liposomes, microwaves, and heat [48,49].

In my opinion, very few nanomedicines are available for cancer chemotherapy that fulfill all the ideal requirements for use in patients, although many candidate nanodrugs are under development [11]. Our prototype polymeric drug, for example, the poly(hydroxypropylacrylamide) conjugate of pirarubicin (P-THP), so far seems to meet these requirements, although it needs approval by a regulatory agency before clinical use [47–51]. Many patients who received P-THP as compassionate use in a hospice mostly with stage IV or terminal disease, showed no apparent toxicity at the therapeutic dose level and responded very well to the treatment. Metastatic bone tumors or tumor nodules in the pleural compartment disappeared as expected ([52,53], and unpublished data]).

3.2. Arterial Infusion of Nanomedicines with Extremely High Accumulation in Tumors

Another option exists for enhanced tumor-targeted drug delivery. This method has not been so widely used because x-ray angiography and arterial infusion using a catheter requires qualified skills. The method involves application of a lipid formulation of lipophilic nanodrugs and trans-arterial infusion into tumor-feeding arteries via a catheter under x-ray monitoring. This modality produces by far the best tumor-targeted drug delivery as well as tumor imaging [31–36] and a tumor/blood ratio of more than 100 can easily be achieved [34,54,55]. We have successfully utilized this technique with SMANCS dissolved in Lipiodol®, and the method was approved for clinical use by the Ministry of Health, Labor, and Welfare of Japan. SMANCS in Lipiodol® solution becomes microparticles as it is pushed into arterial vessels, that is, SMANCS/Lipiodol® selectively extravasates into tumor tissues as microparticles, with results that are based on the EPR effect [31–36].

Arterial infusion of lipophilic drugs dissolved in Lipiodol® can be so selectively targeted to a tumor that the dose of the drug used in the infusion can be far reduced compared with the conventional systemic (i.e., intravenous) dosage. Therefore, we proposed that the doses for such arterial injections should be based on tumor size, not the body surface area or body weight of a patient [56]. Additionally, infusions for particular tumors such as bronchial, lung, or colon require special attention because a targeted area may suffer damage caused by a high concentration of drug and complications may ensue. For this reason, the dose of the drug should be 1/10 of the liver or gallbladder cancer. It is thus not strictly based on the tumor size [36,56]; high drug concentrations in such tissues with neighboring void spaces may cause the tissue to rupture, the results being perforation and bleeding.

4. Enhancement of Cancer Chemotherapy, Utilization of Photodynamic Therapy (PDT), Innovation in Boron Neutron Capture Therapy (BNCT), and Use of Reactive Oxygen Species (ROS)/Reactive Nitrogen Species (RNS) as Scavengers for Cancer and Inflammation via Nanodrugs

4.1. Enhancement of Photodynamic Therapy (PDT)

We and others have reported the many advantages of the EPR effect, primarily for cancer chemotherapy with nanomedicines. However, the usefulness of nanomedicines for photodynamic therapy (PDT) and boron neutron capture therapy (BNCT), which have been known for more than a century and several decades, respectively, would be far greater with nanotechnology when LMW photosensitizers (PSs) as well as boron containing drugs were converted to nanomedicine.

With regard to PSs, one can clearly demonstrate tumor-selective accumulation of polymer-conjugated PSs via in vivo models (Figure 3). We developed polymer conjugates of PEG, SMA, and HPMA to LMW zinc protoporphyrin (ZnPP) [4–6,13,50,57–62] (Figure 3). The PSs yielded fluorescence values above 500 nm and generated singlet oxygen or ROS, which can kill tumor cells. Selective fluorescence can be clearly detected in tumors in vivo (Figure 4A,B). This evidence is clear proof of the EPR effect.

Despite the long history of PDT-use in cancer therapy, its clinical impact has been insignificant. The reasons for this are: (i) most PSs developed so far such as Photofrin and Laserphyrin are of LMW with little EPR effect; and (ii) PSs being used contain a porphyrin chromophore, which is best excited at about 390–450 nm. However, in the past, most human applications used a HeNe laser that emits light only at 633 nm, which is far from the proper excitation wavelength of about 400 nm. Another criticism concerns hemoglobin interference: PSs composed of porphyrin derivatives with excitation wavelengths of about 400 nm will be affected in vivo by hemoglobin, which exists in massive amounts in the blood and will absorb excitation energy that is similar to the wavelength of the PSs being used, so the irradiating light will be absorbed before reaching the PSs. We can assume that the irradiating light will not effectively excite the PSs, which is a consequence of using improper wavelengths (633 nm) to excite PSs. However, this assumption may be true only in heme-rich organs such as the liver, spleen, and blood vessels. In contrast, tumor tissues do not have many blood cells. Red blood cells have a diameter of about 6 μm and cannot easily extravasate into tumor tissues or normal tissues. In addition, some PSs such as HPMA-polymer ZnPP and PEG-conjugated ZnPP have a compact micellar form, so that aromatic rings of the PSs molecules are packed within a close distance of each other. Thus, π–π interactions will quench the fluorescence and no singlet oxygen will be generated (Figure 3B). These PSs will fluoresce after the micelles traverse via endocytosis through cell membranes, which contains the lipid-bilayer into tumor cells and then the micelles disintegrate due to the detergent effect of the lipid bilayer (Figure 3B, in cell, right).

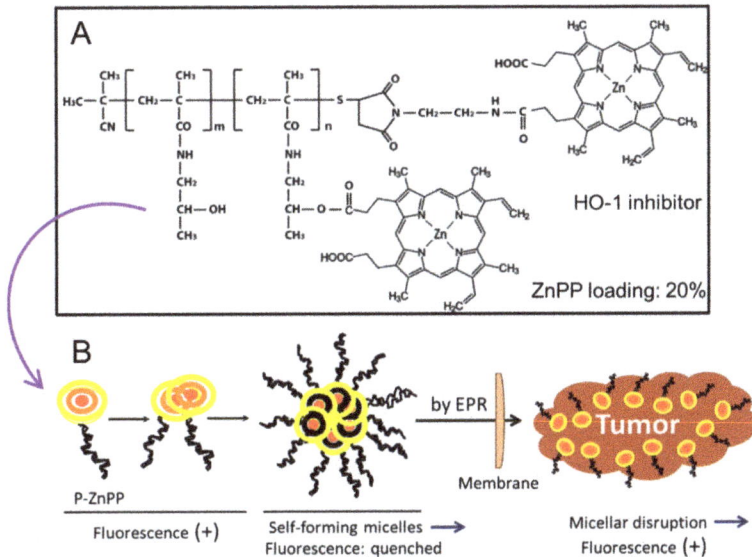

Figure 3. Self-assembling PS polymer conjugates of HPMA and ZnPP. (**A**) Chemical structure of the HPMA-PS polymer conjugate. (**B**) Polymer-ZnPP in solution. Spontaneous micelles were formed. Quenching occurs in the self-forming micellar form of P-ZnPP, which leads to a lack of fluorescence in the micellar form. When tumor cells take up these micelles, the micelles disintegrate during the traversing lipid bilayer due to its amphiphilic nature. Then, fluorescence becomes positive and singlet oxygen (ROS) are generated in the tumor upon light irradiation (**B**). ZnPP itself also inhibits heme oxygenase-1 (HO-1) and suppresses tumors (see text for details).

The therapeutic effect depends on both the PS (polymeric PS) dose and the intensity of the irradiating light (Figure 5B,C). We adapted the light source used for conventional endoscopy for this purpose (Figure 4A).

Drawbacks associated with current conventional PDT will not be seen with nano PSs because of the highly tumor-selective nature of the fluorescent nanoprobe, polymer-conjugated protoporphyrin (P-ZnPP) (Figure 4B,C). One problem involves hyper-sensitivity to light: patients who have undergone injections of conventional PSs are required to stay in a dark environment for a few weeks because of hypersensitivity of the skin: PSs will spread throughout the body including normal tissues, particularly the skin of the face and hands.

Our ZnPP has another beneficial effect. Even without light irradiation, it inhibits heme oxygenase (HO-1) as well as heat shock protein-32, and it downregulates oncogene expression [63–65]. HO-1 generates carbon monoxide and biliverdin/bilirubin as products of heme degradation by heme oxidation. Both carbon monoxide and bilirubin are potent antioxidants and block the actions of ROS/RNS, which are generated to produce a tumoricidal effect by host macrophages and neutrophils as part of the innate immunity mechanism. Therefore, PEG-ZnPP and SMA-ZnPP have antitumor effects themselves by potentiating tumor cell killing by ROS/RNS that are generated by leukocytes [62,66].

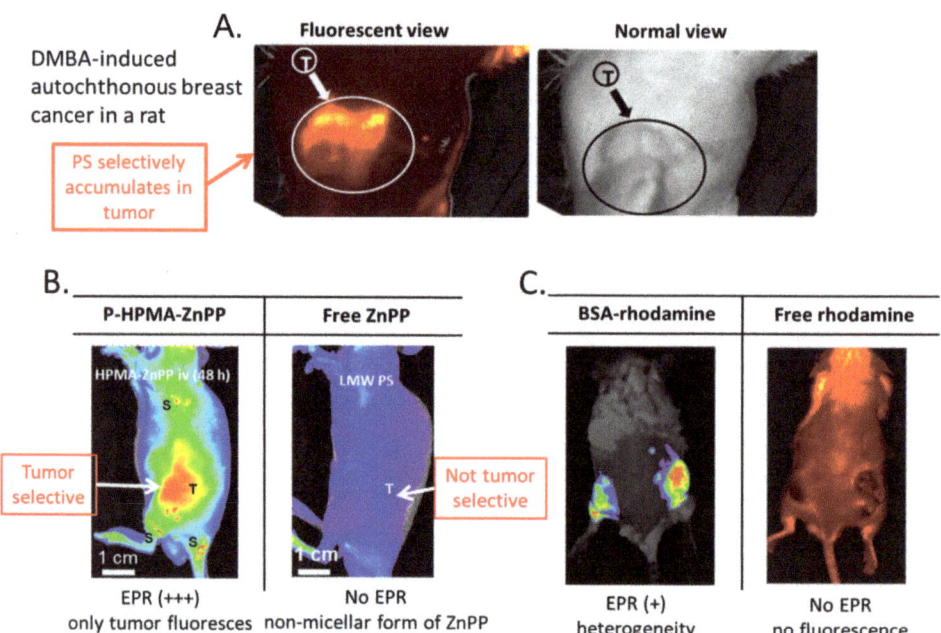

Figure 4. Fluorescence imaging of breast cancer in a rat and of implanted S180 tumor in a mouse, after intravenous injection of P-ZnPP. (**A**) DMBA (7,12-dimethylbenz[*a*]anthracene)-induced breast cancer in a rat. Under fluorescent light (left) and under normal light (right). (**B**) Fluorescent image of nano-PSs: polymeric HPMA-ZnPP (P-HPMA-ZnPP) and free ZnPP. (**C**) Rhodamine-conjugated bovine albumin (BSA) vs. free rhodamine. Images show no accumulation of LMW free PSs in tumors (**B**,**C**). (**A**, adapted from [58]; **B**,**C**, adapted from ref. [4]).

4.2. A Hot Progress in Boron Neutron Capture Therapy (BNCT) with Boron Nanomedicines

BNCT, like PDT, has been poorly developed. BNCT utilizes compounds containing ^{10}B and thermal neutron irradiation generated by a nuclear reactor or an accelerator. In this modality, ^{10}B compounds, as in PDT, must reach the local tumor for the best therapeutic effect without adverse effects. This requirement of tumor selective localization of ^{10}B means that the possibility exists for application of EPR effect-based ^{10}B-containing nanomedicines. In contrast to radiotherapy with x-ray or γ-ray irradiation, which require oxygen that will become effector ROS molecules, the thermal neutrons of BNCT, however, do not need oxygen molecules. The thermal neutrons need to hit ^{10}B atoms, the result being a yield of α-particles and lithium atoms as active principles that can kill cancer cells within a radius of 10 micron (see Figures 6 and 7A′). Current conventional BNCT in clinical settings uses an LMW ^{10}B derivative such as boronophenylalanine (BPA). Similar to the situation with chemotherapy with LMW cytotoxic drugs, BPA is not expected to be tumor selective (Figure 7B′). A continuous intravenous infusion of BPA during neutron irradiation is necessary to maintain an adequate boron concentration in the tumor tissue because its urinary excretion is quite rapid.

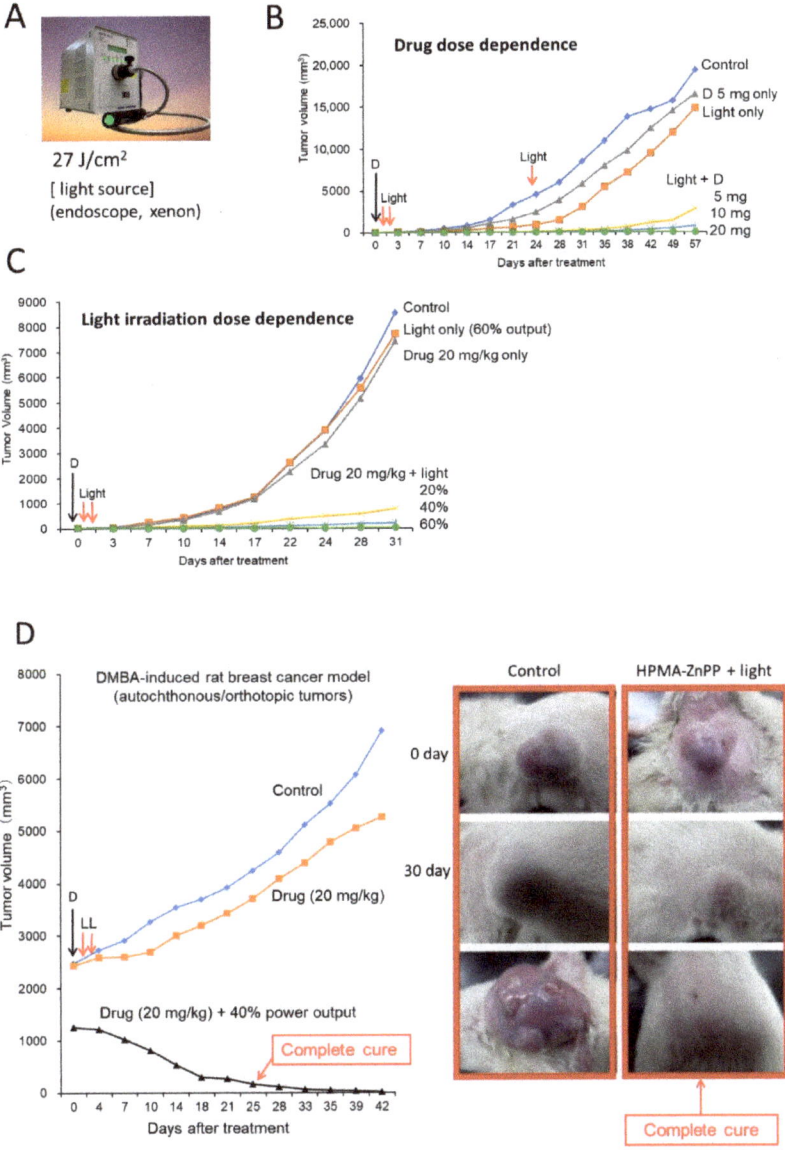

Figure 5. Photodynamic therapy (PDT) with polymeric PSs. (**A**) View of the light source for the endoscope; a xenon lamp was used. (**B**) Dose dependence of P-ZnPP dosage, marked D. (**C**) Dose of light irradiation intensity. The D indicates the time of drug injection of P-ZnPP in B and C. The power of irradiation light (%) is relative to full power output of the endoscope (100%). (**D**) Results of PDT treatment of DMBA-induced breast cancer in rats. L, light irradiation. D, drug injection. Control received only light. Boxed images at right show growth and suppression of tumor after PDT and P-ZnPP treatment (**right**) and tumor without treatment (**left**).

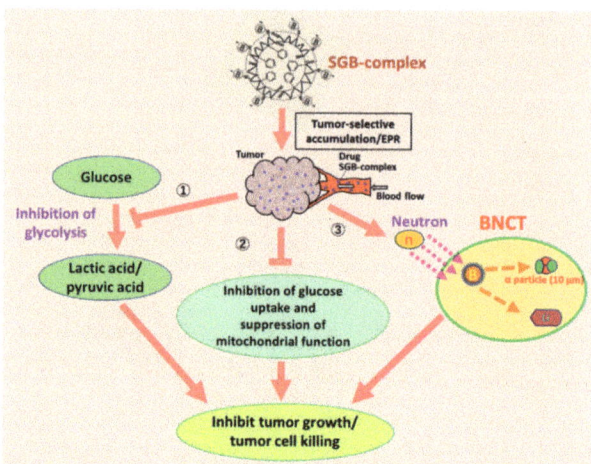

Figure 6. This represents the mode of action of poly(styrene-co-maleic acid) conjugated glucosamine (SGB-complex), which forms complex with boric acid, then forms micelles (~15 nm) and exhibits the EPR effect, about 10 times more boron accumulation in the tumor than other normal tissue [67]. When this SGB-complex is used, it exhibits three different cell killing mechanisms as denoted by "①, ②, and ③" in this figure. By neutron irradiation at right, ③, it elicits the production of α-particles which will kill the tumor cells within 10 micron radius. SGB-complex is rapidly incorporated into the tumor cells and inhibit both glycolysis ① and production of lactic acid; ② it also affects the structural integrity of mitochondria, and its size will shrink and suppress ATP production in the cells (Reprinted with permission from ref. [67]. 2020 Elsevier Ltd.).

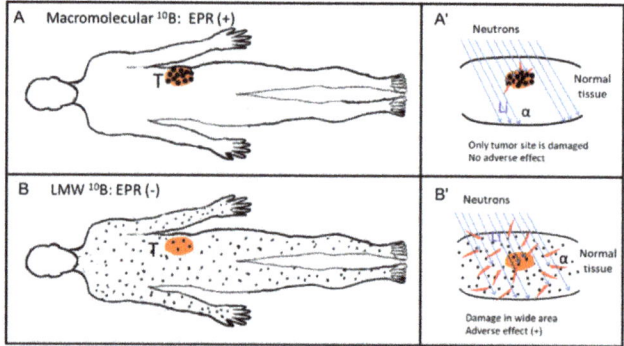

Figure 7. Body distribution of boron-containing drugs. (**A**) Body distribution of a macromolecular ^{10}B compound (e.g., SGB-complex). (**B**) Distribution of an LMW ^{10}B compound. In (**A**), boron-containing micelles such as the SGB-complex accumulates predominantly in tumor tissue (T), with the accumulation being about 10 times greater than that of a LMW compound or all other normal tissues in (**B**). (**A**′,**B**′) at right represent enlarged views of the neutron irradiation sites. In (**A**′), only tumor tissue is damaged: boron micelles (back dots) are evident only in the tumor (T). In (**B**′), neighboring normal tissue to tumor the boron compound are distributed in most normal tissues such as skin, which will be then be damaged. Red specks around black dots indicate the area of emission of α-particles. (**B**′) shows that a wide area of tissue is damaged in (**B**′) (adverse effect).

As Figure 7B illustrates, BPA exists in both normal and cancer tissues. Therefore, BPA may affect normal tissue such as the skin as well as cancer-neighboring normal tissues other than tumor tissue. For instance, when treating an oral cancer with BNCT, vocal cords and superficial skin may be harmed. Use of BNCT thus carries the probability of adverse effects. However, we can avoid this problem by using macromolecular boron derivatives [67].

We recently published a report on such macromolecular boron derivatives in which SMA was first linked with glucosamine (SG) [67]. Glucosamine forms a stable complex with boric acid (SGB complex). Natural boric acid contains about 25–30% of ^{10}B, with the remainder being ^{11}B. ^{10}B-enriched boron derivatives are available, however. The SGB complex forms micelles of about 12 nm, as seen with election microscopy, about 65 kDa in solution (Sephacryl S200), and it can bind with albumin in solution, so that its size increases to more than 120 kDa [67]. This size is ideal for the EPR effect to operate. In experiments with a tumor-bearing mouse model, the accumulation of the SGB complex in tumors was about 10-fold higher than that in all normal tissues including the liver and kidney [67].

The SGB complex has multiple actions in addition to the generation of α-particles such as the inhibition of glycolysis; see reference [67] for details, and Figure 6. Similar to glucosamine, one can conjugate BPA to the SMA polymer, and similar results will be expected, but neither inhibition of glycolysis (suppression of lactic acid formation), nor damage to mitochondria are expected. Preliminary data for neutron irradiation in vitro and in vivo were validated: tumors shrunk without any effects on skin or on toxicity in the liver and kidney, or on blood counts. I can thus envision new possibilities for BNCT with boron nanomedicines, where a new wave is coming.

5. Development of ROS and RNS Generators or Scavengers Utilizing the Advantages of Nanodrugs, and Future Clinical Applications

5.1. Elimination of Toxic Free Radical ROS/RNS in Infection and Cancer by Using Nanomedicines

Oxygen free radicals, or ROS, and RNS cause various diseases. ROS and RNS species are produced primarily at sites of infection, inflammation, and cancer. Maeda et al. demonstrated that excessive generation of ROS and RNS, together with nitric oxide (NO), occurs during influenza virus infection in mice. These species are responsible for the pathogenesis of influenza and influenza-related pneumonia; they are also associated with other microbial infection, and they also further accelerate viral mutations [68–71].

We have investigated the effects of a free radical-scavenging enzyme, superoxide dismutase (SOD; MW about 20 kDa), in influenza virus-infected mice. Intravenously injected native SOD was not effective by itself, because the $t_{1/2}$ of native SOD is too short (<1 h), as discussed above. Conjugating SOD to pyran copolymer (pyran-SOD) considerably improved the pharmacological and therapeutic effects, and diseased mice were cured. Namely, mice that received injections of pyran-SOD had a 95% cure, whereas native SOD had no effect on the survival of the mice [68,69].

ROS have no single source, but are initially derived from macrophages or neutrophils, followed by activation of xanthine dehydrogenase to xanthine oxidase (XO) in diseased tissue such as the lung [68–70]. In contrast, more extensive production NO is derived from the inducible form of NO synthase in macrophages in the inflamed tissue or in cancer. Two of these molecular species, O_2^- and NO, react quite rapidly in situ and form peroxynitrite, which is more reactive than O_2^- and NO and has highly oxidative and nitrative effects on DNA, RNA, proteins, and lipids. A free radical storm (i.e., NO, O_2^-, HClO, $ONOO^-$, etc.) are likely operating behind the scenes in this complicated current COVID-19 pandemic and must be controlled [69–72]. This pandemic may be out of control until we have effective vaccines or antiviral agents as well as control of the ROS/RNS storm [72]. As with ROS, O_2^- is converted to H_2O_2 (a less reactive ROS) by SOD, and when myeloperoxidase in neutrophils is accessible to H_2O_2 and chlorine, HClO (hypochlorite) will be formed, which will also damage DNA, RNA, proteins, and lipids as well as bacteria, tumors, and normal tissues, the consequence being a triggering of many diseases. ROS/RNS generation thus formed in microbial infection will result in the accelerated formation of mutation unless the formation of ROS/RNS is controlled [73–76].

Shashni and Nagasaki prepared a unique polymer conjugate of 4-amino-TEMPO, a redox-cycling nitroxide (4-hydroxy-TEMPO; (4-hydroxy-2,2,6,6-tetramethylpiperidine-1-oxyl)-TEMPO), another free radical scavenger with poor pharmacokinetic properties by itself [77]. When they conjugated this redox-sensitive prosthetic group (amino-TEMPO) to a diblock copolymer (PEG) plus [poly(tetramethyl-piperidine-1-oxyl)aminomethylstyrene], the polymer conjugate was superior, with far better pharmacokinetics and showed suppressive effects on tumor growth (see [77]). The finding of this polymer conjugate may be applied to ROS/RNS-related diseases with inflammation or complicated infections such as COVID-19.

5.2. Using ROS/RNS Generation to Kill Cancers by Means of ROS-Generating Polymer-Conjugated Enzymes, or Rescuing ROS-Caused Damage by Means of Enzyme Replacement Therapy via Conjugation with Synthetic Polymers

An important early use of PEGylated enzymes was enzyme replacement therapy. Use of PEGylated adenosine deaminase (ADA) for congenital disease is well documented [78]; the $t_{1/10}$ in humans was about one month, which may be better than that for the infusion of recombinant lymphocytes with ADA being the $t_{1/2}$ of normal lymphocytes in general is about a month. Additionally, PEG-L-asparaginase has long been used in clinical situations for patients with leukemia [79]. Its $t_{1/2}$ was 3 min and converted to 56 h, and its $t_{1/10}$ was >11 days. In this context, the HPMA-polymer conjugate of protein may be preferable to PEGylated enzymes because it is so far free from immunogenicity or less immunogenic compared with PEGylated enzymes. Namely, PEGylation generates an anti-PEG antibody, which becomes a problem a few weeks later after initial infusion, even in the case of PEG-L-asparaginase. On the basis of a similar principle, we addressed hyper-bilirubinemia (jaundice). High concentration of bilirubin in blood causes jaundice and at higher concentrations, it becomes toxic to many cells. We PEGylated bilirubin oxidase produced by fungus and found that its $t_{1/10}$ became much higher (1.8 min → 48 h in rats) [80].

We also investigated an opposite direction to utilize ROS generation by XO as a possible cancer cure [81,82]. PEGylated XO (PEG-XO) produced significant antitumor activity after three PEG-XO injections in two weeks; each PEG-XO injection was followed by daily injections of its substrate, hypoxanthine. Here again, native XO alone followed by infusion with hypoxanthine resulted in no therapeutic effect, but conjugation of biocompatible PEG improved the pharmacokinetics of XO and exhibited an EPR effect, and therapeutic benefit was improved.

We later applied a similar strategy to D-amino acid oxidase (DAO), which is another ROS (H_2O_2)-generating enzyme. When we injected a D-amino acid such as D-proline or D-alanine to tumor bearing mice i.v., PEGylated-DAO (PEG-DAO) generated H_2O_2 in the tumors because of selective tumor accumulation of PEG-DAO by virtue of the EPR effect; this antitumor strategy worked well to control tumor growth in the mouse [83,84]. In a different investigation, Fang et al. achieved successful therapeutic results with polymer (SMA)-conjugated AHPP (4-amino-6-hydroxypyrazolo[3,4-d]pyrimidine), an XO inhibitor [85] with an anti-inflammatory and antihypersensitivity activity.

More examples may exist of which I am not aware, but so far, no drugs that utilize free radical generation or scavengers are in clinical use.

H_2O_2 generation is an important event in healthy organisms and is essential in that it occurs (predominantly) via NADPH oxidase or other enzymes in leukocytes. Congenital deficiency of NADPH oxidase results in chronic granulomatous disease (CGD), particularly in infant and children because of the lack of H_2O_2 or O_2^- to kill bacteria, and constant or chronic infections will lead to CGD. We therefore prepared PEGylated DAO to deliver PEG-DAO to inflamed sites and thus supply ROS, in parallel with administration of D-proline or D-alanine, the DAO substrates. When H_2O_2 is generated, it will be converted to the more powerful bactericidal molecule. HClO is generated by neutrophils in the presence of both myeloperoxidase and chloride ion, which will kill bacteria [82,83]. Normal healthy cells contain enzymes for defense against ROS, which is catalase for H_2O_2 and SOD for O_2^-.

Many cancer cells lack these anti-oxystress enzymes or have downregulated levels of these enzymes, so they are vulnerable to oxystress. Many advanced cancer cells propagate well under anaerobic conditions, and antioxidant enzymes may be lost [6,7,12,81,82] due to elevated levels of hypoxia due to embolization or clotting in the blood vessels [46,86]. To dissolve fibrin clots to activate plasminogen to plasmin, Mei et al. used redox sensitive polymer conjugate, and made enhanced vascular permeability by newly generated plasmin [87], and also modulate an extra cellular tumor environment [86,88]. Thus far, delivery of ROS-generating or scavenging enzymes conjugated to synthetic polymers may be an intriguing therapeutic strategy.

6. Concluding Remarks

This Special Issue commemorates my 35th year after discovery of the EPR effect [1,2], and therefore this review includes many of my own papers related to this area. I have focused primarily on synthetic and artificial nanomedicines, so I have not included antibody-linked drugs, cytokines such as interferon, interleukin-6, and tumor necrosis factor-β, and liposomes.

The ultimate purpose of personalized medicine is to provide the best benefits for individual patients. The EPR effect is a ubiquitous phenomenon found in almost all solid tumors, with sizes from less than 1 mm to larger than 10 cm; this effect also occurs in inflamed tissues and applies to biocompatible macromolecules. To utilize the EPR effect or the related drug delivery system more effectively, vascular blood flow must be restored and maintained. Nanomedicines are of prime importance for receiving the benefits of the EPR effect. The issues of vascular flow in tumor tissues is a relatively recent issue in cancer therapy [4,7,12,13,45,47,63,86,88], although vascular embolism in cardiology, for example, has been investigated often for some time, but not much in relation to cancer [13,45,67,86,89].

Various advantages of the unique properties of nanomedicines as well as selective drug targeting to tumors and inflamed tissues were easily demonstrated via pharmacokinetics and pharmacodynamics and imaging; the use of EPR effect enhancers exhibit fewer adverse effects and improved therapeutic results are thus expected when combined with nanomedicines compared with conventional medicines in the future. Nanomedicine is therefore worthy of study and challenges for the benefit of patients. Wider applications of PDT and BNCT as well as strategies to control the ubiquitous undesirable molecules like ROS/RNS are future lines of study (e.g., [77]). The growing knowledge of the tumor microenvironment, as discussed by Subrahmanyam and Ghandehari in this volume [86], will provide many clues for the future delivery of nanomedicines and may make use of many intelligent or sophisticated sensors or probes.

Supplementary Materials: The following are available online at https://www.mdpi.com/2075-4426/11/3/229/s1, Figure S1: The bradykinin (kinin)-generating cascade of host animals that is activated by various microbial proteases at different steps and inhibitors.

Funding: The author acknowledges support from the Japan Society for the Promotion of Science (JSPS), a Grant-in-Aid for Scientific Research (KAKENHI) Grant Number 18H04059 to H. Yamamoto/H. Maeda, a Bilateral Joint Research Project between the Czech Academy of Sciences (CAS) and JSPS (29400001) to H. Maeda, and the BioDynamics Research Foundation.

Data Availability Statement: The data that support the findings in this article are available from the corresponding author, H.M. upon reasonable request.

Acknowledgments: The author would like to express his sincere appreciation to his many colleagues: R. Kanamura, J. Takeshita, Y. Matsumura, Y. Noguchi, T. Konno, S. Maki, K. Iwai, T. Sawa, R. Duncan, L. Seymour, J. Wu, K. Ulbrich, T. Etrych, T. Seki, H. Nakamura, M. Kimura, Chiang. Li, C. Christophi, J. Fang, A. Iyer, A. Nagamitsu, K. Sakurai, W. Islam, H. Dozono, S. Ozaki, and H. Yamamoto as well as many others, too many to mention individually. The author also acknowledges Judith Gandy for her excellent and invaluable assistance in English editing and Asami Yamashiro for her excellent secretarial work on the manuscript.

Conflicts of Interest: The authors declare no conflict of interest.

References

1. Matsumura, Y.; Maeda, H. A new concept for macromolecular therapeutics in cancer chemotherapy: Mechanism of tumortropic accumulation of proteins and the antitumor agent SMANCS. *Cancer Res.* **1986**, *46*, 6387–6392.
2. Noguchi, Y.; Wu, J.; Duncan, R.; Strohalm, J.; Ulbrich, K.; Akaike, T.; Maeda, H. Early phase tumor accumulation of macromolecules: A great difference in clearance rate between tumor and normal tissues. *Jpn. J. Cancer Res.* **1998**, *89*, 307–314. [CrossRef] [PubMed]
3. Maeda, H. Tumor-Selective Delivery of Macromolecular Drugs via the EPR Effect: Background and Future Prospects. *Bioconjugate Chem.* **2010**, *21*, 797–802. [CrossRef]
4. Maeda, H. The link between infection and cancer: Tumor vasculature, free radicals, and drug delivery to tumors via the EPR effect. *Cancer Sci.* **2013**, *104*, 779–789. [CrossRef]
5. Maeda, H. Polymer therapeutics and the EPR effect. *J. Drug Target.* **2017**, *25*, 781–785. [CrossRef]
6. Maeda, H.; Tsukigawa, K.; Fang, J. A retrospective 30 years after discovery of the EPR effect of solid tumors: Treatment, imaging, and next-generation PDT—problems, solutions, prospects. *Microcirculation* **2016**, *23*, 173–182. [CrossRef]
7. Maeda, H. Toward a full understanding of the EPR effect in primary and metastatic tumors as well as issues related to its heterogeneity. *Adv. Drug Deliv. Rev.* **2015**, *91*, 3–6. [CrossRef] [PubMed]
8. Fang, J.; Nakamura, H.; Maeda, H. The EPR effect: Unique features of tumor blood vessels for drug delivery, factors involved, and limitations and augmentation of the effect. *Adv. Drug Deliv. Rev.* **2011**, *63*, 136–151. [CrossRef]
9. Germain, M.; Caputo, F.; Metcalfe, S.; Tosi, G.; Spring, K.; Åslund, A.K.; Pottier, A.; Schiffelers, R.; Ceccaldi, A.; Schmid, R. Delivering the power of nanomedicine to patients today. *J. Control. Release* **2020**, *326*, 164–171. [CrossRef] [PubMed]
10. Lammers, T. Drug delivery research in Europe. *J. Control. Release* **2012**, *161*, 151. [CrossRef] [PubMed]
11. Martins, J.P.; Das Neves, J.; De La Fuente, M.; Celia, C.; Florindo, H.; Günday-Türeli, N.; Popat, A.; Santos, J.L.; Sousa, F.; Schmid, R.; et al. The solid progress of nanomedicine. *Drug Deliv. Transl. Res.* **2020**, *10*, 726–729. [CrossRef] [PubMed]
12. Fang, J.; Islam, W.; Maeda, H. Exploiting the dynamics of the EPR effect and strategies to improve the therapeutic effects of nanomedicines by using EPR effect enhancers. *Adv. Drug Deliv. Rev.* **2020**, *157*, 142–160. [CrossRef] [PubMed]
13. Maeda, H.; Khatami, M. Analyses of repeated failures in cancer therapy for solid tumors: Poor tumor-selective drug delivery, low therapeutic efficacy and unsustainable costs. *Clin. Transl. Med.* **2018**, *7*, 11. [CrossRef]
14. Park, K. The beginning of the end of the nanomedicine hype. *J. Control. Release* **2019**, *305*, 221–222. [CrossRef]
15. Wilhelm, S.; Tavares, A.J.; Dai, Q.; Ohta, S.; Audet, J.; Dvorak, H.F.; Chan, W.C.W. Analysis of nano-particle delivery to tumours. *Nat. Rev. Mater.* **2016**, *1*, 16014. [CrossRef]
16. Gabizon, A.; Catane, R.; Uziely, B.; Kaufman, B.; Safra, T.; Cohen, R.; Martin, F.; Huang, A.; Barenholz, Y. Prolonged circulation time and enhanced accumulation in malignant exudates of doxorubicin en-capsulated in polyethylene-glycol coated liposomes. *Cancer Res.* **1994**, *54*, 987–992.
17. Ding, Y.; Xu, Y.; Yang, W.; Niu, P.; Li, X.; Chen, Y.; Li, Z.; Liu, Y.; An, Y.; Liu, Y.; et al. Investigating the EPR effect of nanomedicines in human renal tumors via ex vivo perfusion strategy. *Nano Today* **2020**, *35*, 100970. [CrossRef]
18. Lee, H.; Shields, A.F.; Siegel, B.A.; Miller, K.D.; Krop, I.; Ma, C.X.; Lorusso, P.M.; Munster, P.N.; Campbell, K.; Gaddy, D.F.; et al. 64Cu-MM-302 Positron Emission Tomography Quantifies Variability of Enhanced Permeability and Retention of Nanoparticles in Relation to Treatment Response in Patients with Metastatic Breast Cancer. *Clin. Cancer Res.* **2017**, *23*, 4190–4202. [CrossRef]
19. Matsumoto, K.; Yamamoto, T.; Kamata, R.; Maeda, H. Pathogenesis of Serratial Infection: Activation of the Hageman Factor-Prekallikrein Cascade by Serratial Protease. *J. Biochem.* **1984**, *96*, 739–749. [CrossRef] [PubMed]
20. Kamata, R.; Yamamoto, T.; Matsumoto, K.; Maeda, H. A serratial protease causes vascular permeability reaction by activation of the Hageman factor-dependent pathway in guinea pigs. *Infect. Immun.* **1985**, *48*, 747–753. [CrossRef] [PubMed]
21. Molla, A.; Yamamoto, T.; Akaike, T.; Miyoshi, S.; Maeda, H. Activation of Hageman factor and prekal-likrein and generation of kinin by various microbial proteinases. *J. Biol. Chem.* **1989**, *264*, 10589–10594. [CrossRef]
22. Maruo, K.; Akaike, T.; Inada, Y.; Ohkubo, I.; Ono, T.; Maeda, H. Effect of microbial and mite proteases on low and high molecular weight kininogens. Generation of kinin and inactivation of thiol protease inhibitory activity. *J. Biol. Chem.* **1993**, *268*, 17711–17715. [CrossRef]
23. Maeda, H. The enhanced permeability and retention (EPR) effect in tumor vasculature: The key role of tumor-selective macromolecular drug targeting. *Adv. Enzym. Regul.* **2001**, *41*, 189–207. [CrossRef]
24. Maeda, H.; Wu, J.; Okamoto, T.; Maruo, K.; Akaike, T. Kallikrein–kinin in infection and cancer. *Immunopharmacology* **1999**, *43*, 115–128. [CrossRef]
25. Maeda, H.; Fang, J.; Inutsuka, T.; Kitamoto, Y. Vascular permeability enhancement in solid tumor: Various factors, mechanisms involved and its implications. *Int. Immunopharmacol.* **2003**, *3*, 319–328. [CrossRef]
26. Wu, J.; Akaike, T.; Maeda, H. Modulation of enhanced vascular permeability in tumors by a bradykinin antagonist, a cyclooxygenase inhibitor, and a nitric oxide scavenger. *Cancer Res.* **1998**, *58*, 159–165.
27. Wu, J.; Akaike, T.; Hayashida, K.; Okamoto, T.; Okuyama, A.; Maeda, H. Enhanced vascular permea-bility in solid tumor involving peroxynitrite and matrix metalloproteinase. *Jpn. J. Cancer Res.* **2001**, *92*, 439–451. [CrossRef]
28. Maeda, H.; Matsumura, Y.; Kato, H. Purification and identification of [hydroxyprolyl3]bradykinin in ascitic fluid from a patient with gastric cancer. *J. Biol. Chem.* **1988**, *263*, 16051–16054. [CrossRef]

29. Matsumura, Y.; Kimura, M.; Yamamoto, T.; Maeda, H. Involvement of the Kinin-generating Cascade in Enhanced Vascular Permeability in Tumor Tissue. *Jpn. J. Cancer Res.* **1988**, *79*, 1327–1334. [CrossRef] [PubMed]
30. Matsumura, Y.; Maruo, K.; Kimura, M.; Yamamoto, T.; Konno, T.; Maeda, H. Kinin-generating Cascade in Advanced Cancer Patients andin vitroStudy. *Jpn. J. Cancer Res.* **1991**, *82*, 732–741. [CrossRef] [PubMed]
31. Konno, T.; Maeda, H.; Iwai, K.; Tashiro, S.; Maki, S.; Morinaga, T.; Mochinaga, M.; Hiraoka, T.; Yokoyama, I. Effect of arterial administration of high-molecular-weight anticancer agent SMANCS with lipid lymphographic agent on hepatoma: A preliminary report. *Eur. J. Cancer Clin. Oncol.* **1983**, *19*, 1053–1065. [CrossRef]
32. Maki, S.; Konno, T.; Maeda, H. Image enhancement in computerized tomography for sensitive diagnosis of liver cancer and semiquantitation of tumor selective drug targeting with oily contrast medium. *Cancer* **1985**, *56*, 751–757. [CrossRef]
33. Konno, T.; Maeda, H.; Iwai, K.; Maki, S.; Tashiro, S.; Uchida, M.; Miyauchi, Y. Selective targeting of anti-cancer drug and simultaneous image enhancement in solid tumors by arterially administered lipid contrast medium. *Cancer* **1984**, *54*, 2367–2374. [CrossRef]
34. Maeda, H. Vascular permeability in cancer and infection as related to macromolecular drug delivery, with emphasis on the EPR effect for tumor-selective drug targeting. *Proc. Jpn. Acad. Ser. B Phys. Biol. Sci.* **2012**, *88*, 53–71. [CrossRef]
35. Maeda, H. Macromolecular therapeutics in cancer treatment: The EPR effect and beyond. *J. Control. Release* **2012**, *164*, 138–144. [CrossRef]
36. Nagamitsu, A.; Greish, K.; Maeda, H. Elevating Blood Pressure as a Strategy to Increase Tumor-targeted Delivery of Macromolecular Drug SMANCS: Cases of Advanced Solid Tumors. *Jpn. J. Clin. Oncol.* **2009**, *39*, 756–766. [CrossRef]
37. Prabhakar, U.; Maeda, H.; Jain, R.K.; Sevick-Muraca, E.; Zamboni, W.; Farokhzad, O.C.; Barry, S.T.; Gabizon, A.; Grodzinski, P.; Blakey, D.C. Challenges and key considerations of the enhanced permeability and retention effect (EPR) for nanomedicine drug delivery in oncology. *Cancer Res.* **2013**, *73*, 2412–2417. [CrossRef]
38. Laginha, K.M.; Verwoert, S.; Charrois, G.J.; Allen, T.M. Determination of Doxorubicin Levels in Whole Tumor and Tumor Nuclei in Murine Breast Cancer Tumors. *Clin. Cancer Res.* **2005**, *11*, 6944–6949. [CrossRef] [PubMed]
39. Nakamura, H.; Koziolová, E.; Chytil, P.; Tsukigawa, K.; Fang, J.; Haratake, M.; Ulbrich, K.; Etrych, T.; Maeda, H. Pronounced Cellular Uptake of Pirarubicin versus That of Other Anthracyclines: Comparison of HPMA Copolymer Conjugates of Pirarubicin and Doxorubicin. *Mol. Pharm.* **2016**, *13*, 4106–4115. [CrossRef]
40. Nakamura, H.; Koziolová, E.; Chytil, P.; Etrych, T.; Haratake, M.; Maeda, H. Superior Penetration and Cytotoxicity of HPMA Copolymer Conjugates of Pirarubicin in Tumor Cell Spheroid. *Mol. Pharm.* **2019**, *16*, 3452–3459. [CrossRef]
41. Oda, T.; Sato, F.; Maeda, H. Facilitated internalization of neocarzinostatin and its lipophilic polymer conjugate, SMANCS, into cytosol in acidic pH. *J. Natl. Cancer Inst.* **1987**, *79*, 1205–1211.
42. Oda, T.; Maeda, H. Binding to and internalization by cultured cells of neocarzinostatin and enhance-ment of its actions by conjugation with lipophilic styrene-maleic acid copolymer. *Cancer Res.* **1987**, *47*, 3206–3211. [PubMed]
43. Maeda, H.; Islam, W. Overcoming barriers for tumor-targeted drug delivery: The power of macromo-lecular anticancer drugs with the EPR effect and the modulation of vascular physiology. In *Polymer-Protein Conjugation: From PEGylation and Beyond*; Pasut, G., Zalipsky, S., Eds.; Elsevier: Amsterdam, The Netherlands, 2020; pp. 41–58.
44. Miyamoto, Y.; Oda, T.; Maeda, H. Comparison of the cytotoxic effects of the high- and low-molecular-weight anticancer agents on multidrug-resistant Chinese hamster ovary cells in vitro. *Cancer Res.* **1990**, *50*, 1571–1575.
45. Navi, B.B.; Reiner, A.S.; Kamel, H.; Iadecola, C.; Okin, P.M.; Tagawa, S.T.; Panageas, K.S.; DeAngelis, L.M. Arterial thromboembolic events preceding the diagnosis of cancer in older persons. *Blood* **2019**, *133*, 781–789. [CrossRef] [PubMed]
46. Seki, T.; Fang, J.; Maeda, H. Enhanced delivery of macromolecular antitumor drugs to tumors by nitroglycerin application. *Cancer Sci.* **2009**, *100*, 2426–2430. [CrossRef] [PubMed]
47. Islam, W.; Fang, J.; Imamura, T.; Etrych, T.; Subr, V.; Ulbrich, K.; Maeda, H. Augmentation of the enhanced permeability and retention effect with nitric oxide-generating agents improves the therapeutic effects of nanomedicines. *Mol. Cancer Ther.* **2018**, *17*, 2643–2653. [CrossRef] [PubMed]
48. Nittayacharn, P.; Yuan, H.-X.; Hernandez, C.; Bielecki, P.; Zhou, H.; Exner, A.A. Enhancing Tumor Drug Distribution with Ultrasound-Triggered Nanobubbles. *J. Pharm. Sci.* **2019**, *108*, 3091–3098. [CrossRef] [PubMed]
49. Khan, M.S.; Hwang, J.; Lee, K.; Choi, Y.; Seo, Y.; Jeon, H.; Hong, J.W.; Choi, J. Anti-Tumor Drug-Loaded Oxygen Nanobubbles for the Degradation of HIF-1α and the Upregulation of Reactive Oxygen Species in Tumor Cells. *Cancers* **2019**, *11*, 1464. [CrossRef]
50. Maeda, H.; Nakamura, H.; Fang, J. The EPR effect for macromolecular drug delivery to solid tumors: Improvement of tumor uptake, lowering of systemic toxicity, and distinct tumor imaging in vivo. *Adv. Drug Deliv. Rev.* **2013**, *65*, 71–79. [CrossRef]
51. Nakamura, H.; Etrych, T.; Chytil, P.; Ohkubo, M.; Fang, J.; Ulbrich, K.; Maeda, H. Two step mechanisms of tumor selective delivery of N-(2-hydroxypropyl)methacrylamide copolymer conjugated with pirarubicin via an acid-cleavable linkage. *J. Control. Release* **2014**, *174*, 81–87. [CrossRef]
52. Dozono, H.; Yanazume, S.; Nakamura, H.; Etrych, T.; Chytil, P.; Ulbrich, K.; Fang, J.; Arimura, T.; Douchi, T.; Kobayashi, H.; et al. HPMA Copolymer-Conjugated Pirarubicin in Multimodal Treatment of a Patient with Stage IV Prostate Cancer and Extensive Lung and Bone Metastases. *Target. Oncol.* **2015**, *11*, 101–106. [CrossRef]
53. Okuno, S. Birth of Anticancer Agent Without Adverse Effect. In *Revolution in Cancer Treatment*; (Book in Japanese. Interviews with treated patients of HPMA-polymer conjugated. Follow up by interview with P-THP treated many patients over several months to years); Bungei Shunju Sha: Tokyo, Japan, 2016; pp. 1–284.

54. Iwai, K.; Maeda, H.; Konno, T. Use of oily contrast medium for selective drug targeting to tumor: Enhanced therapeutic effect and X-ray image. *Cancer Res.* **1984**, *44*, 2115–2121.
55. Maeda, H. SMANCS and polymer-conjugated macromolecular drugs: Advantages in cancer chemotherapy. *Adv. Drug Deliv. Rev.* **1991**, *6*, 181–202. [CrossRef]
56. Seymour, L.W.; Olliff, S.P.; Poole, C.J.; De Takats, P.G.; Orme, R.; Ferry, D.R.; Maeda, H.; Konno, T.; Kerr, D.J. A novel dosage approach for evaluation of SMANCS [poly-(styrene-co-maleyl-half-n-butylate)-neocarzinostatin] in the treatment of primary hepatocellular carcinoma. *Int. J. Oncol.* **1998**, *12*, 1217–1240. [CrossRef]
57. Fang, J.; Liao, L.; Yin, H.; Nakamura, H.; Subr, V.; Ulbrich, K.; Maeda, H. Photodynamic therapy and imaging based on tumor-targeted nanoprobe, polymer-conjugated zinc protoporphyrin. *Futur. Sci. OA* **2015**, *1*, fso4. [CrossRef]
58. Maeda, H.; Fang, J.; Nakamura, H. Great expectations for innovative PDT and tumor imaging using fluorescing nanophotosensitizers that utilizes EPR effect. *JSMI Rep.* **2015**, *9*, 3–10.
59. Fang, J.; Tsukigawa, K.; Liao, L.; Yin, H.; Eguchi, K.; Maeda, H. Styrene-maleic acid-copolymer conju-gated zinc protoporphyrin as a candidate drug for tumor-targeted therapy and imaging. *J. Drug Target.* **2016**, *24*, 399–407. [CrossRef] [PubMed]
60. Fang, J.; Vladimir, Š.; Islam, W.; Islam, R.; Ulbrich, K.; Maeda, H. N-(2-Hydroxypropyl) methacrylamide polymer conjugated pyropheophorbide-a, a promising tumor-targeted theranostic probe for photody-namic therapy and imaging. *Eur. J. Pharm. Biopharm.* **2018**, *130*, 165–176. [CrossRef]
61. Nakamura, H.; Liao, L.; Hitaka, Y.; Tsukigawa, K.; Subr, V.; Fang, J.; Ulbrich, K.; Maeda, H. Micelles of zinc protoporphyrin conjugated to N-(2-hydroxypropyl)methacrylamide (HPMA) copolymer for imaging and light-induced antitumor effects in vivo. *J. Control. Release* **2013**, *165*, 191–198. [CrossRef] [PubMed]
62. Fang, J.; Sawa, T.; Akaike, T.; Akuta, T.; Sahoo, S.K.; Khaled, G.; Hamada, A.; Maeda, H. In vivo antitumor activity of pegylated zinc protoporphyrin: Targeted inhibition of heme oxygenase in solid tumor. *Cancer Res.* **2003**, *63*, 3567–3574. [PubMed]
63. Hadzijusufovic, E.; Rebuzzi, L.; Gleixner, K.V.; Ferenc, V.; Peter, B.; Kondo, R.; Gruze, A.; Kneidinger, M.; Krauth, M.-T.; Mayerhofer, M. Targeting of heat-shock protein 32/heme oxygenase-1 in canine mastocytoma cells is associated with reduced growth and induction of apoptosis. *Exp. Hematol.* **2008**, *36*, 1461–1470. [CrossRef]
64. Mayerhofer, M.; Gleixner, K.V.; Mayerhofer, J.; Hoermann, G.; Jaeger, E.; Aichberger, K.J.; Ott, R.G.; Greish, K.; Nakamura, H.; Derdak, S.; et al. Targeting of heat shock protein 32 (Hsp32)/heme oxygenase-1 (HO-1) in leukemic cells in chronic myeloid leukemia: A novel approach to overcome resistance against imatinib. *Blood* **2008**, *111*, 2200–2210. [CrossRef] [PubMed]
65. Herrmann, H.; Kneidinger, M.; Cerny-Reiterer, S.; Rülicke, T.; Willmann, M.; Gleixner, K.V.; Blatt, K.; Hörmann, G.; Peter, B.; Samorapoompichit, P.; et al. The Hsp32 inhibitors SMA-ZnPP and PEG-ZnPP exert major growth-inhibitory effects on CD34+/CD38+ and CD34+/CD38-AML progenitor cells. *Curr. Cancer Drug Targets* **2012**, *12*, 51–63. [CrossRef]
66. Fang, J.; Greish, K.; Qin, H.; Liao, L.; Nakamura, H.; Takeya, M.; Maeda, H. HSP32 (HO-1) inhibitor, copoly(styrene-maleic acid)-zinc protoporphyrin IX, a water-soluble micelle as anticancer agent: In vitro and in vivo anticancer effect. *Eur. J. Pharm. Biopharm.* **2012**, *81*, 540–547. [CrossRef]
67. Islam, W.; Matsumoto, Y.; Fang, J.; Harada, A.; Nidome, T.; Ono, K.; Tsutsuki, H.; Sawa, T.; Sakurai, K.; Fukumitsu, N.; et al. Polymer conjugated glucosamine complexed with boric acid shows tumor-selective accumulation and simultaneous inhibition of glycolysis. *Biomaterials* **2021**, *269*, 120631. [CrossRef]
68. Oda, T.; Akaike, T.; Hamamoto, T.; Suzuki, F.; Hirano, T.; Maeda, H. Oxygen radicals in influen-za-induced pathogenesis and treatment with pyran polymer-conjugated SOD. *Science* **1989**, *244*, 974–976. [CrossRef]
69. Akaike, T.; Ando, M.; Oda, T.; Doi, T.; Ijiri, S.; Araki, S.; Maeda, H. Dependence on O2- generation by xanthine oxidase of pathogenesis of influenza virus infection in mice. *J. Clin. Investig.* **1990**, *85*, 739–745. [CrossRef] [PubMed]
70. Akaike, T.; Suga, M.; Maeda, H. Free radicals in viral pathogenesis: Molecular mechanisms involving superoxide and NO. *Proc. Soc. Exp. Boil. Med.* **1998**, *217*, 64–73. [CrossRef]
71. Akaike, T.; Maeda, H. Nitric oxide and virus infection. *Immunology* **2000**, *101*, 300–308. [CrossRef] [PubMed]
72. Wu, J. Tackle the free radicals damage in COVID-19. *Nitric Oxide* **2020**, *102*, 39–41. [CrossRef]
73. Akaike, T.; Fujii, S.; Kato, A.; Yoshitake, J.; Miyamoto, Y.; Sawa, T.; Okamoto, S.; Suga, M.; Asakawa, M.; Nagai, Y.; et al. Viral mutation accelerated by nitric oxide production during infection in vivo. *FASEB J.* **2000**, *14*, 1447–1454. [CrossRef] [PubMed]
74. Fujii, S.; Akaike, T.; Maeda, H. Role of Nitric Oxide in Pathogenesis of Herpes Simplex Virus Encephalitis in Rats. *Virology* **1999**, *256*, 203–212. [CrossRef]
75. Akaike, T.; Okamoto, S.; Sawa, T.; Yoshitake, J.; Tamura, F.; Ichimori, K.; Miyazaki, K.; Sasamoto, K.; Maeda, H. 8-Nitroguanosine formation in viral pneumonia and its implication for pathogenesis. *Proc. Natl. Acad. Sci. USA* **2003**, *100*, 685–690. [CrossRef]
76. Yoshitake, J.; Akaike, T.; Akuta, T.; Tamura, F.; Ogura, T.; Esumi, H.; Maeda, H. Nitric Oxide as an Endogenous Mutagen for Sendai Virus without Antiviral Activity. *J. Virol.* **2004**, *78*, 8709–8719. [CrossRef]
77. Shashni, B.; Nagasaki, Y. Newly Developed Self-Assembling Antioxidants as Potential Therapeutics for the Cancers. *J. Pers. Med.* **2021**, *11*, 92. [CrossRef] [PubMed]
78. Booth, C.; Gaspar, H.B. Pegademase bovine (PEG-ADA) for the treatment of infants and children with severe combined immunodeficiency (SCID). *Biol. Targets Ther.* **2009**, *3*, 349–358.
79. Kamisaki, Y.; Wada, H.; Yagura, T.; Matsushima, A.; Inada, Y. Reduction in immunogenicity and clearance rate of Escherichia coli L-asparaginase by modification with monomethoxypolyethylene glycol. *J. Pharmacol. Exp. Ther.* **1981**, *216*, 410–414.

80. Kimura, M.; Matsumura, Y.; Miyauchi, Y.; Maeda, H. A New Tactic for the Treatment of Jaundice: An Injectable Polymer-Conjugated Bilirubin Oxidase. *Exp. Biol. Med.* **1988**, *188*, 364–369. [CrossRef] [PubMed]
81. Sawa, T.; Wu, J.; Akaike, T.; Maeda, H. Tumor-targeting chemotherapy by a xanthine oxidase-polymer conjugate that generates oxygen-free radicals in tumor tissue. *Cancer Res.* **2000**, *60*, 666–671. [PubMed]
82. Fang, J.; Deng, D.; Nakamura, H.; Akuta, T.; Quin, H.; Iyer, A.; Greish, K.; Maeda, H. Oxystress in-ducing antitumor therapeutics via tumor-targeted delivery of PEG-conjugated D-amino acid oxidase. *Int. J. Cancer* **2008**, *122*, 1135–1144. [CrossRef]
83. Nakamura, H.; Fang, J.; Maeda, H. Protective role of D-amino acid oxidase against bacterial infection. *Infect. Immun.* **2012**, *80*, 1546–1553. [CrossRef]
84. Nakamura, H.; Fang, J.; Mizukami, T.; Nunoi, H.; Maeda, H. Pegylated D-amino acid oxidase restores bactericidal activity of neutrophils in chronic granulomatous disease via hypochlorite. *Exp. Biol. Med.* **2012**, *237*, 703–708. [CrossRef] [PubMed]
85. Fang, J.; Iyer, A.K.; Seki, T.; Nakamura, H.; Greish, K.; Maeda, H. SMA–copolymer conjugate of AHPP: A polymeric inhibitor of xanthine oxidase with potential antihypertensive effect. *J. Control. Release* **2009**, *135*, 211–217. [CrossRef] [PubMed]
86. Subrahmanyam, N.; Ghandehari, H. Harnessing Extracellular Matrix Biology for Tumor Drug Delivery. *J. Pers. Med.* **2021**, *11*, 88. [CrossRef]
87. Meiab, T.; Shashnia, B.; Maeda, H.; Nagasakiade, Y. Fibrinolytic tissue plasminogen activator installed redox-active nanoparticles (t-PA@iRNP) for cancer therapy. *Biomaterials* **2020**, *259*, 120290. [CrossRef]
88. Daruwalla, J.; Greish, K.; Malconti-Wilson, C.; Muralidharan, V.; Iyer, A.; Maeda, H.; Christophi, C. Styrene maleic acid-pirarubicin disrupts tumor microcirculation and enhances the permeability of col-orectal liver metastases. *J. Vasc. Res.* **2009**, *46*, 218–228. [CrossRef] [PubMed]
89. Daruwalla, J.; Nikfarjam, M.; Greish, K.; Malconti-WilsonI, C.; Muralidharan, V.; Christophi, C.; Maeda, H. In vitro and in vivo evaluation of tumor targeting styrene-maleic acid copolymer-pirarubicin micelles: Survival improvement and inhibition of liver metastases. *Cancer Sci.* **2010**, *101*, 1866–1874. [CrossRef]

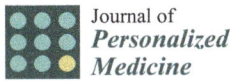

Article

Tumor Environment-Responsive Hyaluronan Conjugated Zinc Protoporphyrin for Targeted Anticancer Photodynamic Therapy

Shanghui Gao [†], Rayhanul Islam [†] and Jun Fang *

Faculty of Pharmaceutical Sciences, Sojo University, Ikeda 4-22-1, Nishi-ku, Kumamoto 860-0082, Japan; g2031d01@m.sojo-u.ac.jp (S.G.); rayhanulislam88@gmail.com (R.I.)
* Correspondence: fangjun@ph.sojo-u.ac.jp; Tel.: +81-96-326-4137
† S.G. and R.I. contributed equally to this work.

Abstract: Targeted tumor accumulation, tumor environment responsive drug release, and effective internalization are critical issues being considered in developing anticancer nanomedicine. In this context, we synthesized a tumor environment-responsive nanoprobe for anticancer photodynamic therapy (PDT) that is a hyaluronan conjugated zinc protoporphyrin via an ester bond (HA-es-ZnPP), and we examined its anticancer PDT effect both in vitro and in vivo. HA-es-ZnPP exhibits high water-solubility and forms micelles of ~40 nm in aqueous solutions. HA-es-ZnPP shows fluorescence quenching without apparent $^1O_2$ generation under light irradiation because of micelle formation. However, $^1O_2$ was extensively generated when the micelle is disrupted, and ZnPP is released. Compared to native ZnPP, HA-es-ZnPP showed lower but comparable intracellular uptake and cytotoxicity in cultured mouse C26 colon cancer cells; more importantly, light irradiation resulted in 10-time increased cytotoxicity, which is the PDT effect. In a mouse sarcoma S180 solid tumor model, HA-es-ZnPP as polymeric micelles exhibited a prolonged systemic circulation time and the consequent tumor-selective accumulation based on the enhanced permeability and retention (EPR) effect was evidenced. Consequently, a remarkable anticancer PDT effect was achieved using HA-es-ZnPP and a xenon light source, without apparent side effects. These findings suggest the potential of HA-es-ZnPP as a candidate anticancer nanomedicine for PDT.

Keywords: EPR effect; tumor targeting; photodynamic; hyaluronan; zinc protoporphyrin

Citation: Gao, S.; Islam, R.; Fang, J. Tumor Environment-Responsive Hyaluronan Conjugated Zinc Protoporphyrin for Targeted Anticancer Photodynamic Therapy. *J. Pers. Med.* **2021**, *11*, 136. https://doi.org/10.3390/jpm11020136

Academic Editor: Hiroshi Maeda

Received: 29 January 2021
Accepted: 12 February 2021
Published: 17 February 2021

Publisher's Note: MDPI stays neutral with regard to jurisdictional claims in published maps and institutional affiliations.

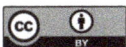

Copyright: © 2021 by the authors. Licensee MDPI, Basel, Switzerland. This article is an open access article distributed under the terms and conditions of the Creative Commons Attribution (CC BY) license (https://creativecommons.org/licenses/by/4.0/).

1. Introduction

Targeted cancer therapy has been recognized as a key issue for achieving a successful anticancer outcome and is becoming a trend for developing anticancer drugs. In the past few decades, molecular target drugs designed to selectively inhibit the oncogene products and other molecules involved in tumor growth have attracted attention, and many such drugs got approved and used in clinics. However, the tumor heterogeneity, diversity, and frequent mutation of tumor-related molecules largely limit the application and availability of molecular target drugs [1,2]. To solve these problems and to increase the efficacy of molecular target drugs, personalized medicine or precision medicine has recently been proposed to intensely focus on the major genes/molecules in a single cancer patient [3]. This strategy is promising. However, there is still a long way to go, and extensive efforts and costs are needed to achieve success.

Recently, an alternative tumor-targeting strategy has drawn considerable interest, which targets the tumor tissues as a whole by using macromolecular drugs or nano-designed drugs, i.e., nanomedicine [4,5]. The principle of tumor tissue targeting is based on the unique phenomenon of tumor vasculature's pathophysiological nature called the enhanced permeability and retention (EPR) effect [6–9]. Compared to normal blood vessels, tumor blood vessels have larger fenestration along with high vascular permeability due to the extensively produced vascular mediators such as nitric oxide (NO), bradykinin (BK), vascular endothelial growth factor (VEGF), etc. These vascular mediators contribute to macromolecules' selective entry and accumulation in tumor tissues [7–9]. Furthermore, because of the dysfunctional lymphatic recovery system in tumors, macromolecules accumulated in tumor tissues could not be removed effectively, resulting in prolonged retention times [7,10]. Thus, by using nanomedicines, one could achieve much higher tumor concentrations of drugs than using conventional low molecular drugs. At the same time, a decreased distribution of nanomedicines in normal tissues could also be achieved because nanomedicines could not cross normal blood vessels, a benefit of their larger size, which is vastly different from conventional low molecular drugs that distribute indiscriminately in normal tissues. Consequently, a superior antitumor effect, as well as greatly lowered side effects, could be achieved for nanomedicines compared to conventional low molecular anticancer drugs [4,5,9,11,12]. To date, many anticancer nanomedicines have been developed, some are approved in the clinic, and more are in clinical trials or under preclinical evaluation [4,5,9].

Photodynamic therapy (PDT) is a promising therapeutic regimen for cancer. Singlet oxygen ($^1O_2$) and other reactive oxygen species (ROS) generated from photosensitizers (PS) upon light irradiation, are the effector molecules of PDT [13,14]. Namely, a PS is first administered, followed by irradiation using light with the appropriate wavelength, where PS in the tumor is excited, and the energy is transferred to molecular oxygen to generate $^1O_2$. As a group of highly reactive molecules, ROS, including $^1O_2$, rapidly react with and damage different biomolecules, including proteins, DNA, and lipids, which leads to the apoptosis of tumor cells [14]. Now PDT is already in use for the treatment of some cancers, for example early-stage lung (bronchogenic) and superficial skin cancers [15–17]. However, to achieve the ideal PDT effect, PS must be delivered selectively into the tumor, otherwise an insufficient tumor concentration of PS will not generate enough ROS to kill cancer cells. Also, an unpreferable distribution may induce adverse side effects. For overcoming this drawback, EPR effect-based nano-designed PS is becoming popular for the targeted delivery of PS to tumor tissues. Many nano-platforms have been utilized to modify PS, including polymer conjugates, polymer micelles, liposomes, and antibody-drug conjugates [18–21]. In our group, by utilizing zinc protoporphyrin (ZnPP) and pyropheophorbide-a as PS, we have developed several polymeric micellar types of nanoprobes for PDT using different polymers, including polyethylene glycol (PEG), styrene maleic acid copolymer (SMA), N-(2-Hydroxypropyl) methacrylamide (HPMA) copolymer, and hyaluronan (HA), all of which showed a superior tumor-selective accumulation and thus therapeutic effect in different murine solid tumor models [22–27].

Among different polymers for preparing nanomedicines, HA as a natural polydisaccharide composed of alternative repeating units of d-glucuronic acid and N-acetyl-d-glucosamine, has attracted substantial interest as a biomaterial for medical applications as well as drug delivery systems because of its high biocompatibility, non-immunogenicity, non-toxicity, biodegradability, high water-solubility, and so on [28]. Many nanomedicines or nanoparticles using HA have been reported for the treatment of various diseases, including cancer and inflammatory diseases [29,30]. In our laboratory, we previously developed a HA conjugated ZnPP through an amide bond (HA-ZnPP), which formed micelles of 156 nm in aqueous solutions [27]. The micelle formation was relatively stable in physiological solution (e.g., circulation), and thus accumulated in tumors more selectively than free ZnPP [27]. Subsequently, after being taken up by tumor cells, the micelle formation was disrupted by lipid components in the cell membrane (i.e., lecithin), consequently fulfilling tumoricidal activity under xenon light irradiation [27]. However, compared to native ZnPP, the in vivo therapeutic effect of HA-ZnPP was not significantly improved, which is considered mostly due to its much lower rate of internalization than native ZnPP [27]. Namely, because of the stable uncleavable amide bond, HA-ZnPP could not release free ZnPP in tumors, thus remaining as a micelle, which quenched the activity of PS (ZnPP) and hindered ROS generation. It is thus of necessity and reasonable to further improve the therapeutic efficacy of HA-ZnPP by modulating the release of free ZnPP in tumor tissues.

In this context, tumor environment responsive release of free drugs from nanomedicines is known as a key issue for the design of anticancer nanomedicines. One focus is on the pH of tumor tissues that is weakly acidic (6~7) compared to the neutral pH (~7.4) of normal tissues [31,32]. Utilization of acidic pH-responsive chemical bonds such as the hydrazone bond is becoming a consensus for the development of anticancer nanomedicines, which have been proven to be an excellent strategy with high tumor targeting and therapeutic efficacy by many research groups and by using different polymers and drugs [12,33]. Another strategy focuses on the proteases in tumors. It is known that many tumors exhibit high levels of various proteinases, such as cathepsin B, cathepsin K, and esterase [13,34]. Thus, a protease/esterase-sensitive linker can be used to increase the tumor-specific release of free drugs, which has been proven as an effective approach in many studies [34,35]. As a proof of concept, in previous studies, we compared PEGylated ZnPP (PEG-ZnPP) with different chemical bonds (i.e., ester bond, ether bond, and amide bond) for the release properties under different conditions and in different tissues, including cancer [36]. The results clearly showed that PEG-ZnPP with ether bond and amide bond rarely released ZnPP derivatives in tumors as well as normal tissues, whereas, in the case of PEG-ZnPP with ester bond, cleaved ZnPP derivatives became the major components in the tumor but not in normal tissues except for liver due to its high esterase expression [36]; consequently, this tumor-responsive cleavage of the free drug resulted in a much stronger anticancer effect than those PEG-ZnPP with ether and amide bonds [36].

Along this line, in this study, we designed and synthesized a HA conjugated ZnPP via ester bond (HA-es-ZnPP) and investigated its potential as a nanoprobe for tumor-targeted PDT, especially focusing on its tumor environment-responsive release properties. Also, the tumor imaging capacity of HA-es-ZnPP toward anticancer theranostics was evaluated and is discussed here.

2. Materials and Methods

2.1. Materials

HA with a mean molecular weight of 30,000 (polydispersity index of 1.212) was purchased from MRC polysaccharide Corp., Ltd (Toyama, Japan). RPMI 1640 medium, 4-dimethylaminopyridine (DMAP) isoflurane, 3-(4,5-Dimethylthiazol-2-yl)-2,5-diphenyltetrazolium bromide (MTT), Tween 20, sodium dodecyl sulfate (SDS) and zinc acetate were purchased from Wako pure chemical (Osaka, Japan). Protoporphyrin IX (PP) and cetyltrimethylammonium bromide (CTA) were from Sigma-Aldrich Chemical (St. Louis, MO, USA). Water-soluble carbodiimide (WSC) was purchased from Dojindo Laboratory, Kumamoto, Japan. Additionally, 2,2,6,6-Tetramethyl-4-piperidone (4-oxo-TEMP) was purchased from Tokyo Chemical Industry (Tokyo, Japan). Esterase from porcine liver was purchased from Roche Diagnostics GmbH (Mannheim, Germany). The other reagents and solvents of a reagent grade were from commercial sources and were used without further purification.

2.2. Synthesis of HA Conjugated ZnPP via Ester Bond (HA-es-ZnPP)

Cetyltrimethylammonium salt of HA (CTA-HA) was first synthesized according to a previous report [37] with some modifications. Briefly, 110 mg of CTA bromide was dissolved in 1.5 mL of deionized water at 40 °C, to which an aqueous solution of HA (100 mg, 0.5% w/v) was added dropwise. The white precipitate thus formed was collected after centrifugation (10,000× g, 5 min), and washed three times with 40 mL of hot water, and finally dried under vacuum.

ZnPP was prepared by inserting zinc into PP as described previously [38]. In brief, a 10-time molar excess of zinc acetate was added to PP in dimethyl sulfoxide (DMSO) and stirred at 60 °C for 24 h. After cooling, cold deionized water was added 5-fold to the volume of DMSO to precipitate the product ZnPP, which was purified by centrifugation to remove excess zinc acetate and washed thrice with cold deionized water.

CTA-HA obtained as described above was dissolved in 20 mL of DMSO, and 10 mg of ZnPP that was dissolved in 1 mL of DMSO was added dropwise, then DMAP (500 mg) and WSC (500 mg) were added to the reaction mixture. The reaction was continued for 3 days at 50 °C. The solution was then subjected to dialysis using a dialysis bag with an average cutoff of 8000 (Wako) against a 1:1 (*v/v*) sodium phosphate buffer (0.3 M, pH = 7.4): DMSO mixture for 1 day, then against 5% sodium bicarbonate for 1 day, and finally against deionized water for 1 day. Each solvent was changed every 8 h. The solution was then lyophilized to give a brown powder. Figure 1 shows the synthetic scheme of HA-es-ZnPP. During the reaction, high-performance liquid chromatography (HPLC) was performed to monitor the reaction by using LC-2000Plus series HPLC system (JASCO, Tokyo, Japan) with an Asahipak GF-310 HQ column (7.5 × 300 mm) (Showa Denko, Tokyo, Japan). Using a mobile phase of 70% methanol/30% DMSO with 0.001% trifluoroacetic acid (Wako) at a flow rate of 0.8 mL/min, the eluate was monitored at 415 nm for ZnPP.

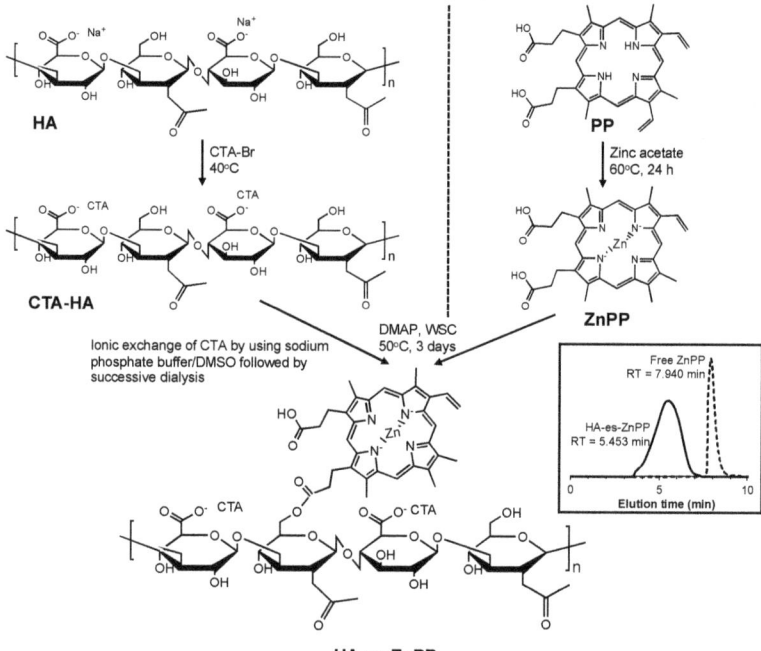

Figure 1. Synthesizing protocol of hyaluronan (HA) conjugated ZnPP through ester bond (HA-es-ZnPP). Inset shows the gel permeation chromatograph of HA-es-ZnPP and free ZnPP, by using a high-performance liquid chromatography (HPLC) system with an Asahipak GF-310 HQ column.

2.3. Characterization of HA-es-ZnPP

2.3.1. UV–Visible Spectrophotometry and Fluorescence Spectroscopy

UV/vis absorption spectra and fluorescence spectrum of ZnPP and HA-es-ZnPP were measured by a spectrophotometer (Hitachi U-3900, Tokyo, Japan), and a spectrofluorometer model FP-6600 (Jasco Corp., Tokyo, Japan), respectively. For spectroscopy, the sample solution was excited at 420 nm, and emissions from 550 to 700 nm were recorded.

2.3.2. Determination of the ZnPP Content in HA-es-ZnPP

Standard ZnPP solutions at 0.05–1 mg/mL and HA-es-ZnPP (1 mg/mL) were prepared in DMSO. The standard curve of ZnPP was then created by measuring the absorbance of samples at 421 nm (absorption maximum of ZnPP), and the content of ZnPP in HA-es-ZnPP was calculated according to the standard curve.

2.3.3. Dynamic Light Scattering (DLS) and Zeta Potential

HA-es-ZnPP was dissolved in phosphate-buffered saline (PBS) at 5 mg/mL and filtered through a 0.45 μm filter. The particle size and surface charge (zeta potential) were measured by using an electrophoretic light-scattering analyzer (ELS-Z2, Otsuka Electronics Co., Ltd., Osaka, Japan).

2.4. Release of ZnPP from HA-es-ZnPP

To investigate the release of ZnPP from HA-es-ZnPP conjugate, HA-es-ZnPP of 5 mg/mL was dissolved in a 0.2 M sodium phosphate buffer (PB) of different pHs (i.e., 6.5, 7.4, 8.5) with 0.5% Tween 20. For the study of an enzymatic effect on drug release, porcine liver esterase solution (10 units/ml) was added to a HA-es-ZnPP solution in a pH 7.4 PB buffer with 0.5% Tween 20. In some experiments, HA-es-ZnPP was added to 100% fetal bovine serum (FBS) or supernatant of tumor homogenate from mouse sarcoma S180 as described below, to the final concentration of 5 mg/mL. All samples (each of 5 mL) were then placed in dialysis tubes with a cutoff of ~8000 Da and were dialyzed against PBS (25 mL) with shaking (1 Hz) at 37 °C. At each indicated time point, 0.1 mL of the solution outside the dialysis bag was collected, which was diluted by 2 mL DMSO followed by fluorescence measurement as described above. The amount of released ZnPP was quantified according to a standard curve using standard ZnPP samples.

O_2 Generation from HA-es-ZnPP as Measured by Electron Spin Resonance (ESR) Spectroscopy

HA-es-ZnPP (40 μg/mL ZnPP equivalent) was dissolved in PBS with/without 0.5% Tween 20, to which 20 mM of 4-oxo-TEMP (spin trapping agent) was added. Samples were placed in a flat quartz cell (Labotec, Tokyo, Japan), and then subjected to light irradiation, using a xenon light source (MAX-303; Asahi Spectra Co. Ltd., Tokyo, Japan) at a wavelength of 400–700 nm. The ESR spectra were recorded by using a JEOL JES FA-100 spectrometer (Tokyo, Japan) at 25 °C, with a microwave power of 1.0 mW, amplitude of 100 kHz, and field modulation width of 0.1 mT.

2.5. Intracellular Uptake of HA-es-ZnPP

Mouse colon cancer C26 cells were seeded in a 12-well plate (5×10^5 cells/well). After overnight pre-incubation, 20 μg/mL (ZnPP equivalent) of ZnPP dissolved in DMSO, or HA-es-ZnPP dissolved in PBS was added to the cells. After washing thrice with cold PBS at the scheduled time point, the cells were harvested, collected, and sonicated (30 W, 30 s, Dr.Hielscher, UP50H homogenizer, tip drip type) in ethanol on ice, followed by centrifugation ($10,000 \times g$, 5 min). The amount of ZnPP/HA-es-ZnPP in the supernatant was quantified by measuring fluorescence intensity as described above.

2.6. In Vitro Cytotoxicity Assay

Mouse colon cancer C26 cells were maintained in RPMI-1640 medium supplemented with 10% fetal bovine serum (FBS, Nichirei Biosciences Inc.,Tokyo, Japan) under 5% CO_2/air at 37 °C. For cytotoxicity assay. Cells were seeded in 96-well plates (3000 cells/well). After overnight incubation, HA-es-ZnPP or free ZnPP of different concentrations was added, and the cells were cultured for 24 h. Irradiation was then carried out by using fluorescent blue light with a peak emission at 420 nm (TL-D; Philips, Eindhoven, The Netherland), at a total energy of 1.0 J/cm^2 (3.3 mW/ cm^2, 5 min). After a further 24 h of culture, cell viability was measured by MTT assay.

2.7. In Vivo Tissue Distribution of HA-es-ZnPP

Male ddY mice that were 6 weeks old were purchased from SLC Inc., Shizuoka, Japan. All animals were maintained at 22 ± 1 °C and a 55% ± 5% relative humidity, with a 12-h light/dark cycle. All of the experiments were approved by the Animal Ethics Committees of Sojo University (no. 2020-P-009, approved on April 01, 2020) and were carried out according to the Laboratory Protocol for Animal Handling of Sojo University.

A mouse sarcoma S180 solid tumor model was established by injecting S180 cells (2×10^6) that were maintained in the ascitic form in the ddY mice into the dorsal skin of the ddY mice. After 10-12 days of tumor cell inoculation, when the tumor grew to ~10 mm in diameter, HA-es-ZnPP (5 mg/kg, ZnPP equivalent) dissolved in physiological saline was injected intravenously (i.v.) via the tail vein. For comparison, free ZnPP (5 mg/kg) that was dissolved in 0.01 N NaOH with 10% DMSO was injected i.v. At 24 h after i.v. injection, mice were killed, and tumors as well as normal tissues (e.g., liver, spleen, kidney, etc.) were collected. Tissues were first subjected to fluorescence imaging using IVIS XR (Caliper Life Science, Hopkinton, MA, USA) with Ex-420 nm/Em-DsRed. Then, to 100 mg of each tissue, 1 mL of DMSO was added, followed by homogenization. After centrifugation ($10,000 \times g$, 10 min), the extracted HA-es-ZnPP in the supernatant was quantified by fluorescence intensity (Ex 420 nm/Em 630 nm).

2.8. In Vivo Antitumor Activity of HA-es-ZnPP

Mouse sarcoma S180 solid tumor model, as described above, was used in this assay. At 7–10 days after tumor inoculation, when the diameters of the tumors became 8–10 mm, HA-es-ZnPP dissolved in physiological saline at indicated concentrations was administered i.v. Physiological saline was used for control mice. At 24 and 48 h after injection of HA-es-ZnPP, irradiation to the tumors was carried out using xenon light (MAX-303; Asahi Spectra) at 400–700 nm for 5 min (36 J/cm^2), under anesthesia with isoflurane gas. The tumor volume (mm^3), which was calculated as ($W^2 \times L$)/2 by measuring the width (W) and length (L) of the tumor, and body weight of mice were recorded every 2–3 days during the study period.

2.9. Statistical Analyses

All data were expressed as means ± SD. Statistical analyses were performed by using GraphPad Prism 8.0 (GraphPad Software, Inc. La Jolla, CA, USA). Data were analyzed by using ANOVA followed by the Bonferroni correction for multiple comparisons (*p*-value was corrected by multiplying it by the number of comparisons), and unpaired Student's *t*-test for dual comparisons. A difference was considered to be statistically significant when $p < 0.05$.

3. Results

3.1. Synthesis and Characterization of HA-es-ZnPP

HA-es-ZnPP was synthesized by using the carboxyl group of ZnPP and hydroxyl group of HA, which forms an ester bond (Figure 1). Gel permeation chromatograph using a HPLC system with an Asahipak GF-310 HQ column as described above, showed a single peak of the product HA-es-ZnPP with a retention time of 5.453 min, whereas ZnPP exhibited a retention time of 7.940 min (inset of Figure 1), suggesting the completion of the conjugation.

The resulted HA-es-ZnPP had a ZnPP loading of 10% (wt/wt, 5–6 ZnPP units in one HA molecule) based on absorbance of ZnPP at 421 nm in DMSO, and showed very good water-solubility (>20 mg/mL). In an aqueous solution, HA-es-ZnPP showed an average particle size of 41.2 nm by DLS with a polydispersity index of 0.012 (Figure 2A), and the zeta potential of HA-es-ZnPP was −37.12 mV. These results indicated the micelle formation of HA-es-ZnPP in which ZnPP creates the hydrophobic core and hydrophilic HA forms the outer surface, as similarly seen in other examples of polymeric ZnPP reported in our previous studies [24,26,27,38–40]. The decreased absorbance of ZnPP supported the micelle formation in PBS compared to that in DMSO (Figure 2B). More pieces of evidence were obtained by quenching of fluorescence from HA-es-ZnPP in an aqueous solution (i.e., PBS) compared to the strong fluorescence of DMSO solution of HA-es-ZnPP (Figure 2C,D). The micelle formation would be disrupted by detergent SDS and Tween 20 in a concentration-dependent manner, as evidenced by the increased fluorescence (Figure 2C,D). However, no apparent change was found in the presence of urea (Figure 2E). These findings suggested the micelle was formed mostly by the hydrophobic interactions, but hydrogen bond is not involved. Moreover, increased fluorescence intensity was found in the presence of 10% FBS, but an increase of FBS concentration did not result in a further increase of fluorescence intensity (Figure 2E), suggesting that micelle formation could be partially disrupted in the circulation.

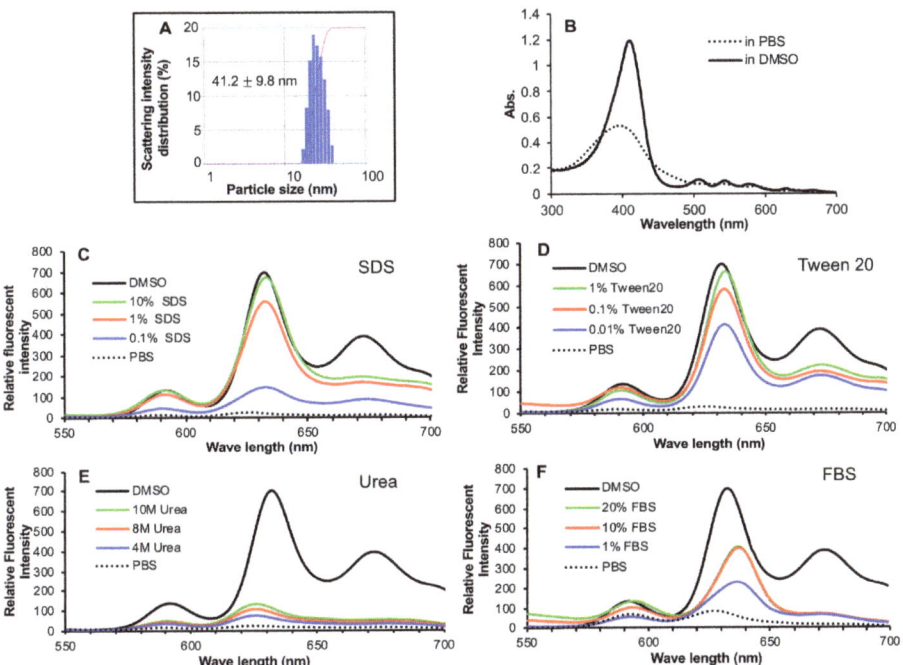

Figure 2. Micelle formation of HA-es-ZnPP. HA-es-ZnPP showed a hydrodynamic diameter in physiological saline of 41.2 nm, as measured by DLS (**A**). The micelle formation was supported by decreased absorbance as seen in UV/vis spectra (**B**), and more importantly, fluorescence quenching, the fluorescence intensity of HA-es-ZnPP in PBS was almost undetectable compared to that in DMSO (**C**,**D**). The micelle formation could be effectively disrupted by detergent SDS (**C**) and Tween 20 (**D**), as evidenced by increased fluorescence, but it could not be affected by urea (**E**). Increased fluorescence intensity/disruption of micelles was also found in the presence of FBS (**F**). See text for details.

3.2. Release Profiles of HA-es-ZnPP

As shown in Figure 3, in PB of physiological pH (7.4) and weak acidic pH (6.5), almost no release of ZnPP from HA-es-ZnPP was found till 12 h, while the release reached to 0.7–1.4% in 36 h. However, in the presence of esterase, a significant increase of ZnPP release was triggered; almost 10% of ZnPP was released in 36 h (Figure 3), which is another side supported that ZnPP was conjugated to HA via an ester bond. In parallel with this finding, in 100% FBS, which is known to exhibit esterase activity [41], increased release was observed, which were 6.5% and 8.6% in 24 h and 48 h, respectively (Figure 3). More importantly, when HA-es-ZnPP was incubated in the homogenate of mouse solid tumor (S180), relatively high levels of ZnPP release were achieved, e.g., 3.5% after 36 h incubation which is about 3-time higher that in PB (Figure 3), suggesting a preferable release behavior of HA-es-ZnPP in the tumor site.

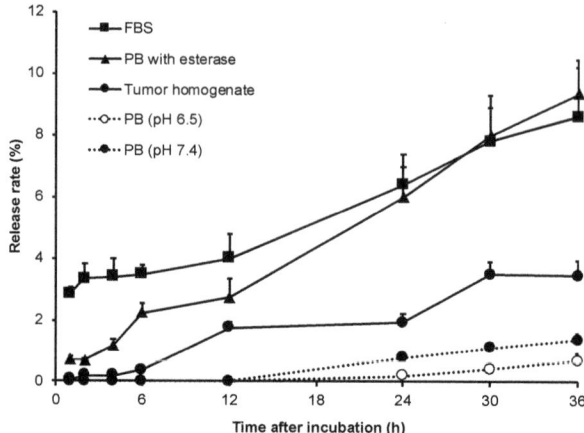

Figure 3. ZnPP release from HA-es-ZnPP at different conditions. In sodium phosphate buffer, almost no ZnPP was released from the conjugate at both physiological pH and weak acidic pH up to 12 h. Much rapid release of ZnPP occurred in presence of either esterase or FBS having esterase activities. A relatively high level of ZnPP release was also found in tumor homogenate.

3.3. Generation of $^1O_2$ from HA-es-ZnPP after Light Irradiation

The capacity of HA-es-ZnPP to generate $^1O_2$ was evaluated by means of ESR spectroscopy under light irradiation using a xenon light source. Similar to our previous studies of polymeric ZnPP using HPMA copolymer [24,27], as the micelle form in aqueous solution (i.e., PBS), no apparent generation of $^1O_2$ was observed even after 6 min of light irradiation (Figure 4). However, when micelle formation was disrupted in the presence of 0.5% of Tween 20, a strong ESR signal of $^1O_2$ was found in an irradiation time-dependent manner (Figure 4). These findings agree with those of fluorescence spectroscopy showing fluorescence quenching in PBS and appearance of fluorescence in Tween 20 (Figure 2D).

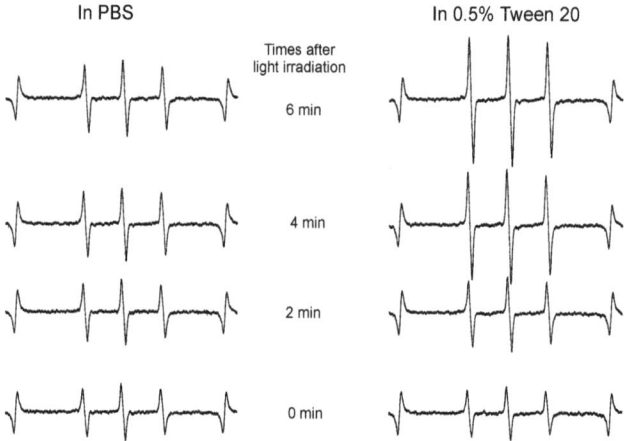

Figure 4. Electron Spin Resonance (ESR) spectra of HA-es-ZnPP in phosphate-buffered saline (PBS) in the presence/absence of Tween 20 under light irradiation. $^1O_2$ generation from HA-es-ZnPP was captured by 4-oxo-TEMP, and triplet 4-oxo-TEMP signal as the indicator of $^1O_2$ was detected by ESR spectra. In the presence of Tween 20, a relatively high level of $^1O_2$ generation was observed in an irradiation time-dependent manner, whereas no $^1O_2$ generation occurred in PBS without Tween 20, in which HA-es-ZnPP behaves as micelles.

3.4. Intracellular Uptake of HA-es-ZnPP

Free ZnPP was rapidly and extensively internalized into C26 colon cancer cells as early as 1 h after incubation and maintained similar levels for up to 8 h (Figure 5A). Compared to free ZnPP, HA-es-ZnPP exhibited a slower but constant uptake by C26 cells, at 8 h after incubation, the intracellular fluorescence from internalized ZnPP in cells treated with HA-es-ZnPP was one-third of that in free ZnPP treated cells (Figure 5A).

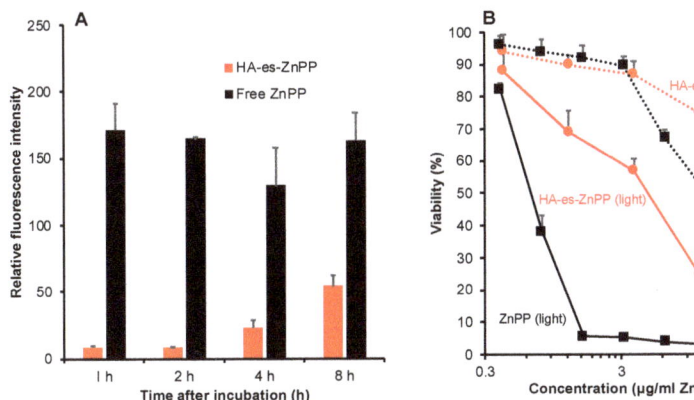

Figure 5. Intracellular uptake (**A**) and in vitro cytotoxicity (**B**) of HA-es-ZnPP in C26 colon cancer cells. (**A**), free ZnPP or HA-es-ZnPP (20 µg/mL ZnPP equivalent) was added to C26 cells for the indicated time. The intracellular ZnPP or HA-es-ZnPP was detected and quantified by measuring fluorescence intensity. (**B**), free ZnPP or HA-es-ZnPP at different concentrations was added into the cells, and the cells were treated for 48 h. In a separate plate, cells were irradiated by using fluorescent blue light (1.0 J/cm^2, 5 min irradiation) at 24 h after HA-es-ZnPP treatment followed by further 24 h incubation. The cell viability was then measured by MTT assay. Data are mean ± SD.

3.5. In Vitro Cytotoxicity of HA-es-ZnPP

In vitro cytotoxicity of HA-es-ZnPP was examined in a C26 colon cancer cell line. As shown in Figure 5B, without light irradiation, ZnPP per se showed a cell-killing effect with an inhibitory concentration (IC$_{50}$) of 12.5 µg/mL, whereas a more than 15-time increased cytotoxicity was achieved after light irradiation, indicating a remarkable PDT effect. Compared to free ZnPP, HA-es-ZnPP itself exhibited lower cytotoxicity with an IC$_{50}$ of 50 µg/ml (ZnPP equivalent). However, after light irradiation, significantly increased cytotoxicity (IC$_{50}$ of 4.5 µg/mL) was observed, which is 10-fold higher than that of HA-es-ZnPP per se (Figure 5B). These results are parallel with the findings of intracellular uptake shown in Figure 5B.

3.6. In Vivo Tissue Distribution of HA-es-ZnPP after I.V. Injection

Tissue distribution of HA-es-ZnPP in mice bearing sarcoma S180 solid tumor at 24 h after i.v. administration of HA-es-ZnPP was shown in Figure 6. Compared with native ZnPP which showed very low or negligible distribution in all tested tissues, including tumor (Figure 7A), HA-es-ZnPP exhibited a significantly prolonged circulation time, while the blood concentration of HA-es-ZnPP was 2.5-times more than that of ZnPP (Figure 7A).

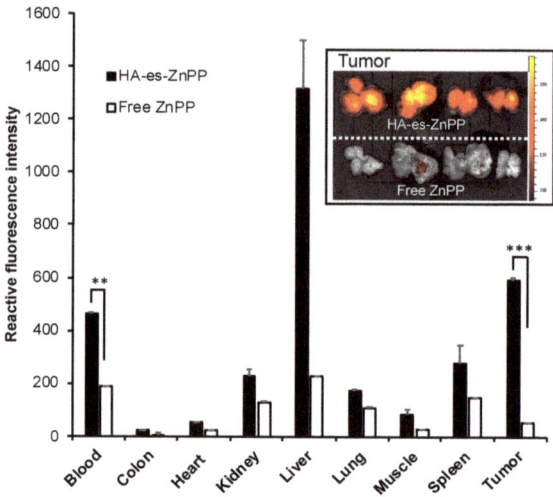

Figure 6. In vivo tissue distribution of HA-es-ZnPP in S180 solid tumor-bearing ddY mice. HA-es-ZnPP or free ZnPP was injected i.v. in the mice. After 24 h, mice were killed, and tissues, including tumors were collected. Tissue samples were homogenated using DMSO, and extracted HA-es-ZnPP or ZnPP in the supernatant was quantified by fluorescence spectroscopy. Inset shows the fluorescence images of mice-tumors treated with free ZnPP or HA-es-ZnPP. The tumors were cut in the middle of tumor nodules, and the cross-sectional views were shown. Data are mean ± SD. **, $p < 0.01$; ***, $p < 0.001$.

More importantly, tumor accumulation of HA-es-ZnPP was 10-times higher than that of free ZnPP (Figure 7A). Moreover, the amount of HA-es-ZnPP in the tumor was higher than those in most of the normal tissues except the liver, which is rich in reticuloendothelial systems and is the primary organ for the protoporphrin metabolism [24,39,42]. These findings suggest a preferentially targeted delivery of HA-es-ZnPP in the tumor by taking advantage of the EPR effect. The tumor-selective delivery of HA-es-ZnPP was also visualized and confirmed by using fluorescence imaging involving detecting the fluorescence from ZnPP, during which much-intensified fluorescence was detected in tumors from mice treated by HA-es-ZnPP compared to those in free ZnPP treated mice (inset of Figure 6). In addition, the pictures shown in the inset of Figure 6 were the cross-sectional view of tumors, which clearly showed a strong fluorescence of HA-es-ZnPP in the core of the tumor (inset of Figure 6).

3.7. In Vivo Antitumor Effect of PDT Using HA-es-ZnPP

The in vivo therapeutic effect of PDT using HA-es-ZnPP was evaluated in a mouse sarcoma S180 solid tumor model. Irradiation was carried out twice at 24 h and 48 h after HA-es-ZnPP administration using a xenon light source, at 36 J/cm^2, which is a relatively low irradiation dose [25]. By using this protocol, a dose-dependent PDT effect was observed, i.e., one round of treatment resulted in a slight suppression of tumor growth, whereas significantly delayed tumor growth was found when the treatment protocol was repeated 3 times (Figure 7A). Moreover, three injections of HA-es-ZnPP alone without light irradiation, or light irradiation alone without HA-es-ZnPP did not show apparent tumor suppression (Supplemental data Figure S1). In addition, a weight gain but no loss of body weight was observed in all groups during the treatment (Figure 7B).

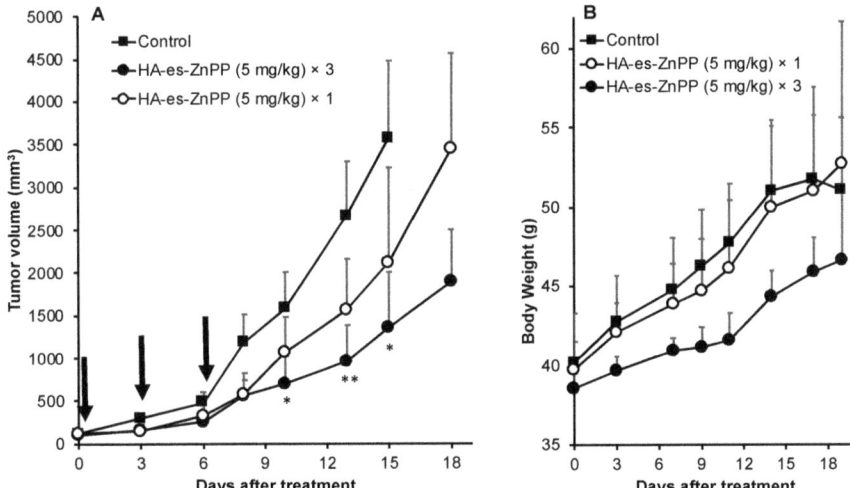

Figure 7. In vivo therapeutic effect of HA-es-ZnPP based PDT. In a mouse sarcoma S180 solid tumor model, HA-es-ZnPP (5 mg/kg, ZnPP equivalent) was injected i.v. when the tumor grew to 8–10 mm in diameter. At 24 and 48 h after injection of HA-es-ZnPP, irradiation to the tumors was carried out using xenon light (MAX-303; Asahi Spectra) at 400–700 nm for 5 min (36 J/cm^2). This treatment protocol was carried out 1 time or 3 times in different groups. The tumor volume (**A**) and body weight (**B**) of mice were recorded every 2–3 days during the study period. Arrows indicate the PDT treatments. Data are mean ± SD. *, $p < 0.05$; **, $p < 0.01$.

4. Discussion

For the development of anticancer nanomedicine, several critical issues must be considered. The first necessary step is the EPR effect-based tumor accumulation. For this aim, nanomedicine must be stable enough in circulation to ensure there is a sufficient circulation time that is essential for achieving the EPR effect. Otherwise, disruption of unstable nano-formulation in circulation will result in similar behaviors to those of small molecular drugs [10,12,43]. In this context, HA-es-ZnPP behaves as micelles of ~40 nm (Figure 2A) and maintains the stable micelle formation in an aqueous solution as evidenced by the fluorescence quenching (Figure 2C,D). In the presence of FBS, though fluorescence quenching was partly liberated, complete disruption of micelles was not seen (Figure 2F), indicating HA-es-ZnPP could maintain at least a partially stable micelle formation in circulation. As a consequence, relatively large amount of HA-es-ZnPP remained in circulation compared to ZnPP at 24 h after i.v. injection, indicating a much longer blood half-life of HA-es-ZnPP than native ZnPP (Figure 6). In accordance with this finding, HA-es-ZnPP remarkably accumulated in the tumor, which showed a 10-times higher concentration than that of native ZnPP (Figure 6). Moreover, when we cut the tumors, we found stronger fluorescence (HA-es-ZnPP) in the tumor center than in the peripheral area (inset of Figure 6). It is known that the core of tumors is usually poor in blood vessels with many necroses, while the peripheral areas are actively growing parts with rich vasculature. This finding suggests that HA-es-ZnPP could penetrate tumor tissue effectively after extravasation from tumor blood vessels, which is probably due to its relatively small size (i.e., 40 nm) as demonstrated by Kataoka's group; smaller nano micelles (i.e., 30 nm) penetrate much deeper into tumor tissues than larger micelles (i.e., 80 nm) [44]. Together, these findings strongly indicate the preferable properties of HA-es-ZnPP as a nanomedicine to target tumors by the EPR effect.

However, nanomedicine should quickly and effectively unload active pharmaceutical ingredients (API) to fulfill a therapeutical effect after reaching the tumor in a way that benefitted from the EPR effect. Otherwise, too stable nanomedicines with little API release in tumor sites will suffer from insufficient therapeutic activity [10,12,45]. In this context, nanomedicines with tumor environment responsive linkers have attracted more and more attention. Many strategies have been developed by utilizing, as examples, acidic pH-sensitive bond (e.g., hydrazone bond) or a protease cleavable peptide linker [31,32,34,35], as described above in "Introduction". Besides, other strategies such as using magnetically responsive peptide [46], thermosensitive nano-platform [47], and Arg-Gly-Asp (RGD) linker [48] have been challenged which showed promising results. In the present study, we focused on the relatively high esterase activity in tumors [36], and designed a HA conjugated ZnPP with ester bond, i.e., HA-es-ZnPP. As expected, the covalent bond of HA-es-ZnPP ensures little release of ZnPP in water solutions, but ZnPP release could be triggered in the presence of esterase as well as FBS (Figure 3), indicating that HA-es-ZnPP will release ZnPP in circulation and more importantly, in tumor tissues. However, it should also be noted that the release of ZnPP in FBS was less than 10% in 36 h (Figure 3), which again supported that HA-es-ZnPP behaves as a relatively stable nano-micelles in circulation.

Intracellular uptake of API released from nanomedicines is also a critical matter for achieving a satisfactory anticancer effect, because in most cases, entering the cell and accessing the cellular components are necessary for anticancer drugs' actions. Regarding this issue, low molecular weight hydrophobic drugs usually show rapid and extensive internalization. In contrast, most nano-drugs modified with hydrophilic polymers such as PEG suffer from the low cellular absorption and thus therapeutic effect, as known as "PEG dilemma" [49]. Our previous studies also showed that polymer conjugated ZnPP with covalent bonds exhibited much lower intracellular uptake than the corresponding native drugs [24,50]. Given this situation, the release of API from nanomedicine in the tumor site is an important matter of concern for developing anticancer nanomedicines, as described above. By use of the ester bond, in this study, we found that although the intracellular uptake of HA-es-ZnPP was slower and lower than free ZnPP, the uptake increased gradually in a time-dependent manner, which reached a level of one-third of that of ZnPP after 8 h (Figure 5). This result is partly parallel with the release profiles in the presence of FBS (Figure 3), suggesting that effective internalization of active drug (ZnPP) could be achieved in HA-es-ZnPP by benefiting from the esterase-dependent cleavage of ester bond and release of ZnPP. In addition, it is well known that CD44, the primary membrane receptor of HA, is highly expressed in many tumor cells [51]; thus, the CD44 mediated endocytosis may also contribute to the internalization of HA-es-ZnPP. As a consequence, HA-es-ZnPP alone showed relatively potent cytotoxicity to tested cancer cells with a IC_{50} of 50 μg/mL, which is one fourth the cytotoxicity of free ZnPP (12.5 μg/mL) (Figure 5B), and is much more potent than polymer conjugate of ZnPP using uncleavable bonds previously developed in our laboratory (i.e., IC_{50} > 100 μg/mL for HPMA conjugated ZnPP) [24].

More importantly, after light irradiation, the cytotoxicities of both free ZnPP and HA-es-ZnPP were remarkably (10–15 times) augmented (Figure 5B). The increased cytotoxicity was attributed to the generation of $^1O_2$, i.e., PDT effect, which was confirmed in ESR measurement as indicated by the time-dependent intensified spin-polarized triplet signal (Figure 4). One concern about anticancer PDT is the off-target generation of toxic $^1O_2$, namely, generation of $^1O_2$ in normal tissues will induce adverse side effects. This could be substantially improved by nano-designed PS to target tumor tissue by taking advantage of the EPR effect as discussed in "Introductions". In this regard, HA-es-ZnPP, as a micellar type nanomedicine, exhibited much higher accumulation in tumors than most normal tissues, which could not be seen in case of small molecule free ZnPP (Figure 6). In addition, interestingly, we found that HA-es-ZnPP in micellar form did not emit $^1O_2$ as well as fluorescence under light irradiation (Figures 2 and 4). This was probably due to a π–π stacked structure of ZnPP in the core of micelles, in which excited fluorochrome dissipates the energy [24]. This property will further ensure the safety of anticancer PDT using HA-es-ZnPP. Namely, in circulation HA-es-ZnPP behaves mostly as micelles with relative stability, so no or largely reduced $^1O_2$ will be generated under ambient light. During circulation, HA-es-ZnPP will accumulate and retain in the tumor due to the EPR effect, during which micelles will be gradually disrupted and free ZnPP is released and is then taken up by tumor cells. The following light irradiation will thus trigger the generation of $^1O_2$ mostly in the tumor to fulfill the anticancer effect, whereas less side effects to normal tissues and organs will be induced. Thus, the PDT using HA-es-ZnPP will confer a superior therapeutic effect over conventional PDT using low molecular weight PS as well the improved safety of the treatment and quality of life in patients. As expected, we found significant suppression of tumor growth by PDT using HA-es-ZnPP (Figure 7A), whereas we did not observe body weight loss in this treatment regimen that indicates no apparent side effects (Figure 7B). It should be noted that the dose of HA-es-ZnPP (i.e., 5 mg/kg) and intensity of light irradiation (36 J/cm^2) are relatively low compared to many other studies [25]; we thus believe the therapeutic effect could be optimized by modulating the dosing/irradiation regimen which will be investigated in future studies.

Compared to other polymeric PS, HA-es-ZnPP also potentially has some other advantages beyond the PDT effect. Besides the EPR effect-based tumor targeting and CD44-driven tumor targeting as described above [52], HA could also work in a tumor microenvironment to trigger the reprogramming of tumor-associated macrophages towards anti-tumor M1 type macrophages. Thus, a synergistic anticancer effect could be achieved using HA-based nanomedicine [53]. Moreover, because of the extensive tumor accumulation of HA-es-ZnPP (Figure 6), it may become possible to visualize tumors, especially tiny metastatic tumor nodules and disseminated cancer by using fluorescence imaging, as indicated in Figure 6 (inset). Namely, HA-es-PDT could be a theranostic nanoprobe for PDT as well as for photodynamic diagnosis, which warrants further investigations.

Taken together, in this study, we successfully synthesized a HA conjugated ZnPP via an ester bond, (Figure 1), which exhibits high water-solubility and forms micelles in aqueous solutions (Figure 2). As micellar formation, HA-es-ZnPP shows fluorescence quenching, and $^1O_2$ generation does not occur under light irradiation. However, it is extensively generated when the micelle is disrupted, and ZnPP is released (Figure 4). On the other hand, the micelle formation imposes a prolonged circulation time and tumor-selective accumulation upon HA-es-ZnPP based on the EPR effect (Figure 6). Consequently, a remarkable anticancer PDT effect is achieved both in vitro (Figure 5) and in vivo (Figure 7), suggesting the potential of HA-es-ZnPP as a candidate anticancer nanomedicine for PDT.

Supplementary Materials: The following are available online at https://www.mdpi.com/2075-4426/11/2/136/s1, Figure S1: Tumor environment-responsive hyaluronan conjugated zinc protoporphyrin for targeted anticancer photodynamic therapy.

Author Contributions: Conceptualization, J.F.; Data curation, S.G. and R.I.; Formal analysis, S.G., R.I., and J.F.; Funding acquisition, J.F.; Investigation, S.G., R.I., and J.F.; Methodology, S.G. and J.F.; Project administration, J.F.; Resources, J.F.; Software, S.G.; Validation, S.G. and R.I.; Visualization, S.G. and R.I.; Writing—original draft, J.F.; Writing—review & editing, R.I. and J.F. All authors have read and agreed to the published version of the manuscript.

Funding: This research was funded by Japan Society for the Promotion of Science (JSPS) KAKENHI grant number JP22700927 and JP25430162.

Institutional Review Board Statement: The animal study was conducted according to the guidelines of the Laboratory Protocol for Animal Handling of Sojo University, and approved by the Animal Ethics Committees of Sojo University (no. 2020-P-009, approved on 1 April 2020).

Informed Consent Statement: Not applicable.

Data Availability Statement: The data presented in this study are available on request from the corresponding author.

Conflicts of Interest: The authors declare no conflict of interest.

References

1. Vogelstein, B.; Papadopoulos, N. Cancer genome landscapes. *Science* **2013**, *339*, 1546–1558. [CrossRef] [PubMed]
2. Gerlinger, M.; Rowan, A.J. Intratumor heterogeneity and branched evolution revealed by multiregion sequencing. *N. Engl. J. Med.* **2012**, *366*, 883–892. [CrossRef] [PubMed]
3. Cutler, D.M. Early returns from the era of precision medicine. *JAMA* **2020**, *323*, 109–110. [CrossRef] [PubMed]
4. Germain, M.; Caputo, F. Delivering the power of nanomedicine to patients today. *J. Control. Release* **2020**, *326*, 164–171. [CrossRef]
5. Lammers, T.; Ferrari, M. The success of nanomedicine. *Nano Today* **2020**, *31*, 100853. [CrossRef]
6. Matsumura, Y.; Maeda, H. A new concept for macromolecular therapeutics in can- cer chemotherapy: Mechanism of tumoritropic accumulation of proteins and the antitumor agent smancs. *Cancer Res.* **1986**, *46*, 6387–6392.
7. Fang, J.; Nakamura, H. The EPR effect: Unique features of tumor blood vessels for drug delivery, factors involved, and limitations and augmentation of the effect. *Adv. Drug Deliv. Rev.* **2011**, *63*, 136–151. [CrossRef]
8. Maeda, H. Toward a full understanding of the EPR effect in primary and metastatic tumors as well as issues related to its heterogeneity. *Adv. Drug Deliv. Rev.* **2015**, *91*, 3–6. [CrossRef]
9. Fang, J.; Islam, W. Exploiting the dynamics of the EPR effect and strategies to improve the therapeutic effects of nanomedicines by using EPR effect enhancers. *Adv. Drug Deliv. Rev.* **2020**, *157*, 142–160. [CrossRef]
10. Noguchi, Y.; Wu, J. Early phase tumor accumulation of macromolecules: A great difference in clearance rate between tumor and normal tissues. *Jpn. J. Cancer Res* **1998**, *89*, 307–314. [CrossRef]
11. Duncan, R.; Vicent, M.J. Polymer therapeutics-prospects for 21st century: The end of the beginning. *Adv. Drug Deliv. Rev.* **2013**, *65*, 60–70. [CrossRef] [PubMed]
12. Hare, J.I.; Lammers, T. Challenges and strategies in anti-cancer nanomedicine development: An industry perspec- tive. *Adv. Drug Deliv. Rev.* **2017**, *108*, 25–38. [CrossRef] [PubMed]
13. Dolmans, D.E.; Fukumura, D. Photodynamic therapy for cancer. *Nat. Rev. Cancer* **2003**, *3*, 380–387. [CrossRef]
14. Wilson, B.C.; Can, J. Photodynamic therapy for cancer: Principles. *Gastroenterology* **2020**, *16*, 393–396. [CrossRef] [PubMed]
15. Tsukagoshi, S. Development of a novel photosensitizer, talaporfin sodium, for the photodynamic therapy (PDT). *Gan Kagaku Ryoho* **2004**, *31*, 979–985.
16. Usuda, J.; Kato, H. Photodynamic therapy (PDT) for lung cancers. *J. Thorac. Oncol.* **2006**, *1*, 489–493. [CrossRef]
17. Del Duca, E.; Manfredini, M. Daylight Photodynamic Therapy with 5-aminolevulinic acid 5% gel for the treatment of mild-to-moderate inflammatory acne. *G Ital. Derm. Venereol.* **2019**, 12.
18. Sibani, S.A.; McCarron, P.A. Photosensitiser delivery for photodynamic therapy. Part 2: Systemic carrier platforms. *Expert Opin. Drug Deliv.* **2008**, *5*, 1241–1254. [CrossRef]
19. Nishiyama, N.; Morimoto, Y. Design and development of dendrimer photosensitizer-incorporated polymeric micelles for enhanced photodynamic therapy. *Adv. Drug Deliv. Rev.* **2009**, *61*, 327–338. [CrossRef]
20. Ghosh, S.; Carter, K.A. Liposomal formulations of photosensitizers. *Biomaterials* **2009**, *218*, 119341. [CrossRef]
21. Kobayashi, H.; Choyke, P.L. Near-Infrared Photoimmunotherapy of Cancer. *Acc. Chem. Res.* **2019**, *52*, 2332–2339. [CrossRef]
22. Regehly, M.; Greish, K. Water-soluble polymer conjugates of ZnPP for photodynamic tumor therapy. *Bioconjug. Chem.* **2007**, *18*, 494–499. [CrossRef]
23. Iyer, A.K.; Greish, K. Polymeric micelles of zinc protoporphyrin for tumor targeted delivery based on EPR effect and singlet oxygen generation. *Drug Target* **2007**, *15*, 496–506. [CrossRef]
24. Nakamura, H.; Liao, L. Micelles of zinc protoporphyrin conjugated to N-(2-hydroxypropyl) methacrylamide (HPMA) copolymer for imaging and light- induced antitumor effects in vivo. *J. Control. Release* **2013**, *165*, 191–198. [CrossRef]
25. Fang, J.; Liao, L. Photodynamic therapy and imaging based on tumor-targeted nanoprobe, polymer-conjugated zinc protopor- phyrin. *Future Sci. OA* **2015**, 1. [CrossRef]
26. Fang, J.; Šubr, V. N-(2-hydroxypropyl) methacrylamide polymer conjugated pyropheophorbide-a, a promising tumor-targeted theranostic probe for photodynamic therapy and imaging. *Pharm. Biopharm.* **2018**, *130*, 165–176. [CrossRef] [PubMed]
27. Eguchi, K.; Nakamura, H. Hyaluronic Acid-zinc Protoporphyrin Conjugates for Photodynamic Antitumor Therapy. *Nanomed. Nanotechnol.* **2007**, *8*, 100400.
28. Choi, K.Y.; Saravanakumar, G. Hyaluronic acid-based nanocarriers for intracellular targeting: Interfacial interactions with proteins in cancer. *Colloids Surf. B Biointerfaces* **2012**, *99*, 82–94. [CrossRef]
29. Rao, N.V.; Rho, J.G. Hyaluronic acid nanoparticles as nanomedicine for treatment of inflammatory diseases. *Pharmaceutics* **2020**, *12*, 931. [CrossRef] [PubMed]
30. Lee, S.Y.; Kang, M.S. Hyaluronic acid-based theranostic nanomedicines for targeted cancer therapy. *Cancers* **2020**, *12*, 940. [CrossRef] [PubMed]
31. Racker, E. Bioenergetics and the Problem of Tumor Growth: An understanding of the mechanism of the generation and control of biological energy may shed light on the problem of tumor growth. *Am. Sci.* **1972**, *60*, 56–63.
32. Fang, J.; Quinones, Q.J. The H+-linked monocarboxylate transporter (MCT1/SLC16A1): A potential therapeutic target for high-risk neuroblastoma. *Mol. Pharmacol.* **2006**, *70*, 2108–2115. [CrossRef] [PubMed]
33. Bae, Y.; Nishiyama, N. Preparation and biological characterization of polymeric micelle drug carriers with intracellular pH-triggered drug release property: Tumor permeability, controlled subcellular drug distribution, and enhanced in vivo antitumor efficacy. *Bioconjug. Chem.* **2005**, *16*, 122–130. [CrossRef] [PubMed]

34. Duncan, R.; Sat-Klopsch, Y.N. Validation of tumour models for use in anticancer nanomedicine evaluation: The EPR effect and cathepsin B-mediated drug release rate. *Cancer Chemother. Pharmacol.* **2013**, *72*, 417–427. [CrossRef] [PubMed]
35. Pola, O.; Janoušková, T. Etrych, The pH-dependent and enzymatic release of cytarabine from hydrophilic polymer conjugates. *Physiol. Res* **2016**, *65*, S225–S232. [CrossRef]
36. Tsukigawa, K.; Nakamura, H. Effect of different chemical bonds in pegylation of zinc protoporphyrin that affects drug release, intracellular uptake, and therapeutic effect in the tumor. *Pharm. Biopharm.* **2015**, *89*, 259–270. [CrossRef]
37. Pravata, L.; Braud, C. New amphiphilic lactic acid oligomer-hyaluronan conjugates: Synthesis and physicochemical characterization. *Biomacromolecules* **2008**, *9*, 340–348. [CrossRef]
38. Iyer, A.K.; Greish, K. High-loading nanosized micelles of copoly(styrene-maleic acid)-zinc protoporphyrin for targeted delivery of a potent heme oxygenase inhibitor. *Biomaterials* **2007**, *28*, 1871–1881. [CrossRef]
39. Fang, J.; Tsukigawa, K. Styrene-maleic acid-copolymer conjugated zinc protoporphyrin as a candidate drug for tumor-targeted therapy and imaging. *Drug Target* **2016**, *24*, 399–407. [CrossRef]
40. Sahoo, S.K.; Sawa, T. Pegylated zinc protoporphyrin: A water-soluble heme oxygenase inhibitor with tumor-targeting capacity. *Bioconjug. Chem.* **2002**, *13*, 1031–1038. [CrossRef]
41. Cordova, J.; Ryan, J.D. Esterase activity of bovine serum albumin up to 160 degrees C: A new benchmark for biocatalysis. *Enzym. Microb. Technol.* **2008**, *42*, 278–283. [CrossRef]
42. Fang, J.; Sawa, T. In vivo antitumor activity of pegylated zinc protoporphyrin: Targeted inhibition of heme oxygenase in solid tumor. *Cancer Res.* **2003**, *63*, 3567–3574.
43. Matsumura, Y.; Hamaguchi, T. Phase I clinical trial and pharmacokinetic evaluation of NK911, a micelle-encapsulated doxorubicin. *Br. J. Cancer* **2004**, *91*, 1775–1781. [CrossRef]
44. Cabral, H.; Matsumoto, Y. Accumulation of sub-100 nm polymeric micelles in poorly permeable tumours depends on size. *Nat. Nanotechnol.* **2011**, *6*, 815–823. [CrossRef] [PubMed]
45. Barenholz, Y. Doxil®-the first FDA-approved nano-drug: Lessons learned. *J. Control. Release* **2012**, *160*, 117–134. [CrossRef] [PubMed]
46. Lim, Z.W.; Varma, V.B.; Ramanujan, R.V.; Miserez, A. Magnetically responsive peptide coacervates for dual hyperthermia and chemotherapy treatments of liver cancer. *Acta Biomater.* **2020**, *110*, 221–230. [CrossRef] [PubMed]
47. Pradhan, L.; Srivastava, R.; Bahadur, D. pH- and thermosensitive thin lipid layer coated mesoporous magnetic nanoassemblies as a dual drug delivery system towards thermochemotherapy of cancer. *Acta Biomater.* **2014**, *10(7)*, 2976–2987. [CrossRef] [PubMed]
48. Lin, W.; Ma, G.; Kampf, N.; Yuan, Z.; Chen, S. Development of Long-Circulating Zwitterionic Cross-Linked Micelles for Active-Targeted Drug Delivery. *Biomacromolecules* **2016**, *17*, 2010–2018. [CrossRef] [PubMed]
49. Hatakeyama, H.; Akita, H. The polyethyleneglycol dilemma: Advantage and disadvantage of PEGylation of liposomes for systemic genes and nucleic acids delivery to tumors. *Biol Pharm Bull* **2013**, *36*, 892–899. [CrossRef]
50. Nakamura, H.; Fang, J. Intracellular uptake and behavior of two types zinc protoporphyrin (ZnPP) micelles, SMA-ZnPP and PEG-ZnPP as anticancer agents; unique intracellular disintegration of SMA micelles. *J. Control Release* **2011**, *155*, 367–375. [CrossRef]
51. Bayer, I.S. Hyaluronic Acid and Controlled Release: A Review. *Molecules* **2020**, *25*, 2649. [CrossRef] [PubMed]
52. Luo, Z.; Dai, Y. Development and application of hyaluronic acid in tumor targeting drug delivery. *Acta Pharm. Sin. B* **2019**, *9*, 1099–1112. [CrossRef] [PubMed]
53. Ai, X.; Hu, M. Enhanced Cellular Ablation by Attenuating Hypoxia Status and Reprogramming Tumor-Associated Macrophages via NIR Light-Responsive Upconversion Nanocrystals. *Bioconjug. Chem.* **2018**, *29*, 928–938. [CrossRef] [PubMed]

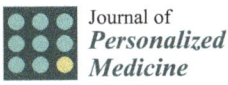

Review

Nanodrug Delivery Systems Modulate Tumor Vessels to Increase the Enhanced Permeability and Retention Effect

Dong Huang [1,2], Lingna Sun [1,2], Leaf Huang [3] and Yanzuo Chen [1,2,*]

1. Shanghai Key Laboratory of Functional Materials Chemistry, East China University of Science and Technology, Shanghai 200237, China; y53200022@mail.ecust.edu.cn (D.H.); y30191353@mail.ecust.edu.cn (L.S.)
2. Engineering Research Centre of Pharmaceutical Process Chemistry, Ministry of Education, Shanghai Key Laboratory of New Drug Design, School of Pharmacy, East China University of Science and Technology, Shanghai 200237, China
3. Division of Pharmacoengineering and Molecular Pharmaceutics, Eshelman School of Pharmacy, University of North Carolina, Chapel Hill, NC 27599, USA; leafh@email.unc.edu
* Correspondence: chenyz@ecust.edu.cn; Tel.: +86-21-64252449

Abstract: The use of nanomedicine for antitumor therapy has been extensively investigated for a long time. Enhanced permeability and retention (EPR) effect-mediated drug delivery is currently regarded as an effective way to bring drugs to tumors, especially macromolecular drugs and drug-loaded pharmaceutical nanocarriers. However, a disordered vessel network, and occluded or embolized tumor blood vessels seriously limit the EPR effect. To augment the EPR effect and improve curative effects, in this review, we focused on the perspective of tumor blood vessels, and analyzed the relationship among abnormal angiogenesis, abnormal vascular structure, irregular blood flow, extensive permeability of tumor vessels, and the EPR effect. In this commentary, nanoparticles including liposomes, micelles, and polymers extravasate through the tumor vasculature, which are based on modulating tumor vessels, to increase the EPR effect, thereby increasing their therapeutic effect.

Keywords: nanoparticles; tumor vascular regulation; EPR effect; angiogenesis; blood perfusion; vascular permeability

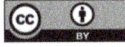

1. Introduction

Solid tumors are the major cause of death worldwide and their treatment remains a challenge [1–3]. Chemotherapy is one of the few treatment options available for metastasized tumors which cannot be removed surgically; however, the effectiveness of this therapeutic modality is not yet satisfactory [4]. This problem mainly stems from the lack of tumor selectivity by these agents; hence, the occurrence of severe adverse effects limits the usage of chemotherapy [5]. Nanomedicines have been designed to guide drugs more precisely to tumor cells and away from sites of toxicity. These agents have numerous theoretical advantages over low-molecular-weight drugs, including high drug loading, specific targeting, and the ability to protect the payload from degradation and release the drug in a controlled or sustained manner [6]. Theoretically, nanomedicines with larger particle size leak more slowly from blood vessels compared with most chemotherapy drugs. Fortunately, vascular leakage is a major feature of the vasculature of solid tumors. Specifically, tumor neovasculature has larger lumens and wider fenestrations (200 nm to 1.2 μm in diameter) due to its lack of a smooth muscle layer and pericytes [7]. When injected intravenously, nanomedicines ranging in size from 10 to 500 nm tend to circulate for a long time and can preferentially access the tumor tissue through the leaky tumor vasculature; subsequently, they are retained in the tumor bed due to reduced lymphatic drainage [8–12]. This pathophysiological phenomenon based on abnormal tumor angiogenesis to increase the delivery of nanomedicines in tumors is known as "the enhanced permeability and retention" (EPR) effect [10–13]. Matsumura and Maeda first reported the EPR effect in

1986 [11]. Follow-up studies rigorously verified that the EPR effect can be observed using macromolecules with an apparent molecular size >45 kDa (the threshold for renal clearance) and a longer plasma half-life. In recent years, Ding et al. conducted real-time research on human kidney tumors using X-ray computed tomography to confirm the existence of the EPR effect in humans. The results showed that the significant EPR effect can be found in >87% of human kidney tumors [14]. However, low-molecular-weight contrast agents do not stay in the tumor and can be washed out in a minute from tumor, which greatly differs from macromolecular drug retention in tumors. Therefore, Maeda et al. reported a more distinct method to prove the EPR effect in human by conjugating lipiodol with a macromolecular nanodrug [15]. This method lasts longer than X-ray computed tomography, and it can be used to further explore the significant difference between the EPR effect of macromolecular drugs and low-molecular-weight counterparts.

Nanodrug delivery is based on the accumulation of drugs in tumors due to the EPR effect, and the subsequent release of the therapeutic payload [11,16]. However, the EPR effect is inadequate in tumors; this inadequacy can be attributed to the high interstitial fluid pressure (IFP), the dense extracellular matrix (ECM), and the occluded or embolized tumor blood vessels [12,17,18]. Moreover, the prolonged circulation of the drug increases the ability of extravasation into the tumor through the EPR effect. Clinically, it has been demonstrated that the function of long-circulating liposomes, for example, doxorubicin (DOX)-loaded polyethylene glycol (PEG)ylated liposomes (Doxil), reduces opsonization and premature clearance, increases the blood circulation time, and potentially enhances drug accumulation in the tumor [19]. However, when the EPR effect is insufficient, the drug may extravasate and bring more toxicity into normal tissues. Thus, there is an urgent need to identify the physiological barriers that affect the EPR effect of tumors. The aim of such research would be the development of methods to enhance tumor penetration and retention, thereby improving tumor targeting and the therapeutic effect. In this review, we analyzed the barriers to drug delivery, focusing on the influence of tumor vasculature on the EPR effect. Moreover, we discussed the method utilized for the regulation of tumor blood vessels through the nanodrug delivery system to enhance the EPR effect [20–24].

2. Abnormal Vascular Functions Affect the Tumor EPR Effect

To satisfy the overgrowth of tumor cells, solid tumors need to induce and maintain a dedicated tumor blood supply, which is termed neovascularization. Under inflammatory or hypoxic tumor conditions, cells such as vascular endothelial cells release vascular permeability mediators, resulting in more enhanced tumor vascular permeability than in normal tissue, which can be demonstrated by angiography [25]. However, due to their short half-life and the rapid dilution in the bloodstream, these mediators mainly affect tumor vessels, but not normal tissue blood vessels. In such regions, macromolecules ranging from 10 to 500 nm (e.g., macromolecular anticancer agent, albumin, immunoglobulin, micelles, liposomes, and protein–polymer conjugates) can selectively leak out from the vascular bed and accumulate inside the interstitial space. However, in solid tumors, the EPR effect exhibits great heterogeneity. Tumors show different EPR effects regardless of their types and sizes, patients, or their developmental stages. Tumors with high blood vessel density (e.g., hepatocellular carcinoma) show a strong EPR effect, whereas others with low vascular density (e.g., pancreatic cancer) show a weak EPR effect [5]. Therefore, accurate monitoring and evaluation of the EPR effects in different tumors is essential for the development of personalized EPR-mediated plans for the treatment of tumors.

In principle, due to the widespread presence of EPR in tumors, nanomedicines based on the EPR effect show great promise for improving the efficacy of systemic anticancer drug therapy. However, their full anticancer potential has been hindered because of biological and pathophysiological barriers [26]. Obviously, the vascular system of tumors, which exhibit different vessel density, maturity, perfusion, and pore cutoff size, could be considered one of the main factors that affect the EPR effect [27]. In this review, we summarize the three main approaches through which abnormal tumor blood vessels affect the EPR effect and the related vascular mediators (Table 1).

Table 1. Relationship between tumor vascular-related mediators and three typical vascular characteristics.

Features	Vascular Mediators	Functions	Tumors with This Substance	Reference
Abnormal angiogenesis	Vascular endothelial growth factor (VEGF)	Key factors in angiogenesis, VEGFs bind to the kinase function of VEGF receptor (VEGFR)-activated receptors, triggering a variety of downstream signaling cascades, such as increased capillary permeability, nitric oxide (NO) production (relaxation of vascular smooth muscle), endothelial cell (EC) proliferation, migration, and survival under stress.	Overexpression in most solid tumors	[28–30]
	Tumor necrosis factor (TNF)-α	TNF-α mediates monocyte differentiation into angiogenic cells that support tumor angiogenesis. It is also a multipotent proinflammatory cytokine with vascular permeability activity, which can enhance vascular leakage by disrupting the EC adhesion junction VE-cadherin.		[22,31–36]
	Acidic fibroblast growth factor (FGF)/FGF-1	Interacts with receptor tyrosine kinase subtypes to induce EC proliferation and maintain tumor angiogenesis.		[37]
	Basic FGF/FGF-2	Controls angiogenesis by inducing the expression of VEGF through paracrine and endocrine mechanisms.		[38–40]
	Platelet-derived growth factor (PDGF)	PDGF signals through two cell-surface tyrosine kinase receptors, PDGF receptor α (PDGFRα) and PDGFRβ, and induces angiogenesis by upregulating the production of VEGF and regulating the proliferation and recruitment of perivascular cells.		[41–43]
	Placenta growth factor (PLGF)	PLGF only binds to VEGFR-1 and induces tumor angiogenesis, promoting the survival of ECs in tumor-associated blood vessels.		[44]
	Epidermal growth factor (EGF)	A key EGF receptor (EGFR) ligand is one of many growth factors that drive the expression of VEGF.		[45]
	Hepatocyte growth factor (HGF)	Stimulates cell motility and the secretion of proteinases and plays an important role in tumor invasion and progression.		[46]
	Hypoxia-inducible factor (HIF)-1α	Upregulates VEGF gene expression by hypoxia response element binding to the promoter region of VEGF.		[47–51]
	Transforming growth factor (TGF)-β	Induces strong VEGF production in recruited hematopoietic cells, leading to activated angiogenesis and vascular remodeling. Low TGF-β levels contribute to angiogenesis, and high levels of TGF-β can inhibit EC growth.		[52–54]

Table 1. *Cont.*

Features	Vascular Mediators	Functions	Tumors with This Substance	Reference
	Interleukin (IL)-1β	Induces angiogenesis indirectly by activating the expression of VEGF in smooth muscle cells.		[55]
	IL-3	Stimulates EC movement and promotes the formation of new blood vessels in vivo. It also stimulates migration and proliferation of vascular smooth muscle cells.		[56]
	IL-6	Regulates the synthesis of VEGF and influences tumor angiogenesis by inducing the production of VEGF.		[57]
	IL-8	Enhances EC survival, proliferation, and matrix metalloproteinase production, and regulates angiogenesis.		[58]
	Neuropilin 1 and 2	Regulates receptor–ligand interactions of the VEGF family.		[59]
	Adrenomedullin	Promotes angiogenesis, protects cells from apoptosis and vascular injury, and affects vascular tone and permeability.		[60]
	Stromal cell-derived factor 1 (SDF-1), a chemokine	Synergizes with VEGF to induce angiogenesis in human ovarian cancer tumors. Furthermore, in invasive breast cancer, stromal fibroblast-derived SDF-1 promotes angiogenesis by recruiting bone marrow-derived endothelial precursors. It plays an angiogenic role through the receptor CXC motif chemokine receptor type 4.		[61]
	Endostatin	Inhibits cell cycle control and antiapoptotic genes in proliferating ECs, thus inhibiting angiogenesis.		[62]
	Integrin	Adhesion molecules such as $\alpha_6\beta_1$ and $\alpha_6\beta_4$ integrins mediate VEGF-induced angiogenesis, which regulates the adhesion of ECs to the ECM, thereby promoting the migration and survival of tumor vasculature. Other integrins (e.g., $\alpha_v\beta_3$, $\alpha_v\beta_5$, and $\alpha_5\beta_1$) have also been shown to mediate angiogenesis.		[63,64]
	Pigment epithelium-derived factor	Inhibits angiogenesis via downregulation of VEGF.		[65]
	Nuclear factor kappa-B (NF-κB)	Activated NF-κB can bind to DNA, promote cell proliferation, regulate cell apoptosis, promote angiogenesis, and stimulate invasion and metastasis.		[66]
	Thyroid hormone	Thyroid hormones have proangiogenic effects on ECs and vascular smooth muscle cells initiated by integrin $\alpha_v\beta_3$ extracellular domain hormone cell-surface receptors.		[67]

Table 1. *Cont.*

Features	Vascular Mediators	Functions	Tumors with This Substance	Reference
	Matrix metalloproteinases (MMPs)	Involved in the process of angiogenesis through its proteolytic role in tissue remodeling, as well as the growth of new blood vessels and the release of angiogenic factors sequestered in the matrix.		[68]
	Endogenous carbon monoxide (CO) and heme oxygenase (HO)	Play an important role in regulating vascular tension and inducing angiogenesis, and can significantly increase vascular permeability and blood flow.		[69–73]
	Angiogenin	Undergoes nuclear translocation in ECs where it stimulates ribosomal RNA transcription and cell proliferation.		[74]
	Angiopoietin 1	Activates matrix-degrading enzymes, including plasminogen activators and MMPs, to loosen the matrix and promote ECs migration.		[75]
	Vashohibin-1	A novel angiogenesis inhibitory protein regulates angiogenesis, inhibits pathological angiogenesis, and promotes tumor vascular maturation by negative feedback.	High expression in liver cancer, prostate cancer, renal cancer, and colorectal cancer	[76,77]
Vascular permeability	VEGF (VEGF-A/B/C/D)	As mentioned above.	Overexpression in most solid tumors	[28–30]
	Bradykinin (BK)	Activates EC-derived NO synthase, which leads to an increase in NO and plays a role in increasing vascular permeability.		[78,79]
	Hydroxyprolyl3 BK	As mentioned above.	Advanced cancer	[80–82]
	Inducible nitric oxide synthase (iNOS) and NO	NO is an effective endothelium-derived vascular regulator, which plays an important role in vascular permeability, cell proliferation, and extravasation (EPR effect), inducing vasodilation and increasing blood flow.		[83–85]
	Prostaglandin E1 and I2	Usually involved in inflammation and cancer, it has similar effects as NO and can enhance extravasation and EPR effects.		[83,86]
	TNF-α	As mentioned above.		[22,31–36]
	Angiotensin receptor type 2 (AGTR2)	AGTR2 can induce vasoconstriction in healthy tissues and increase systemic blood pressure, and is an effective substance to enhance blood flow and promote vascular permeability in tumors.		[87]
	IL-2	Increased vascular permeability by inducing NO production		[76,77]
	Endothelin-1 (Et-A, Et-B)	Endothelin is an endogenous long-acting vasoconstrictor regulator.		[76,77]
Irregular blood flow	AGTR2	As mentioned above.		[87]
	Endogenous CO and HO	As mentioned above.		[69–73]

2.1. Abnormal Angiogenesis

Angiogenesis is essential for the continuous growth and development of solid tumors. Tumor vessels provide oxygen and nutrients and remove waste products, supply a favorable niche for cancer stem cells, and serve as a conduit for tumor cell metastatic spread and immune cell infiltration. Unlike normal blood vessels, tumor blood vessels with abnormal structure and function impede the delivery of adequate and effective oxygen, as well as therapeutic drugs to cancer cells [88,89]. In cancer progression, the overexpression of proangiogenic factors drives the pathological angiogenesis. An imbalance between local proangiogenic and antiangiogenic factors may lead to the proliferation, migration, and new vessel formation of endothelial cells (EC). Furthermore, pericyte coverage of EC is often absent in the tumor vasculature. Compared with normal tissue with an organized microvasculature with regular branching order, the vascular organization of tumor tissue is disorganized and lacks the conventional hierarchy. Abnormal angiogenesis may lead to structural and functional abnormalities of the vascular system, which are often characterized by tortuous, unorganized, and excessive leakage [90,91]. This feature contributes to the vascular permeability of fluids and the escape of metastatic cancer cells [92,93]. Furthermore, the solid pressure generated by the proliferation of cancer cells compresses the blood and lymphatic vessels in the tumor, further impairing blood and lymphatic flows. These abnormal vascular structures collectively lead to an abnormal tumor microenvironment (TME), characterized by high IFP, hypoxia, and acidosis [88,94,95]. A physiological consequence of these vascular abnormalities is heterogeneity of tumor blood flow, which can interfere with the EPR effect and the uniform distribution of drugs within the tumor.

Tumor cells can promote blood vessel sprouting by releasing angiogenic molecules that bind to their respective receptors in adjacent cells or by paracrine signals [96,97]. Vascular endothelial growth factor (VEGF) appears to play the most critical role in physiological and pathological angiogenesis among all the known angiogenic molecules. It is overexpressed in the majority of solid tumors [28,29] and can promote the survival and proliferation of ECs, increase the display of adhesion molecules on these cells, and increase vascular permeability. By downregulating VEGF signaling in solid tumors, the vasculature may return to a more "normal" state, accompanied by decreased IFP, increased tumor oxygenation, and improved drug permeability in these tumors [98].

In addition to VEGF, other factors and proteins can also promote the abnormal formation of tumor blood vessels. Thus far, 28 proangiogenic factors/genes have been found to mediate tumor angiogenesis [76,77], including the fibroblast growth factor (FGF), hypoxia-inducible factor (HIF), platelet-derived growth factor-B (PDGF-B), tumor necrosis factor-α (TNF-α), chemokines, integrins, and transforming growth factor-β (TGF-β), as well as their receptors [76,99–103]. Acidic and basic FGF (FGF1 and FGF2) have the ability to induce angiogenesis [39]. FGFs stimulate the proliferation and migration of ECs, as well as the production of collagenase and plasminogen activator (PDGF), which stimulate angiogenesis and are related to the aging process of the tumor vasculature in vivo [42,43]. TGF-β possesses dual pro- and antiangiogenic properties. At low levels, TGF-β participates in the switch of angiogenesis by upregulating angiogenic factors and proteinases. At high levels, it can inhibit EC growth, stimulate the differentiation and recruitment of smooth muscle cells, and promote the reorganization of the basement membrane [52]. Moreover, as effective angiogenic factors, chemokines can induce the migration and proliferation of ECs, and they have pro- or antiangiogenic activities [104]. As an angiogenic factor, HIF cooperates with TNF inhibitors to initiate angiogenesis under hypoxic conditions [48–51]. It activates the signaling pathway and upregulates the expression of VEGF. Growth factors generated by this pathway activate the mitogen-activated protein kinase and protein kinase B signaling pathways, leading to increased levels of HIF-1 protein, thereby promoting tumor angiogenesis. Adhesion molecules (e.g., $\alpha_6\beta_1$ and $\alpha_6\beta_4$ integrins) mediate VEGF-induced angiogenesis, which regulates the adhesion of ECs to the ECM, thereby promoting the migration and survival of tumor vasculature. Other integrins (e.g., $\alpha_v\beta_3$, $\alpha_v\beta_5$, and $\alpha_5\beta_1$) also mediate angiogenesis [63,64].

2.2. Irregular Blood Flow

Compared with normal vessels, newly formed tumor vessels are irregular or inconsistent [87]. It has been reported that tumor vessels are insensitive to angiotensin receptor type 2 (AGTR2). In addition, there is intermittent flow (only one flow in 15–20 min) and reverse flow of blood at the tumor site [105,106]. Moreover, blood often flows in the opposite direction. Irregular blood flow in the tumor is usually caused by irregular vascular structure. Unlike normal tissues, angiogenic factors in tumors at the late stage of vascular maturation will continue to be activated, leading to vascular abnormalities, which are characterized by irregular vascular structure and spatiotemporal heterogeneity [107]. Tumor vessels with irregular structure are characterized by a curved vascular shape, filling of the EC septum, and damage of the basement membrane. These effects lead to distortion of the vascular morphology and high permeability of the vascular EC space [31,108–110]. The distortion of blood vessels increases the geometric resistance of blood flow. The high permeability of blood vessels increases the hematocrit of tumor blood, thus increasing the blood viscosity [111]. In addition, the phenomenon of rapid proliferation of tumor cells in a finite space and excessive deposition of ECM can lead to large solid stress between adjacent cells and matrix components. The continuous accumulation of solid stress can lead to the compression of tumor blood vessels and the reduction of cross-sectional area and pressure difference in the direction of blood vessels [112]. The increase in vascular resistance and blood viscosity and the compression of accumulated solid stress significantly increases the resistance to blood perfusion. The increased resistance of tumor vessels to blood perfusion results in a low blood perfusion rate and a slow blood flow rate [113]. The change in blood flow velocity on the transport of nanoparticles through blood vessels has been investigated. A computer simulation explained the effect of blood flow velocity on the transport of nanoparticles. The results showed that the pressure at the vessel wall and the pressure gradient between the vascular wall and interstitial tissue increase in turn with the increase of fluid velocity in the vascular domain. Moreover, the trans-vascular transport efficiency of nanoparticles initially increases and subsequently decreases [114]. In addition, driven by the difference in pressure along the vascular direction, blood perfusion has the characteristics of convection–diffusion. Convection–diffusion differs between tumor blocks and depends on the local pressure gradient and flow resistance due to the heterogeneity of tumor blood vessels [115].

In addition to an irregular structure, the abnormal blood vessels of tumors also exhibit spatiotemporal heterogeneity [116,117]. This heterogeneity indicates the differing distribution of tumor vessels in various parts of the tumor or during the proliferation period. This is mainly indicated by the fact that the distribution of vessels in the periphery of the tumor is usually very rich, while their extension into the interior of the tumor gradually decreases. Therefore, this uneven distribution complicates the delivery of nanodrugs to the tumor center, which seriously hinders the penetration and extravascular transport of such agents. Of note, the high heterogeneity of tumor vessels in experimental mice and humans reduces the antitumor effects of some nanomedicines [26,118].

2.3. Extensive Vascular Permeability

Increased vascular permeability is widely found in endothelium discontinuous tumor vessels such as neovessels and immature vessels, as well as in other pathological tissues with disturbed vascular function. Compared with normal blood vessels, macromolecular drugs can reach the tumor stroma through the leaky vessel wall with large pores without hindrance [12]. However, excessive vascular leakage can cause plasma escape and hemoconcentration. This results in flow stasis and high IFP, which greatly hinder the extravasation of drugs and their movement to the tumor parenchyma. Furthermore, deposited clots of fibrin transiently promote the formation of blood vessels and ECM and prevent the penetration of antitumor therapeutic agents. The vascular media affecting the tumor vascular permeability are summarized below.

Bradykinin (BK) is of great importance in elevating the permeability of inflammatory sites and tumor tissues, thereby maintaining tumor growth [79,81]. Overexpression of BK receptors in solid tumors has been observed, resulting in defective vascular architecture with large intracellular gaps [119]. Kinin can activate EC-derived nitric oxide (NO) synthase, leading to increased levels of NO, a well-established and effective endothelium-derived vascular modulator [85,120,121]. NO is of great significance in vascular permeability, cell proliferation and extravasation (EPR effect), blood vessel dilation, and elevation of blood flow [83,84]. For example, NO generated from L-arginine under the action of NO synthase induces tumor vascular permeability. It has been demonstrated that the inhibition of NO generation can decrease vascular permeability, thereby weakening the EPR effect. This further confirms that NO is inextricably linked to vascular permeability in solid tumors [84,85]. Prostaglandins E1 and I2 are commonly involved in inflammation and cancer, exert similar effects to those of NO, and can enhance extravasation and EPR effects [83,86]. In summary, vascular permeability in tumors is often directly or indirectly related to kinins.

In addition, it has been shown that several vascular mediators, such as vascular permeability factor (VPF), which is important in tumor angiogenesis, TNF-α, and others elevate the vascular permeability of tumors [31]. EC survival and vascular permeability are closely related to the level of VPF/VEGF, as increasing this level can lead to upregulation of the corresponding receptors on ECs. [34,35]. TNF-α, a multifunctional proinflammatory cytokine with vascular permeabilizing effects [22], can enhance vascular leakiness via disrupting the EC adherence junction vascular endothelial cadherin [36]. TNF-α can increase the sensitivity to nanoparticles through serving as a vascular disrupting agent (VDA). At low levels, TNF-α may promote angiogenesis; however, at higher concentrations, it destroys the tumor vessels and increases the accumulation of drug in tumors [122].

3. Nanoparticles for Enhancing the Tumor EPR Effect

The EPR effect is an effective way for nanoparticles to passively target tumor cells. As opposed to passive drug targeting, nanoparticles based on the use of targeting ligands are termed "active drug targeting". Actively targeted nanomedicines have failed to demonstrate benefit at the clinical level. This failure can be attributed to the fact that nanomedicines may face an insufficient endothelial vascular gap and a number of physiological barriers, such as high cellular density within solid malignancies and high IFP. Consequently, actively targeted nanoparticles have difficulties in identifying target cells due to the inadequate EPR effect. Therefore, enhancing the EPR effect through the use of nanoparticles can provide a better platform for subsequent treatment by elevating blood pressure, or conjugating with antibodies or EPR enhancers such as NO-generating agents. Several techniques have been employed to enhance the EPR effect, including the inhibition of angiogenesis, upregulation of tumor blood perfusion, and disruption of vascular or enhancement of vessel penetration to modulate the tumor vasculature [15,79,109,123,124]. Moreover, Ojha et al. described several pharmacological strategies for vascular regulation (Figure 1). Combined with nanoparticles, these strategies can enhance the EPR effect and improve treatment (Table 2).

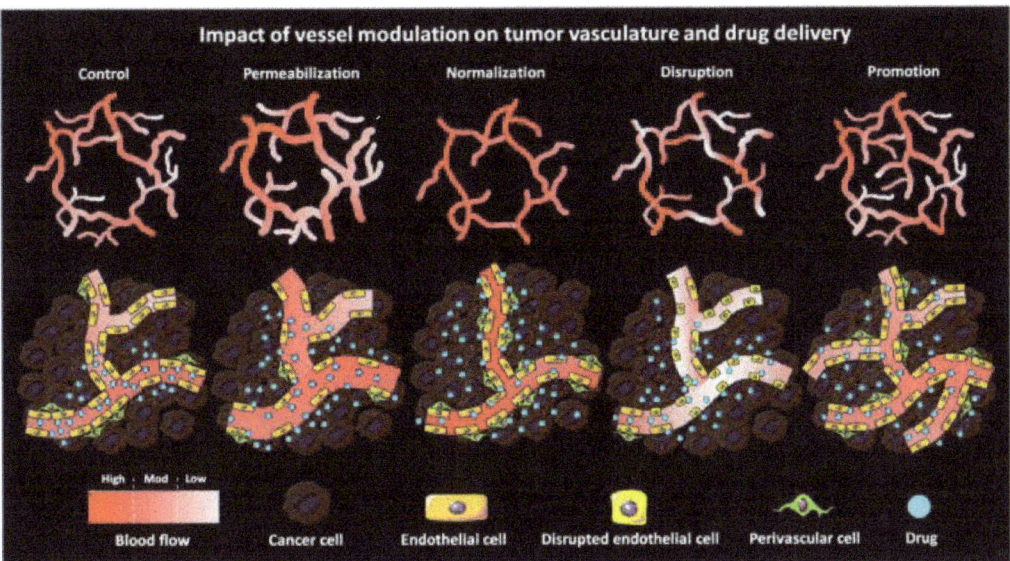

Figure 1. Schematic illustration of the impact of pharmacological vascular regulation strategies on tumor vasculature and tumor-targeted drug delivery. Vascular permeability enlarges the gap between ECs by vasodilating and increasing the gap between ECs and perivascular cells. Vascular normalization promotes vascular maturation and improves vascular perfusion, thereby restoring the morphology and function of tumor vasculature to a certain extent. Vascular rupture enhances vascular permeability by disrupting the endothelial lining while reducing perfusion (especially in immature vessels). Vascular facilitation increases relative blood volume in tumors by increasing vascular density and distribution. Reproduced from Ojha [20].

Table 2. Nanoparticles for enhancing the tumor enhanced permeability and retention (EPR) effect.

Types of Nanoparticles	Size Range	Types of Tumor	Active Ingredients	Mechanisms for Enhancing EPR Effect	Reference
Polyetherimide–*g*–PEG–RGD	~200 nm	CT-26 colon adenocarcinoma	sFLT1 protein and siRNA	Inhibiting tumor-specific VEGF	[125,126]
Tetraiodothyroacetic acid (tetrac) combined with poly(lactide-*co*-glycolic acid) nanoparticles	~200 nm	Drug-resistant breast cancer orthotopic tumor	tetrac	Suppressing angiogenesis	[127–130]
Hydralazine (HDZ)–liposomes	88 ± 4 nm	Desmoplastic melanoma	HDZ	Expanding blood vessels	[131]
Captopril combined with paclitaxel-loaded nanoparticles	~100 nm	Human glioma (U87)	Captopril	Increasing tumor blood perfusion and enlarging endothelial gaps in tumor blood vessels	[132]
Cisplatin–sildenafil co-loaded nanoparticles	~200 nm	Murine melanoma	Sildenafil	Inducing vasodilation	[133]
Tissue plasminogen activator (t-PA)-installed redox-active nanoparticles	48 ± 2 nm	Mouse colorectal carcinoma	t-PA	Increasing drug delivery near the solid tumor through fibrin degradation and blood flow restoration.	[134]

Table 2. Cont.

Types of Nanoparticles	Size Range	Types of Tumor	Active Ingredients	Mechanisms for Enhancing EPR Effect	Reference
(Losartan+ DOX) @ hollow mesoporous prussian blue nanoparticles	~187 nm	Mouse breast cancer	Losartan + DOX	Near-infrared spectroscopy-activated losartan in Prussian blue nanoparticles to degrade ECM, which improved the penetration of most nanoparticles	[135]
Nanocells (comprises a nuclear nanoparticle within an extranuclear PEGylated lipid envelope)	80–120 nm	Melanomas or Lewis lung carcinoma	DOX and combretastatin A4 phosphate	Enhancing vessel penetration	[136]
Platelet membrane-coated mesoporous silica nanoparticles (MTD@P)	~130 nm	Mouse colorectal carcinoma (CT26)	Tirapazamine and 5,6-dimethylxanthenone-4-acetic acid (DMXAA)	Increasing vascular permeability, through the tumor vessel disrupting effect of DMXAA.	[137]
Leukolike vector (LLV) modified nanoporous silicon particles	-	BALB/c 4T1 breast cancer	LLV	Activating the endothelial receptor intercellular adhesion molecule-1 (ICAM-1) pathway, and leading to increased vascular permeability through the phosphorylation of vascular endothelial cadherin	[138]
radiofrequency-assisted gadofullerene nanocrystals (GFNCs)	140–170 nm	Human liver hepatocellular carcinoma (HepG2-luc cells)	GFNCs	Significantly downregulating tumor vascular endothelial cadherin, leading to vascular collapse and destruction, thereby increasing vascular penetration	[139]
PEGylated ^{131}I labeled bovine serum albu-min (^{131}I-BSA)-liposomes	<200 nm	4T1 murine breast cancer	^{131}I-BSA	Increasing vascular permeability by damaging tumor vascular ECs	[140]
Temperature-sensitive liposomes	~200 nm	Human squamous cell carcinoma and B16BL6 melanomas	DOX	Enhancing vessel penetration	[141]

3.1. Antiangiogenesis

VEGF, FGF and their receptors, matrix metalloproteinases (MMPs), tubulin, and integrins are closely related to tumor survival, migration, metastasis, and angiogenesis [49,142,143]. It has been reported that drugs targeting these factors can inhibit tumor angiogenesis, thereby increasing blood perfusion and reducing the IFP [21,98,144]. Antiangiogenic agents, to some extent, can restore the pressure gradient between the vascular wall and tumor interstitium. Subsequently, they decrease the blood flow stasis to allow more nanoparticles to penetrate the blood vessels and reach the interstitial tissue [29,98,145]. Hence, antiangiogenesis improves the delivery of the therapeutic entities via maintaining the integrity of the EPR effect and reducing the IFP. Numerous different types of nanoparticles have been extensively investigated to facilitate the delivery of antiangiogenic agents [62,125,127].

Several studies have shown the potential effectiveness of soluble VEGF receptors on inhibiting pathological tumor angiogenesis. Nanoparticles are able to carry VEGF inhibitors to vascular EC. These inhibitors block pathological angiogenesis and promote tumor cell apoptosis, thereby inhibiting tumor growth and metastasis. Although nanoparticles are potentially applicable to antiangiogenesis, better delivery carriers that can improve the targeting activity are urgently sought. The arginylglycylaspartic acid (RGD) peptide can specifically bind to the integrin receptor of tumor vascular ECs with high affinity [146,147]. Grafting RGD onto nanoparticles may improve their active targeting ability and increase the drug transfection efficiency under conditions of sufficient EPR. However, Storm et al. stated that the potential of RGD-conjugate tumor targeting should not be overestimated due to the RGD receptors being widely distributed on blood vessels, which can induce the less tumor selectivity [148,149].

Some RNA interference (RNAi) strategies that require entry into tumor cells to function, such as small interfering RNA (siRNA) and short hairpin RNA (shRNA), are ideal for tumor-specific VEGF inhibition. The strategy of silencing VEGF by RNAi has achieved satisfactory results in some solid tumor models [150–154]. The angiogenesis of VEGF is mediated by binding to two endothelium-specific receptor tyrosine kinases with high affinity, namely, FLT1 (VEGFR1) and FLK1/KDR (VEGFR2). The use of homologous tyrosine kinase receptor soluble FLT1 (sFLT1) gene therapy has illustrated that the transduced sFLT1 protein can bind to VEGF and inhibit its activity, and this binding is similarly characterized by high affinity. Kim et al. reported an angiogenic EC-targeted polymeric gene vehicle, polyetherimide-g-polyethylene glycol (PEG)–RGD, which contained sFLT1 protein and siRNA [125,126]. These nanoparticles can effectively transfer therapeutic genes to angiogenic ECs, but not to nonangiogenic cells, and effectively inhibit the proliferation of VEGF-responsive ECs by the delivered genes. Kanazawa et al. prepared the amphiphilic and cationic triblock copolymer as an siRNA carrier to efficiently deliver small interfering VEGF into tumor tissues and significantly inhibit tumor growth because of the suppression of VEGF secretion from tumor tissues [155].

Some other vascular mediators are also involved in tumor angiogenesis. Targeting these mediators can also effectively inhibit abnormal tumor angiogenesis. Endostatin, a peptide cleaved from the carboxy terminus of collagen XVIII, suppresses the cell cycle and expression of antiapoptosis genes in proliferating ECs, thereby suppressing angiogenesis. To assess the endostatin gene therapy, Oga et al. prepared polyvinylpyrrolidone–pentostatin nanoparticles which exhibit a strong antiangiogenic effect and effective inhibition of metastatic growth in the brain [62]. Moreover, the combined use of sFLT1 with endostatin could be an effective antiangiogenic approach to the treatment of unresectable hepatocellular carcinoma [156]. Pigment epithelium-derived factor is a type of glycoprotein that plays a universally acknowledged role in the inhibition of angiogenesis via downregulation of VEGF [65]. The cyclic RGD–PEG–polyetherimide exhibited increased gene transfection efficiency in human umbilical vein ECs via binding to $\alpha_v\beta_3$, and significantly inhibited tumor growth and angiogenesis [157]. The binding of activated NF-κB to DNA can promote angiogenesis in addition to its role in facilitating cell proliferation, regulating apoptosis, facilitating angiogenesis, and stimulating invasion and metastasis [66]. Xiao et al. inhibited the growth and metastasis of breast cancer through delivering p65 shRNA into cells with a bioreducible polymer to block the signaling of NF-κB [158]. The proangiogenic effects of thyroid hormone on ECs and vascular smooth cells are initiated from the cell surface receptor for the hormone on the extracellular domain of integrin $\alpha_v\beta_3$ [67]. Tetraiodothyroacetic acid (tetrac) is a deamination product of L-thyroxine that blocks thyroid hormone binding with the integrin receptor [159]. Therefore, tetrac combined with liposomes and poly(lactide-co-glycolic acid) nanoparticles can achieve tetrac targeting of cell membrane integrin $\alpha_v\beta_3$ receptors and significantly inhibit angiogenesis [127–130]. MMPs participate in the process of angiogenesis in tissue reconstruction and neovascular growth through their proteolytic effect. Moreover, they release angiogenic factors residing in the matrix. Therefore, MMP inhibitors decrease angiogenesis and the migration of tumor cells, leading to slower progression of transplanted tumors [68]. Indeed, the antitumor efficacy of angiostatin and tissue inhibitor of metalloproteinases (TIMPs) has been demonstrated in various types of solid tumors [160,161]. Dendrimers containing plasmids of angiostatin and TIMP-2 showed high antitumor and antiangiogenic activity [162]. Nevertheless, antiangiogenic drugs also reduce the gap between tumor vascular ECs. Hence, the size of nanoparticles has to be strictly controlled if antiangiogenic drugs are employed to enhance the EPR effect [114].

3.2. Upregulated Tumor Blood Perfusion

The main obstacle of blood perfusion in intravascular transport is due to irregular vascular structure and accumulated solid stress. Therefore, in accordance with the above two points, the blood perfusion of tumor vessels can be upregulated by vascular normalization and decompression, respectively (Figure 2). Yang et al. concluded that the former can use angiogenesis inhibitors to improve blood perfusion, so as to reduce the transport resistance of nanoparticles [115,163]. The latter can effectively reduce the solid stress through ablation of cells or the ECM, thus increasing the diameter of blood vessels to promote intravascular transport. Reduced blood flow directly limits the perfusion of nanoparticles into the tumor site [164]. In addition, the proliferating cancer cells in the center of the tumor tissue will form excessive pressure and compress the blood vessels and lymphatic vessels, leading to vascular collapse [88,94,95]. This results in an abundance and scarcity of functional blood vessels and lymphatic vessels in the periphery and center of the tumor, respectively [165]. This uneven distribution of blood vessels further worsens the relatively weak penetration ability of nanoparticles.

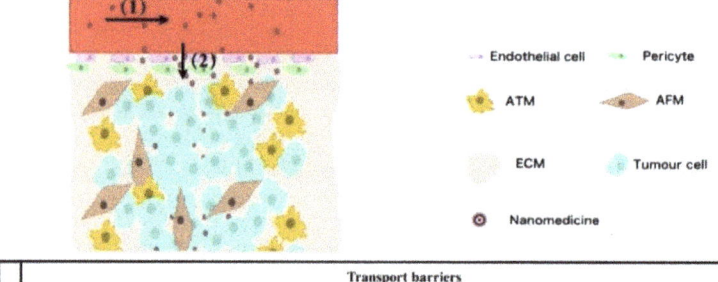

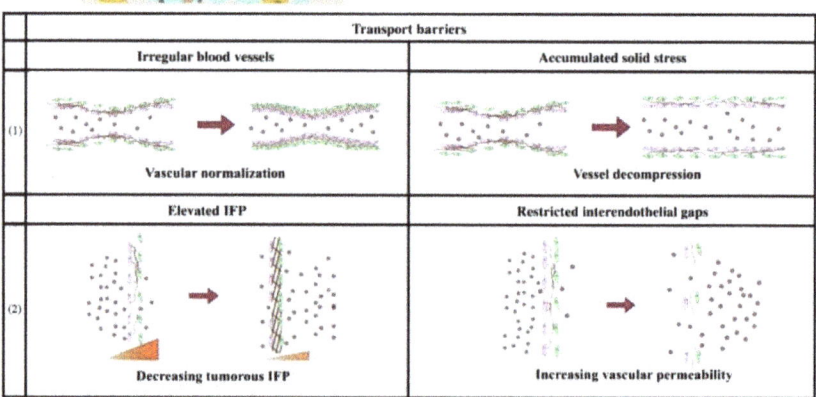

Figure 2. Schematic representation of vascular-related problems and countermeasures faced in the process of nanodrug penetration. (1) Intravascular transport: vascular irregularity and cumulative solid stress are resolved by normalization and decompression, respectively. (2) Trans-vascular transport: elevated interstitial fluid pressure (IFP) and limited endothelial space are improved by decreasing intertumoral IFP and increasing vascular permeability, respectively. Adapted from Yang et al. [115].

Vascular promotion is a vascular regulation strategy that addresses the issue of poor accumulation and distribution of drugs in tumors via increasing the vascular density and upregulating blood perfusion. Induction of angiogenesis appears to promote tumor growth. However, moderate induction of angiogenesis or vascular promotion may also contribute to better enrichment and distribution of anticancer drugs and improve their anticancer efficacy in some tumor models [20]. Among the recently developed strategies, the use of vasodilator-encapsulated nanoparticles for tumor angiectasis has been investigated as a potential option for promoting the extravasation of nanoparticles in tumors. Some vasodilator formulation nanoparticles have been employed, including angiotensin inhibitor, antihypertensive agents, gaseous vascular mediator-generating vasodilators, and ECM degradation agents.

The change of angiotensin I to angiotensin II mediated via carboxypeptidase can be inhibited by angiotensin-converting enzyme inhibitors (ACEI). AGTR2 is an effective agent in enhancing blood flow and promoting vascular permeability in tumors due to its vasoconstrictive function in healthy tissues, as well as increasing the systemic blood pressure. It has been shown that the perfusion of tumor vessels is gradually shifted from poor to good after slow systemic administration of AGTR2 [87]. An increase in BK levels leads to the activation of endothelial NO synthase. ACEIs (e.g., captopril) inhibit the degradation of BK, thereby increasing its local concentration in tumor tissues. Captopril, an ACEI, acts by downregulating the expression of AGTR2, thereby dilating blood vessels and lowering blood pressure. A combination of captopril with paclitaxel-loaded nanoparticles has been employed to simultaneously ameliorate tumor perfusion and expand EC gaps, thus enhancing nanodrug delivery to cancer cells [132]. Meanwhile, losartan is an angiotensin II receptor antagonist that increases nanodrug delivery through two mechanisms [166]. Losartan can lower solid stress that compresses blood vessels, thus improving vessel perfusion and drug delivery. However, it also increases the intratumoral penetration of the intraperitoneally or intravenously injected nanoparticles into the tumors by decreasing the ECM [167].

In addition to AGTR2, other drugs may also expand blood vessels. Hydralazine (HDZ), a drug applied to hypertension and heart failure therapy, has been used as a tumor vasodilator to modulate the TME. It is thought that HDZ functions by dilating blood vessels. Therefore, Chen et al. prepared HDZ-encapsulated liposomes which can expand tumor vessels and strengthen tumor permeability. These liposomes also ameliorated the accumulation and permeation of nanoparticles inside the tumor. Compared with free HDZ, intravenous injection of these liposomes in desmoplastic tumor-bearing mice prolonged the blood circulation time of HDZ. Moreover, its vasodilation effect increased the penetration and accumulation of nanoparticles into tumors mediated by the EPR effect to some extent [131]. Of note, in vivo and in vitro studies have shown that HDZ exerts certain antiangiogenesis effects [168]. Therefore, such nanomedicines have great potential in upregulating tumor blood perfusion. Sildenafil, a conventional medicine utilized for pulmonary hypertension therapy, can be utilized for developing effective and tumor-selective angiectasis approaches. Sildenafil can be encapsulated into the hydrophobic core of a cisplatin-incorporated polymeric micelle to form a nanoparticle with a hydrophobic center and a dense PEG shell. This polymeric micelle is effective in dilating tumor vessels and boosting the accumulation of cisplatin–sildenafil coloaded nanoparticles in tumors [133].

Endogenous signal molecule endogenous carbon monoxide (CO) and heme oxygenase (HO) play an important role in regulating vascular tension and inducing angiogenesis [69,70]. Fang et al. clearly demonstrated that vascular permeability and blood flow were significantly increased after using CO donors or HO-1 inducers (PEGylated heme) [72]. They designed two CO generators with tumor selectivity. The first was the CO external donor tricarbonyldichlororuthenium (II) dimer nanomicelle, which can slowly enhance the release characteristics and selective accumulation of tumors mediated by the EPR effect [71]. The second was the HO-1 inducer (PEGylated hemin), which can be selectively enriched in tumors after injection and produce CO by inducing HO-1 expression in tumors [72,73]. In solid tumor models, both nanodrugs exhibited higher selectivity for CO production in tumor tissues versus normal tissues, which resulted in augmented tumor blood flow recovery [72].

Platelets preserve tumor vessel integrity and prevent nanomedicines from diffusing into solid tumors. Previous findings have shown that the specific depletion of tumor-associated platelets may be a potent approach for disrupting vascular barriers and enhancing the extravasation of nanoparticles from tumor vessels [169–171]. Nie et al. showed that drug delivery can be facilitated via functionalizing nanoparticles, thereby locally depleting tumor-associated platelets that normally restore the leaky vessels [172]. They developed a polymer lipid peptide nanoparticle core consisting of a charged amphiphilic polymer where the positively charged region adsorbs the antibody R300. The platelet-specific R300 antibody can bind to platelets, leading to their micro-aggregation and subsequent removal by macrophages, and further increasing the intratumoral accumulation and retention of drugs.

Excessive constituents of ECM, such as collagen, fibrin, laminin, elastin, and aggregated platelet in the TME, deposit in the tumor vessels [173]. This hinders the blood supply, impairing the delivery of drugs to the tumor site and reducing efficacy. However, degradation of ECM components by enzymatic treatment (e.g., collagenase) can improve the vascular properties and upregulate blood perfusion at tumor sites [174,175]. Tissue plasminogen activator (t-PA) binds to drug carriers to degrade fibrin. Mei et al. developed t-PA-assembled redox-active nanoparticles (T-PA@iRNP) by degrading fibrin to reduce the pressure on tumor blood vessels, thereby increasing the perfusion of blood and nanomedicines in tumors (Figure 3). When applied to colon cancer models, T-PA@iRNP degradation of deposited fibrin enhances the infiltration of iRNP and immune cells into tumor tissues through an increase in blood flow. This enhances the EPR effect and consequently amplifies the inhibitory effect on tumor growth [134]. Zhang et al. encapsulated DOX and near-infrared spectroscopy-activated losartan in hollow mesoporous Prussian blue nanoparticles to degrade the ECM. The results showed that losartan-containing nanoparticles can enhance the penetration of DOX, and exhibit a good tumor inhibition effect under the synergistic action of photothermal therapy/chemotherapy [135].

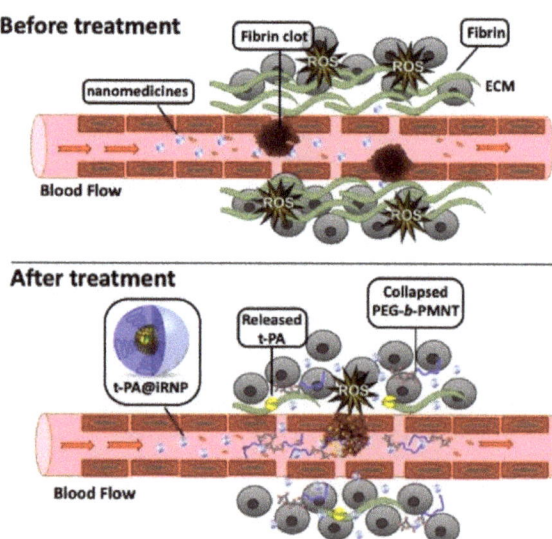

Figure 3. Schematic representation of transmission and action in the microenvironment of large amounts of fibrin around colon tumors and their tissues. Compared with free tissue plasminogen activator (t-PA), using t-PA-assembled redox-active nanoparticles (T-PA@iRNP) can effectively relieve the compressed tumor vessels and upregulate blood perfusion, and improve the poor distribution of nanodrugs in tumors. Reproduced from Mei [134].

3.3. Enhanced Vessel Penetration

The gap in tumor vascular ECs is one of the important bases of the EPR effect. However, in some tumors with poor permeability, the size and rate limitation of large-scale nanodrugs by the vascular endothelial space cannot achieve the purpose of trans-vascular transport [115]. Therefore, augmenting the permeability of tumor vessels and even destroying the vascular system can effectively promote extravasation [176,177]. Nanodrugs with a size <10 nm can effectively permeate inside tumors via trans- and extravascular transport. However, the rapid clearance by the kidneys is a problem, resulting in an insufficient EPR effect. Nanodrugs, with size ranging 50–200 nm, can realize long-time circulation and passively target the tumor site by intravascular transport. However, due to the existence of various barriers, they often have difficulty in reaching the core of the tumor. Therefore, nanodrugs of variable size can be used to simultaneously achieve long-time circulation, good passive targeting, and high permeability [178–183].

Integrating VDAs in nanomedicines is a promising therapy for meliorating vascular permeability and the EPR effect. Several VDAs have been evaluated; for example, combretastatin A4 phosphate (CA4P) is a tubulin-binding agent which induces vessel disruption by suppressing tubulin polymerization. Furthermore, flavonoid acetic acid-based agent 5,6-dimethylxanthenone-4-acetic acid (DMXAA) increases the levels of NO and serotonin, resulting in weak endothelial function. Sengupta et al. introduced poly(lactide-co-glycolic acid) nanoparticles conjugated to DOX, which were trapped in a phospholipid block-copolymer membrane containing CA4P [136]. The nanoparticles were designed to first release CA4P, which initially induces vessel disruption, thereby creating a niche for the release of DOX. This approach was linked to significant tumor inhibition and improvement in overall survival. VDAs and other physiological agents are commonly used to enhance vascular permeability and, thus, promote the extravasation of nanoparticles. Zhang et al. developed a bioinspired nanodesign, which combined vasculature-destructive DMXAA and hypoxia-activated tirapazamine with a mesoporous silica nanoparticle core, as well as a hidden platelet membrane shell [137]. The platelet membrane can be continuously "recruited" by the tumors with characteristics of artificial blood vessel destruction. The results indicated that disruption of the tumor vasculature caused by DMXAA and the platelet membrane-mediated targeting of the intratumoral disrupted vasculature were beneficial to each other and strengthened mutually. Studies have shown that the EPR effect of nanoparticles is induced by rupture of blood vessels, which is closely related to tumor density and the speed of blood flow [176]. As mentioned above, the tumor vasculature consists of only a single layer of ECs with a missing or incomplete basement membrane [184]. Furthermore, the vasculature is closely related to the blood supply of tumor cells [185,186]. Destruction of the vasculature can significantly improve the EPR effect and, if the vasculature is inadequate, the tumor tissue will undergo programmed death [187–189].

The development of strategies for interacting with ECs or destroying vascular EC connections is another effective approach to improving vascular permeability. Inspired by this, Palomba et al. transferred the purified leukocyte membrane onto nanoporous silicon particles to produce a type of leukolike vector (LLV) [138]. Multiple receptors on LLV can interact with ECs and reduce the vascular barrier function. The investigators also demonstrated that the leukocyte plasma membrane on the surface of LLV can effectively interact with the overexpressed intercellular adhesion molecule-1 (ICAM-1) in the tumor vasculature, activate the endothelial receptor ICAM-1 pathway, and boost vascular permeability through the phosphorylation of vascular endothelial cadherin. Li et al. found that phase-induced size expansion through radiofrequency-assisted gadofullerene nanocrystals (GFNCs) can destroy abnormal tumor vasculature. Biocompatible GFNCs with a nanoparticle size were designed to penetrate the leaking tumor blood vessel. With the assistance of radiofrequency, the phase transition occurs when GFNCs spill over the tumor vessels. In addition, the abrupt and drastic changes in nanoparticle structure caused by phase transition directly disrupt the abnormal tumor blood vessels (Figure 4). Treatment with this method can cause rapid ischemia, necrosis, and atrophy of tumor tissues, while significantly reducing the toxic and side effects of other antivascular treatments [139,190].

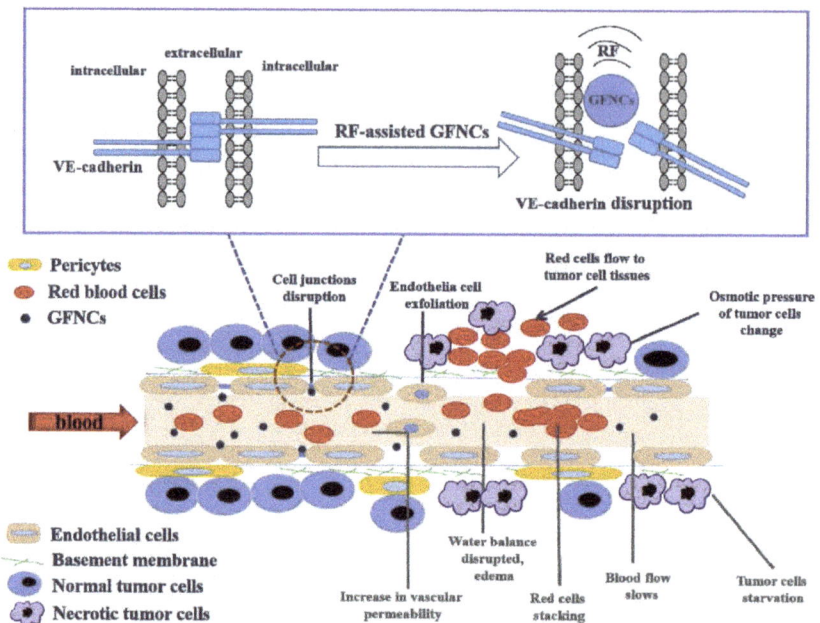

Figure 4. Schematic diagram of the mechanism of tumor vascular rupture after radiofrequency-assisted gadofullerene nanocrystal (GFNC) treatment. GFNC particles injected intravenously into tumor-bearing mice penetrate the vulnerability of tumor vascular ECs. When radiofrequency irradiation is applied, the sudden volume expansion of GFNCs can lead to the destruction of vascular endothelial cadherin at the junction of endothelial adhesion bodies of tumor vessels, thereby increasing vascular permeability and realizing the destruction of tumor vessels. Reproduced from Li and Zhen et al. [139,190].

In addition to chemotherapy, some physical therapies can also significantly enhance blood vessel penetration and improve the effects of antitumor treatment. Ionizing irradiation can increase vascular leakiness by inducing EC apoptosis and enhancing the expression of VEGF and FGF [191]. Liang et al. designed a radioisotope therapy by encapsulating the radioisotope iodine-131 (^{131}I)-labeled bovine serum albumin (BSA) in liposomes. ^{131}I-BSA-liposomes were intravenously injected into 4T1 tumor-bearing mice. Compared with untreated mice, those treated with ^{131}I-BSA-liposomes showed high retention in the tumor site, demonstrating enhanced tumor vascular permeability and improved EPR effect [140]. Koukourakis et al. underlined the value of combining radiotherapy with drug delivery systems based on nanomedicines [192]. Patients were treated with radiolabeled PEGylated liposomal DOX, and achieved an overall remission rate >70%. This is an effective anticancer treatment modality for inducing hyperthermia in tumors. This generally leads to an increase in blood flow and vascular permeability in tumors, thus promoting drug and oxygen supply to tumors [193]. Hyperthermia can be applied to increase the EPR effect, particularly in nonleaky tumors with low baseline levels of nanomedicine accumulation [194]. Temperature-sensitive liposomes have developed into an ideal nanocarrier for coadministration with hyperthermia, enabling triggered drug release locally at the heated tumor site. Several studies have demonstrated that drug delivery and intratumoral distribution can be ameliorated through combining temperature-sensitive liposomes with modest hyperthermia. It was found that the human ovarian carcinoma tumor model was rather impermeable to liposomes with a size of 100 nm at room temperature. However, as the temperature increased, the release of liposomes was significantly elevated [195]. Manzoor et al. established temperature-sensitive liposomes containing DOX, which can enhance blood vessel penetration and liposome accumulation [141].

4. Conclusions and Future Perspectives

The EPR effect, which involves the pathophysiological mediators and unique anatomical architecture of tumor tissues, is becoming a promising avenue for targeted anti-tumor therapy. Thus, the tumor-selective delivery of anticancer nanomedicines based on the EPR effect is becoming possible. However, the EPR effect can be highly heterogeneous. Specifically, in the complex tumor environment, it is difficult for nanoparticles to diffuse into vascular areas of the tumor due to high IFP, abnormal ECM, and massive interaction sites in the tumor. Hence, in the last couple of years, on the basis of the EPR effect, scientists have investigated other mechanisms of nanoparticle entry into solid tumors [196]. Recently, Sindhwani et al. proposed that most of the tumor vasculature is continuous and does not have sufficient EC gaps to explain the accumulation of nanoparticles in tumors. Moreover, they stated that most nanoparticles can reach the interior of the tumor via active trans-endothelial pathways rather than passive transport via gaps [197]. Although they found that the trans-endothelial pathways play a significant role in the accumulation of nanoparticles in tumor sites, their experimental method had certain limitations. Firstly, they only utilized PEGylated gold nanoparticles as simulated nanoparticles to examine the accumulation in the tumor, and could not cover the accumulation of other nanoparticles in tumors. Secondly, they used a Zombie mouse model to distinguish the contribution of the passive gap from active trans-endothelial transport. This model could deactivate active mechanisms and retain the passive way that fixed the mouse by transcardiac perfusion and relied on a peristaltic pump to retain a physiologically relevant flow rate. This could not simulate the blood vessels and blood flow under normal physiological conditions. Lastly, the blood driven by the peristaltic pump only circulated for a short period of time (15 and 60 min). In summary, trans-endothelial pathways may be a reason for the accumulation of nanoparticles in tumor sites; nevertheless, the EPR effect remains the basis of nanodrug delivery to tumors. Furthermore, nanoparticles which can improve tumor vessel penetration, reduce IFP, and degrade the ECM can be applied to enhance the EPR effect [26].

Herein, we summarized the mechanism of abnormal vascular functions, such as tumor angiogenesis, irregular blood flow, and extensive vascular permeability, as well as their influence on the EPR effect. In addition, we analyzed some nanoparticles developed to facilitate the EPR effect in tumors in response to the above factors. In terms of antiangiogenesis, gene therapy nanomedicines targeting angiogenic growth factors and their receptors are the most widely studied, and offer another approach to directly inhibiting tumor angiogenesis early in the process. Its diverse nanocarrier form provides a rich selection for delivery to different types of tumors. For irregular blood flow caused by abnormal vascular morphology and structure, blood perfusion can be effectively upregulated by slight vascular facilitation, vasodilation, or removal of excessive ECM in the TME. Nanoparticles encapsulated with different types of drugs exhibit the diversity and universality of nanocarriers, providing more possibilities for the selection of nanodrugs. However, EPR effect-based drug delivery strategies continue to be characterized by numerous problems and limitations. For example, enhancing the EPR effect may help maintain nutrient and oxygen transport, thereby accelerating tumor growth. Therefore, when designing such nanoparticles, it is particularly important to properly balance the relationship between tumor killing or inhibition and tumor growth promotion caused by the EPR effect.

Author Contributions: Conceptualization, L.H. and Y.C.; writing, review, and editing, Y.C., D.H., and L.S.; preparation of tables and figures, D.H. and L.S.; revision, Y.C., L.H., and L.S.; funding acquisition, L.H. and Y.C. All authors have read and agreed to the published version of the manuscript.

Funding: This work of L.H. was funded by the Carolina Center for Cancer Nanotechnology Excellence, United States (NIH grant CA198999). Y.C. is supported by the Natural Science Foundation of Shanghai (19ZR1472500).

Conflicts of Interest: The authors declare no conflict of interest.

Abbreviations

ACEI	angiotensin-converting enzyme inhibitor
AGTR2	angiotensin receptor type 2
BK	bradykinin
BSA	bovine serum albumin
CA4P	combretastatin A4 phosphate
CO	carbon monoxide
DMXAA	5,6-dimethylxanthenone-4-acetic acid
DOX	doxorubicin
EC	endothelial cell
ECM	extracellular matrix
EGF	epidermal growth factor
EGFR	epidermal growth factor receptor
EPR	enhanced permeability and retention
Et-A/B	endothelin-A/B
FGF	fibroblast growth factor
FLK1/KDR	vascular endothelial growth factor receptor 2
FLT1	vascular endothelial growth factor receptor 1
GFNC	gadofullerene nanocrystal
HDZ	hydralazine
HGF	hepatocyte growth factor
HIF	hypoxia-inducible factor
HO	heme oxygenase
^{131}I	iodine-131
ICAM-1	intercellular adhesion molecule-1
IFP	interstitial fluid pressure
IL	interleukin
iNOS	inducible nitric oxide synthase
LLV	leukolike vector
MMP	matrix metalloproteinase
NO	nitric oxide
NF-κB	nuclear factor kappa-B
PDGF	platelet-derived growth factor
PDGFR	platelet-derived growth factor receptor
PEG	polyethylene glycol
PLGF	placenta growth factor
RGD	arginylglycylaspartic acid
RNAi	RNA interference
SDF-1	stromal cell-derived factor 1
sFLT1	soluble vascular endothelial growth factor receptor 1
shRNA	short hairpin RNA
siRNA	small interfering RNA
tetrac	tetraiodothyroacetic acid
TGF-β	transforming growth factor-β
TIMP	tissue inhibitor of metalloproteinase
TME	tumor microenvironment
TNF-α	tumor necrosis factor-α
t-PA	tissue plasminogen activator
VDA	vascular disrupting agent
VEGF	vascular endothelial growth factor
VEGFR	vascular endothelial growth factor receptor
VPF	vascular permeability factor

References

1. Sudhakar, A. History of Cancer, Ancient and Modern Treatment Methods. *J. Cancer Sci. Ther.* **2009**, *1*, 1–4. [CrossRef]
2. Siegel, R.L.; Miller, K.D.; Jemal, A. Cancer statistics, 2020. *CA Cancer J. Clin.* **2020**, *70*, 7–30. [CrossRef] [PubMed]
3. Bray, F.; Ferlay, J.; Soerjomataram, I.; Siegel, R.L.; Torre, L.A.; Jemal, A. Global cancer statistics 2018: GLOBOCAN estimates of incidence and mortality worldwide for 36 cancers in 185 countries. *CA Cancer J. Clin.* **2018**, *68*, 394–424. [CrossRef] [PubMed]
4. Gotwals, P.; Cameron, S.; Cipolletta, D.; Cremasco, V.; Crystal, A.; Hewes, B.; Mueller, B.; Quaratino, S.; Sabatos-Peyton, C.; Petruzzelli, L.; et al. Prospects for combining targeted and conventional cancer therapy with immunotherapy. *Nat. Rev. Cancer* **2017**, *17*, 286–301. [CrossRef] [PubMed]
5. Kalyane, D.; Raval, N.; Maheshwari, R.; Tambe, V.; Kalia, K.; Tekade, R.K. Employment of enhanced permeability and retention effect (EPR): Nanoparticle-based precision tools for targeting of therapeutic and diagnostic agent in cancer. *Mater. Sci. Eng. C Mater. Biol. Appl.* **2019**, *98*, 1252–1276. [CrossRef] [PubMed]
6. Tekade, R.K.; Maheshwari, R.; Soni, N.; Tekade, M.; Chougule, M.B. Chapter 1 -Nanotechnology for the Development of Nanomedicine. In *Nanotechnology-Based Approaches for Targeting and Delivery of Drugs and Genes*; Academic Press: Cambridge, MA, USA, 2017; pp. 3–61. [CrossRef]
7. Nagy, J.A.; Chang, S.H.; Dvorak, A.M.; Dvorak, H.F. Why are tumour blood vessels abnormal and why is it important to know? *Br. J. Cancer* **2009**, *100*, 865–869. [CrossRef] [PubMed]
8. Maeda, H.; Nakamura, H.; Fang, J. The EPR effect for macromolecular drug delivery to solid tumors: Improvement of tumor uptake, lowering of systemic toxicity, and distinct tumor imaging in vivo. *Adv. Drug Deliv. Rev.* **2013**, *65*, 71–79. [CrossRef] [PubMed]
9. Prabhakar, U.; Maeda, H.; Jain, R.K.; Sevick-Muraca, E.M.; Zamboni, W.; Farokhzad, O.C.; Barry, S.T.; Gabizon, A.; Grodzinski, P.; Blakey, D.C. Challenges and key considerations of the enhanced permeability and retention effect for nanomedicine drug delivery in oncology. *Cancer Res.* **2013**, *73*, 2412–2417. [CrossRef]
10. Greish, K. Enhanced permeability and retention effect for selective targeting of anticancer nanomedicine: Are we there yet? *Drug Discov. Today Technol.* **2012**, *9*, 71–174. [CrossRef]
11. Matsumura, Y.; Maeda, H. A new concept for macromolecular therapeutics in cancer chemotherapy: Mechanism of tumoritropic accumulation of proteins and the antitumor agent smancs. *Cancer Res.* **1986**, *46*, 6387–6392.
12. Fang, J.; Nakamura, H.; Maeda, H. The EPR effect: Unique features of tumor blood vessels for drug delivery, factors involved, and limitations and augmentation of the effect. *Adv. Drug Deliv. Rev.* **2011**, *63*, 136–151. [CrossRef]
13. Folkman, J. What is the evidence that tumors are angiogenesis dependent? *J. Natl. Cancer Inst.* **1990**, *82*, 4–6. [CrossRef]
14. Ding, Y.; Xu, Y.; Yang, W.; Niu, P.; Li, X.; Chen, Y.; Li, Z.; Liu, Y.; An, Y.; Liu, Y.; et al. Investigating the EPR effect of nanomedicines in human renal tumors via ex vivo perfusion strategy. *Nano Today* **2020**, *35*. [CrossRef]
15. Nagamitsu, A.; Greish, K.; Maeda, H. Elevating blood pressure as a strategy to increase tumor-targeted delivery of macromolecular drug SMANCS: Cases of advanced solid tumors. *Jpn J. Clin. Oncol.* **2009**, *39*, 756–766. [CrossRef]
16. Satchi-Fainaro, R.; Duncan, R.; Barnes, C.M. Polymer Therapeutics for Cancer: Current Status and Future Challenges. In *Polymer Therapeutics II*; Springer: Berlin/Heidelberg, Germany, 2006; pp. 1–65. [CrossRef]
17. Jain, R.K.; Stylianopoulos, T. Delivering nanomedicine to solid tumors. *Nat. Rev. Clin. Oncol.* **2010**, *7*, 653–664. [CrossRef]
18. Danquah, M.K.; Zhang, X.A.; Mahato, R.I. Extravasation of polymeric nanomedicines across tumor vasculature. *Adv. Drug Deliv. Rev.* **2011**, *63*, 623–639. [CrossRef]
19. Barenholz, Y. Doxil(R)—The first FDA-approved nano-drug: Lessons learned. *J. Control. Release* **2012**, *160*, 117–134. [CrossRef] [PubMed]
20. Ojha, T.; Pathak, V.; Shi, Y.; Hennink, W.E.; Moonen, C.T.W.; Storm, G.; Kiessling, F.; Lammers, T. Pharmacological and physical vessel modulation strategies to improve EPR-mediated drug targeting to tumors. *Adv. Drug Deliv. Rev.* **2017**, *119*, 44–60. [CrossRef] [PubMed]
21. Chauhan, V.P.; Stylianopoulos, T.; Martin, J.D.; Popovic, Z.; Chen, O.; Kamoun, W.S.; Bawendi, M.G.; Fukumura, D.; Jain, R.K. Normalization of tumour blood vessels improves the delivery of nanomedicines in a size-dependent manner. *Nat. Nanotechnol.* **2012**, *7*, 383–388. [CrossRef] [PubMed]
22. Seki, T.; Carroll, F.; Illingworth, S.; Green, N.; Cawood, R.; Bachtarzi, H.; Subr, V.; Fisher, K.D.; Seymour, L.W. Tumour necrosis factor-alpha increases extravasation of virus particles into tumour tissue by activating the Rho A/Rho kinase pathway. *J. Control. Release* **2011**, *156*, 381–389. [CrossRef] [PubMed]
23. Batchelor, T.T.; Gerstner, E.R.; Emblem, K.E.; Duda, D.G.; Kalpathy-Cramer, J.; Snuderl, M.; Ancukiewicz, M.; Polaskova, P.; Pinho, M.C.; Jennings, D.; et al. Improved tumor oxygenation and survival in glioblastoma patients who show increased blood perfusion after cediranib and chemoradiation. *Proc. Natl. Acad. Sci. USA* **2013**, *110*, 19059–19064. [CrossRef] [PubMed]
24. Satterlee, A.B.; Rojas, J.D.; Dayton, P.A.; Huang, L. Enhancing Nanoparticle Accumulation and Retention in Desmoplastic Tumors via Vascular Disruption for Internal Radiation Therapy. *Theranostics* **2017**, *7*, 253–269. [CrossRef]
25. Ganten, D.; Ruckpaul, K. Tumor Angiogenesis. In *Encyclopedic Reference of Genomics and Proteomics in Molecular Medicine*; Springer: Berlin/Heidelberg, Germany, 2006; p. 1930. [CrossRef]
26. Danhier, F. To exploit the tumor microenvironment: Since the EPR effect fails in the clinic, what is the future of nanomedicine? *J. Control. Release* **2016**, *244*, 108–121. [CrossRef] [PubMed]

27. Koukourakis, M.I.; Koukouraki, S.; Giatromanolaki, A.; Archimandritis, S.C.; Skarlatos, J.; Beroukas, K.; Bizakis, J.G.; Retalis, G.; Karkavitsas, N.; Helidonis, E.S. Liposomal doxorubicin and conventionally fractionated radiotherapy in the treatment of locally advanced non-small-cell lung cancer and head and neck cancer. *J. Clin. Oncol.* **1999**, *17*, 3512–3521. [CrossRef]
28. Ferrara, N.; Hillan, K.J.; Gerber, H.P.; Novotny, W. Discovery and development of bevacizumab, an anti-VEGF antibody for treating cancer. *Nat. Rev. Drug Discov.* **2004**, *3*, 391–400. [CrossRef] [PubMed]
29. Tong, R.T.; Boucher, Y.; Kozin, S.V.; Winkler, F.; Hicklin, D.J.; Jain, R.K. Vascular normalization by vascular endothelial growth factor receptor 2 blockade induces a pressure gradient across the vasculature and improves drug penetration in tumors. *Cancer Res.* **2004**, *64*, 3731–3736. [CrossRef] [PubMed]
30. Roskoski, R., Jr. Vascular endothelial growth factor (VEGF) signaling in tumor progression. *Crit. Rev. Oncol. Hematol.* **2007**, *62*, 179–213. [CrossRef] [PubMed]
31. Maeda, H.; Fang, J.; Inutsuka, T.; Kitamoto, Y. Vascular permeability enhancement in solid tumor: Various factors, mechanisms involved and its implications. *Int. Immunopharmacol.* **2003**, *3*, 319–328. [CrossRef]
32. Li, B.; Vincent, A.; Cates, J.; Brantley-Sieders, D.M.; Polk, D.B.; Young, P.P. Low Levels of Tumor Necrosis Factor α Increase Tumor Growth by Inducing an Endothelial Phenotype of Monocytes Recruited to the Tumor Site. *Cancer Res.* **2009**, *69*, 338–348. [CrossRef] [PubMed]
33. Mantovani, A.; Allavena, P.; Sica, A.; Balkwill, F. Cancer-related inflammation. *Nature* **2008**, *454*, 436–444. [CrossRef] [PubMed]
34. Papapetropoulos, A.; Garcia-Cardena, G.; Madri, J.A.; Sessa, W.C. Nitric oxide production contributes to the angiogenic properties of vascular endothelial growth factor in human endothelial cells. *J. Clin. Investig.* **1997**, *100*, 3131–3139. [CrossRef]
35. Murohara, T.; Horowitz, J.R.; Silver, M.; Tsurumi, Y.; Chen, D.; Sullivan, A.; Isner, J.M. Vascular endothelial growth factor/vascular permeability factor enhances vascular permeability via nitric oxide and prostacyclin. *Circulation* **1998**, *97*, 99–107. [CrossRef]
36. Friedl, J.; Puhlmann, M.; Bartlett, D.L.; Libutti, S.K.; Turner, E.N.; Gnant, M.F.; Alexander, H.R. Induction of permeability across endothelial cell monolayers by tumor necrosis factor (TNF) occurs via a tissue factor-dependent mechanism: Relationship between the procoagulant and permeability effects of TNF. *Blood* **2002**, *100*, 1334–1339. [CrossRef]
37. Compagni, A.; Wilgenbus, P.; Impagnatiello, M.-A.; Cotten, M.; Christofori, G. Fibroblast Growth Factors Are Required for Efficient Tumor Angiogenesis. *Cancer Res.* **2000**, *60*, 7163–7169.
38. Seghezzi, G.; Patel, S.; Ren, C.J.; Gualandris, A.; Pintucci, G.; Robbins, E.S.; Shapiro, R.L.; Galloway, A.C.; Rifkin, D.B.; Mignatti, P. Fibroblast growth factor-2 (FGF-2) induces vascular endothelial growth factor (VEGF) expression in the endothelial cells of forming capillaries: An autocrine mechanism contributing to angiogenesis. *J. Cell Biol.* **1998**, *141*, 1659–1673. [CrossRef] [PubMed]
39. Ornitz, D.M.; Itoh, N. Fibroblast growth factors. *Genome Biol.* **2001**, *2*, 1–12. [CrossRef] [PubMed]
40. Millauer, B.; Wizigmann-Voos, S.; Schnurch, H.; Martinez, R.; Moller, N.P.; Risau, W.; Ullrich, A. High affinity VEGF binding and developmental expression suggest Flk-1 as a major regulator of vasculogenesis and angiogenesis. *Cell* **1993**, *72*, 835–846. [CrossRef]
41. Laschke, M.W.; Elitzsch, A.; Vollmar, B.; Vajkoczy, P.; Menger, M.D. Combined inhibition of vascular endothelial growth factor (VEGF), fibroblast growth factor and platelet-derived growth factor, but not inhibition of VEGF alone, effectively suppresses angiogenesis and vessel maturation in endometriotic lesions. *Hum. Reprod* **2006**, *21*, 262–268. [CrossRef]
42. Andrae, J.; Gallini, R.; Betsholtz, C. Role of platelet-derived growth factors in physiology and medicine. *Genes Dev.* **2008**, *22*, 1276–1312. [CrossRef] [PubMed]
43. Yang, X.P.; Pei, Z.H.; Ren, J. Making up or breaking up: The tortuous role of platelet-derived growth factor in vascular ageing. *Clin. Exp. Pharmacol. Physiol.* **2009**, *36*, 739–747. [CrossRef]
44. Taylor, A.P.; Rodriguez, M.; Adams, K.; Goldenberg, D.M.; Blumenthal, R.D. Altered tumor vessel maturation and proliferation in placenta growth factor-producing tumors: Potential relationship to post-therapy tumor angiogenesis and recurrence. *Int. J. Cancer* **2003**, *105*, 158–164. [CrossRef]
45. Ellis, L.M. Epidermal growth factor receptor in tumor angiogenesis. *Hematol. Oncol. Clin. N. Am.* **2004**, *18*, 1007–1021. [CrossRef] [PubMed]
46. Tamatani, T.; Hattori, K.; Iyer, A.; Tamatani, K.; Oyasu, R. Hepatocyte growth factor is an invasion/migration factor of rat urothelial carcinoma cells in vitro. *Carcinogenesis* **1999**, *20*, 957–962. [CrossRef] [PubMed]
47. Forsythe, J.A.; Jiang, B.H.; Iyer, N.V.; Agani, F.; Leung, S.W.; Koos, R.D.; Semenza, G.L. Activation of vascular endothelial growth factor gene transcription by hypoxia-inducible factor 1. *Mol. Cell Biol.* **1996**, *16*, 4604–4613. [CrossRef] [PubMed]
48. Du, R.; Lu, K.V.; Petritsch, C.; Liu, P.; Ganss, R.; Passegue, E.; Song, H.; Vandenberg, S.; Johnson, R.S.; Werb, Z.; et al. HIF1alpha induces the recruitment of bone marrow-derived vascular modulatory cells to regulate tumor angiogenesis and invasion. *Cancer Cell* **2008**, *13*, 206–220. [CrossRef]
49. Jain, R.K. Antiangiogenesis strategies revisited: From starving tumors to alleviating hypoxia. *Cancer Cell* **2014**, *26*, 605–622. [CrossRef] [PubMed]
50. Dulloo, I.; Phang, B.H.; Othman, R.; Tan, S.Y.; Vijayaraghavan, A.; Goh, L.K.; Martin-Lopez, M.; Marques, M.M.; Li, C.W.; Wang de, Y.; et al. Hypoxia-inducible TAp73 supports tumorigenesis by regulating the angiogenic transcriptome. *Nat. Cell Biol.* **2015**, *17*, 511–523. [CrossRef]
51. Palucka, A.K.; Coussens, L.M. The Basis of Oncoimmunology. *Cell* **2016**, *164*, 1233–1247. [CrossRef]
52. Carmeliet, P. Angiogenesis in health and disease. *Nat. Med.* **2003**, *9*, 653–660. [CrossRef] [PubMed]

53. Ferrari, G.; Cook, B.D.; Terushkin, V.; Pintucci, G.; Mignatti, P. Transforming growth factor-beta 1 (TGF-β1) induces angiogenesis through vascular endothelial growth factor (VEGF)-mediated apoptosis. *J. Cell Physiol.* **2009**, *219*, 449–458. [CrossRef]
54. Jeon, S.-H.; Chae, B.-C.; Kim, H.-A.; Seo, G.-Y.; Seo, D.-W.; Chun, G.-T.; Kim, N.-S.; Yie, S.-W.; Byeon, W.-H.; Eom, S.-H.; et al. Mechanisms underlying TGF-β1-induced expression of VEGF and Flk-1 in mouse macrophages and their implications for angiogenesis. *J. Leukoc Biol.* **2007**, *81*, 557–566. [CrossRef] [PubMed]
55. Fan, F.; Stoeltzing, O.; Liu, W.; McCarty, M.F.; Jung, Y.D.; Reinmuth, N.; Ellis, L.M. Interleukin-1β Regulates Angiopoietin-1 Expression in Human Endothelial Cells. *Cancer Res.* **2004**, *64*, 3186–3190. [CrossRef] [PubMed]
56. Dentelli, P.; Sorbo, L.D.; Rosso, A.; Molinar, A.; Garbarino, G.; Camussi, G.; Pegoraro, L.; Brizzi, M.F. Human IL-3 Stimulates Endothelial Cell Motility and Promotes In Vivo New Vessel Formation. *J. Immunol.* **1999**, *163*, 2151–2159.
57. Loeffler, S.; Fayard, B.; Weis, J.; Weissenberger, J. Interleukin-6 induces transcriptional activation of vascular endothelial growth factor (VEGF) in astrocytes in vivo and regulates VEGF promoter activity in glioblastoma cells via direct interaction between STAT3 and Sp1. *Int. J. Cancer* **2005**, *115*, 202–213. [CrossRef]
58. Li, A.; Dubey, S.; Varney, M.L.; Dave, B.J.; Singh, R.K. IL-8 Directly Enhanced Endothelial Cell Survival, Proliferation, and Matrix Metalloproteinases Production and Regulated Angiogenesis. *J. Immunol.* **2003**, *170*, 3369–3376. [CrossRef]
59. Roy Choudhury, S.; Karmakar, S.; Banik, N.L.; Ray, S.K. Targeting Angiogenesis for Controlling Neuroblastoma. *J. Oncol.* **2012**, *2012*, 782020. [CrossRef] [PubMed]
60. Oehler, M.K.; Hague, S.; Rees, M.C.P.; Bicknell, R. Adrenomedullin promotes formation of xenografted endometrial tumors by stimulation of autocrine growth and angiogenesis. *Oncogene* **2002**, *21*, 2815–2821. [CrossRef]
61. Orimo, A.; Gupta, P.B.; Sgroi, D.C.; Arenzana-Seisdedos, F.; Delaunay, T.; Naeem, R.; Carey, V.J.; Richardson, A.L.; Weinberg, R.A. Stromal Fibroblasts Present in Invasive Human Breast Carcinomas Promote Tumor Growth and Angiogenesis through Elevated SDF-1/CXCL12 Secretion. *Cell* **2005**, *121*, 335–348. [CrossRef]
62. Oga, M.; Takenaga, K.; Sato, Y.; Nakajima, H.; Koshikawa, N.; Osato, K.; Sakiyama, S. Inhibition of metastatic brain tumor growth by intramuscular administration of the endostatin gene. *Int. J. Oncol.* **2003**, *23*, 73–79. [CrossRef] [PubMed]
63. Imanishi, Y.; Hu, B.; Jarzynka, M.J.; Guo, P.; Elishaev, E.; Bar-Joseph, I.; Cheng, S.Y. Angiopoietin-2 stimulates breast cancer metastasis through the alpha(5)beta(1) integrin-mediated pathway. *Cancer Res.* **2007**, *67*, 4254–4263. [CrossRef]
64. Srivastava, K.; Hu, J.; Korn, C.; Savant, S.; Teichert, M.; Kapel, S.S.; Jugold, M.; Besemfelder, E.; Thomas, M.; Pasparakis, M.; et al. Postsurgical Adjuvant Tumor Therapy by Combining Anti-Angiopoietin-2 and Metronomic Chemotherapy Limits Metastatic Growth. *Cancer Cell* **2014**, *26*, 880–895. [CrossRef]
65. Zhang, Y.; Han, J.D.; Yang, X.; Shao, C.K.; Xu, Z.M.; Cheng, R.; Cai, W.B.; Ma, J.X.; Yang, Z.H.; Gao, G.Q. Pigment epithelium-derived factor inhibits angiogenesis and growth of gastric carcinoma by down-regulation of VEGF. *Oncol. Rep.* **2011**, *26*, 681–686. [CrossRef]
66. Wu, Y.; Deng, J.; Rychahou, P.G.; Qiu, S.M.; Evers, B.M.; Zhou, B.P.H. Stabilization of Snail by NF-kappa B Is Required for Inflammation-Induced Cell Migration and Invasion. *Cancer Cell* **2009**, *15*, 416–428. [CrossRef] [PubMed]
67. Davis, F.B.; Mousa, S.A.; O'Connor, L.; Mohamed, S.; Lin, H.Y.; Cao, H.J.; Davis, P.J. Proangiogenic action of thyroid hormone is fibroblast growth factor-dependent and is initiated at the cell surface. *Circ. Res.* **2004**, *94*, 1500–1506. [CrossRef]
68. Itoh, T.; Tanioka, M.; Yoshida, H.; Yoshioka, T.; Nishimoto, H.; Itohara, S. Reduced angiogenesis and tumor progression in gelatinase A-deficient mice. *Cancer Res.* **1998**, *58*, 1048–1051.
69. Motterlini, R.; Otterbein, L.E. The therapeutic potential of carbon monoxide. *Nat. Rev. Drug Discov.* **2010**, *9*, 728–743. [CrossRef]
70. Abraham, N.G.; Kappas, A. Pharmacological and clinical aspects of heme oxygenase. *Pharmacol. Rev.* **2008**, *60*, 79–127. [CrossRef] [PubMed]
71. Yin, H.Z.; Fang, J.; Liao, L.; Nakamura, H.; Maeda, H. Styrene-maleic acid copolymer-encapsulated CORM2, a water-soluble carbon monoxide (CO) donor with a constant CO-releasing property, exhibits therapeutic potential for inflammatory bowel disease. *J. Control. Release* **2014**, *187*, 14–21. [CrossRef] [PubMed]
72. Fang, J.; Qin, H.; Nakamura, H.; Tsukigawa, K.; Shin, T.; Maeda, H. Carbon monoxide, generated by heme oxygenase-1, mediates the enhanced permeability and retention effect in solid tumors. *Cancer Sci.* **2012**, *103*, 535–541. [CrossRef] [PubMed]
73. Fang, J.; Qin, H.B.; Seki, T.; Nakamura, H.; Tsukigawa, K.; Shin, T.; Maeda, H. Therapeutic Potential of Pegylated Hemin for Reactive Oxygen Species-Related Diseases via Induction of Heme Oxygenase-1: Results from a Rat Hepatic Ischemia/Reperfusion Injury Model. *J. Pharmacol. Exp. Ther.* **2011**, *339*, 779–789. [CrossRef]
74. Moroianu, J.; Riordan, J.F. Nuclear translocation of angiogenin in proliferating endothelial cells is essential to its angiogenic activity. *Proc. Natl. Acad. Sci. USA* **1994**, *91*, 1677–1681. [CrossRef]
75. Eilken, H.M.; Adams, R.H. Dynamics of endothelial cell behavior in sprouting angiogenesis. *Curr. Opin. Cell Biol.* **2010**, *22*, 617–625. [CrossRef]
76. Rolny, C.; Mazzone, M.; Tugues, S.; Laoui, D.; Johansson, I.; Coulon, C.; Squadrito, M.L.; Segura, I.; Li, X.J.; Knevels, E.; et al. HRG Inhibits Tumor Growth and Metastasis by Inducing Macrophage Polarization and Vessel Normalization through Downregulation of PlGF. *Cancer Cell* **2011**, *19*, 31–44. [CrossRef]
77. Facciabene, A.; Peng, X.H.; Hagemann, I.S.; Balint, K.; Barchetti, A.; Wang, L.P.; Gimotty, P.A.; Gilks, C.B.; Lal, P.; Zhang, L.; et al. Tumour hypoxia promotes tolerance and angiogenesis via CCL28 and T-reg cells. *Nature* **2011**, *475*, 226–230. [CrossRef]
78. Yu, H.S.; Lin, T.H.; Tang, C.H. Involvement of intercellular adhesion molecule-1 up-regulation in bradykinin promotes cell motility in human prostate cancers. *Int. J. Mol. Sci.* **2013**, *14*, 13329–13345. [CrossRef] [PubMed]

79. Kou, R.; Greif, D.; Michel, T. Dephosphorylation of endothelial nitric-oxide synthase by vascular endothelial growth factor. Implications for the vascular responses to cyclosporin A. *J. Biol. Chem.* **2002**, *277*, 29669–29673. [CrossRef]
80. Matsumura, Y.; Kimura, M.; Yamamoto, T.; Maeda, H. Involvement of the kinin-generating cascade in enhanced vascular permeability in tumor tissue. *Jpn J. Cancer Res.* **1988**, *79*, 1327–1334. [CrossRef] [PubMed]
81. Maeda, H.; Matsumura, Y.; Kato, H. Purification and identification of [hydroxyprolyl3]bradykinin in ascitic fluid from a patient with gastric cancer. *J. Biol. Chem.* **1988**, *263*, 16051–16054. [CrossRef]
82. Matsumura, Y.; Maruo, K.; Kimura, M.; Yamamoto, T.; Konno, T.; Maeda, H. Kinin-generating cascade in advanced cancer patients and in vitro study. *Jpn J. Cancer Res.* **1991**, *82*, 732–741. [CrossRef]
83. Wu, J.; Akaike, T.; Maeda, H. Modulation of enhanced vascular permeability in tumors by a bradykinin antagonist, a cyclooxygenase inhibitor, and a nitric oxide scavenger. *Cancer Res.* **1998**, *58*, 159–165. [CrossRef] [PubMed]
84. Wu, J.; Akaike, T.; Hayashida, K.; Okamoto, T.; Okuyama, A.; Maeda, H. Enhanced vascular permeability in solid tumor involving peroxynitrite and matrix metalloproteinases. *Jpn J. Cancer Res.* **2001**, *92*, 439–451. [CrossRef]
85. Maeda, H.; Noguchi, Y.; Sato, K.; Akaike, T. Enhanced vascular permeability in solid tumor is mediated by nitric oxide and inhibited by both new nitric oxide scavenger and nitric oxide synthase inhibitor. *Jpn J. Cancer Res.* **1994**, *85*, 331–334. [CrossRef] [PubMed]
86. Tanaka, S.; Akaike, T.; Wu, J.; Fang, J.; Sawa, T.; Ogawa, M.; Beppu, T.; Maeda, H. Modulation of tumor-selective vascular blood flow and extravasation by the stable prostaglandin 12 analogue beraprost sodium. *J. Drug Target.* **2003**, *11*, 45–52. [CrossRef]
87. Hori, K.; Suzuki, M.; Tanda, S.; Saito, S.; Shinozaki, M.; Zhang, Q.H. Fluctuations in tumor blood flow under normotension and the effect of angiotensin II-induced hypertension. *Jpn. J. Cancer Res.* **1991**, *82*, 1309–1316. [CrossRef] [PubMed]
88. Omidi, Y.; Barar, J. Targeting tumor microenvironment: Crossing tumor interstitial fluid by multifunctional nanomedicines. *Bioimpacts* **2014**, *4*, 55–67. [CrossRef] [PubMed]
89. Tredan, O.; Galmarini, C.M.; Patel, K.; Tannock, I.F. Drug resistance and the solid tumor microenvironment. *J. Natl. Cancer Inst.* **2007**, *99*, 1441–1454. [CrossRef]
90. Nagy, J.A.; Vasile, E.; Feng, D.; Sundberg, C.; Brown, L.F.; Detmar, M.J.; Lawitts, J.A.; Benjamin, L.; Tan, X.L.; Manseau, E.J.; et al. Vascular permeability factor/vascular endothelial growth factor induces lymphangiogenesis as well as angiogenesis. *J. Exp. Med.* **2002**, *196*, 1497–1506. [CrossRef]
91. Huang, Y.H.; Yuan, J.P.; Righi, E.; Duda, D.G.; Fukumura, D.; Poznanasky, M.C.; Jain, R.K. Vascular normalization as an emerging strategy to enhance cancer immunotherapy. *Cancer Res.* **2013**, *73*, 2943–2948. [CrossRef]
92. Cooke, V.G.; LeBleu, V.S.; Keskin, D.; Khan, Z.; O'Conne, J.T.; Teng, Y.; Duncan, M.B.; Xie, L.; Maeda, G.; Vong, S.; et al. Pericyte Depletion Results in Hypoxia-Associated Epithelial-to-Mesenchymal Transition and Metastasis Mediated by Met Signaling Pathway. *Cancer Cell* **2012**, *21*, 66–81. [CrossRef] [PubMed]
93. Chen, X.L.; Nam, J.O.; Jean, C.; Lawson, C.; Walsh, C.T.; Goka, E.; Lim, S.T.; Tomar, A.; Tancioni, I.; Uryu, S.; et al. VEGF-Induced Vascular Permeability Is Mediated by FAK. *Dev. Cell* **2012**, *22*, 146–157. [CrossRef] [PubMed]
94. Jain, R.K. Normalization of tumor vasculature: An emerging concept in antiangiogenic therapy. *Science* **2005**, *307*, 58–62. [CrossRef] [PubMed]
95. Padera, T.P.; Stoll, B.R.; Tooredman, J.B.; Capen, D.; di Tomaso, E.; Jain, R.K. Pathology: Cancer cells compress intratumour vessels. *Nature* **2004**, *427*, 695. [CrossRef] [PubMed]
96. Sheldon, H.; Heikamp, E.; Turley, H.; Dragovic, R.; Thomas, P.; Oon, C.E.; Leek, R.; Edelmann, M.; Kessler, B.; Sainson, R.C.; et al. New mechanism for Notch signaling to endothelium at a distance by Delta-like 4 incorporation into exosomes. *Blood* **2010**, *116*, 2385–2394. [CrossRef]
97. Oon, C.E.; Bridges, E.; Sheldon, H.; Sainson, R.C.A.; Jubb, A.; Turley, H.; Leek, R.; Buffa, F.; Harris, A.L.; Li, J.L. Role of Delta-like 4 in Jagged1-induced tumour angiogenesis and tumour growth. *Oncotarget* **2017**, *8*, 40115–40131. [CrossRef] [PubMed]
98. Lee, C.G.; Heijn, M.; di Tomaso, E.; Griffon-Etienne, G.; Ancukiewicz, M.; Koike, C.; Park, K.R.; Ferrara, N.; Jain, R.K.; Suit, H.D.; et al. Anti-vascular endothelial growth factor treatment augments tumor radiation response under normoxic or hypoxic conditions. *Cancer Res.* **2000**, *60*, 5565–5570.
99. Luttun, A.; Tjwa, M.; Carmeliet, P. Placental growth factor (PlGF) and its receptor Flt-1 (VEGFR-1)—Novel therapeutic targets for angiogenic disorders. *Ann. N. Y. Acad. Sci.* **2002**, *979*, 80–93. [CrossRef]
100. Shahneh, F.Z.; Baradaran, B.; Zamani, F.; Aghebati-Maleki, L. Tumor angiogenesis and anti-angiogenic therapies. *Hum. Antibodies* **2013**, *22*, 15–19. [CrossRef]
101. Ribatti, D. The discovery of angiogenic growth factors: The contribution of Italian scientists. *Vasc. Cell* **2014**, *6*, 8–14. [CrossRef]
102. Peterson, T.; Kirkpatrick, N.; Huang, Y.H.; Farrar, C.; Marjit, K.; Kloepper, J.; Datta, M.; Amoozgar, Z.; Seano, G.; Jung, K.; et al. Dual Inhibition of Ang-2 and Vegf Receptors Normalizes Tumor Vasculature and Prolongs Survival in Glioblastoma by Altering Macrophages. *Proc. Natl. Acad. Sci. USA* **2016**, *113*, 4470–4475. [CrossRef]
103. Carmeliet, P.; Jain, R.K. Molecular mechanisms and clinical applications of angiogenesis. *Nature* **2011**, *473*, 298–307. [CrossRef]
104. Chow, M.T.; Luster, A.D. Chemokines in cancer. *Cancer Immunol. Res.* **2014**, *2*, 1125–1131. [CrossRef] [PubMed]
105. Suzuki, M.; Hori, K.; Abe, I.; Saito, S.; Sato, H. A new approach to cancer chemotherapy: Selective enhancement of tumor blood flow with angiotensin II. *J. Natl. Cancer Inst.* **1981**, *67*, 663–669. [CrossRef]
106. Hori, K.; Saito, S.; Takahashi, H.; Sato, H.; Maeda, H.; Sato, Y. Tumor-selective blood flow decrease induced by an angiotensin converting enzyme inhibitor, temocapril hydrochloride. *Jpn. J. Cancer Res.* **2000**, *91*, 261–269. [CrossRef] [PubMed]

107. Chauhan, V.P.; Stylianopoulos, T.; Boucher, Y.; Jain, R.K. Delivery of Molecular and Nanoscale Medicine to Tumors: Transport Barriers and Strategies. *Annu. Rev. Chem. Biomol. Eng.* **2011**, *2*, 281–298. [CrossRef]
108. Fang, J.; Sawa, T.; Maeda, H. Factors and mechanism of "EPR" effect and the enhanced antitumor effects of macromolecular drugs including SMANCS. *Adv. Exp. Med. Biol.* **2003**, *519*, 29–49. [CrossRef]
109. Greish, K.; Fang, J.; Inutsuka, T.; Nagamitsu, A.; Maeda, H. Macromolecular therapeutics: Advantages and prospects with special emphasis on solid tumour targeting. *Clin. Pharmacokinet* **2003**, *42*, 1089–1105. [CrossRef] [PubMed]
110. Daruwalla, J.; Greish, K.; Malcontenti-Wilson, C.; Muralidharan, V.; Iyer, A.; Maeda, H.; Christophi, C. Styrene maleic acid-pirarubicin disrupts tumor microcirculation and enhances the permeability of colorectal liver metastases. *J. Vasc. Res.* **2009**, *46*, 218–228. [CrossRef]
111. Sun, C.; Jain, R.K.; Munn, L.L. Non-uniform plasma leakage affects local hematocrit and blood flow: Implications for inflammation and tumor perfusion. *Ann. Biomed. Eng.* **2007**, *35*, 2121–2129. [CrossRef] [PubMed]
112. Stylianopoulos, T.; Jain, R.K. Combining two strategies to improve perfusion and drug delivery in solid tumors. *Proc. Natl. Acad. Sci. USA* **2013**, *110*, 18632–18637. [CrossRef]
113. Jain, R.K. Molecular regulation of vessel maturation. *Nat. Med.* **2003**, *9*, 685–693. [CrossRef]
114. Gao, Y.; Shi, Y.; Fu, M.; Feng, Y.; Lin, G.; Kong, D.; Jiang, B. Simulation study of the effects of interstitial fluid pressure and blood flow velocity on transvascular transport of nanoparticles in tumor microenvironment. *Comput. Methods Programs Biomed.* **2020**, *193*, 105493. [CrossRef] [PubMed]
115. Yang, H.; Tong, Z.; Sun, S.; Mao, Z. Enhancement of tumour penetration by nanomedicines through strategies based on transport processes and barriers. *J. Control. Release* **2020**, *328*, 28–44. [CrossRef]
116. Dewhirst, M.W.; Secomb, T.W. Transport of drugs from blood vessels to tumour tissue. *Nat. Rev. Cancer* **2017**, *17*, 738–750. [CrossRef] [PubMed]
117. Dagogo-Jack, I.; Shaw, A.T. Tumour heterogeneity and resistance to cancer therapies. *Nat. Rev. Clin. Oncol.* **2018**, *15*, 81–94. [CrossRef]
118. Hare, J.I.; Lammers, T.; Ashford, M.B.; Puri, S.; Storm, G.; Barry, S.T. Challenges and strategies in anti-cancer nanomedicine development: An industry perspective. *Adv. Drug Deliv. Rev.* **2017**, *108*, 25–38. [CrossRef] [PubMed]
119. Plendl, J.; Snyman, C.; Naidoo, S.; Sawant, S.; Mahabeer, R.; Bhoola, K.D. Expression of tissue kallikrein and kinin receptors in angiogenic microvascular endothelial cells. *Biol. Chem.* **2000**, *381*, 1103–1115. [CrossRef]
120. Seki, T.; Fang, J.; Maeda, H. Enhanced delivery of macromolecular antitumor drugs to tumors by nitroglycerin application. *Cancer Sci.* **2009**, *100*, 2426–2430. [CrossRef]
121. Maeda, H.; Tsukigawa, K.; Fang, J. A Retrospective 30 Years After Discovery of the Enhanced Permeability and Retention Effect of Solid Tumors: Next-Generation Chemotherapeutics and Photodynamic Therapy—Problems, Solutions, and Prospects. *Microcirculation* **2016**, *23*, 173–182. [CrossRef] [PubMed]
122. Shenoi, M.M.; Iltis, I.; Choi, J.; Koonce, N.A.; Metzger, G.J.; Griffin, R.J.; Bischof, J.C. Nanoparticle delivered vascular disrupting agents (VDAs): Use of TNF-alpha conjugated gold nanoparticles for multimodal cancer therapy. *Mol. Pharm.* **2013**, *10*, 1683–1694. [CrossRef]
123. Fukuto, J.M.; Cho, J.Y.; Switzer, C.H. Chapter 2—The Chemical Properties of Nitric Oxide and Related Nitrogen Oxides. In *Nitric Oxide*; Ignarro, L.J., Ed.; Academic Press: San Diego, CA, USA, 2000; pp. 23–40. [CrossRef]
124. Jordan, B.F.; Misson, P.; Demeure, R.; Baudelet, C.; Beghein, N.; Gallez, B. Changes in tumor oxygenation/perfusion induced by the no donor, isosorbide dinitrate, in comparison with carbogen: Monitoring by EPR and MRI. *Int. J. Radiat. Oncol. Biol. Phys.* **2000**, *48*, 565–570. [CrossRef]
125. Kim, W.J.; Yockman, J.W.; Jeong, J.H.; Christensen, L.V.; Lee, M.; Kim, Y.H.; Kim, S.W. Anti-angiogenic inhibition of tumor growth by systemic delivery of PEI-g-PEG-RGD/pCMV-sFlt-1 complexes in tumor-bearing mice. *J. Control. Release* **2006**, *114*, 381–388. [CrossRef] [PubMed]
126. Kim, J.; Kim, S.W.; Kim, W.J. PEI-g-PEG-RGD/small interference RNA polyplex-mediated silencing of vascular endothelial growth factor receptor and its potential as an anti-angiogenic tumor therapeutic strategy. *Oligonucleotides* **2011**, *21*, 101–107. [CrossRef]
127. Bharali, D.J.; Yalcin, M.; Davis, P.J.; Mousa, S.A. Tetraiodothyroacetic acid-conjugated PLGA nanoparticles: A nanomedicine approach to treat drug-resistant breast cancer. *Nanomedicine* **2013**, *8*, 1943–1954. [CrossRef] [PubMed]
128. Rebbaa, A.; Chu, F.; Davis, F.B.; Davis, P.J.; Mousa, S.A. Novel function of the thyroid hormone analog tetraiodothyroacetic acid: A cancer chemosensitizing and anti-cancer agent. *Angiogenesis* **2008**, *11*, 269–276. [CrossRef] [PubMed]
129. Mousa, S.A.; Bergh, J.J.; Dier, E.; Rebbaa, A.; O'Connor, L.J.; Yalcin, M.; Aljada, A.; Dyskin, E.; Davis, F.B.; Lin, H.Y.; et al. Tetraiodothyroacetic acid, a small molecule integrin ligand, blocks angiogenesis induced by vascular endothelial growth factor and basic fibroblast growth factor. *Angiogenesis* **2008**, *11*, 183–190. [CrossRef]
130. Rajabi, M.; Sudha, T.; Darwish, N.H.E.; Davis, P.J.; Mousa, S.A. Synthesis of MR-49, a deiodinated analog of tetraiodothyroacetic acid (tetrac), as a novel pro-angiogenesis modulator. *Bioorg. Med. Chem. Lett.* **2016**, *26*, 4112–4116. [CrossRef]
131. Chen, Y.; Song, W.; Shen, L.; Qiu, N.; Hu, M.; Liu, Y.; Liu, Q.; Huang, L. Vasodilator Hydralazine Promotes Nanoparticle Penetration in Advanced Desmoplastic Tumors. *ACS Nano* **2019**, *13*, 1751–1763. [CrossRef] [PubMed]

132. Zhang, B.; Jiang, T.; Tuo, Y.Y.; Jin, K.; Luo, Z.M.; Shi, W.; Mei, H.; Hu, Y.; Pang, Z.Q.; Jiang, X.G. Captopril improves tumor nanomedicine delivery by increasing tumor blood perfusion and enlarging endothelial gaps in tumor blood vessels. *Cancer Lett.* **2017**, *410*, 12–19. [CrossRef] [PubMed]
133. Zhang, P.; Zhang, Y.; Ding, X.Y.; Xiao, C.S.; Chen, X.S. Enhanced nanoparticle accumulation by tumor-acidity-activatable release of sildenafil to induce vasodilation. *Biomater. Sci.* **2020**, *8*, 3052–3062. [CrossRef] [PubMed]
134. Mei, T.; Shashni, B.; Maeda, H.; Nagasaki, Y. Fibrinolytic tissue plasminogen activator installed redox-active nanoparticles (t-PA@iRNP) for cancer therapy. *Biomaterials* **2020**, *259*, 120290. [CrossRef]
135. Zhang, Y.; Liu, Y.; Gao, X.; Li, X.; Niu, X.; Yuan, Z.; Wang, W. Near-infrared-light induced nanoparticles with enhanced tumor tissue penetration and intelligent drug release. *Acta Biomater.* **2019**, *90*, 314–323. [CrossRef]
136. Sengupta, S.; Eavarone, D.; Capila, I.; Zhao, G.; Watson, N.; Kiziltepe, T.; Sasisekharan, R. Temporal targeting of tumour cells and neovasculature with a nanoscale delivery system. *Nature* **2005**, *436*, 568–572. [CrossRef] [PubMed]
137. Zhang, M.K.; Ye, J.J.; Xia, Y.; Wang, Z.Y.; Li, C.X.; Wang, X.S.; Yu, W.Y.; Song, W.; Feng, J.; Zhang, X.Z. Platelet-Mimicking Biotaxis Targeting Vasculature-Disrupted Tumors for Cascade Amplification of Hypoxia-Sensitive Therapy. *ACS Nano* **2019**, *13*, 14230–14240. [CrossRef]
138. Palomba, R.; Parodi, A.; Evangelopoulos, M.; Acciardo, S.; Corbo, C.; de Rosa, E.; Yazdi, I.K.; Scaria, S.; Molinaro, R.; Furman, N.E.T.; et al. Biomimetic carriers mimicking leukocyte plasma membrane to increase tumor vasculature permeability. *Sci. Rep.* **2016**, *6*, 34422. [CrossRef]
139. Li, X.; Zhen, M.; Deng, R.; Yu, T.; Li, J.; Zhang, Y.; Zou, T.; Zhou, Y.; Lu, Z.; Guan, M.; et al. RF-assisted gadofullerene nanoparticles induces rapid tumor vascular disruption by down-expression of tumor vascular endothelial cadherin. *Biomaterials* **2018**, *163*, 142–153. [CrossRef]
140. Liang, C.; Chao, Y.; Yi, X.; Xu, J.; Feng, L.; Zhao, Q.; Yang, K.; Liu, Z. Nanoparticle-mediated internal radioisotope therapy to locally increase the tumor vasculature permeability for synergistically improved cancer therapies. *Biomaterials* **2019**, *197*, 368–379. [CrossRef] [PubMed]
141. Manzoor, A.A.; Lindner, L.H.; Landon, C.D.; Park, J.Y.; Simnick, A.J.; Dreher, M.R.; Das, S.; Hanna, G.; Park, W.; Chilkoti, A.; et al. Overcoming limitations in nanoparticle drug delivery: Triggered, intravascular release to improve drug penetration into tumors. *Cancer Res.* **2012**, *72*, 5566–5575. [CrossRef] [PubMed]
142. Srinivasan, M.; Rajabi, M.; Mousa, S.A. Chapter 3—Nanobiomaterials in cancer therapy. In *Nanobiomaterials in Cancer Therapy*; Grumezescu, A.M., Ed.; William Andrew Publishing: Bucharest, Romania, 2016; pp. 57–89. [CrossRef]
143. Yoncheva, K.; Momekov, G. Antiangiogenic anticancer strategy based on nanoparticulate systems. *Expert Opin. Drug Deliv.* **2011**, *8*, 1041–1056. [CrossRef]
144. Fukumura, D.; Kloepper, J.; Amoozgar, Z.; Duda, D.G.; Jain, R.K. Enhancing cancer immunotherapy using antiangiogenics: Opportunities and challenges. *Nat. Rev. Clin. Oncol.* **2018**, *15*, 325–340. [CrossRef] [PubMed]
145. Huber, P.E.; Bischof, M.; Jenne, J.; Heiland, S.; Peschke, P.; Saffrich, R.; Gröne, H.J.; Debus, J.; Lipson, K.E.; Abdollahi, A. Trimodal cancer treatment: Beneficial effects of combined antiangiogenesis, radiation, and chemotherapy. *Cancer Res.* **2005**, *65*, 3643–3655. [CrossRef]
146. Kok, R.J.; Schraa, A.J.; Bos, E.J.; Moorlag, H.E.; Asgeirsdottir, S.A.; Everts, M.; Meijer, D.K.; Molema, G. Preparation and functional evaluation of RGD-modified proteins as alpha(v)beta(3) integrin directed therapeutics. *Bioconjug. Chem.* **2002**, *13*, 128–135. [CrossRef]
147. Hynes, R.O. A reevaluation of integrins as regulators of angiogenesis. *Nat. Med.* **2002**, *8*, 918–921. [CrossRef]
148. Sakae, M.; Ito, T.; Yoshihara, C.; Iida-Tanaka, N.; Yanagie, H.; Eriguchi, M.; Koyama, Y. Highly efficient in vivo gene transfection by plasmid/PEI complexes coated by anionic PEG derivatives bearing carboxyl groups and RGD peptide. *Biomed. Pharmacother.* **2008**, *62*, 448–453. [CrossRef] [PubMed]
149. Kunjachan, S.; Pola, R.; Gremse, F.; Theek, B.; Ehling, J.; Moeckel, D.; Hermanns-Sachweh, B.; Pechar, M.; Ulbrich, K.; Hennink, W.E.; et al. Passive versus Active Tumor Targeting Using RGD- and NGR-Modified Polymeric Nanomedicines. *Nano Lett.* **2014**, *14*, 972–981. [CrossRef] [PubMed]
150. Huang, Z.; Dong, L.; Chen, J.; Gao, F.B.; Zhang, Z.P.; Chen, J.N.; Zhang, J.F. Low-molecular weight chitosan/vascular endothelial growth factor short hairpin RNA for the treatment of hepatocellular carcinoma. *Life Sci.* **2012**, *91*, 1207–1215. [CrossRef]
151. Guo, J.F.; Ogier, J.R.; Desgranges, S.; Darcy, R.; O'Driscoll, C. Anisamide-targeted cyclodextrin nanoparticles for siRNA delivery to prostate tumours in mice. *Biomaterials* **2012**, *33*, 7775–7784. [CrossRef] [PubMed]
152. Kim, W.J.; Chang, C.W.; Lee, M.; Kim, S.W. Efficient siRNA delivery using water soluble lipopolymer for anti-angiogenic gene therapy. *J. Control. Release* **2007**, *118*, 357–363. [CrossRef] [PubMed]
153. Chen, Y.; Gu, H.; Zhang, D.S.; Li, F.; Liu, T.; Xia, W. Highly effective inhibition of lung cancer growth and metastasis by systemic delivery of siRNA via multimodal mesoporous silica-based nanocarrier. *Biomaterials* **2014**, *35*, 10058–10069. [CrossRef]
154. Chen, Y.; Wang, X.; Liu, T.; Zhang, D.S.; Wang, Y.; Gu, H.; Di, W. Highly effective antiangiogenesis via magnetic mesoporous silica-based siRNA vehicle targeting the VEGF gene for orthotopic ovarian cancer therapy. *Int. J. Nanomed.* **2015**, *10*, 2579–2594. [CrossRef]
155. Kanazawa, T.; Sugawara, K.; Tanaka, K.; Horiuchi, S.; Takashima, Y.; Okada, H. Suppression of tumor growth by systemic delivery of anti-VEGF siRNA with cell-penetrating peptide-modified MPEG-PCL nanomicelles. *Eur. J. Pharm. Biopharm.* **2012**, *81*, 470–477. [CrossRef] [PubMed]

156. Graepler, F.; Verbeek, B.; Graeter, T.; Smirnow, I.; Kong, H.L.; Schuppan, D.; Bauer, M.; Vonthein, R.; Gregor, M.; Lauer, U.M. Combined endostatin/sFlt-1 antiangiogenic gene therapy is highly effective in a rat model of HCC. *Hepatology* **2005**, *41*, 879–886. [CrossRef]
157. Li, L.; Yang, J.; Wang, W.W.; Yao, Y.C.; Fang, S.H.; Dai, Z.Y.; Hong, H.H.; Yang, X.; Shuai, X.T.; Gao, G.Q. Pigment epithelium-derived factor gene loaded in cRGD-PEG-PEI suppresses colorectal cancer growth by targeting endothelial cells. *Int. J. Pharm.* **2012**, *438*, 1–10. [CrossRef] [PubMed]
158. Xiao, J.S.; Duan, X.P.; Yin, Q.; Miao, Z.H.; Yu, H.J.; Chen, C.Y.; Zhang, Z.W.; Wang, J.; Li, Y.P. The inhibition of metastasis and growth of breast cancer by blocking the NF-kappa B signaling pathway using bioreducible PEI-based/p65 shRNA complex nanoparticles. *Biomaterials* **2013**, *34*, 5381–5390. [CrossRef] [PubMed]
159. Tang, H.Y.; Lin, H.Y.; Zhang, S.L.; Davis, F.B.; Davis, P.J. Thyroid hormone causes mitogen-activated protein kinase-dependent phosphorylation of the nuclear estrogen receptor. *Endocrinology* **2004**, *145*, 3265–3272. [CrossRef]
160. Indraccolo, S.; Minuzzo, S.; Gola, E.; Habeler, W.; Carrozzino, F.; Noonan, D.; Albini, A.; Santi, L.; Amadori, A.; Chieco-Bianchi, L. Generation of expression plasmids for angiostatin, endostatin and TIMP-2 for cancer gene therapy. *Int. J. Biol. Markers* **1999**, *14*, 251–256. [CrossRef]
161. Li, H.; Lindenmeyer, F.; Grenet, C.; Opolon, P.; Menashi, S.; Soria, C.; Yeh, P.; Perricaudet, M.; Lu, H. AdTIMP-2 inhibits tumor growth, angiogenesis, and metastasis, and prolongs survival in mice. *Hum. Gene Ther.* **2001**, *12*, 515–526. [CrossRef] [PubMed]
162. Vincent, L.; Varet, J.; Pille, J.Y.; Bompais, H.; Opolon, P.; Maksimenko, A.; Malvy, C.; Mirshahi, M.; Lu, H.; Soria, J.P.V.C.; et al. Efficacy of dendrimer-mediated angiostatin and TIMP-2 gene delivery on inhibition of tumor growth and angiogenesis: In vitro and in vivo studies. *Int. J. Cancer* **2003**, *105*, 419–429. [CrossRef]
163. Steins, A.; Klaassen, R.; Jacobs, I.; Schabel, M.C.; van Lier, M.G.J.T.B.; Ebbing, E.A.; Hectors, S.J.; Tas, S.W.; Maracle, C.X.; Punt, C.J.A.; et al. Rapid stromal remodeling by short-term VEGFR2 inhibition increases chemotherapy delivery in esophagogastric adenocarcinoma. *Mol. Oncol.* **2020**, *14*, 704–720. [CrossRef] [PubMed]
164. Chauhan, V.P.; Martin, J.D.; Liu, H.; Lacorre, D.A.; Jain, S.R.; Kozin, S.V.; Stylianopoulos, T.; Mousa, A.S.; Han, X.X.; Adstamongkonkul, P.; et al. Angiotensin inhibition enhances drug delivery and potentiates chemotherapy by decompressing tumour blood vessels. *Nat. Commun.* **2013**, *4*, 2516–2528. [CrossRef]
165. Jain, R.K. Normalizing Tumor Microenvironment to Treat Cancer: Bench to Bedside to Biomarkers. *J. Clin. Oncol.* **2013**, *31*, 2205–2210. [CrossRef]
166. Farahani, A.; Azimi, S.; Tajaddodi, A.; Docoslis, A.; Tashakori, C. Screen-printed anion-exchange solid-phase extraction: A new strategy for point-of-care determination of angiotensin receptor blockers. *Talanta* **2021**, *222*, 121518. [CrossRef]
167. Zhao, Y.X.; Cao, J.H.; Melamed, A.; Worley, M.; Gockley, A.; Jones, D.; Nia, H.T.; Zhang, Y.L.; Stylianopoulos, T.; Kumar, A.S.; et al. Losartan treatment enhances chemotherapy efficacy and reduces ascites in ovarian cancer models by normalizing the tumor stroma. *Proc. Natl. Acad. Sci. USA* **2019**, *116*, 2210–2219. [CrossRef]
168. Zhang, Q.; Lin, Z.; Yin, X.; Tang, L.; Luo, H.; Li, H.; Zhang, Y.; Luo, W. In vitro and in vivo study of hydralazine, a potential anti-angiogenic agent. *Eur. J. Pharmacol.* **2016**, *779*, 138–146. [CrossRef] [PubMed]
169. Demers, M.; Wagner, D.D. Targeting platelet function to improve drug delivery. *Oncoimmunology* **2012**, *1*, 100–102. [CrossRef] [PubMed]
170. Demers, M.; Ho-Tin-Noe, B.; Schatzberg, D.; Yang, J.J.; Wagner, D.D. Increased efficacy of breast cancer chemotherapy in thrombocytopenic mice. *Cancer Res.* **2011**, *71*, 1540–1549. [CrossRef] [PubMed]
171. Li, Z.; Di, C.; Li, S.; Yang, X.; Nie, G. Smart Nanotherapeutic Targeting of Tumor Vasculature. *Acc. Chem. Res.* **2019**, *52*, 2703–2712. [CrossRef] [PubMed]
172. Li, S.; Zhang, Y.; Wang, J.; Zhao, Y.; Ji, T.; Zhao, X.; Ding, Y.; Zhao, X.; Zhao, R.; Li, F.; et al. Nanoparticle-mediated local depletion of tumour-associated platelets disrupts vascular barriers and augments drug accumulation in tumours. *Nat. Biomed. Eng.* **2017**, *1*, 667–679. [CrossRef] [PubMed]
173. Netti, P.A.; Berk, D.A.; Swartz, M.A.; Grodzinsky, A.J.; Jain, R.K. Role of extracellular matrix assembly in interstitial transport in solid tumors. *Cancer Res.* **2000**, *60*, 2497–2503.
174. Eikenes, L.; Bruland, O.S.; Brekken, C.; Davies, C.D.L. Collagenase increases the transcapillary pressure gradient and improves the uptake and distribution of monoclonal antibodies in human osteosarcoma xenografts. *Cancer Res.* **2004**, *64*, 4768–4773. [CrossRef]
175. McKee, T.D.; Grandi, P.; Mok, W.; Alexandrakis, G.; Insin, N.; Zimmer, J.P.; Bawendi, M.G.; Boucher, Y.; Breakefield, X.O.; Jain, R.K. Degradation of fibrillar collagen in a human melanoma xenograft improves the efficacy of an oncolytic herpes simplex virus vector. *Cancer Res.* **2006**, *66*, 2509–2513. [CrossRef]
176. Matsumoto, Y.; Nichols, J.W.; Toh, K.; Nomoto, T.; Cabral, H.; Miura, Y.; Christie, R.J.; Yamada, N.; Ogura, T.; Kano, M.R.; et al. Vascular bursts enhance permeability of tumour blood vessels and improve nanoparticle delivery. *Nat. Nanotechnol.* **2016**, *11*, 533–538. [CrossRef] [PubMed]
177. Duan, L.; Yang, L.; Jin, J.; Yang, F.; Liu, D.; Hu, K.; Wang, Q.X.; Yue, Y.B.; Gu, N. Micro/nano-bubble-assisted ultrasound to enhance the EPR effect and potential theranostic applications. *Theranostics* **2020**, *10*, 462–483. [CrossRef] [PubMed]
178. Yu, W.Q.; Liu, R.; Zhou, Y.; Gao, H.L. Size-Tunable Strategies for a Tumor Targeted Drug Delivery System. *ACS Cent. Sci.* **2020**, *6*, 100–116. [CrossRef] [PubMed]

179. Dai, L.L.; Li, X.; Yao, M.J.; Niu, P.Y.; Yuan, X.C.; Li, K.; Chen, M.W.; Fu, Z.X.; Duan, X.L.; Liu, H.B.; et al. Programmable prodrug micelle with size-shrinkage and charge-reversal for chemotherapy-improved IDO immunotherapy. *Biomaterials* **2020**, *241*, 119901. [CrossRef]
180. Jin, Y.; Wu, Z.M.; Wu, C.C.; Zi, Y.X.; Chu, X.Y.; Liu, J.P.; Zhang, W.L. Size-adaptable and ligand (biotin)-sheddable nanocarriers equipped with avidin scavenging technology for deep tumor penetration and reduced toxicity. *J. Control. Release* **2020**, *320*, 142–158. [CrossRef]
181. Wang, K.W.; Tu, Y.L.; Yao, W.; Zong, Q.Y.; Xiao, X.; Yang, R.M.; Jiang, X.Q.; Yuan, Y.Y. Size-Switchable Nanoparticles with Self-Destructive and Tumor Penetration Characteristics for Site-Specific Phototherapy of Cancer. *ACS Appl. Mater. Interfaces* **2020**, *12*, 6933–6943. [CrossRef]
182. Chen, L.; Zhao, T.C.; Zhao, M.Y.; Wang, W.X.; Sun, C.X.; Liu, L.; Li, Q.; Zhang, F.; Zhao, D.Y.; Li, X.M. Size and charge dual-transformable mesoporous nanoassemblies for enhanced drug delivery and tumor penetration. *Chem. Sci.* **2020**, *11*, 2819–2827. [CrossRef]
183. Song, C.F.; Li, Y.G.; Li, T.L.; Yang, Y.M.; Huang, Z.C.; de la Fuente, J.M.; Ni, J.; Cui, D.X. Long-Circulating Drug-Dye-Based Micelles with Ultrahigh pH-Sensitivity for Deep Tumor Penetration and Superior Chemo-Photothermal Therapy. *Adv. Funct. Mater.* **2020**, *30*, 1462–1474. [CrossRef]
184. Nagy, J.A.; Feng, D.; Vasile, E.; Wong, W.H.; Shih, S.C.; Dvorak, A.M.; Dvorak, H.F. Permeability properties of tumor surrogate blood vessels induced by VEGF-A. *Lab. Investig.* **2006**, *86*, 767–780. [CrossRef]
185. Siemann, D.W. The unique characteristics of tumor vasculature and preclinical evidence for its selective disruption by Tumor-Vascular Disrupting Agents. *Cancer Treat. Rev.* **2011**, *37*, 63–74. [CrossRef]
186. Yang, Y.L.; Zhang, Y.; Iwamoto, H.; Hosaka, K.; Seki, T.; Andersson, P.; Lim, S.; Fischer, C.; Nakamura, M.; Abe, M.; et al. Discontinuation of anti-VEGF cancer therapy promotes metastasis through a liver revascularization mechanism. *Nat. Commun.* **2016**, *7*, 12680. [CrossRef]
187. Ferrara, N.; Kerbel, R.S. Angiogenesis as a therapeutic target. *Nature* **2005**, *438*, 967–974. [CrossRef]
188. Kunjachan, S.; Detappe, A.; Kumar, R.; Ireland, T.; Cameron, L.; Biancur, D.E.; Motto-Ros, V.; Sancey, L.; Sridhar, S.; Makrigiorgos, G.M.; et al. Nanoparticle Mediated Tumor Vascular Disruption: A Novel Strategy in Radiation Therapy. *Nano Lett.* **2015**, *15*, 7488–7496. [CrossRef]
189. Song, C.H.; Zhang, Y.J.; Li, C.Y.; Chen, G.C.; Kang, X.F.; Wang, Q.B. Enhanced Nanodrug Delivery to Solid Tumors Based on a Tumor Vasculature-Targeted Strategy. *Adv. Funct. Mater.* **2016**, *26*, 4192–4200. [CrossRef]
190. Zhen, M.M.; Shu, C.Y.; Li, J.; Zhang, G.Q.; Wang, T.S.; Luo, Y.; Zou, T.J.; Deng, R.J.; Fang, F.; Lei, H.; et al. A highly efficient and tumor vascular-targeting therapeutic technique with size-expansible gadofullerene nanocrystals. *Sci. China Mater.* **2015**, *58*, 799–810. [CrossRef]
191. Park, J.-S.; Su, Z.-Z.; Hinman, D.; Willoughby, K.; McKinstry, R.; Yacoub, A.; Duigou, G.; Young, C.; Grant, S.; Hagan, M.; et al. Ionizing radiation modulates vascular endothelial growth factor (VEGF) expression through multiple mitogen activated protein kinase dependent pathways. *Oncogene* **2001**, *20*, 3266–3280. [CrossRef] [PubMed]
192. Koukourakis, M.I.; Koukouraki, S.; Giatromanolaki, A.; Kakolyris, S.; Georgoulias, V.; Velidaki, A.; Archimandritis, S.; Karkavitsas, N.N. High intratumoral accumulation of stealth liposomal doxorubicin in sarcomas–rationale for combination with radiotherapy. *Acta Oncol.* **2000**, *39*, 207–211. [CrossRef] [PubMed]
193. Burd, R.; Dziedzic, T.S.; Xu, Y.; Caligiuri, M.A.; Subjeck, J.R.; Repasky, E.A. Tumor cell apoptosis, lymphocyte recruitment and tumor vascular changes are induced by low temperature, long duration (fever-like) whole body hyperthermia. *J. Cell Physiol.* **1998**, *177*, 137–147. [CrossRef]
194. Lammers, T.; Peschke, P.; Kuhnlein, R.; Subr, V.; Ulbrich, K.; Debus, J.; Huber, P.; Hennink, W.; Storm, G. Effect of radiotherapy and hyperthermia on the tumor accumulation of HPMA copolymer-based drug delivery systems. *J. Control. Release* **2007**, *117*, 333–341. [CrossRef] [PubMed]
195. Kong, G.; Braun, R.D.; Dewhirst, M.W. Characterization of the effect of hyperthermia on nanoparticle extravasation from tumor vasculature. *Cancer Res.* **2001**, *61*, 3027–3032. [PubMed]
196. Islam, W.; Fang, J.; Imamura, T.; Etrych, T.; Subr, V.; Ulbrich, K.; Maeda, H. Augmentation of the Enhanced Permeability and Retention Effect with Nitric Oxide–Generating Agents Improves the Therapeutic Effects of Nanomedicines. *Mol. Cancer Ther.* **2018**, *17*, 2643–2653. [CrossRef] [PubMed]
197. Sindhwani, S.; Syed, A.M.; Ngai, J.; Kingston, B.R.; Maiorino, L.; Rothschild, J.; MacMillan, P.; Zhang, Y.W.; Rajesh, N.U.; Hoang, T.; et al. The entry of nanoparticles into solid tumours. *Nat. Mater.* **2020**, *19*, 566–575. [CrossRef] [PubMed]

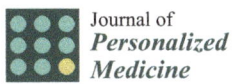

Review

HPMA Copolymer-Based Nanomedicines in Controlled Drug Delivery

Petr Chytil, Libor Kostka and Tomáš Etrych *

Institute of Macromolecular Chemistry, Czech Academy of Sciences, Heyrovsky Sq. 2, 162 06 Prague, Czech Republic; chytil@imc.cas.cz (P.C.); kostka@imc.cas.cz (L.K.)
* Correspondence: etrych@imc.cas.cz; Tel.: +420-296-809-231

Abstract: Recently, numerous polymer materials have been employed as drug carrier systems in medicinal research, and their detailed properties have been thoroughly evaluated. Water-soluble polymer carriers play a significant role between these studied polymer systems as they are advantageously applied as carriers of low-molecular-weight drugs and compounds, e.g., cytostatic agents, anti-inflammatory drugs, antimicrobial molecules, or multidrug resistance inhibitors. Covalent attachment of carried molecules using a biodegradable spacer is strongly preferred, as such design ensures the controlled release of the drug in the place of a desired pharmacological effect in a reasonable time-dependent manner. Importantly, the synthetic polymer biomaterials based on *N*-(2-hydroxypropyl) methacrylamide (HPMA) copolymers are recognized drug carriers with unique properties that nominate them among the most serious nanomedicines candidates for human clinical trials. This review focuses on advances in the development of HPMA copolymer-based nanomedicines within the passive and active targeting into the place of desired pharmacological effect, tumors, inflammation or bacterial infection sites. Specifically, this review highlights the safety issues of HPMA polymer-based drug carriers concerning the structure of nanomedicines. The main impact consists of the improvement of targeting ability, especially concerning the enhanced and permeability retention (EPR) effect.

Keywords: HPMA copolymers; EPR effect; drug delivery; controlled release; nanomedicines

Citation: Chytil, P.; Kostka, L.; Etrych, T. HPMA Copolymer-Based Nanomedicines in Controlled Drug Delivery. *J. Pers. Med.* **2021**, *11*, 115. https://doi.org/10.3390/jpm11020115

Academic Editor: Hiroshi Maeda
Received: 18 January 2021
Accepted: 8 February 2021
Published: 10 February 2021

Publisher's Note: MDPI stays neutral with regard to jurisdictional claims in published maps and institutional affiliations.

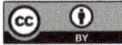

Copyright: © 2021 by the authors. Licensee MDPI, Basel, Switzerland. This article is an open access article distributed under the terms and conditions of the Creative Commons Attribution (CC BY) license (https://creativecommons.org/licenses/by/4.0/).

1. Introduction

Generally, polymer nanomedicines are macromolecule-based water-soluble, particular or micellar constructs with the 1–100 nm size range in at least one dimension that can load or attach active molecules, e.g., drugs, to a carrier to enable targeted delivery and/or site-specific controlled release of biologically active molecules [1]. Polymer nanomedicines are generally employed for the delivery of a variety of drugs, but their most important research applications fall in the field of anti-inflammatory, antibiotics, and mainly anticancer drug delivery [2,3]. Nanomedicines delivering antibiotics, anti-inflammatory, or anticancer drugs substantially reduce the overall toxicity of carried chemotherapeutics, accumulate in the inflamed or solid tumor tissue, and highly improve drug solubility, stability against degradation and biotransformation, and pharmacokinetics [4,5]. "Impeccable" nanomedicines deliver drugs directly into the target cells and their compartments with minimal drug release in the bloodstream, and thus reducing side effects on healthy tissue.

Polymer-based nanomedicines are intensively studied for several decades, and the concept of polymer-drug constructs became generally accepted and thoroughly studied [6]. Polymer nanomedicines restrain much of the drawbacks associated with the application of conventional low-molecular-weight chemotherapeutics, such as short circulation time, a low area under the curve, and significant systemic toxicity. Moreover, polymer-based nanomedicines enable targeted delivery and controlled drug release in the treated tissue. Although the application of polymer-based nanomedicines is wide, in this review, we focus mainly only on polymer-drug conjugates intended for cancer treatment with the possible application also to anti-inflammatory compounds or antibiotics delivery. A potent anticancer efficacy devoid of substantial systemic toxicity has been thoroughly documented in tumor-targeted therapies based on conjugates containing various consisting of N-(2-hydroxypropyl) methacrylamide (HPMA) copolymers (pHPMAs). They are biocompatible, non-toxic, and non-immunogenic and enable the attachment of the drug to the carrier via suitable biodegradable spacer responsive to various tumor- or inflammation-site associated stimuli. Importantly, pHPMA or other water-soluble polymers are used in drug delivery due to their hydrophilic nature of the polymer backbone, which hydration, i.e., tightly bound water layer, increases the energetic barrier of protein or other biomacromolecules adsorption during the blood circulation [7,8]. Moreover, the binding of active compounds to the pHPMA can solubilize water-insoluble drugs, dramatically improve pharmacokinetics, and eliminate the side effects of drugs. Recently, many examples of polymer prodrugs showed prolonged blood clearance, enhanced localization in solid tumors via the enhanced and permeability retention (EPR) effect [9], followed by controlled release of the active drug in target tumor tissues or cells. For example, an excellent antitumor activity of polymer prodrugs containing cytostatics, e.g., doxorubicin (Dox), pirarubicin (THP), or docetaxel bound by pH-sensitive spacer stable during circulation in the blood (pH 7.4), but rapidly hydrolysable in tumors upon pH decrease to pH 6 in the tumor microenvironment or pH 5–5.5 in endosomes/lysosomes of target cancer cells, was shown repeatedly [10–12].

Polymer design, including polymer structure, molecular weight, spacer structure, etc., strongly influences the overall therapeutic activity. An enormous effort has been pushed on the development of pHPMA-based nanomedicines taking advantage of the EPR effect. Their high molecular weight (HMW) prevents fast blood clearance of carried drugs and thus enables their increased uptake in solid tumors. The extent of accumulated polymer carriers primarily depends on their molecular weight [13]. Nevertheless, there is an upper limit in molecular weights due to the slower extravasation of polymers with quite high M_w. For example, the star-like pHPMA-Dox conjugate with M_w = 1,000,000 g/mol was accumulated much lower than the conjugate with M_w = 600,000 g/mol [14]. To prevent the undesired accumulation of carriers in the body, which can lead to serious long-term side-effects, the elimination of carriers after fulfilling their role must be ensured.

The polymer biomaterial serving as the carrier should be removed from the body after the carried cargo is delivered to the target tissue and released. The clearance of polymer carriers by glomerular filtration is mainly controlled by the size of the polymer coil in solution, which is correlated to polymer M_w. Non-charged copolymers with a size smaller than the size of glomerular pores can permeate through them, resulting in the elimination of polymers from the body by urine. Polymer carriers with biodegradable backbone, e.g., poly (glutamic acid) [15], can be hydrolyzed and degraded directly in the body. Nevertheless, methacrylamide-based polymer biomaterials are non-degradable in general; thus, their direct biodegradation cannot be taken into consideration. Polymer carriers consisted of non-degradable polymers that undergo renal filtration only up to a certain limit of M_w, which differs for various types of polymers. For example, for the vinylic type of polymers, it is known that this limit is about 50,000 g/mol [16]. Nevertheless, a thorough study using various water-soluble HPMA polymer-Dox conjugates showed that even linear polymers with M_w around 70,000 g/mol had been found in the urine [17]. Interestingly, star conjugates with M_w around 50,000 g/mol have been found in urine, nicely illustrating the role of flexibility or vice versa rigidity of polymer carriers. Here, more flexible linear polymer chains above 50,000 g/mol were able to penetrate through glomerular pores (although slower than that below this value), rather rigid branched star polymer structures could not.

Hence, HMW pHPMA carriers exhibiting the significant EPR effect should contain biodegradable linkages between single non-degradable polymer chains with M_w below the limit of renal filtration to increase passive targeting and to allow the following elimination of the carrier fragment from the body. Alternatively, HMW supramolecular structures such as micelles formed by self-assembly of amphiphilic copolymers with a molecular weight below the limit of the renal threshold have been proposed. The variety of such HMW polymer carriers is described in Chapter 3.

The EPR effect is a vascular issue that is dynamic and flexible. Vascular dilatation by various mediators or tumor-selective passive gap opening augment the EPR effect and thus enhance the accumulation of nanomedicines in tumor tissue. Such modulation of therapy using nanomedicines is discussed in Chapter 4. The effectiveness and applicability of nanomedicines designed for passive versus active tumor targeting are considered in Chapter 5. Nevertheless, prior demonstration of the variety of pHPMA carriers, let us focus on safety issues related to HPMA homopolymer in the following chapter.

2. Safety Features of HPMA Polymers Per Se

The pHPMAs have been "invited to the stage" of drug delivery in the early 1970s. In 1974 two patent applications were filed, which covered the synthesis of N-substituted (meth) acrylamides containing oligopeptide sequences and their application as drug and other biologically active compounds carriers [18,19]. The HPMA polymer was originally developed as a fully synthetic plasma expander under the commercial name Duxon™ [20–22]. Therefore, early in the 1980s, HPMA polymer was also tested in vitro as well as in vivo in several animal models [23–28] for biocompatibility and immunogenicity.

Selected types of cell lines have been used to evaluate the toxicity of Duxon™ (HeLa, L-cells, WI-38), and none of the tested cell lines showed any toxicity. Moreover, Duxon™ in saline solution was completely apirogenic, as was demonstrated in guinea pigs after intraperitoneal administration of 5 mL of the 5% solution of Duxon™ in saline [22,23]. As a further test of HPMA polymer biocompatibility, an attempt to heal experimental implants of pHPMA crosslinked with 1 mol% methylene-bis-acrylamide subcutaneously implanted in experimental rats and pigs was chosen. Macroscopically, the implant was well tolerated by the organism in all groups and at all time intervals, both in rats and pigs, and did not elicit any adverse reaction [29]. The implant was encapsulated with a fine fibrous sheath. Microscopically, in the first days after implantation, the implant was surrounded by a border of polynuclear leukocytes and fibrin. On the tenth day after implantation, in most cases, the polynuclear leukocytes disappear, and the implant was surrounded by a sheath of fine collagen fibers and fibrocytes. Importantly, the sheath was highly vascularized. At longer intervals, the collagen fibers became coarser, and the sheath was less cellular. The vascularization of the capsule persists. The histological picture does not change from the tenth day after implantation [25,30].

Šprincl et al. in 1976 observed that, in some organs (spleen, lymph nodes), the amount of the polymer first decreases and then increases again, which was attributed to the release and trapping of the polymer in RES. More pronounced accumulation was observed in organs with phagocytic activity. The usual histological examination did not reveal any changes in the individual organs [21]. Říhová et al. concluded that HPMA homopolymer is not recognized as a foreign macromolecule in any of the five inbred strains of mice, and no detectable antibodies were formed against it [31].

3. Structural Aspects

The preferable way of pHPMA carrier elimination is renal filtration; thus, the molecular weight of non-degradable polymer carriers or fragments remaining after biodegradation of HMW polymer carriers must be below the limit of renal filtration. The pHPMA carrier, which does not meet such criterium, could be excluded from the organism by a very slow process through the hepatobiliary pathway, as documented elsewhere [32,33]. However, this option is not ideal and generally preferred as the slow clearance of even biocompatible polymer carrier could cause in the long term in the body adverse effects unnoticed in the experiments focusing on the acute toxicity of the used polymer biomaterial.

This chapter is divided into three subchapters. The first chapter is focused on the employment of linear polymer with M_w reaching the limit of renal filtration. The influence of the synthetic method on the properties of pHPMA nanomedicines is shown in detail. The second chapter presents various HMW polymer constructs containing biodegradable linkages in their structure. Moreover, the third part introduces HMW supramolecular structures formed by self-assembly of amphiphilic pHPMAs.

3.1. Linear Polymer Carriers

The improvement of controlled polymerization techniques in the last two decades enabled the synthesis of polymer carriers with quite narrow dispersity. Specifically, the reversible addition–fragmentation transfer (RAFT) polymerization has been successfully employed for the synthesis of HPMA copolymers and their drug conjugates [34–36]. Recently, also Cu-RDRP polymerization (part of atom transfer radical polymerization (ATRP) technique family) was employed for successful HPMA polymerization and copolymerization. Here, the reaction was optimized with respect to monomer conversion (82–99%), product dispersity (<1.25), and M_w control (from 20,000 up to 100,000 g/mol). For this purpose, different chlorine-based initiators in conjunction with a $CuCl/CuCl_2$/PMDETA catalytic system have been used. The utility of the optimized method was exemplified in the preparation of the pHPMA carrier having the anticancer drug Dox conjugated through a pH-sensitive hydrazone bond [37].

A preliminary study comparing pHPMA-drug conjugates bearing Dox bound by pH-sensitive hydrazone bond differing in the dispersity of polymer carriers showed the potential of low-dispersed conjugates prepared using RAFT polymerization [38]. While the polymer precursors have the same M_w, about 30,000 g/mol, the dispersity was highly different ($Đ$ = 1.13, or 1.75) due to the utilization of controlled RAFT or free radical polymerization, respectively. The higher antitumor activity of the low-dispersed conjugate could be ascribed to an enhanced tumor accumulation due to the retention of polymer chains with sufficient molecular weights and vice versa the absence of fraction of polymer chains with lower molecular, which are fast cleared from the blood circulation and removed by urine. Therefore, it can be expected that such polymer–drug conjugates will be efficient in the treatment of solid tumors and still capable of carrier removal from the body.

The following more detailed study using fluorescently- or ^{89}Zr-labeled polymer carriers differing in dispersity and also in M_w showed similar results [39]. The pHPMA characterized by low dispersity ($Đ$ = 1.1) and M_w close to renal threshold ($M_w \approx 45$ kg/mol) prepared by RAFT polymerization exhibited the slowest blood clearance and the highest tumor accumulation, as was demonstrated by positron emission tomography (PET) on Figure 1.

Recently, also a thorough comparative study between polymer conjugates with THP bound by hydrazone bond differing in M_w (38,200 vs. 51,700 g/mol) and $Đ$ (1.92 vs. 1.17) showed approximately two times higher accumulation in sarcoma S-180 tumors in the majority of time intervals for the low-dispersed conjugate with M_w about the renal threshold [40]. Importantly, a quite high amount of polymer was found in urine within the first hour in the case of the high-dispersed polymer conjugate. Consequently, prolonged blood circulation and higher accumulation resulted in higher antitumor activity. Nevertheless, although the trend was repeatedly documented in these studies, the increase was not always significant. It was found that both polymer conjugates, despite their different accumulation rate in tumors, exhibited a similar therapeutic effect on early-stage tumors (initial volume about 40 mm^3), which have highly active angiogenesis and show better EPR effect. However, the efficacy of the low-dispersed conjugate was significantly higher than that of the high-dispersed conjugate during the treatment of well-developed S-180 tumors (initial volume about 150–250 mm^3).

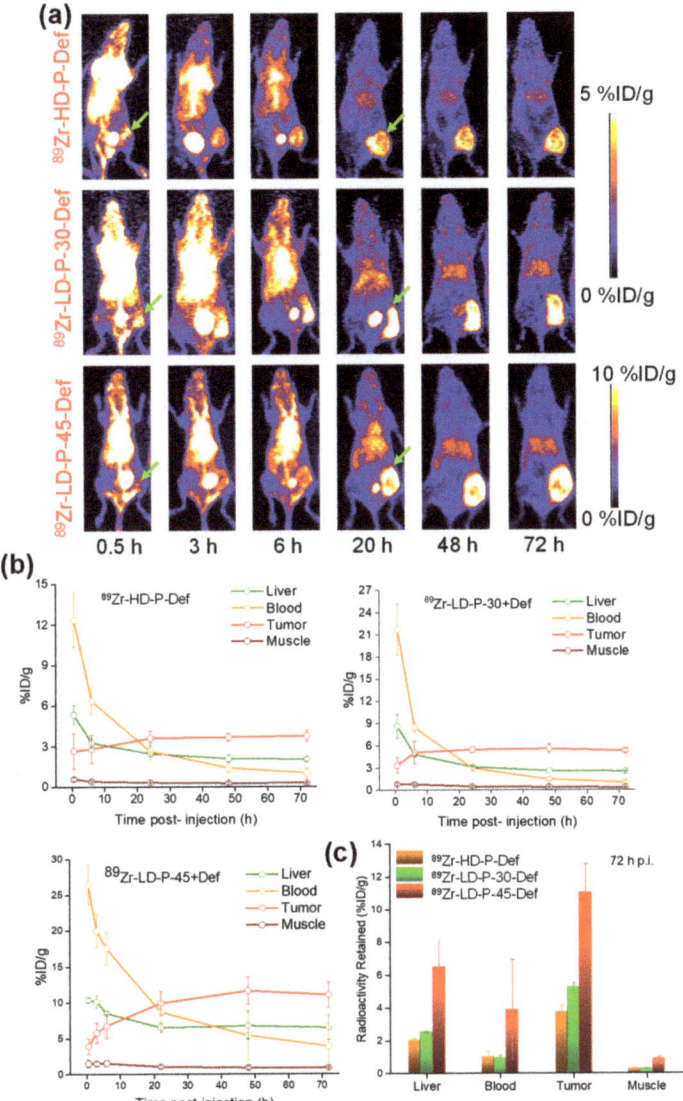

Figure 1. In vivo positron emission tomography (PET) imaging and biodistribution study: (**a**) serial maximum intensity projection (MIP) images, (**b**) time–activity curves, (**c**) and comparison of radioactivity retained in liver, blood, tumor and muscle of ^{89}Zr-labeled linear pHPMAs; HD-P + Def (M_w = 27,800 g/mol, Đ = 1.74), ^{89}Zr-LD-P-30 + Def (M_w = 33,300 g/mol, Đ = 1.06) and ^{89}Zr-LD-P-45 + Def (M_w = 45,200 g/mol, Đ = 1.07). Reprinted with permission from [39]. Copyright (2017) The Royal Society of Chemistry.

It can be concluded that pHPMAs characterized by quite low Đ and M_w near the limit of renal filtration is very promising carriers of imaging agents and/or drugs for highly efficient solid tumor treatment and diagnostics with minimal side effects.

Recently, linear pHPMAs have also been employed for the targeted delivery of anti-inflammatory drug dexamethasone [41,42]. Preferable accumulation of dexamethasone carrying nanomedicines within the inflamed tissue was detected, showing the potential of these nanomedicines to be passively accumulated within the inflammation tissue upon intravenous or intraperitoneal injection. Importantly, the intraperitoneal injection of these nanomedicines led to the highly elevated anti-inflammatory effect in the treatment of induced rheumatoid arthritis in mice or rats.

3.2. Biodegradable HMW Polymer Carriers

After it was recognized that pHPMAs accumulate in solid tumors due to the EPR effect in a molecular weight-dependent manner, various HMW biodegradable conjugates differing in the inner structure and biodegradability have been designed and synthesized. Four basic types of HMW nanomedicines have been designed and studied in detail, in, which diblock [43], multiblock [44–47], grafted [48], or star [49–52] structure was employed. All the HMW pHPMA constructs can be synthesized directly using modern controlled polymerization techniques [37,47] or by multiple-step synthesis. Star-shaped systems with high molecular weight could be synthesized via grafting-from approach utilizing the RAFT polymerization or via grafting to approach [52] employing the pre-prepared polymers for controlled grafting procedure.

As we discussed above in the Introduction, the effective extravasation of nanomedicines in solid tumors cannot be achieved above a certain limit. For example, star pHPMA above 600,000 g/mol, which corresponds to hydrodynamic size around 50 nm, exhibited markedly reduced accumulation in EL-4 lymphoma [14]. Moreover, also, there is a limit to renal filtration. While more flexible linear pHPMAs with M_w up to 70,000 g/mol can be excreted by the urine, more rigid star pHPMAs have a lower renal threshold of around 50,000 g/mol [17].

Biodegradable linear diblock or multiblock pHPMA drug carriers have been synthesized with the aim to create nanomedicines with prolonged blood circulation, and enhanced drug accumulation in solid tumors or inflamed tissues than that achieved previously by simple linear pHPMA. Disulfide spacers that are degraded reductively in the cytoplasm or GFLG spacers that are degraded enzymatically in lysosomes were positioned between polymer blocks, enabling intracellular polymer carrier degradation and the subsequent elimination of the resulting shorter degradation fragments. Importantly, the size of the polymer coil in solution controls the rate of polymer elimination by glomerular filtration rather than the polymer's M_w per se, although the M_w is a convenient and easily calculated measure and is often used as a characteristic for the elimination limit of polymers. The resulting long-circulating carriers have been used to deliver potent drugs (Dox [53], THP [54], gemcitabine [55], paclitaxel [44], prostaglandin [53]) and also proved its suitability for combination therapy, thus delivering a combination of drugs [56–58]. Biodegradation of the diblock conjugates in solution modeling the intracellular condition resulted in the formation of polymeric degradation products with M_w values below the renal threshold [59]. Another HMW biodegradable multiblock carriers and conjugates have been synthesized using well-defined diblocks as a click reaction substrate. Diblock precursors have been synthesized via RAFT polymerization using a specific GFLG oligopeptide containing chain-transfer agent, [45,47,60] Figure 2. All these diblock and multiblock conjugates have been summarized and reviewed last year by Kopeček and Yang [61].

A new simplified approach for the synthesis of biodegradable diblock carriers was published recently. In the novel synthetic route, the diblock copolymers are directly formed from linear pHPMAs with TTc end groups during the removal of these groups with butylamine in water. The molar ratio of butylamine and the TTc group (20:1) was selected to reach a high reaction yield. The formed thiol groups on the polymer ends in situ reacted with each other to form a disulfide bond between polymer chains. The conversion reached its maximum after 1 h (from 80 up to 90% of diblock was formed) [63].

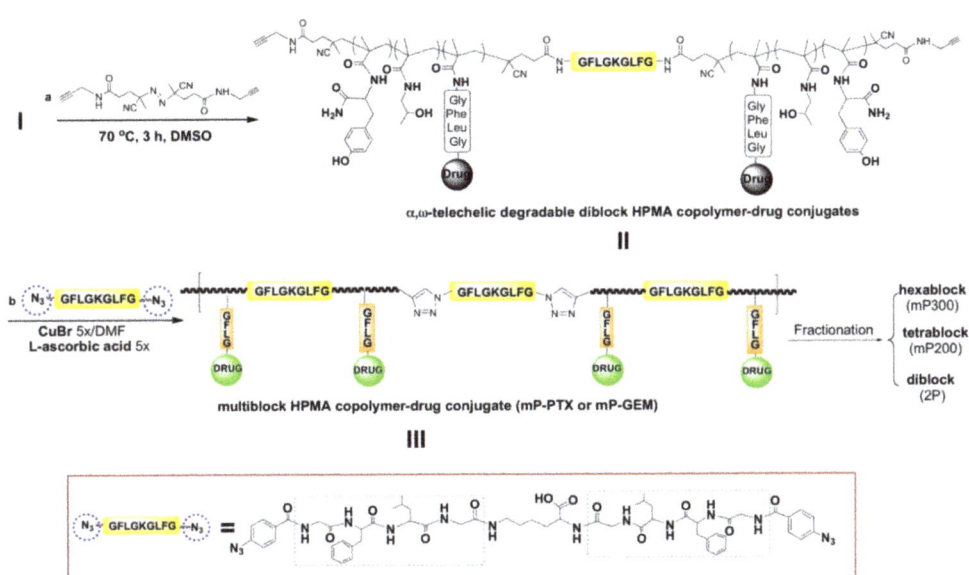

Figure 2. Synthesis of multiblock biodegradable *N*-(2-hydroxypropyl) methacrylamide (HPMA) copolymer (pHPMA)–drug conjugates. Reprinted with permission from [62]. Copyright (2017) American Chemical Society.

Grafted and branched polymer carriers received great attention in the 1990s and in the first decade of the current century. Today, they are out of the main interest of researchers and have been replaced by diblock or star-shaped structures due to controlled polymerization techniques. The results of grafted and branched pHPMA carriers have been partially summarized in a recent review [64].

The effect of size and 3D structure of pHPMA biomaterials on in vitro transport and in vivo organ accumulation was investigated thoroughly by Pearce et al. [65]. Through aqueous RAFT polymerization, they successfully produced a set of polymer materials spanning a size range from 5 to 60 nm, with the linear, hyperbranched, star, or self-assembling micellar structures and investigated the contribution of the structure, size and degradability on in vivo distribution by maintaining the same materials chemistry throughout. The results showed promising behavior of pHPMA biomaterials as stealth carriers both in vitro and in vivo. In vitro macrophage uptake studies demonstrated significantly different behaviors governed by surface zeta potential and size. The small hyperbranched structures were taken up by macrophages to a significantly lower degree than the larger hyperbranched and star constructs, which was in concordance with reduced mononuclear phagocytic system uptake and increased renal clearance in vivo. Hyperbranched and star carriers have been conjugated with anticancer drug Dox and showed improved efficacy over free drug in 2D and 3D cell culture models as well as in an aggressive orthotopic model of human triple-negative breast cancer in mice.

The newest members of the HMW conjugate family are the star-like conjugates. Star-shaped carriers based on pHPMA have been recently summarized in two reviews [64,66]. The newest generation of star-shaped nanomedicines based on pHPMA was synthesized with the grafting to approach using a biodegradable hyperbranched polyester core based on 2,2-bis (hydroxymethyl)propionic acid (bisMPA), described first by Kostková et al. [67]. In general, also the grafting from approach could be employed along with the development of novel controlled RAFT polymerization techniques, Figure 3. The HMW star system containing hydrolytically degradable ester bonds on a bis-MPA core was constructed as a long-circulating polymer carrier, enabling prolonged drug circulation with highly enhanced accumulation in solid tumors. The time-dependent hydrolytic biodegradation of the HMW system in normoxic physiologic conditions in model buffers and human plasma ensures the safe elimination of polymer carriers from the body after fulfilling their function. Moreover, the pH-sensitive release of the active drug Dox in a hypoxic tumor microenvironment showed the stimuli-responsive behavior of the star polymer conjugates.

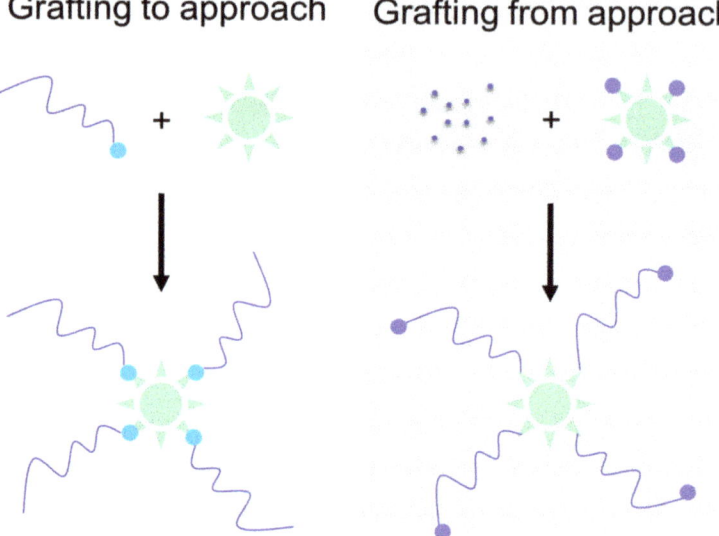

Figure 3. Schematic description of pHPMA-based star-like nanomedicine synthesis. The grafting-to approach is based on the covalent one-point attachment of semitelechelic polymer precursors (the light blue dot is reactive group on main chain end of polymer) onto the core (green star) containing functional groups. The grafting-from approach is employing the reversible addition–fragmentation transfer (RAFT) polymerization using the core containing several chain-transfer agents (violet dots) leading to the growth of the polymer chain from monomers (small violet dots) directly on the core.

Recently, a whole library of star materials based on semitelechelic pHPMAs and bisMPA cores was described, and the biological behavior in mice tumor models was determined, Figure 4 [52]. The hydrodynamic diameter of the star copolymer biomaterials was tuned from 13 to 31 nm, with corresponding molar mass ranged from 87 to 720 kg/mol. Therefore, the star nanomedicines and their size could be adjusted to a given purpose by a proper selection of the bisMPA dendritic core type and generation and by considering the semitelechelic copolymer M_w and polymer-to-core molar ratio. The hydrolytic degradation was proved for both the star copolymers containing either dendron or dendrimer core, in aqueous buffers and plasma in vitro and in vivo using PET imaging. An excellent clearance from the body was shown in vivo for the dendron-based material, with more than 60% of biomaterial mass eliminated after 7 days. It has been shown unequivocally that the therapy by the biodegradable star conjugate with attached Dox strongly the tumor growth in mice and was fully curative in most of the treated animals at a dose corresponding approximately to one-fourth of the maximum tolerated dose (MTD). The newly developed biodegradable star nanomedicines showed superior efficacy and tumor accumulation over the first generation of star copolymers containing a non-degradable PAMAM core.

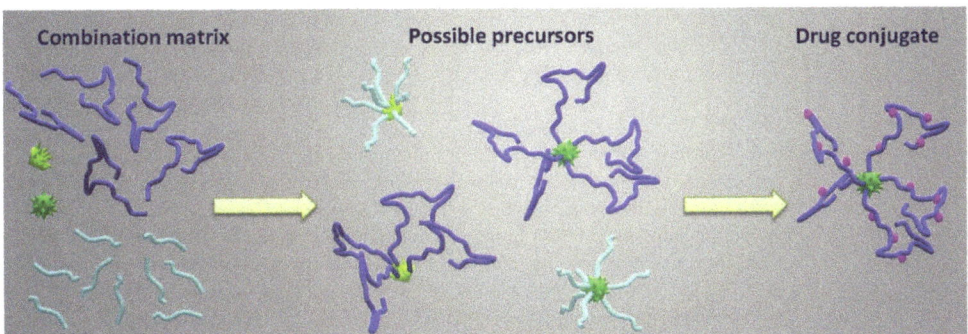

Figure 4. Schematic sketch of the formation of adjustable star-shaped nanomedicine based on semitelechelic pHPMAs and polyester-based core. Green stars are bisMPA cores, light and dark blue lines are polymers, violet dots represent drugs.

Indeed, the tumor spheroid penetration study showed identical penetration through spheroids of linear and star-like pHPMA and their constructs with pirarubicin. Nevertheless, the THP penetration after application of pHPMA conjugated THP was considerably deeper than for free THP, thus proving the benefits of polymer carriers, notwithstanding their inner structure [68]. Moreover, the cytotoxicity of THP conjugates against tumor cell spheroids was nearly the same as for free THP, whereas the 2D cell cytotoxicity of the pHPMA-conjugated drug is usually lower. Star-shape nanomedicines contain β- or γ-cyclodextrins as the biodegradable core have also been described recently [69]. Two synthetic approaches differing in the method of polymer grafting have been employed with the aim to obtain similar polymer carriers with different degradation rates.

3.3. Self-Assembled HMW Polymer Carriers

Another approach of how to prepare long-circulating HMW polymer carriers to consist of the utilization of self-assembled supramolecular structures, e.g., polymer micelles. Recently, micellar pHPMA nanomedicines with controlled degradation have been reviewed in detail [6,70]. Generally, amphiphilic copolymers self-assemble into supramolecular structures, usually termed as micelles, with a size exceeding the limit of the renal filtration. Moreover, polymer micelles disintegrate under their critical micellar concentration (CMC) into individual polymer chains, unimers, whose M_w should be under the limit of the renal threshold. The micelle-forming polymer carriers do not need to comprise any biodegradable linkages to enable their elimination from the body. It is a known fact that any shift in hydrophilicity of polymer carriers to a more hydrophobic nature could lead to undesired accumulation in the organism, often in the liver or other organs. Thus, there have been several attempts to disintegrate supramolecular structures after they deliver their cargo to the target tissue and facilitate their elimination from the body.

Typical structures of amphiphilic copolymers are block or graft copolymers. The hydrophobic blocks or molecules constitute the micelle core, which is surrounded by a hydrophilic shell formed by an HPMA homopolymer or copolymer, which should protect the micellar carrier from undesired interactions with proteins in blood and recognition by RES [6].

Amphiphilic block copolymers can be comprised of various diblock or triblock copolymers where the hydrophobic block consists of e.g., poly (laurylmethacrylate) [71], poly (ε-caprolactone) [72], poly (L-lactide) [73], poly (propyleneoxide) [74]. Moreover, the hydrophobic block can also be formed by pHPMA modified with valproate [75], or monolactate, dilactate, or benzoyl [76] on the hydroxyl group of HPMA. After hydrolyzes of these ester bonds, the hydrophilicity of the polymer carrier increased, and the micellar structure disintegrates. Similar behavior is also expected in the case of hydrolytically degradable polyesters core-containing amphiphilic copolymers mentioned above. Indeed, amphiphilic copolymers can also be designed as graft copolymers. Recently, semitelechelic pHPMA have been grafted to poly (ε-caprolactone) by azide-alkyne click reaction leading to the formation of amphiphilic copolymer self-assembling to micelles enabling both the physical entrapment of hydrophobic drugs, i.e., venetoclax, and covalent attachment via pH-sensitive hydrazone bond, i.e., Dox [77].

Another approach consists in the "decorating" of a hydrophilic polymer chain with rather small hydrophobic molecules. Oleyl, dodecyl, or various cholesterol-derived moieties have been attached to linear pHPMAs and used as carriers of Dox [78–80]. Alternatively, a hydrophobic moiety can be introduced into the hydrophilic polymer main chain end. For example, the presence of hexaleucine oligopeptide resulted in the formation of micelles [81]. Interestingly, hydrophobic moieties have been bound to pHPMA by means of a pH-sensitive hydrazone bond, enabling the tumor low pH-driven disintegration of supramolecular structure, Figure 5 [79,82]. In this case, the stability of the micellar structure at neutral pH strongly influenced the extent of their accumulation in solid tumors. The overall stability of micelles can be additionally improved by core crosslinking using, e.g., disulfide bridges [83] or hydrazone linkages [80], which can be further reduced by glutathione, or hydrolyzed in tumor cells, respectively. Another important feature for the successful utilization of amphiphilic polymer drug carriers in medicine is the absence of interaction with serum proteins, i.e., non-fouling behavior. Such proof was described for albumin and several other proteins and cholesterol-based pHPMA micelles [84–86].

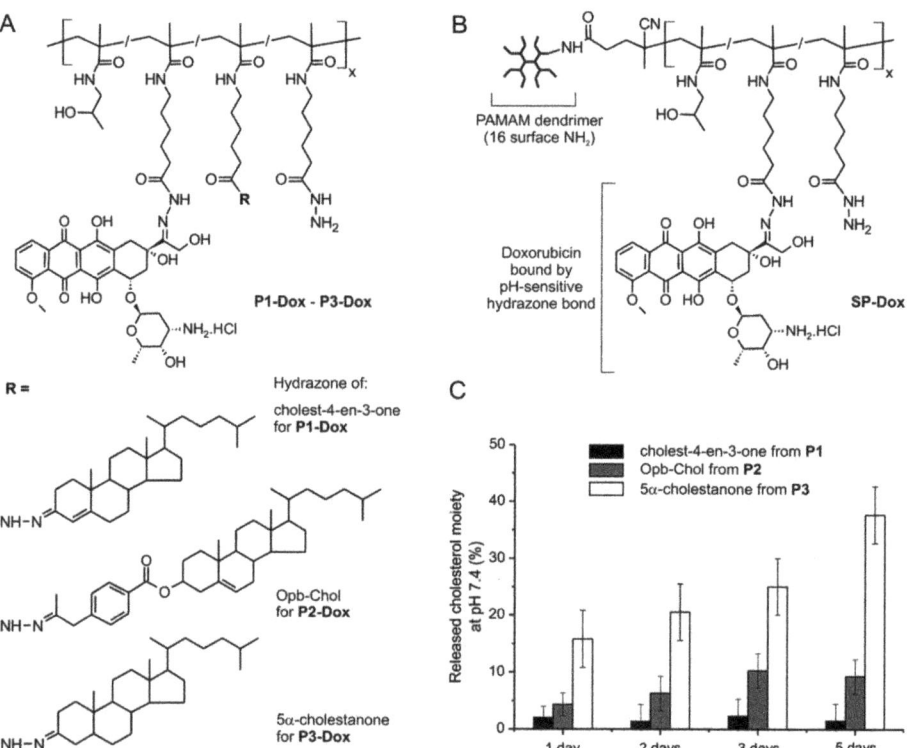

Figure 5. Schematic structure of amphiphilic pHPMA−doxorubicin (Dox) conjugates P1–P3 differing in the hydrophobic moiety (**A**) and star pHPMA−Dox conjugate (**B**). Release of cholesterol moieties from copolymers P1–P3 at pH 7.4 and 37 °C, mimicking the bloodstream environment (**C**). Reprinted with permission from [82]. Copyright© American Chemical Society (2018).

Generally, drugs can be entrapped in the micellar core or bound by biodegradable bonds, which can enable precise control over drug release. Often, the covalent attachment of hydrophobic drugs switched the physicochemical properties of the conjugates to a more hydrophobic or amphiphilic nature according to the content and chemical structure of drugs. For example, the polymer coil of linear polymer conjugates with Dox bound by the hydrazone bond collapsed with the increasing content of the drug [87]. The second virial coefficient changed to negative at about 13 wt %, and at about 18 wt %, the formation of dynamic aggregates was observed. Such behavior was found even for different drugs, e.g., docetaxel, dexamethasone [11,56]. However, in the case of a much more hydrophobic drug, betulinic acid, the formation of micelles was determined [88]. Here, the micelles were disintegrated after the drug derivative release in an acidic condition of tumor cells and thus facilitated polymer carrier elimination.

A specific part of micelle-forming polymer carriers represents thermoresponsive copolymers that are characterized by low critical solution temperature. They form micelles above a certain temperature, while they are fully soluble as polymer coils at room temperature, which is important for the simple and define preparation of micellar samples. Block or statistical copolymers of HPMA and N-isopropylacrylamide (NIPAM) [89], 2-(2-methoxyethoxy) ethyl methacrylate (DEGMA) [90,91], or HPMA-dilactate [92] have been synthesized and transition temperature set by tuning of monomer ratio.

4. Augmentation of the Passive Accumulation in Solid Tumors

Current clinical results of conventional chemotherapy are still not appropriate even they are used in clinical practice for more than 60 years [93]. The major issue in the insufficient anticancer efficacy is driven by the lack of tumor selectivity of such anticancer drugs. Thus, the development of selective tumor-targeted drug systems, i.e., nanomedicines, is an urgent need in current anticancer therapy. Within the last decades, molecular drugs have attracted serious attention, as they target important particular molecules, growth factors, and/or specific oncogenes highly expressed by tumor cells. Their preclinical results were highly positive, showing their serious potential to treat tumor cells of various origins. Nevertheless, recently described results of the clinical investigation have not fully confirmed the positive expectations. These investigations showed unsatisfactory results in the efficacy of molecular target drugs, especially for solid tumors [94]. There are several pieces of evidence that the intrinsic heterogeneity of tumors and several mutations in individual patients may lead to the failure of these treatments [95]. It is believed that the intratumor heterogeneity, associated with heterogeneous protein function, can cause and foster tumor adaptation and therapeutic failure through a Darwinian selection of tumor cells.

Moreover, even nanomedicines showing excellent efficacy in mice models when intravenously injected do not effectively reach the tumors due to the biological barriers in the body [96]. Importantly, the use of nanomedicines in humans often resulted in a lack of overall patient response and survival [97]. The PEGylated liposomal Dox nanoformulations (Doxil®) generally reached safety improvements, but not an increase in efficacy compared to the standard therapies [98]. Recently, considerable effort has been expended to develop advanced nanomedicines alternative to the approved liposomal formulations; unfortunately, their clinical translation has been frequently depleted by various technical, cost, and efficacy-related issues. Thus, skepticism about the use of nanomedicines increased in the scientific community in recent years [99].

Extensive angiogenesis is the key factor in tumorigenesis of early growth stages of solid tumors, thus enabling accelerated tumor growth as the cancer cells are fully supplied by nutrients and oxygen. As a consequence, the early-staged solid tumors are often endowed with higher vascular density compared with normal healthy tissues. Indeed, for large-size tumors, more precisely in late-stages, the vascular blood flow is, on the contrary, seriously obstructed. In that case, the needs of tumor cells are not fulfilled, as the vascular oxygen supply and nutrients are not sufficiently delivered, and tumor tissues become strongly hypoxic, the tumor cells are dying, and tumors become avascular [100].

Nevertheless, most clinical tumors are large and advanced or late-stage tumors, and their structure is known for the necrotic and avascular areas that lead to an insufficient EPR effect [101]. Recently, it was found that tumor tissue coagulation or thrombogenicity was highly enhanced as tumors grew up [102,103], which lead to the occlusion and blocking of tumor blood vessels and consequently to a poor EPR effect, highly depleting the success of cancer chemotherapy in advanced cancer. Moreover, tumor interstitial fluid pressure (IFP) has become an important barrier to efficient drug delivery via the EPR effect [104]. Most solid tumors are connected with increased IFP, which is most probably linked to the osmotic pressure of the extravasated fluid and the dysfunctional lymphatic system of tumor tissues. Importantly, the rapid growth of tumors reporting a short doubling time of 24 h to 1 week will, in addition, enhance the physical and mechanical pressure that can be even summed up with osmotic pressure, which is caused by increases in tumor mass [93]. In summary, advanced large tumors are frequently heterogeneous containing regions of defective vasculature and highly restricted blood flow, which finally deplete the EPR effect and linked drug delivery to tumors.

Recently, a novel approach based on the augmentation of the EPR effect was described [101,105]. Various vascular mediators, the nitric oxide (NO) generators nitroglycerin (NG) [106], hydroxyurea [107], and L-arginine [105], have been studied as potential enhancers of the EPR effect in order to improve the therapeutic effect of nanomedicines (Figure 6). It was described that all the studied compounds are able to generate the NO with relatively high selectivity in solid tumors [105]. The augmentation of therapeutic effect via the EPR effect enhancement was studied in detail using pHPMA nanomedicines carrying cytostatic drug THP, or photodynamic therapy (PDT) nanoprobes pyropheophorbide-a, or zinc protoporphyrin. Interestingly, the NO-donor–base augmentation significantly increased, almost twice, the tumor accumulation of nanomedicines and nanoprobes in various solid tumor models. As a consequence, the antitumor effects, either cytostatic or PDT-based, were also markedly improved, showing the potential for further clinical application. Indeed, in a murine autochthonous colon tumor, NO donors markedly enhanced the therapeutic effects of THP bearing pHPMA even after one single administration, and the therapy outcome was comparable with those achieved with three weekly nanomedicines treatments. Moreover, a similar positive effect of the NO donors was described in the compassionate use in human trials. Nitroglycerine was used to increase the efficacy of the THP bearing polymer conjugates in a patient with stage IV prostate cancer [108]. The augmentation of the EPR effect, in this case, led to the enhanced efficacy proving even the remission of the lung and bone metastasis.

Similarly, carbon monoxide (CO) was utilized as a potential enhancer of the EPR effect. Recently, Fang et al. employed two CO generating agents, either extrinsic CO donor micelle containing tricarbonyldichlororuthenium (II) dimer or endogenous CO donor using PEGylated hemin inducing heme oxygenase-1 [109]. It was proved that the agents induced the generation of CO selectively in solid tumors, thus enhanced the EPR effect leading to a two- to three-fold increased tumor accumulation of used nanomedicines. Importantly, the CO enhancers worked similarly for the pHPMA nanomedicines containing THP as well as for the pHPMA nanoprobe with pyropheophorbide-a. The application of CO generators altogether with anticancer nanomedicines resulted in a significant increase of efficacy in various transplanted solid tumor models.

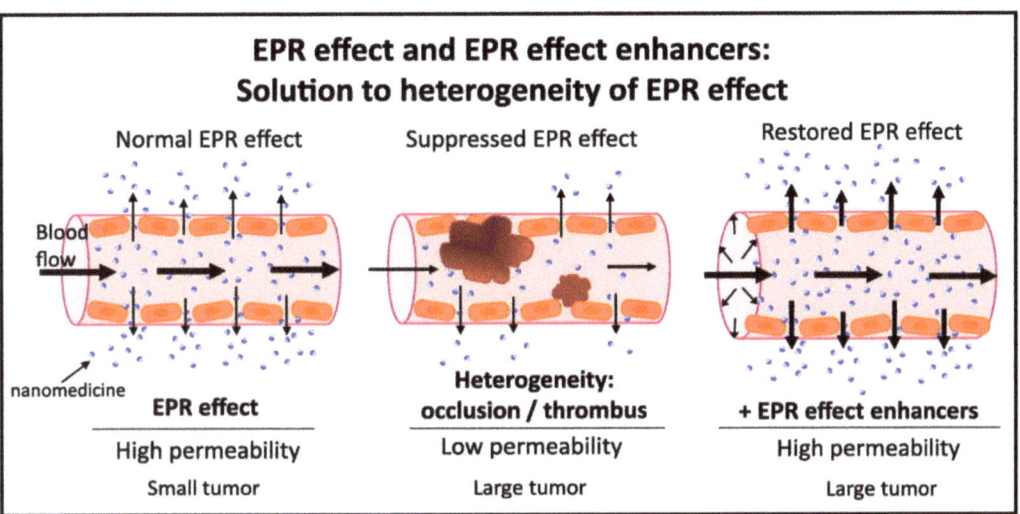

Figure 6. Schematic description of the enhanced and permeability retention (EPR) effect and application of EPR effect enhancers for the solution of heterogenicity of tumor tissue. Reprinted with permission from [101]. Copyright (2020) Elsevier B.V. (Amsterdam, Netherlands).

As mentioned above, the utilization of low-molecular-weight NO and CO donors leads to the enhancement of nanomedicine accumulation and efficacy in the treatment of various solid tumor models. Nevertheless, the use of small NO and CO donors could also cause vasodilatation in healthy organs leading in combination with nanomedicines to some obstructions. Thus, another approach based on the binding of the organic nitrate precursor of NO to a water-soluble pHPMAs was published [110], Figure 7. Four different pHPMA-bound NO donors differing in structure and hydrolytic stability have been investigated. These polymer-bound NO donors have been able to overcome some drawbacks related to low-molecular-weight NO-releasing compounds, namely systemic toxicity, lack of site-specificity, and fast blood clearance.

A significant increase in the EPR effect was found for pHPMA-Dox conjugate in a murine lymphoma model. The augmentation of the EPR effect enhanced the therapeutic outcome of Dox-containing nanomedicines, but not of free Dox. Similarly, the study using an S-nitrosated human serum albumin dimer was recently published, showing the synergistic effect when used as a pretreatment agent in albumin-bound paclitaxel nanoparticle (Abraxane®) therapy carried on various tumor models [111,112]. Interestingly, in the C26 murine colon cancer, the NO-generating dimer enhanced tumor selectivity of paclitaxel containing nanoparticle and attenuated myelosuppression. Augmentation of the tumor growth inhibition during the treatment by paclitaxel bearing nanoparticles was also seen in the low vascular permeable B16 murine melanoma model. In summary, the tumor-site localized augmentation of the EPR effect via the polymer-bound NO delivery system is recognized as a highly promising strategy to a highly potentiate nanomedicines-based tumor therapy without increasing systemic toxicity. The proper selection of delivering vectors altogether with the proper NO release profile should be investigated for further development.

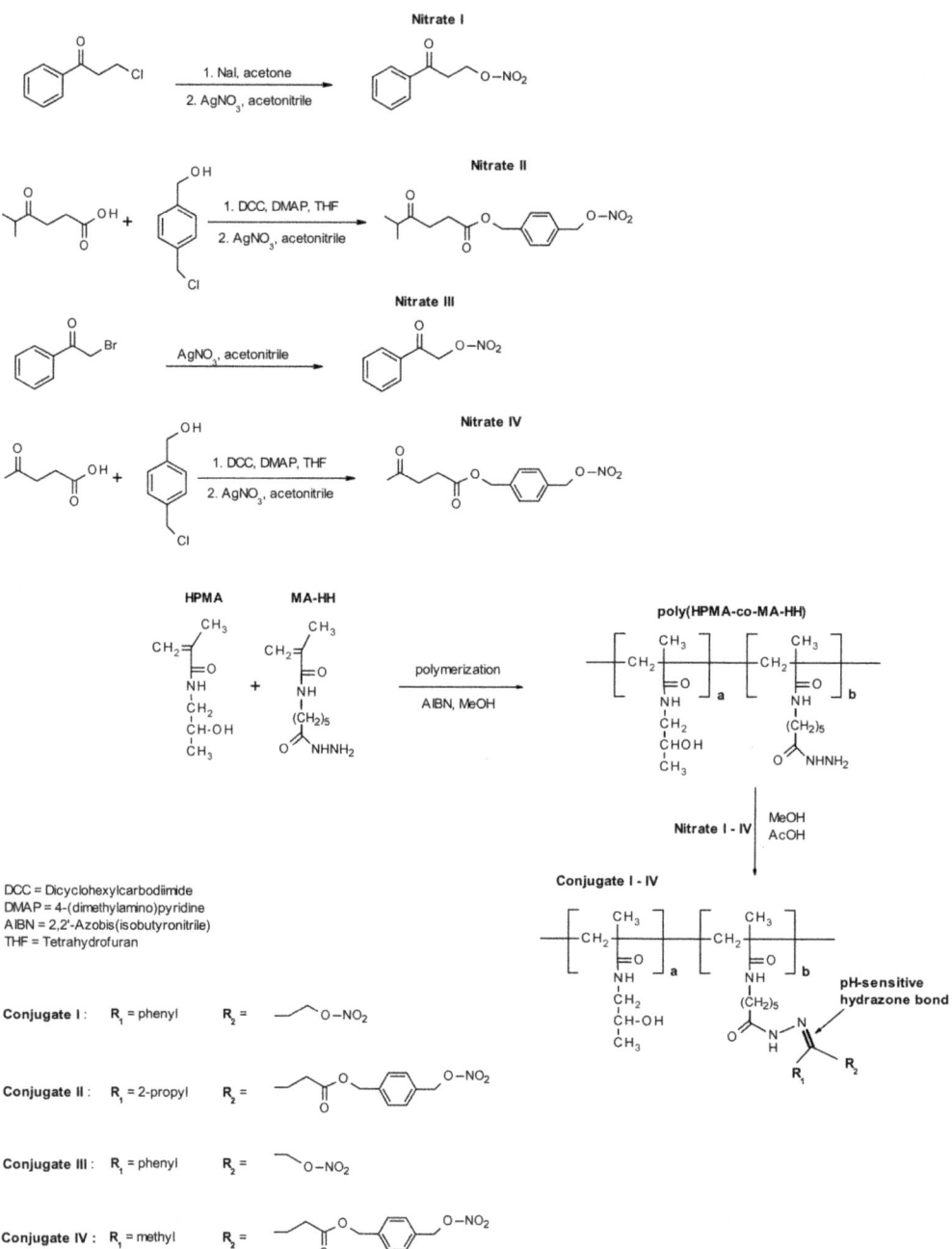

Figure 7. Synthesis of polymer-bound nitric oxide (NO) donors. Reprinted with permission from [110]. Copyright (2018) Elsevier B.V. (Amsterdam, Netherlands).

5. Active Targeting Versus Passive Accumulation of pHPMA Nanomedicines

Generally, targeted nanomedicines have several advantages, which lays mainly in the protection of healthy cells during the treatment, serious reduction of the side adverse effects, and overcoming various biological barriers making the cancer cells highly resistant to the treatment [6]. Highly specific characteristics of the tumor tissue in general and of its microenvironment made it possible to design nanomedicines that are able to deliver biologically active molecules, e.g., drugs, to tumors [113]. Conventional anticancer drugs show inappropriate pharmacokinetics and are localized within the body nonspecifically. Thus, it is impossible to solely reach the target tumor tissue, and their use is associated with serious side effects. The development of nanomedicines enabled more favorable pharmacokinetics and enhanced tumor accumulation. It has been generally accepted that nanomedicines can reach solid tumors through the leaky vasculature utilizing the above-mentioned EPR effect. Nevertheless, specific targeting of the tumor tissue is still a remaining challenge for researchers around the world, especially in the case of poorly vascularized and dispersed tumors. The interest has been focused on nanomedicines bearing specific molecules enabling to mediate the active targeting by selective interaction to the receptors overexpressed on the cancer cells or tumor endothelium. Recently, a huge number of reviews was published discussing the possibility and pros and cons of passive nanomedicine accumulation and active targeting [114,115].

Already in the 1990s, Seymour et al. described the influence of M_w of pHPMA on passive accumulation in tumors, namely sarcoma 180 or B16F10 melanoma models [116]. From this time, an enormous number of reports describing the dependence of passive accumulation of polymers onto their structure, M_w and size was published [5,117,118]. The tumor-selective accumulation was improved either by the synthesis of more complex structures, e.g., grafted, multiblock, or star polymers, or by the controlled self-assembly of the amphiphilic HPMA copolymers [66,70], or by the utilization of various EPR effect enhancers as we discussed in previous chapters.

On the other hand, many attempts have been made to design and synthesize actively targeted pHPMA nanomedicines. Various targeting ligands, e.g., monoclonal antibodies, immunoglobulins, peptides, lectins, saccharides, have been employed and studied in detail [6]. In general, the two targeting approaches have been employed, i.e., direct targeting to cell receptors overexpressed on the tumor cell or tumor endothelium as the final destination of the targeting ligand. Generally, the targeting efficacy was found significantly higher for the monoclonal antibodies in contrast to smaller molecular weight targeting ligands. Even in the case of multiple presentations of oligopeptides originated from the active site of antibodies, it is not able to reach the same affinity to their target ligands [119]. Recently, the targeting efficacy of antibody-targeted pHPMA nanomedicines was reviewed in detail [120].

Importantly, H. Maeda recently analyzed repeated failures in cancer therapy for solid tumors [93]. Regardless of the huge financial support of bullet-like therapies targeting site-specific cancers, i.e., molecular drugs for the depletion of specific enzymes such as kinases or inhibitors of growth factor receptors, the therapeutic results are unsatisfactory and disappointing. The main scientific reasons leading to the malfunction of the mentioned drug development approaches should be linked to the infinite number of genetic mutations in a chaotic molecular environment of solid tumor tissue. It was found, the outcome failure rates of approximately 90% on current therapeutic approaches for solid tumors are estimated. Partial success was achieved with drugs such as Gleevec or few other molecules that are used for treating patients with hematopoietic cancers and soft tissue or seminoma. Similar to the new molecular therapies, the active targeting in the case of solid tumors reach the limitation of a huge number of genetic mutations in the tumor environment, which strongly suppresses the overall targeting ability of solid tumors. Nevertheless, the antibody-targeted pHPMA nanomedicines reached significant benefits in the treatment efficacy in the case of various hematological malignancies studies in vivo. Various lymphomas [121,122] and leukemias [123,124] have been efficiently eradicated by the antibody-targeted pHPMA conjugates, showing the potential of the active targeting in the case of hematological malignancies, which are known for low genetic mutations in contrast to other solid tumors [93].

Indeed, the efficacy of the active targeting was also thoroughly studied in a time-dependent manner to prove the potential benefit of the active targeting. Either epidermal growth factor (EGF)-based [125] or tumor endothelium-based targeting [119] have been employed to study the time dependence of the active targeting. In both cases, it was observed that the active targeting is worth being effective in short times up to the 1 or 4 h, respectively. After that time, the passive accumulation of nanomedicines with similar hydrodynamic sizes reach the same accumulation as the actively targeted polymer conjugates. Specifically, in mice bearing both highly leaky CT26 and poorly leaky BxPC3 tumors, it was observed that tumor vascular endothelium could be targeted effectively, showing the rapid and efficient early binding to tumor blood vessels [125]. Nevertheless, over a short period of time, the passive targeting based on the EPR-driven accumulation highly prevailed, leading to a higher overall accumulation. Similarly, the EGF-targeting to FaDu head and neck carcinoma in mice showed a short time effective prevalence of the active targeting showing the rapid accumulation in tumors within 15 min. Nevertheless, after 4 h, the nontargeted star-like nanosystems reached the same accumulation of similarly sized antibody-targeted conjugates [119].

In summary, the active targeting seems to be suitable for the design of highly effective nanomedicines, especially against the hematological malignancies, where in the last decade, several antibody–drug conjugates have been approved for clinical use [120]. In the case of solid tumors of other origins, it seems that the passive targeting based on the tumor microenvironment abnormalities is more favorable and should be taken into consideration more frequently.

6. Future Prospects

Within the last three decades, a serious number of structures of pHPMA prodrugs have been designed, synthesized and their properties have been described. Even though most of them showed highly promising therapeutic activity or imaging properties in animal models during preclinical development, only a few of them came to any clinical evaluation. Unfortunately, none of them have been approved so far for clinics and marketed yet.

Nevertheless, for future prospects, the application of novel controlled polymerization techniques and advanced synthetic routes, including click chemistry and oriented binding, should enlarge the potential of the wider exploitation of pHPMA-prodrug-based nanomedicines, as shown recently in compassionate clinical use [108]. Employment of tailored tumor-, inflammation- or bacteria-linked stimuli-sensitive spacers should enlarge the importance of the controlled drug release. Similarly, controlled biodegradability of novel pHPMA structures should lead to the next-generation of pHPMA nanomedicines with higher clinical potential. Thus, to sum up, the design of tailor-made pHPMA nanomedicines with increased specificity of tissue- or cell-specific drug delivery is a promising step in terms of future applicability of these prodrugs.

It was shown that the efficacy of passively targeted nanomedicines could be highly improved by the controlled application of various EPR-effect enhanced, both the low-molecular-weight compounds and polymer-based enhancers. Most probably, the application combining the augmentation of the EPR effect with tailored nanomedicines will improve the therapeutic efficacy of such polymer–drug conjugates and thus even their clinical usefulness. Last, but not least, the strong potential is envisioned also in controlled drug delivery for the treatment of specific inflammatory diseases, i.e., site-specific rheumatic musculoskeletal diseases or bacterial infections.

Nevertheless, recently a study showing that the interendothelial gaps in the tumor endothelium are not responsible for the transport of nanoparticles into solid tumors was published [126]. Importantly, the authors found that up to 97% of nanoparticles are entering tumors using an active process through endothelial cells. These results could open a new paradigm for developing cancer nanomedicines and could suggest novel approaches using the understanding of these active pathways to unlock strategies to enhance tumor accumulation.

Author Contributions: P.C., L.K., T.E. contributed to writing the manuscript. P.C., T.E. was responsible for funding, T.E. was responsible for leadership. All authors reviewed and edited the manuscript. All authors have read and agreed to the published version of the manuscript.

Funding: This work was supported by the Czech Science Foundation (projects 20-04790S and 17-08084S) and by the Ministry of Health of the Czech Republic (project NU20-08-00255).

Institutional Review Board Statement: Not applicable.

Informed Consent Statement: Not applicable.

Conflicts of Interest: The authors declare no conflict of interest.

References

1. Farokhzad, O.C.; Langer, R. Impact of nanotechnology on drug delivery. *ACS Nano* **2009**, *3*, 16–20. [CrossRef] [PubMed]
2. Ulbrich, K.; Šubr, V. Structural and chemical aspects of HPMA copolymers as drug carriers. *Adv. Drug Deliv. Rev.* **2010**, *62*, 150–166. [CrossRef] [PubMed]
3. Chytil, P.; Koziolová, E.; Etrych, T.; Ulbrich, K. HPMA Copolymer-Drug Conjugates with Controlled Tumor-Specific Drug Release. *Macromol. Biosci.* **2018**, *18*. [CrossRef] [PubMed]
4. Venditto, V.J.; Szoka, F.C. Cancer nanomedicines: So many papers and so few drugs! *Adv. Drug Deliv. Rev.* **2013**, *65*, 80–88. [CrossRef] [PubMed]
5. Chytil, P.; Kostka, L.; Etrych, T. Structural design and synthesis of polymer prodrugs. In *Polymers for Biomedicine: Synthesis, Characterization, and Applications*; Scholz, C., Ed.; John Wiley and Sons: Hoboken, NJ, USA, 2017; p. 624.
6. Ulbrich, K.; Holá, K.; Šubr, V.; Bakandritsos, A.; Tuček, J.; Zbořil, R. Targeted Drug Delivery with Polymers and Magnetic Nanoparticles: Covalent and Noncovalent Approaches, Release Control, and Clinical Studies. *Chem. Rev.* **2016**, *116*, 5338–5431. [CrossRef] [PubMed]
7. Bag, M.A.; Valenzuela, L.M. Impact of the Hydration States of Polymers on Their Hemocompatibility for Medical Applications: A Review. *Int. J. Mol. Sci.* **2017**, *18*, 1422. [CrossRef] [PubMed]
8. Lin, W.; Klein, J. Control of surface forces through hydrated boundary layers. *Curr. Opin. Colloid Interface Sci.* **2019**, *44*, 94–106. [CrossRef]
9. Maeda, H.; Nakamura, H.; Fang, J. The EPR effect for macromolecular drug delivery to solid tumors: Improvement of tumor uptake, lowering of systemic toxicity, and distinct tumor imaging in vivo. *Adv. Drug Deliv. Rev.* **2013**, *65*, 71–79. [CrossRef] [PubMed]
10. Šírová, M.; Mrkvan, T.; Etrych, T.; Chytil, P.; Rossmann, P.; Ibrahimová, M.; Kovář, L.; Ulbrich, K.; Říhová, B. Preclinical Evaluation of Linear HPMA-Doxorubicin Conjugates with pH-Sensitive Drug Release: Efficacy, Safety, and Immunomodulating Activity in Murine Model. *Pharm. Res.* **2010**, *27*, 200–208. [CrossRef]
11. Etrych, T.; Šírová, M.; Starovoytova, L.; Říhová, B.; Ulbrich, K. HPMA Copolymer Conjugates of Paclitaxel and Docetaxel with pH-Controlled Drug Release. *Mol. Pharm.* **2010**, *7*, 1015–1026. [CrossRef]
12. Nakamura, H.; Etrych, T.; Chytil, P.; Ohkubo, M.; Fang, J.; Ulbrich, K.; Maeda, H. Two step mechanisms of tumor selective delivery of N-(2-hydroxypropyl)methacrylamide copolymer conjugated with pirarubicin via an acid-cleavable linkage. *J. Control. Release* **2014**, *174*, 81–87. [CrossRef]
13. Noguchi, Y.; Wu, J.; Duncan, R.; Strohalm, J.; Ulbrich, K.; Akaike, T.; Maeda, H. Early Phase Tumor Accumulation of Macromolecules: A Great Difference in Clearance Rate between Tumor and Normal Tissues. *Jpn. J. Cancer Res.* **1998**, *89*, 307–314. [CrossRef]
14. Etrych, T.; Kovář, L.; Strohalm, J.; Chytil, P.; Říhová, B.; Ulbrich, K. Biodegradable star HPMA polymer-drug conjugates: Biodegradability, distribution and anti-tumor efficacy. *J. Control. Release* **2011**, *154*, 241–248. [CrossRef]
15. Duncan, R.; Vicent, M.J. Polymer therapeutics-prospects for 21st century: The end of the beginning. *Adv. Drug Deliv. Rev.* **2013**, *65*, 60–70. [CrossRef]
16. Seymour, L.W.; Duncan, R.; Strohalm, J.; Kopeček, J. Effect of Molecular-Weight (Mw) of N-(2-Hydroxypropyl)Methacrylamide Copolymers on Body Distribution and Rate of Excretion after Subcutaneous, Intraperitoneal, and Intravenous Administration to Rats. *J. Biomed. Mater. Res.* **1987**, *21*, 1341–1358. [CrossRef]
17. Etrych, T.; Šubr, V.; Strohalm, J.; Šírová, M.; Říhová, B.; Ulbrich, K. HPMA copolymer-doxorubicin conjugates: The effects of molecular weight and architecture on biodistribution and in vivo activity. *J. Control. Release* **2012**, *164*, 346–354. [CrossRef]
18. Drobník, J.; Kopecek, J.; Labský, J.; Rejmanová, P.; Exner, J.; Kálal, J. Preparation of Biologically Active Substances Bearing NH2 Groups in a Form Releasable by Enzymatic Cleavage. U.S. Patent 4 097,470, 27 June 1978.

19. Kopeček, J.; Ulbrich, K.; Vacík, J.; Strohalm, J.; Chytrý, V.; Drobník, J.; Kálal, J. Copolymers Based on N-Substituted Acrylamides, N-Substituted Methacrylamides and N,N-Disubstituted Acrylamides and the Method of Their Manufacturing. U.S. Patent 4,062,831, 13 December 1977.
20. Štěrba, O.; Uhlířová, Z.; Petz, R. Duxon—A new Czechoslovak-made infusion solution—An experimental contribution to biological evaluation. *Cas. Lek. Cesk.* **1980**, *119*, 994–997.
21. Šprincl, L.; Exner, J.; Štěrba, O.; Kopeček, J. New types of synthetic infusion solutions. III. Elimination and retention of poly-[N-(2-hydroxypropyl)methacrylamide] in a test organism. *J. Biomed. Mater. Res.* **1976**, *10*, 953–963. [CrossRef]
22. Uhlířová, Z.; Jirásek, A.; Štěrba, O. Newly developed Czechoslovak colloid infusion solution Duxon. Preclinical trial. *Cas. Lek. Cesk.* **1981**, *120*, 1553–1556.
23. Cinátl, J.; Štěrba, O.; Paluska, E. New types of synthetic infusion solutions. The effect of Duxon on the proliferation of cells in vitro. *Cesko-Slov. Farm.* **1980**, *29*, 134–138.
24. Korcáková, L.; Paluska, E.; Hašková, V.; Kopeček, J. A simple test for immunogenicity of colloidal infusion solutions; the draining lymph node activation. *Z. Immun.* **1976**, *151*, 219–223. [CrossRef]
25. Paluska, E.; Cinátl, J.; Korcáková, L.; Štěrba, O.; Kopeček, J.; Hrubá, A.; Nezvalová, J.; Staněk, R. Immunosuppressive Effects of a Synthetic-Polymer Poly N-(2-Hydroxypropyl)Methacrylamide (Duxon). *Folia Biol-Prague* **1980**, *26*, 304–311.
26. Petz, R.; Štěrba, O.; Jirásek, A.; Foltinská, Z.; Kostírová, D.; Kopeček, J. Pharmacological evaluation of the toxicity after repeated administration of synthetic colloid solution of Duxon. *Cas. Lek. Cesk.* **1988**, *127*, 553–555. [PubMed]
27. Štěrba, O.; Paluska, E.; Jozová, O. New types of synthetic infusion solutions. Basic biological properties of poly(N-(2 hydroxypropyl) methacrylamide) (Czech). *Cas. Lek. Cesk.* **1975**, *114*, 1268–1270. [PubMed]
28. Uhlířová, Z.; Štěrba, O.; Petz, R.; Viktora, L. Czechoslovak infusion solution Duxon—Preclinical tests. Effect on the haemogram of some laboratory animals (author's transl). *Cas. Lek. Cesk.* **1980**, *119*, 1091–1094.
29. Štěrba, O.; Paluska, E.; Jozová, O.; Spunda, J.; Nezvalová, J.; Šprincl, L.; Kopeček, J.; Cinátl, J. New types of synthetic infusion solutions. Basic biological properties of poly N (2 hydroxypropyl) methacrylamide. *Rev. Czech. Med.* **1976**, *22*, 152–156.
30. Paluska, E.; Hrubá, A.; Štěrba, O.; Kopeček, J. Effect of a synthetic poly N-(2-hydroxypropyl)methacrylamide (Duxon) on haemopoiesis and graft-versus-host reaction. *Folia Biol-Prague* **1986**, *32*, 91–102.
31. Říhová, B.; Kopeček, J.; Ulbrich, K.; Pospíšil, M.; Mančal, P. Effect of the chemical structure of N-(2-hydroxypropyl) methacrylajnide copolymers on their ability to induce antibody formation in inbred strains of mice. *Biomaterials* **1984**, *5*, 143–148. [CrossRef]
32. Hoffmann, S.; Vystrčilová, L.; Ulbrich, K.; Etrych, T.; Caysa, H.; Mueller, T.; Mäder, K. Dual Fluorescent HPMA Copolymers for Passive Tumor Targeting with pH-Sensitive Drug Release: Synthesis and Characterization of Distribution and Tumor Accumulation in Mice by Noninvasive Multispectral Optical Imaging. *Biomacromolecules* **2012**, *13*, 652–663. [CrossRef]
33. Chytil, P.; Hoffmann, S.; Schindler, L.; Kostka, L.; Ulbrich, K.; Caysa, H.; Mueller, T.; Mader, K.; Etrych, T. Dual fluorescent HPMA copolymers for passive tumor targeting with pH- sensitive drug release II: Impact of release rate on biodistribution. *J. Control. Release* **2013**, *172*, 504–512. [CrossRef]
34. Liu, X.-M.; Quan, L.-D.; Tian, J.; Alnouti, Y.; Fu, K.; Thiele, G.; Wang, D. Synthesis and Evaluation of a Well-defined HPMA Copolymer–Dexamethasone Conjugate for Effective Treatment of Rheumatoid Arthritis. *Pharm. Res.* **2008**, *25*, 2910–2919. [CrossRef]
35. Pan, H.; Sima, M.; Kopečková, P.; Wu, K.; Gao, S.; Liu, J.; Wang, D.; Miller, S.C.; Kopeček, J. Biodistribution and Pharmacokinetic Studies of Bone-Targeting N-(2-Hydroxypropyl)methacrylamide Copolymer—Alendronate Conjugates. *Mol. Pharm.* **2008**, *5*, 548–558. [CrossRef]
36. Chytil, P.; Etrych, T.; Kříž, J.; Šubr, V.; Ulbrich, K. N-(2-Hydroxypropyl)methacrylamide-based polymer conjugates with pH-controlled activation of doxorubicin for cell-specific or passive tumour targeting. Synthesis by RAFT polymerisation and physicochemical characterisation. *Eur. J. Pharm. Sci.* **2010**, *41*, 473–482. [CrossRef] [PubMed]
37. Raus, V.; Kostka, L. Optimizing the Cu-RDRP of N-(2-hydroxypropyl) methacrylamide toward biomedical applications. *Polym. Chem.* **2019**, *10*, 564–568. [CrossRef]
38. Chytil, P.; Šírová, M.; Koziolová, E.; Ulbrich, K.; Říhová, B.; Etrych, T. The Comparison of In Vivo Properties of Water-Soluble HPMA-Based Polymer Conjugates with Doxorubicin Prepared by Controlled RAFT or Free Radical Polymerization. *Physiol. Res.* **2015**, *64*, S41–S49. [CrossRef]
39. Koziolová, E.; Goel, S.; Chytil, P.; Janoušková, O.; Barnhart, T.E.; Cai, W.B.; Etrych, T. A tumor-targeted polymer theranostics platform for positron emission tomography and fluorescence imaging. *Nanoscale* **2017**, *9*, 10906–10918. [CrossRef]
40. Randárová, E.; Nakamura, H.; Islam, R.; Studenovský, M.; Mamoru, H.; Fang, J.; Chytil, P.; Etrych, T. Highly effective anti-tumor nanomedicines based on HPMA copolymer conjugates with pirarubicin prepared by controlled RAFT polymerization. *Acta Biomater.* **2020**, *106*, 256–266. [CrossRef]
41. Quan, L.D.; Zhang, Y.J.; Crielaard, B.J.; Dusad, A.; Lele, S.M.; Rijcken, C.J.F.; Metselaar, J.M.; Kostková, H.; Etrych, T.; Ulbrich, K.; et al. Nanomedicines for Inflammatory Arthritis: Head-to-Head Comparison of Glucocorticoid-Containing Polymers, Micelles, and Liposomes. *ACS Nano* **2014**, *8*, 458–466. [CrossRef]
42. Libánská, A.; Randárová, E.; Lager, F.; Renault, G.; Scherman, D.; Etrych, T. Polymer Nanomedicines with pH-Sensitive Release of Dexamethasone for the Localized Treatment of Inflammation. *Pharmaceutics* **2020**, *12*, 700. [CrossRef]

43. Etrych, T.; Šubr, V.; Laga, R.; Říhová, B.; Ulbrich, K. Polymer conjugates of doxorubicin bound through an amide and hydrazone bond: Impact of the carrier structure onto synergistic action in the treatment of solid tumours. *Eur. J. Pharm. Sci.* **2014**, *58*, 1–12. [CrossRef]
44. Zhang, R.; Luo, K.; Yang, J.; Sima, M.; Sun, Y.; Janát-Amsbury, M.M.; Kopeček, J. Synthesis and evaluation of a backbone biodegradable multiblock HPMA copolymer nanocarrier for the systemic delivery of paclitaxel. *J. Control. Release* **2013**, *166*, 66–74. [CrossRef]
45. Luo, K.; Yang, J.; Kopečková, P.; Kopeček, J. Biodegradable Multiblock Poly[N-(2-hydroxypropyl)methacrylamide] via Reversible Addition−Fragmentation Chain Transfer Polymerization and Click Chemistry. *Macromolecules* **2011**, *44*, 2481–2488. [CrossRef]
46. Larson, N.; Yang, J.Y.; Ray, A.; Cheney, D.L.; Ghandehari, H.; Kopeček, J. Biodegradable multiblock poly(N-2-hydroxypropyl)methacrylamide gemcitabine and paclitaxel conjugates for ovarian cancer cell combination treatment. *Int. J. Pharm.* **2013**, *454*, 435–443. [CrossRef]
47. Pan, H.Z.; Yang, J.Y.; Kopečková, P.; Kopeček, J. Backbone Degradable Multiblock N-(2-Hydroxypropyl)methacrylamide Copolymer Conjugates via Reversible Addition-Fragmentation Chain Transfer Polymerization and Thiol-ene Coupling Reaction. *Biomacromolecules* **2011**, *12*, 247–252. [CrossRef]
48. Etrych, T.; Chytil, P.; Mrkvan, T.; Šírová, M.; Říhová, B.; Ulbrich, K. Conjugates of doxorubicin with graft HPMA copolymers for passive tumor targeting. *J. Control. Release* **2008**, *132*, 184–192. [CrossRef]
49. Etrych, T.; Strohalm, J.; Chytil, P.; Černoch, P.; Starovoytova, L.; Pechar, M.; Ulbrich, K. Biodegradable star HPMA polymer conjugates of doxorubicin for passive tumor targeting. *Eur. J. Pharm. Sci.* **2011**, *42*, 527–539. [CrossRef]
50. Wang, D.; Kopečková, P.; Minko, T.; Nanayakkara, V.; Kopeček, J. Synthesis of starlike N-(2-hydroxypropyl)methacrylamide copolymers: Potential drug carriers. *Biomacromolecules* **2000**, *1*, 313–319. [CrossRef]
51. Chytil, P.; Koziolová, E.; Janoušková, O.; Kostka, L.; Ulbrich, K.; Etrych, T. Synthesis and Properties of Star HPMA Copolymer Nanocarriers Synthesised by RAFT Polymerisation Designed for Selective Anticancer Drug Delivery and Imaging. *Macromol. Biosci.* **2015**, *15*, 839–850. [CrossRef]
52. Kostka, L.; Kotrchová, L.; Šubr, V.; Libánská, A.; Ferreira, C.A.; Malátová, I.; Lee, H.J.; Barnhart, T.E.; Engle, J.W.; Cai, W.B.; et al. HPMA-based star polymer biomaterials with tuneable structure and biodegradability tailored for advanced drug delivery to solid tumours. *Biomaterials* **2020**, *235*, 119728. [CrossRef]
53. Pan, H.Z.; Sima, M.; Yang, J.Y.; Kopeček, J. Synthesis of Long-Circulating, Backbone Degradable HPMA CopolymerDoxorubicin Conjugates and Evaluation of Molecular-Weight-Dependent Antitumor Efficacy. *Macromol. Biosci.* **2013**, *13*, 155–160. [CrossRef]
54. Etrych, T.; Tsukigawa, K.; Nakamura, H.; Chytil, P.; Fang, J.; Ulbrich, K.; Otagiri, M.; Maeda, H. Comparison of the pharmacological and biological properties of HPMA copolymer-pirarubicin conjugates: A single-chain copolymer conjugate and its biodegradable tandem-diblock copolymer conjugate. *Eur. J. Pharm. Sci.* **2017**, *106*, 10–19. [CrossRef]
55. Duan, Z.; Zhang, Y.; Zhu, H.; Sun, L.; Cai, H.; Li, B.; Gong, Q.; Gu, Z.; Luo, K. Stimuli-Sensitive Biodegradable and Amphiphilic Block Copolymer-Gemcitabine Conjugates Self-Assemble into a Nanoscale Vehicle for Cancer Therapy. *ACS Appl. Mater. Interfaces* **2017**, *9*, 3474–3486. [CrossRef] [PubMed]
56. Krakovičová, H.; Etrych, T.; Ulbrich, K. HPMA-based polymer conjugates with drug combination. *Eur. J. Pharm. Sci.* **2009**, *37*, 405–412. [CrossRef]
57. Kostková, H.; Etrych, T.; Říhová, B.; Ulbrich, K. Synergistic effect of HPMA copolymer-bound doxorubicin and dexamethasone in vivo on mouse lymphomas. *J. Bioact. Compat. Polym.* **2011**, *26*, 270–286. [CrossRef]
58. Říhová, B.; Etrych, T.; Šírová, M.; Kovář, L.; Hovorka, O.; Kovář, M.; Benda, A.; Ulbrich, K. Synergistic Action of Doxorubicin Bound to the Polymeric Carrier Based on N-(2-Hydroxypropyl)methacrylamide Copolymers through an Amide or Hydrazone Bond. *Mol. Pharm.* **2010**, *7*, 1027–1040. [CrossRef]
59. Yang, J.; Kopeček, J. Macromolecular therapeutics. *J. Control. Release* **2014**, *190*, 288–303. [CrossRef] [PubMed]
60. Yang, J.; Luo, K.; Pan, H.; Kopečková, P.; Kopeček, J. Synthesis of biodegradable multiblock copolymers by click coupling of RAFT-generated heterotelechelic polyHPMA conjugates. *React. Funct. Polym.* **2011**, *71*, 294–302. [CrossRef] [PubMed]
61. Kopeček, J.; Yang, J.Y. Polymer nanomedicines. *Adv. Drug Deliv. Rev.* **2020**, *156*, 40–64. [CrossRef]
62. Yang, J.Y.; Zhang, R.; Pan, H.Z.; Li, Y.L.; Fang, Y.X.; Zhang, L.B.; Kopeček, J. Backbone Degradable N-(2-Hydroxypropyl)methacrylamide Copolymer Conjugates with Gemcitabine and Paclitaxel: Impact of Molecular Weight on Activity toward Human Ovarian Carcinoma Xenografts. *Mol. Pharm.* **2017**, *14*, 1384–1394. [CrossRef]
63. Koziolová, E.; Kostka, L.; Kotrchová, L.; Šubr, V.; Konefal, R.; Nottelet, B.; Etrych, T. N-(2-Hydroxypropyl)methacrylamide-Based Linear, Diblock, and Starlike Polymer Drug Carriers: Advanced Process for Their Simple Production. *Biomacromolecules* **2018**, *19*, 4003–4013. [CrossRef]
64. Kostka, L.; Etrych, T. High-Molecular-Weight HPMA-Based Polymer Drug Carriers for Delivery to Tumor. *Physiol. Res.* **2016**, *65*, S179–S190. [CrossRef]
65. Pearce, A.K.; Anane-Adjei, A.B.; Cavanagh, R.J.; Monteiro, P.F.; Bennett, T.M.; Taresco, V.; Clarke, P.A.; Ritchie, A.A.; Alexander, M.R.; Grabowska, A.M.; et al. Effects of Polymer 3D Architecture, Size, and Chemistry on Biological Transport and Drug Delivery In Vitro and in Orthotopic Triple Negative Breast Cancer Models. *Adv. Healthc. Mater.* **2020**, *9*, 2000892. [CrossRef] [PubMed]
66. Kotrchová, L.; Kostka, L.; Etrych, T. Drug carriers with star polymer structures. *Physiol. Res.* **2018**, *67*, S293–S303. [CrossRef]
67. Kostková, H.; Schindler, L.; Kotrchová, L.; Kovář, M.; Šírová, M.; Kostka, L.; Etrych, T. Star Polymer-Drug Conjugates with pH-Controlled Drug Release and Carrier Degradation. *J. Nanomater.* **2017**, *2017*, 8675435. [CrossRef]

68. Kudláčová, J.; Kotrchová, L.; Kostka, L.; Randárová, E.; Filipová, M.; Janoušková, O.; Fang, J.; Etrych, T. Structure-to-Efficacy Relationship of HPMA-Based Nanomedicines: The Tumor Spheroid Penetration Study. *Pharmaceutics* 2020, *12*, 1242. [CrossRef]
69. Kotrchová, L.; Etrych, T. Synthesis of Water-Soluble Star Polymers Based on Cyclodextrins. *Physiol. Res.* 2018, *67*, S357–S365. [CrossRef]
70. Talelli, M.; Rijcken, C.J.F.; van Nostrum, C.F.; Storm, G.; Hennink, W.E. Micelles based on HPMA copolymers. *Adv. Drug Deliv. Rev.* 2010, *62*, 231–239. [CrossRef]
71. Barz, M.; Tarantola, M.; Fischer, K.; Schmidt, M.; Luxenhofer, R.; Janshoff, A.; Theato, P.; Zentel, R. From Defined Reactive Diblock Copolymers to Functional HPMA-Based Self-Assembled Nanoaggregates. *Biomacromolecules* 2008, *9*, 3114–3118. [CrossRef]
72. Lele, B.S.; Leroux, J.C. Synthesis and micellar characterization of novel Amphiphilic A-B-A triblock copolymers of N-(2-hydroxypropyl)methacrylamide or N-vinyl-2-pyrrolidone with poly(is an element of-caprolactone). *Macromolecules* 2002, *35*, 6714–6723. [CrossRef]
73. Barz, M.; Wolf, F.K.; Canal, F.; Koynov, K.; Vicent, M.J.; Frey, H.; Zentel, R. Synthesis, Characterization and Preliminary Biological Evaluation of P(HPMA)-*b*-P(LLA) Copolymers: A New Type of Functional Biocompatible Block Copolymer. *Macromol. Rapid Commun.* 2010, *31*, 1492–1500. [CrossRef]
74. Braunová, A.; Kostka, L.; Sivák, L.; Cuchalová, L.; Hvězdová, Z.; Laga, R.; Filippov, S.; Černoch, P.; Pechar, M.; Janoušková, O.; et al. Tumor-targeted micelle-forming block copolymers for overcoming of multidrug resistance. *J. Control. Release* 2017, *245*, 41–51. [CrossRef] [PubMed]
75. Alfurhood, J.A.; Sun, H.; Kabb, C.P.; Tucker, B.S.; Matthews, J.H.; Luesch, H.; Sumerlin, B.S. Poly(N-(2-hydroxypropyl)methacrylamide)–valproic acid conjugates as block copolymer nanocarriers. *Polym. Chem.* 2017, *8*, 4983–4987. [CrossRef] [PubMed]
76. Naksuriya, O.; Shi, Y.; van Nostrum, C.F.; Anuchapreeda, S.; Hennink, W.E.; Okonogi, S. HPMA-based polymeric micelles for curcumin solubilization and inhibition of cancer cell growth. *Eur. J. Pharm. Biopharm.* 2015, *94*, 501–512. [CrossRef] [PubMed]
77. Bláhová, M.; Randárová, E.; Konefal, R.; Nottelet, B.; Etrych, T. Graft copolymers with tunable amphiphilicity tailored for efficient dual drug deliveryviaencapsulation and pH-sensitive drug conjugation. *Polym. Chem.* 2020, *11*, 4438–4453. [CrossRef]
78. Chytil, P.; Etrych, T.; Koňák, Č.; Šírová, M.; Mrkvan, T.; Bouček, J.; Říhová, B.; Ulbrich, K. New HPMA copolymer-based drug carriers with covalently bound hydrophobic substituents for solid tumour targeting. *J. Control. Release* 2008, *127*, 121–130. [CrossRef] [PubMed]
79. Chytil, P.; Etrych, T.; Kostka, L.; Ulbrich, K. Hydrolytically Degradable Polymer Micelles for Anticancer Drug Delivery to Solid Tumors. *Macromol. Chem. Phys.* 2012, *213*, 858–867. [CrossRef]
80. Zhou, Z.; Li, L.; Yang, Y.; Xu, X.; Huang, Y. Tumor targeting by pH-sensitive, biodegradable, cross-linked N-(2-hydroxypropyl) methacrylamide copolymer micelles. *Biomaterials* 2014, *35*, 6622–6635. [CrossRef]
81. Koziolová, E.; Machová, D.; Pola, R.; Janoušková, O.; Chytil, P.; Laga, R.; Filippov, S.K.; Šubr, V.; Etrych, T.; Pechar, M. Micelle-forming HPMA copolymer conjugates of ritonavir bound via a pH-sensitive spacer with improved cellular uptake designed for enhanced tumor accumulation. *J. Mater. Chem. B* 2016, *4*, 7620–7629. [CrossRef]
82. Chytil, P.; Šírová, M.; Kudláčová, J.; Říhová, B.; Ulbrich, K.; Etrych, T. Bloodstream Stability Predetermines the Antitumor Efficacy of Micellar Polymer-Doxorubicin Drug Conjugates with pH-Triggered Drug Release. *Mol. Pharm.* 2018, *15*, 3654–3663. [CrossRef]
83. Jia, Z.; Wong, L.; Davis, T.P.; Bulmus, V. One-Pot Conversion of RAFT-Generated Multifunctional Block Copolymers of HPMA to Doxorubicin Conjugated Acid- and Reductant-Sensitive Crosslinked Micelles. *Biomacromolecules* 2008, *9*, 3106–3113. [CrossRef]
84. Klepac, D.; Kostková, H.; Petrova, S.; Chytil, P.; Etrych, T.; Kereiche, S.; Raska, I.; Weitz, D.A.; Filippov, S.K. Interaction of spin-labeled HPMA-based nanoparticles with human blood plasma proteins—The introduction of protein-corona-free polymer nanomedicine. *Nanoscale* 2018, *10*, 6194–6204. [CrossRef]
85. Janisová, L.; Gruzinov, A.; Zaborova, O.V.; Velychkivska, N.; Vaněk, O.; Chytil, P.; Etrych, T.; Janoušková, O.; Zhang, X.H.; Blanchet, C.; et al. Molecular Mechanisms of the Interactions of N-(2-Hydroxypropyl)methacrylamide Copolymers Designed for Cancer Therapy with Blood Plasma Proteins. *Pharmaceutics* 2020, *12*, 106. [CrossRef]
86. Zhang, X.H.; Niebuur, B.J.; Chytil, P.; Etrych, T.; Filippov, S.K.; Kikhney, A.; Wieland, D.C.F.; Svergun, D.I.; Papadakis, C.M. Macromolecular pHPMA-Based Nanoparticles with Cholesterol for Solid Tumor Targeting: Behavior in HSA Protein Environment. *Biomacromolecules* 2018, *19*, 470–480. [CrossRef]
87. Etrych, T.; Mrkvan, T.; Chytil, P.; Koňák, Č.; Říhová, B.; Ulbrich, K. N-(2-hydroxypropyl)methacrylamide-based polymer conjugates with pH-controlled activation of doxorubicin. I. New synthesis, physicochemical characterization and preliminary biological evaluation. *J. Appl. Polym. Sci.* 2008, *109*, 3050–3061. [CrossRef]
88. Lomkova, E.A.; Chytil, P.; Janoušková, O.; Mueller, T.; Lucas, H.; Filippov, S.K.; Trhlíková, O.; Aleshunin, P.A.; Skorik, Y.A.; Ulbrich, K.; et al. Biodegradable Micellar HPMA-Based Polymer-Drug Conjugates with Betulinic Acid for Passive Tumor Targeting. *Biomacromolecules* 2016, *17*, 3493–3507. [CrossRef]
89. Luan, B.; Muir, B.W.; Zhu, J.; Hao, X. A RAFT copolymerization of NIPAM and HPMA and evaluation of thermo-responsive properties of poly(NIPAM-co-HPMA). *RSC Adv.* 2016, *6*, 89925–89933. [CrossRef]
90. Laga, R.; Janoušková, O.; Ulbrich, K.; Pola, R.; Blažková, J.; Filippov, S.K.; Etrych, T.; Pechar, M. Thermoresponsive Polymer Micelles as Potential Nanosized Cancerostatics. *Biomacromolecules* 2015, *16*, 2493–2505. [CrossRef]
91. Truong, N.P.; Whittaker, M.R.; Anastasaki, A.; Haddleton, D.M.; Quinn, J.F.; Davis, T.P. Facile production of nanoaggregates with tuneable morphologies from thermoresponsive P(DEGMA-*co*-HPMA). *Polym. Chem.* 2016, *7*, 430–440. [CrossRef]

92. Shi, Y.; van den Dungen, E.T.A.; Klumperman, B.; van Nostrum, C.F.; Hennink, W.E. Reversible Addition–Fragmentation Chain Transfer Synthesis of a Micelle-Forming, Structure Reversible Thermosensitive Diblock Copolymer Based on the N-(2-Hydroxy propyl) Methacrylamide Backbone. *ACS Macro Lett.* **2013**, *2*, 403–408. [CrossRef]
93. Maeda, H.; Khatami, M. Analyses of repeated failures in cancer therapy for solid tumors: Poor tumor-selective drug delivery, low therapeutic efficacy and unsustainable costs. *Clin. Transl. Med.* **2018**, *7*, 11. [CrossRef]
94. Sosman, J.A.; Kim, K.B.; Schuchter, L.; Gonzalez, R.; Pavlick, A.C.; Weber, J.S.; McArthur, G.A.; Hutson, T.E.; Moschos, S.J.; Flaherty, K.T.; et al. Survival in BRAF V600–Mutant Advanced Melanoma Treated with Vemurafenib. *N. Engl. J. Med.* **2012**, *366*, 707–714. [CrossRef] [PubMed]
95. Gerlinger, M.; Rowan, A.J.; Horswell, S.; Larkin, J.; Endesfelder, D.; Gronroos, E.; Martinez, P.; Matthews, N.; Stewart, A.; Tarpey, P.; et al. Intratumor Heterogeneity and Branched Evolution Revealed by Multiregion Sequencing. *N. Engl. J. Med.* **2012**, *366*, 883–892. [CrossRef]
96. Hernández-Camarero, P.; Amezcua-Hernández, V.; Jiménez, G.; García, M.A.; Marchal, J.A.; Perán, M. Clinical failure of nanoparticles in cancer: Mimicking nature's solutions. *Nanomedicine* **2020**, *15*, 2311–2324. [CrossRef]
97. He, H.L.; Liu, L.S.; Morin, E.E.; Liu, M.; Schwendeman, A. Survey of Clinical Translation of Cancer Nanomedicines-Lessons Learned from Successes and Failures. *Acc. Chem. Res.* **2019**, *52*, 2445–2461. [CrossRef]
98. Hare, J.I.; Lammers, T.; Ashford, M.B.; Puri, S.; Storm, G.; Barry, S.T. Challenges and strategies in anti-cancer nanomedicine development: An industry perspective. *Adv. Drug Deliv. Rev.* **2017**, *108*, 25–38. [CrossRef]
99. Shi, J.J.; Kantoff, P.W.; Wooster, R.; Farokhzad, O.C. Cancer nanomedicine: Progress, challenges and opportunities. *Nat. Rev. Cancer* **2017**, *17*, 20–37. [CrossRef] [PubMed]
100. Folkman, J. What Is the Evidence That Tumors Are Angiogenesis Dependent? *JNCI J. Natl. Cancer Inst.* **1990**, *82*, 4–7. [CrossRef]
101. Fang, J.; Islam, W.; Maeda, H. Exploiting the dynamics of the EPR effect and strategies to improve the therapeutic effects of nanomedicines by using EPR effect enhancers. *Adv. Drug Deliv. Rev.* **2020**, *157*, 142–160. [CrossRef] [PubMed]
102. Navi, B.B.; Reiner, A.S.; Kamel, H.; Iadecola, C.; Okin, P.M.; Tagawa, S.T.; Panageas, K.S.; DeAngelis, L.M. Arterial thromboembolic events preceding the diagnosis of cancer in older persons. *Blood* **2019**, *133*, 781–789. [CrossRef] [PubMed]
103. Young, A.; Chapman, O.; Connor, C.; Poole, C.; Rose, P.; Kakkar, A.K. Thrombosis and cancer. *Nat. Rev. Clin. Oncol.* **2012**, *9*, 437–449. [CrossRef]
104. Jain, R.K. Transport of molecules across tumor vasculature. *Cancer Metastasis Rev.* **1987**, *6*, 559–593. [CrossRef]
105. Islam, W.; Fang, J.; Imamura, T.; Etrych, T.; Šubr, V.; Ulbrich, K.; Maeda, H. Augmentation of the Enhanced Permeability and Retention Effect with Nitric Oxide–Generating Agents Improves the Therapeutic Effects of Nanomedicines. *Mol. Cancer Ther.* **2018**, *17*, 2643–2653. [CrossRef]
106. Seki, T.; Fang, J.; Maeda, H. Enhanced delivery of macromolecular antitumor drugs to tumors by nitroglycerin application. *Cancer Sci.* **2009**, *100*, 2426–2430. [CrossRef]
107. Jiang, J.; Jordan, S.J.; Barr, D.P.; Gunther, M.R.; Maeda, H.; Mason, R.P. In Vivo Production of Nitric Oxide in Rats after Administration of Hydroxyurea. *Mol. Pharm.* **1997**, *52*, 1081–1086. [CrossRef] [PubMed]
108. Dozono, H.; Yanazume, S.; Nakamura, H.; Etrych, T.; Chytil, P.; Ulbrich, K.; Fang, J.; Arimura, T.; Douchi, T.; Kobayashi, H.; et al. HPMA Copolymer-Conjugated Pirarubicin in Multimodal Treatment of a Patient with Stage IV Prostate Cancer and Extensive Lung and Bone Metastases. *Target Oncol.* **2016**, *11*, 101–106. [CrossRef]
109. Fang, J.; Islam, R.; Islam, W.; Yin, H.Z.; Šubr, V.; Etrych, T.; Ulbrich, K.; Maeda, H. Augmentation of EPR Effect and Efficacy of Anticancer Nanomedicine by Carbon Monoxide Generating Agents. *Pharmaceutics* **2019**, *11*, 343. [CrossRef] [PubMed]
110. Studenovský, M.; Sivák, L.; Sedláček, O.; Konefal, R.; Horková, V.; Etrych, T.; Kovář, M.; Říhová, B.; Šírová, M. Polymer nitric oxide donors potentiate the treatment of experimental solid tumours by increasing drug accumulation in the tumour tissue. *J. Control. Release* **2018**, *269*, 214–224. [CrossRef] [PubMed]
111. Kinoshita, R.; Ishima, Y.; Chuang, V.T.G.; Nakamura, H.; Fang, J.; Watanabe, H.; Shimizu, T.; Okuhira, K.; Ishida, T.; Maeda, H.; et al. Improved anticancer effects of albumin-bound paclitaxel nanoparticle via augmentation of EPR effect and albumin-protein interactions using S-nitrosated human serum albumin dimer. *Biomaterials* **2017**, *140*, 162–169. [CrossRef] [PubMed]
112. Kang, Y.; Kim, J.; Lee, Y.M.; Im, S.; Park, H.; Kim, W.J. Nitric oxide-releasing polymer incorporated ointment for cutaneous wound healing. *J. Control. Release* **2015**, *220*, 624–630. [CrossRef]
113. Danhier, F.; Feron, O.; Préat, V. To exploit the tumor microenvironment: Passive and active tumor targeting of nanocarriers for anti-cancer drug delivery. *J. Control. Release* **2010**, *148*, 135–146. [CrossRef]
114. Samuli, H.; Catherine, P.; Jean-Pierre, B. Passive and Active Tumour Targeting with Nanocarriers. *Curr. Drug Discov. Technol.* **2011**, *8*, 188–196. [CrossRef]
115. Attia, M.F.; Anton, N.; Wallyn, J.; Omran, Z.; Vandamme, T.F. An overview of active and passive targeting strategies to improve the nanocarriers efficiency to tumour sites. *J. Pharm. Pharmacol.* **2019**, *71*, 1185–1198. [CrossRef]
116. Seymour, L.W.; Miyamoto, Y.; Maeda, H.; Brereton, M.; Strohalm, J.; Ulbrich, K.; Duncan, R. Influence of molecular weight on passive tumour accumulation of a soluble macromolecular drug carrier. *Eur. J. Cancer* **1995**, *31*, 766–770. [CrossRef]
117. Kopeček, J.; Kopečková, P. HPMA copolymers: Origins, early developments, present, and future. *Adv. Drug Deliv. Rev.* **2010**, *62*, 122–149. [CrossRef]
118. Yang, J.; Kopeček, J. Design of smart HPMA copolymer-based nanomedicines. *J. Control. Release* **2016**, *240*, 9–23. [CrossRef]

119. Pola, R.; Böhmová, E.; Filipová, M.; Pechar, M.; Pankrác, J.; Větvička, D.; Olejár, T.; Kabešová, M.; Poučková, P.; Šefc, L.; et al. Targeted Polymer-Based Probes for Fluorescence Guided Visualization and Potential Surgery of EGFR-Positive Head-and-Neck Tumors. *Pharmaceutics* **2020**, *12*, 31. [CrossRef] [PubMed]
120. Randárová, E.; Kudláčová, J.; Etrych, T. HPMA copolymer-antibody constructs in neoplastic treatment: An overview of therapeutics, targeted diagnostics, and drug-free systems. *J. Control. Release* **2020**, *325*, 304–322. [CrossRef]
121. Ulbrich, K.; Šubr, V.; Strohalm, J.; Plocová, D.; Jelínková, M.; Říhová, B. Polymeric drugs based on conjugates of synthetic and natural macromolecules I. Synthesis and physico-chemical characterisation. *J. Control. Release* **2000**, *64*, 63–79. [CrossRef]
122. Lidický, O.; Klener, P.; Machová, D.; Vočková, P.; Pokorná, E.; Helman, K.; Mavis, C.; Janoušková, O.; Etrych, T. Overcoming resistance to rituximab in relapsed non-Hodgkin lymphomas by antibody-polymer drug conjugates actively targeted by anti-CD38 daratumumab. *J. Control. Release* **2020**, *328*, 160–170. [CrossRef] [PubMed]
123. Kovář, M.; Mrkvan, T.; Strohalm, J.; Etrych, T.; Ulbrich, K.; Šťastný, M.; Říhová, B. HPMA copolymer-bound doxorubicin targeted to tumor-specific antigen of BCL1 mouse B cell leukemia. *J. Control. Release* **2003**, *92*, 315–330. [CrossRef]
124. Kovář, M.; Strohalm, J.; Etrych, T.; Ulbrich, K.; Říhová, B. Star structure of antibody-targeted HPMA copolymer-bound doxorubicin: A novel type of polymeric conjugate for targeted drug delivery with potent antitumor effect. *Bioconj. Chem.* **2002**, *13*, 206–215. [CrossRef] [PubMed]
125. Kunjachan, S.; Pola, R.; Gremse, F.; Theek, B.; Ehling, J.; Moeckel, D.; Hermanns-Sachweh, B.; Pechar, M.; Ulbrich, K.; Hennink, W.E.; et al. Passive versus Active Tumor Targeting Using RGD- and NGR-Modified Polymeric Nanomedicines. *Nano Lett.* **2014**, *14*, 972–981. [CrossRef] [PubMed]
126. Sindhwani, S.; Syed, A.M.; Ngai, J.; Kingston, B.R.; Maiorino, L.; Rothschild, J.; MacMillan, P.; Zhang, Y.; Rajesh, N.U.; Hoang, T.; et al. The entry of nanoparticles into solid tumours. *Nat. Mater.* **2020**, *19*, 566–575. [CrossRef] [PubMed]

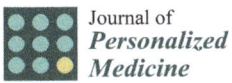

Review

Newly Developed Self-Assembling Antioxidants as Potential Therapeutics for the Cancers

Babita Shashni [1] and Yukio Nagasaki [1,2,3,*]

1. Department of Materials Science, Graduate School of Pure and Applied Sciences, University of Tsukuba, Tennoudai 1-1-1, Tsukuba, Ibaraki 305-8573, Japan; shashni@ims.tsukuba.ac.jp
2. Master's School of Medical Sciences, Graduate School of Comprehensive Human Sciences, University of Tsukuba, Tennoudai 1-1-1, Tsukuba, Ibaraki 305-8573, Japan
3. Center for Research in Isotopes and Environmental Dynamics (CRiED), University of Tsukuba, Tennoudai 1-1-1, Tsukuba, Ibaraki 305-8573, Japan
* Correspondence: happyhusband@nagalabo.jp; Fax: +81-(0)29-853-5750

Abstract: Elevated reactive oxygen species (ROS) have been implicated as significant for cancer survival by functioning as oncogene activators and secondary messengers. Hence, the attenuation of ROS-signaling pathways in cancer by antioxidants seems a suitable therapeutic regime for targeting cancers. Low molecular weight (LMW) antioxidants such as 2,2,6,6-tetramethylpyperidine-1-oxyl (TEMPO), although they are catalytically effective in vitro, exerts off-target effects in vivo due to their size, thus, limiting their clinical use. Here, we discuss the superior impacts of our TEMPO radical-conjugated self-assembling antioxidant nanoparticle (RNP) compared to the LMW counterpart in terms of pharmacokinetics, therapeutic effect, and adverse effects in various cancer models.

Keywords: cancer; reactive oxygen species; antioxidant; self-assembling drug

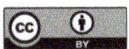

1. Introduction

Reactive oxygen species (ROS) are intracellular free oxygen radicals with one or more unpaired electrons in their valency shell. These unpaired electrons are capable of independent existence and are highly reactive, who tend to stabilize their shell by donating or extracting electron(s) from the oxidizable molecules. These target oxidizable molecules become a radical entity, which further starts a chain reaction of damaging other molecules [1]. The concept of organic free radical began in 1900 by Gomberg, who speculated the presence of triphenyl methyl radical (Ph3C$^{\bullet}$) in the living system. In 1954, a free radical theory was proposed by Gershman, who pointed out the toxicity of oxygen and its reduced forms due to the highly oxidizing power [2,3]. In 1969, McCord and Fridovich discovered the first cellular antioxidant enzyme, superoxide dismutase (SOD) [4].

ROS are broadly classified into radical and non-radical species. Radical species involve entities with unpaired electron(s) such as superoxide ($O_2^{\bullet-}$), hydroxyl radical ($OH^{\bullet-}$), oxygen biradicals ($O_2^{\bullet\bullet}$), peroxyl radicals ($ROO^{\bullet}$), and alkoxy-radicals ($RO^{\bullet}$). In contrast, non-radical species include entities that do not contain an unpaired electron but can easily convert to free radicals in the living system. The primary reported species are hydrogen peroxide (H_2O_2), hypochlorous acid (HOCl), ozone (O_3), singlet oxygen ($^1O_2$), organic peroxides (ROOH), aldehydes (RCHO), and so on [5]. ROS can be produced both through endogenous and exogenous sources. Endogenous sources of ROS are mitochondria, peroxisomes, endoplasmic reticulum, and activated inflammatory neutrophils. Large amount of ROS is generated in mitochondria via several enzymatic reactions such as an electron transport chain, NADH dehydrogenase, and ubiquinone cytochrome C reductase, etc. Several enzymatic reactions generate ROS in peroxisomes (β-oxidation of fatty acids; acyl CoA oxidase, uric acid metabolism; urate oxidase, xanthine metabolism; xanthine oxidase, D-proline metabolism; D-amino acid oxidase), and in the endoplasmic reticulum (cytochrome P450, b5 enzymes, diamine oxidase, thiol oxidase enzyme Erop1p). Activated inflammatory cells such as neutrophils also produce numerous ROS in the inflammatory sites.

In contrast, exogenous sources include pesticides, ultraviolet light, air, and water pollution, metals such as iron, copper, cobalt, cadmium, arsenic, etc. [6,7]. Under normal conditions, a small amount of ROS escapes during the intracellular processes regulated by the enzymatic antioxidant system, viz., superoxide dismutase, catalase, peroxiredoxins, glutathione peroxidases, glutathiones, bilirubin, etc. [6]. Although antioxidant systems maintain a tightly controlled redox homeostasis in the normal cells, irreversible or non-repairable oxidative damage to nuclear and mitochondrial DNA, protein, and lipids are inevitable due to their prolonged overexposure to exogenous ROS producers. These over-produced ROS lead to oxidative stress-related diseases such as cancer, cardiovascular diseases, diabetes, rheumatoid arthritis, neurogenerative diseases, liver disease, and ischemic and post-ischemic pathologies [6–8]. Exogenous oxidative stress or prolonged chronic endogenous oxidative stress such as inflammation has been linked to tumor initiation, promotion and progression, which are evident from the fact that cancer cells are under constant oxidative stress, a hallmark of cancerous phenotype [8,9]. Considering a continuous elevated ROS level in the tumor environment, which is crucial for tumorigenesis, metastasis, and angiogenesis, antioxidant therapies seem to be the most intuitive and apt intervention to attenuate various cancers. Although various low molecular weight (LMW) antioxidants such as vitamin C, vitamin E, selenium, and TEMPOL, showed effectiveness in vitro and in some cases in vivo; however, clinically, they failed to show any conclusive efficacy [10]. Their clinical failure may be attributed to their metabolism and rapid excretion, preventing them from reaching the target ROS production site of the tumor cells in enough amount to scavenge ROS to a critical level to have sufficient anti-cancer efficacy. Another significant and severe problem of the LMW antioxidants is that they internalize in the healthy cells and disturb their redox homeostasis, including the mitochondrial electron transport chain. Here, we conceptualized new antioxidants, "self-assembling antioxidants", which significantly vary in their pharmacokinetic characteristics and reduce undesired adverse side effects related to the LMW antioxidants. In this review, an implication of ROS in cancer, the status of antioxidant cancer therapies using LMW compounds and the precedence of self-assembling antioxidants (we abbreviate them as redox nanoparticle hereafter; RNP) over LMW antioxidant compounds for the cancer therapeutics will be discussed in detail.

2. Oxidative Stress and Cancer

As described in the above section, evidence from the clinical and bench studies indicate that the elevated intracellular ROS contributes to cancer initiation, promotion and progression [8,9]. The intracellular antioxidant system can quench the overproduced ROS generated through the exogenous source or chronic inflammation in the normal cells to some extent and under their capacity. However, ROS that could not be completely eliminated could be mutagenic and induce carcinogenesis [9,11,12]. For instance, white blood cells convert to neutrophils and invade the inflamed colon in ulcerative colitis. These activated neutrophils generate ROS such as $O_2^{\bullet-}$ and HOCl, which are known to stimulate mutagenesis and cause colon cancer [13,14]. Similarly, constant exposure to free radical producers such as ultraviolet, tobacco smoke, and metal ions may stimulate mutagenesis and induce melanoma, bronchogenic carcinoma, and colorectal cancer, respectively [8].

Tumor initiation is triggered by damaging cellular genes, mainly by the oxidation with ROS. It is reported that about 10,000 oxidative hits to DNA per cell are observed daily in humans [15], which are eventually recovered by the cellular repairing system. However, sometimes, when oxidative stress damage is beyond their repair capacity, DNA base adduct with non-scavenged ROS may be observed [8,16]. For instance, one of ROS, hydroxide radical (•OH) attacks the guanine (G) base at the eighth position to become 8-OH-G, which leads to Guanine-Cytosine to Thymine-Adenine transversion, called point mutation [8,16,17]. In addition, DNA helix alterations such as single or double-strand breaks and inter-strand crosslinks are also observed upon damage by free radicals generated through ultraviolet or ionizing lights [18,19]. Such alteration in the DNA results in genomic instability, which may further modulate transcription and transduction pathways favoring carcinogenesis and tumor progression [20,21].

ROS in tumors participates in the intracellular signaling and regulation by acting as secondary messengers [6–8]. Ras protein family, one of the membrane-bound G protein families, regulates transcription, cell growth, and apoptosis [22]. Ras is activated by ROS derived from ultraviolet radiation and metal ions and is known to be frequently mutated in humans cancers such as skin, liver, and colon cancers [22]. It should be noted that Ras-dependent cell proliferation requires ROS, which is unconditionally elevated in cancers [23].

Another tumor suppressor protein, p53, a transcriptional factor, is known to be involved in cell cycle arrest, senescence, apoptosis, DNA repair, and redox homeostasis [24–26]. Upon oxidative stress by ionizing radiation or genotoxic insults, DNA lesions are accumulated, which are repaired before the DNA replication by arresting the cell cycle. Once the DNA lesion is repaired, the normal cell resumes cell division. p53, known as "the guardian of the genome", preserves this DNA integrity [27]. However, when the TP53 gene is mutated, the DNA damage is carried down to several cell divisions, leading to chromosomal rearrangement [28]. TP53 gene is often known to be mutated in various solid cancers [27].

Another popular redox-sensitive transcription factor is NF-kB, which is reported to be involved in cell survival, differentiation, growth, angiogenesis, and inflammation [29,30]. NF-kB is activated by carcinogenic stimuli such as ultraviolet radiation, phorbol esters, toxic metals, and asbestos, all of which are oxidative stress inducers [31]. Although it is evident from several reports that ROS activates NF-kB, recent studies confirm the bidirectional regulation by ROS, which is not clearly understood [30]. Nonetheless, it is reported that the NF-kB pathway is often excessively activated in tumor tissues, promoting tumor cell proliferation and survival [32].

It is reported that ROS also activates protein kinases C (PKCs), critical for cancer proliferation, by increasing the cytosolic calcium concentration and the cysteine oxidization of their regulatory domains [33,34]. This activates downstream cell proliferation, differentiation, and apoptosis pathways, involving mitogen-activated protein kinases (MAPKs) such as extracellular-regulated (ERKs), c-jun-NH_2-terminal kinase (JNKs), and p38 MAPK [35]. Furthermore, ROS also regulates hypoxia-inducible factor, HIF-1, in tumors, which further modulates many cancer-related genes, such as VEGF, involved in tumor progression and angiogenesis [36]. Other ROS-sensitive regulatory proteins such as AP-1 and nuclear factor of activated T cells are also known to be involved in tumorigenesis [37–39]. Interestingly, ROS also regulates pro-proliferative signaling in tumors and prevent apoptosis by activation of proto-oncogene BCL-2, which is an anti-apoptotic protein. BCL-2 family is overexpressed in many cancers such as breast, lung, colorectal, and melanoma, which not only prevents tumor cell death but also promotes their migration, invasion, and metastasis [40].

From the evidence stated above, it is obvious that oxidative stress is critical for tumor initiation and growth by inducing genomic instability and acting as signaling molecules to modulate factors favoring tumorigenesis, angiogenesis, and metastasis, respectively. Since the critical roles of the elevated ROS-signaling pathways are revealed in various cancers, the antioxidant therapies seem to be the most appropriate strategy to impede their growth. The next section will discuss the status of conventional antioxidants for cancer therapy.

3. Conventional Antioxidants for Potential Cancer Therapy

As mentioned above, since ROS is strongly associated with carcinogenesis, tumorigenesis, and metastasis, antioxidant treatments to inhibit cancers have been investigated. Sharma et al. reported that patients with locally advanced squamous cell carcinoma of the tongue had significantly elevated plasma lipid peroxidation levels and conjugated dienes. At the same time, primary endogenous antioxidants such as glutathione, vitamin C, vitamin E, glutathione peroxidase, and superoxide dismutase were significantly decreased, as compared to the healthy controls, implying that oxidative stress plays an essential role in the pathophysiology of tongue cancer [41]. Considering the critical role of ROS in tumors, various antioxidants, including natural antioxidants have been tested to dampen the ROS levels as therapeutic interventions. Numerous natural and synthetic antioxidants have been investigated as potential anti-cancer drugs. These investigations have shown positive effects in vitro and/or in vivo against various cancer models. For example, one of the famous synthetic antioxidants, N-acetylcysteine (NAC), has shown the anti-cancer effect on prostate carcinoma, PC-3 cells (in vitro) and human tongue squamous carcinoma, HSC-3 cells (in vivo) [42,43]. Natural vitamins are also reported to exert anti-cancer effects. For instance, vitamin C inhibited invasion and metastasis of breast cancer cells (in vivo) and impaired tumor growth and eradicated liver cancer stem cells in the xenograft model of a hepatocellular carcinoma cell line [44,45]. Vitamin E analog, RRR-α-tocopherol succinate, is known to induce apoptosis mediated death in MDA-MB435, MDA-MB231, and SKBR-3 human breast cancer cells [46,47]. Quercetin, a bioflavonoid, is also known to inhibit cancer growth by arresting the cell cycle and induced apoptosis in breast cancer, prostate cancer and colorectal cancer [48–50].

TEMPOL, a redox-cycling nitroxide (4-hydroxy-TEMPO; 4-hydroxy-2,2,6,6-tetramethylpiperidine-1-oxyl), is known as a probe of electron spin resonance due to the presence of unpaired electron in the compound. Since this unpaired spin is stable because of the steric hindrance of the surrounding four methyl groups, so they do not react to each other. However, it is known that TEMPOL can rapidly react with free radicals of ROS. Thus, they can be regarded as one of the most potent antioxidants, like a superoxide dismutase [51]. Luo et al. reported a comparative superoxide inhibition activity of TEMPOL and several other antioxidants in angiotensin II-stimulated preglomerular vascular smooth muscle cells assessed by lucigenin-enhanced chemiluminescence. They confirmed that PEGylated-SOD and TEMPOL exhibited the maximum catalytic actions to scavenge $O_2^{\bullet -}$ than NAC, vitamin C and E analogues such as ascorbate, α-tocopherol and 6-hydroxy-2,5,7,8-tetramethylkroman-2-carboxy acid (Trolox) and other uncharacterized antioxidants; 5,10,15,20-tetrakis (4-sulphonatophenyl)porphyrinate iron (III)(Fe-TTPS), 2-phenyl-1,2-benzisoselenazol-3(2H)-one (ebselen), nitroblue tetrazolium (NBT) and (−)-cis-3,3′,4′,5,7-pentahydroxyflavane (2R,3R)-2-(3,4-dihydroxyphenyl)-3,4-dihydro-1(2H)-benzopyran-3,5,7-triol(-epicatechin) [51,52]. With such high catalytic activity, TEMPOL has been the most preferred choice for antioxidant-based therapy for various oxidative stress-related models such as fibrosis, diabetes, neurodegenerative diseases, radio-protection, ischemia-reperfusion injury and inflammation, hypertension, and cancer [53]. Several studies have demonstrated that TEMPOL inhibits tumor growth and decreases tumor incidence. For instance, TEMPOL induced apoptotic cell death in MDA-MB231 breast cancer cell line [54]. Gariboldi et al. reported the inhibitory effects of TEMPOL on the growth of neoplastic than non-neoplastic cell lines such as breast cancer cell line MCF-7, p53-negative human leukemia cell line HL60, and C6 glioma cells [55–57]. Schubert et al. reported that dietary TEMPOL administration to ataxia telangiectasia mutated (ATM)-deficient young mice (develop tumors), prolonged latency to tumors, decreased ROS and oxidative damage, and increased their life span [58]. Corroborating this, Mitchell et al. confirmed that long-term TEMPOL treatment decreased spontaneous tumorigenesis in C3H mice [59]. TEMPO (2,2,6,6-tetramethylpiperidine-1-oxyl) administration into LNCaP tumor-bearing mice also showed significant inhibition to prostate tumor growth [60].

As described above, there are many publications about antioxidant-based cancer chemotherapy. Although numerous antioxidants have been proposed as an efficient anticancer agent in vitro and in vivo, these antioxidants failed to show any cumulative effect clinically on healthy, at-risk, and cancer population [10]. For instance, daily supplementation with selenium (200 µg) and/or Vitamin E (400 IU) did not reduce the incidence of prostate or other cancers. Instead, vitamin E supplementation resulted in 17% increase in prostate cancer incidence [61,62]. Corroborating this, daily supplementation of β-carotene (50 mg) also did not reduce the incidence of prostate cancer or other cancers [63]. However, daily supplementation of beta-carotene (15 mg), alpha-tocopherol (30 mg), and selenium (50 μg) to Chinese at-risk population of developing esophageal cancer and gastric cancer reduced cancer mortality associated with gastric cancer, no effect was seen in esophageal cancer suffering population [64]. In another clinical study, a population who were occupationally exposed to asbestos were supplemented with β-carotene (30 mg) and retinyl palmitate (25,000 IU) daily, which tended to associate with increased lung cancer incidence and mortality [65].

Such contrasting effects of conventional antioxidants in tumorigenesis and inconclusive clinical trials indicate that these conventional antioxidants cannot be used for anti-cancer therapy. Because several elegant studies confirmed the role of elevated ROS in cancer, it is striking to see the failure of antioxidant-based cancer therapy. Their clinical failure could be attributed to several factors such as the level and the location of ROS scavenged and the tumor stage at which antioxidants were introduced. In addition, since most conventional antioxidants are LMW, their extremely rapid renal clearance and very low bioavailability may have led to their insufficient accumulation in the tumors resulting in low efficacy.

Another significant problem with the conventional antioxidants is their molecular size-based adverse effects. Mitochondria in the healthy cells generate ATP via an electron transport chain by oxidation of glucose. During this process, a considerable amount of ROS is produced. LMW antioxidants can rapidly spread to the entire body and internalize into the healthy cells, which causes the dysfunction of the essential redox homeostasis, including the electron transport chain, known as "Mithohormesis" [66]. It is reported that treatment with beta carotene, vitamin A, and vitamin E increased mortality in a randomized clinical investigation of more than 230,000 participants [67]. This means that high dose of LMW antioxidants cannot be administered due to their ability to damage mitochondria. Contrarily, the limited dose of the LMW antioxidants may scavenge low ROS sufficiently to stimulate the survival and proliferation of tumor cells rather than impeding it. This was evident in the studies by Gal et al., who reported that administration of NAC and Trolox, Vitamin E analog, increased lymph node metastasis of malignant melanoma [68]. Furthermore, due to the limited dose and poor pharmacokinetic properties, it is also possible that in clinical trials, LMW antioxidants did not reach the target location to quench crucial ROS, e.g., mitochondria of cancer cells. Porporato et al. reported that mitochondrial superoxide promotes migration, invasion, and clonogenicity of tumor cells, which was prevented upon its scavenging [69].

As mentioned above, most antioxidants are small molecules, which contributes to poor bioavailability, prevents target accumulation and causes mitochondrial damage. To overcome these limitations of LMW antioxidants, a delivery platform (nanoparticle) to modulate their pharmacokinetics property has been employed. Nanoparticles-based delivery of antioxidants may scavenge ROS below critical levels in tumors to inhibit their growth due to their higher bioavailability and enhanced permeability and retention (EPR) effects as compared to their LMW counterparts [70]. Several groups have reported the use of antioxidants with various delivery (drug delivery system; DDS) platforms. For example, quercetin-encapsulated liposomes showed in vitro anti-proliferation effect on the breast cancer cells, MCF-7 [71]. Nanoparticles with intrinsic redox ability also showed anti-proliferative and anti-tumor effects, such as mesoporous silica nanoparticles and cerium oxide nanoparticles [72,73]. However, several antioxidant-based delivery platforms have shown practical inhibitory effects in vitro with limited or no in vivo application. Furthermore, silica and cerium oxide have been reported to exert toxicity in mice models with biodegradability issues, thereby limiting their further use [72,74]. One of the major problems with conventional DDS is that the physically encapsulated drug leaks out of the system before reaching their target, which diminishes their efficacy and increases adverse effects. In order to achieve effective antioxidant cancer chemotherapy, a new strategy should be required to overcome the limitation of nanoparticles with physically encapsulated antioxidants. For the last decade, we have devoted a novel designed self-assembling antioxidants to treat oxidative stress-related diseases. The next section will discuss the design, structure, and advantages of our newly developed self-assembling antioxidants for cancer therapy.

4. Novel Self-Assembling Antioxidants; Nitroxide Radical-Containing Nanoparticle (RNP)

4.1. Design and Structure of RNPs

Although TEMPO is one the most potent antioxidants known, similar to the antioxidant enzyme, SOD, its clinical use is greatly limited due to its off-target effects, which can be attributed to its poor pharmacokinetic properties as stated above. In order to improve the pharmacokinetic properties to obtain high efficacy with negligible off-target effects, we have functionalized TEMPO and developed two different types of nitroxide radical-containing nanoparticles (RNPs); pH-sensitive (RNP^N) and pH-insensitive (RNP^O), and evaluated their ROS-reduction mediated anti-cancer effect in various in vitro and in vivo models of cancers as stand-alone or as adjuvants to reduce the aggressiveness or sensitize several cancers for the chemotherapy (Figure 1). Since TEMPO possesses an unpaired electron, it is an electron spin resonance (ESR) active species, which could be used for magnetic resonance imaging and pharmacokinetic studies. This property along with its powerful ROS scavenging ability, prompted us to employ TEMPO over other LMW antioxidants for developing self-assembling antioxidants for the biomedical applications [53,75,76].

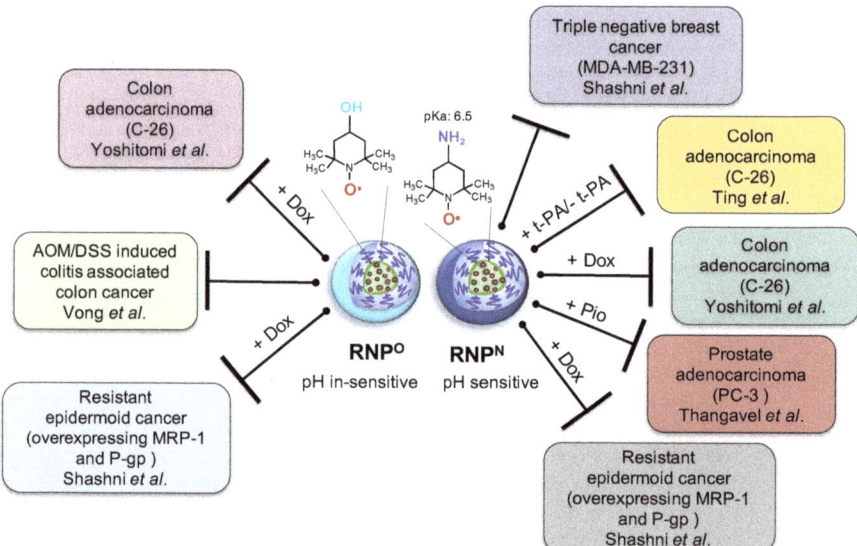

Figure 1. Illustration displaying the therapeutic efficacy of pH sensitive redox nanoparticle $(RNP)^N$ and pH in-sensitive RNP^O in various cancer models as stand-alone or as adjuvants with conventional anti-cancer drugs; doxorubicin (Dox) and pioglitazone (Pio).

RNPs are comprised of self-assembling amphiphilic block copolymer consisting of a hydrophilic poly (ethylene glycol) (PEG) segment and a hydrophobic poly (chloromethylstyrene) (PCMS) segment (Figure 2a). The chloromethyl groups of the PCMS segment are converted to TEMPO via the substitution of PEG-b-PCMS polymer with either 4-amino-TEMPO or with 4-hydroxyl-TEMPO to form base polymers: PEG-b-PMNT and PEG-b-PMOT, respectively [75–78]. Under physiological conditions, the block copolymer assembles into a core shell-type micelles with the hydrophobic segment (PMNT or PMOT, which contains TEMPO moieties as a side chain) in the core and hydrophilic PEG in the shell (cumulative average diameter of approximately 20–50 nm).

Since TEMPO moiety conjugates via ether linkage to the PMOT segment, PEG-*b*-PMOT gives a pH-insensitive RNP^O. In contrast, PEG-*b*-PMNT gives pH-sensitive RNP^N, because TEMPO conjugates to the PMNT segment via the amine linkage, which protonates under the acidic environment and changes its water solubility. Since the pKa of the amino group of the PMNT segment is ca. 6.5, most of the amino groups in RNP^N are not protonated under physiological conditions. However, under the acidic conditions, the protonated amine in the PMNT segment increases, converts their hydrophobic character to the hydrophilic, which weakens the core-coagulation force, leading to the collapse the micelle. Since the inflamed area such as the tumor environment, is known as decreased pH, we anticipated an increase in their antioxidant capacity by the exposure of TEMPO moiety due to collapsed RNP^N (Figure 2b,c). This means that both pH-insensitive RNP^O and pH-sensitive RNP^N will remain intact as a nano-sized self-assembling structure in the blood (pH 7.4). In contrast, under a low pH environment, e.g., cancer, only pH-sensitive RNP^N will collapse into individual polymers and show higher ROS scavenging potential than its intact micelle structure and RNP^O [78].

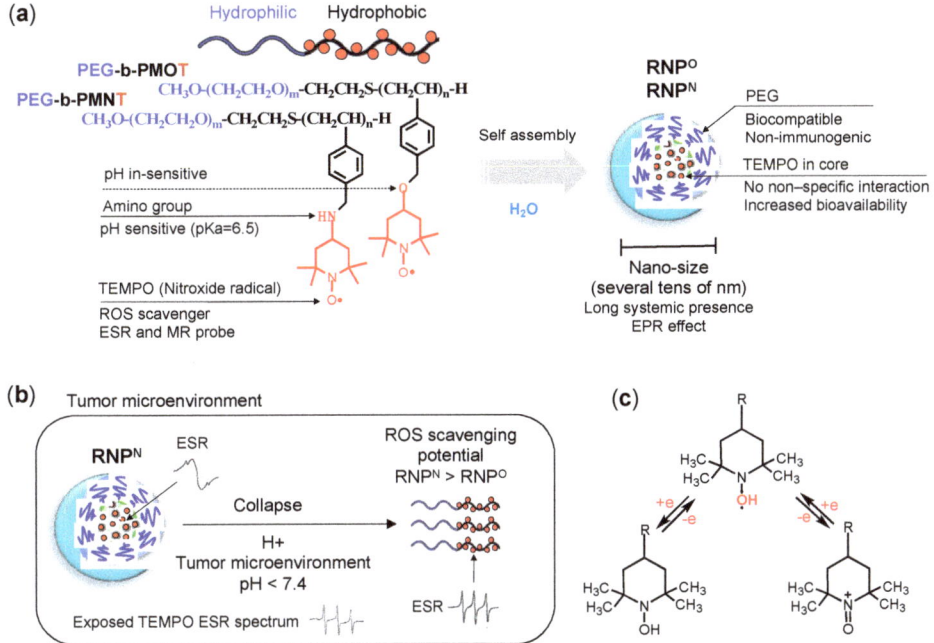

Figure 2. (**a**) Design and structure of antioxidant amphiphilic block copolymers, PEG-*b*-PMOT and PEG-*b*-PMNT, which self-assembles in aqueous media to form nano-sized micelles: pH-insensitive RNP^O and pH-sensitive RNP^N, respectively, used for cancer therapy. (**b**) Illustration showcasing pH-sensitive characteristic of RNP^N in the diseased environment (tumor); the amino groups of antioxidant TEMPO moieties in the copolymer (pKa 6.5) is protonated under the low pH in the tumor environment, leading to collapse of RNP^N micelle, which enhances its ROS scavenging potential than pH-insensitive RNP^O. The exposed radical of TEMPO can be detected by Electron Spin Resonance (ESR) as sharp triplet peaks, but when it is in the core of stable RNP^N, the ESR signal of TEMPO broadens. At low pH, due to disassembly of RNP^N, TEMPO radical is exposed and displays characteristic sharp triplet peaks of TEMPO. This ESR sensitive characteristic is essential for the pharmacokinetics studies of RNPs. (**c**) Reduction and oxidization reaction equations of TEMPO.

Following are the characteristics of RNPs validating its suitability for their use in in vivo applications.

i. Structure: RNP, a polymeric micelle made of amphipathic block copolymers, can stably disperse in in vivo harsh conditions due to the entanglement of hydrophobic segments in its core (Figure 2a) [79]. It is reported that PEG imparts biocompatible characteristic to nanoparticle by inhibiting electrostatic and hydrophobic interactions with proteins and cells sterically, thereby increasing the stability of nanoparticle [80]. Unpaired radical in TEMPO is stable by preventing the coupling with each other due to the protection by four methyl groups surrounding it. However, since ROS are small molecular radical species, they rapidly react with TEMPO's nitroxide radical. Although TEMPO is a highly reactive radical, it is conjugated via covalent linkage in the nanoparticle core; hence, non-specific interaction like LMW TEMPOL can be avoided upon administration. These characteristics potentially improve their accumulation in the target site via the EPR effect, which increases their therapeutic effects and prevents their premature renal excretion.

ii. Size: Core-shell type polymer micelles with several tens of nanometer in size (20–50 nm) ensures efficient accumulation in target intestinal mucosa (oral administration; colon cancer) or tumor vicinity (intravenous administration: breast cancer), additionally supported by the EPR effect [70,81,82]. It should be noted that the size range of RNP used in various anti-cancer studies, were small enough to prevent activation of the phagocytic system ($\leq$100 nm cutoff size). Conversely, RNPs were large enough to evade rapid renal clearance ($\geq$5.5 nm cutoff size) [83,84].

iii. Stability: Dynamic light scattering studies confirmed that RNP^O is stable under various pH 4–8.5, whereas pH-sensitive RNP^N was stable at pH 7.4 but decreased with a decrease in pH, confirming its collapse at low pH (diseased condition; tumor) (Figure 3a). Nonetheless, both the micelles maintained structural integrity at physiological pH 7.4, confirming the structural stability in the blood [77]. Furthermore, in ex vivo spiking experiments, we demonstrated that RNP do not internalize in the blood cells and prevents blood cell aggregation on the glass beads, which was in sharp contrast to TEMPOL (Figure 3b,c) [85]. This inert characteristic of RNPs with blood is extremely important for the systemic administration of nanoparticles.

iv. ESR active properties: ESR measurement shows a characteristics sharp triplet peak of the exposed TEMPO radical (an interaction between ^{14}N nuclei and the unpaired electron), but when confined in the core of RNP, the ESR signal of TEMPO broadens at the same magnetic field, due to restricted mobility of the radicals in RNP's solid core (Figure 2b) [75]. Due to this characteristic, it is very convenient to confirm the integrity and collapse of RNP and localization of RNPs for the pharmacokinetics studies.

RNPs have shown remarkable therapeutic effects with characteristics mentioned above than LMW antioxidant, TEMPOL, in various oxidative stress-related diseases such as cancer, colitis, cerebral hemorrhage, acute renal injury, Alzheimer's disease and so on, attributed to their favorable pharmacokinetic properties [86].

4.2. Safety of RNPs

It was previously reported that TEMPOL induces apoptosis by impairing the oxidative phosphorylation and targeting complex I of the respiratory system affecting mitochondrial membrane potential in HL-60 cells [87]. In our studies, similar findings confirmed that LMW TEMPOL exerts adverse effects in various models, potentially caused due to its facile internalization into the normal cells and disruption of critical redox balance attributed to highly reactive nitroxide radicals. On the other hand, due to their higher molecular weight (ca. 10 kDa) and the self-assembling size (ca. 20–50 nm), RNPs avoid internalization into the normal cells and prevents disruption of their redox homeostasis [85,88]. For instance, as shown in Figure 3d, when zebrafish were maintained in 3 mM and 30 mM TEMPOL solution, they died within five days of TEMPOL addition. In contrast, in 30 mM

RNP^O-treated group, more than 95% of zebrafish survived at day 5, confirming low toxicity of RNPs. This safety was further confirmed by the negligible damage to zebrafish mitochondria in the RNP-treated group, while the elevated damage was observed in the TEMPOL-treated group (Figure 3e) [88]. In the ex vivo blood spiking experiment, we also confirmed that RNPs do not interact and internalize into the healthy blood cells (Figure 3c) and disrupt mitochondrial membrane potential of blood cells, which was in sharp contrast to TEMPOL [85]. In addition, the median lethal dose (LD$_{50}$) of TEMPOL in C3H mice was 341 mg/kg through intravenous administration, whereas for RNP^N, LD$_{50}$ value was higher than 600 mg/kg (960 mmol N/kg) in ICR mice [77,89]. Extremely low toxicity of RNPs than LMW TEMPOL confirms that the confinement of conjugated TEMPO in the core of several tens of nanometer-sized self-assembled nanoparticles is necessary to avoid off-target effects and attain enhanced accumulation in the target tissue, leading to higher therapeutic effect.

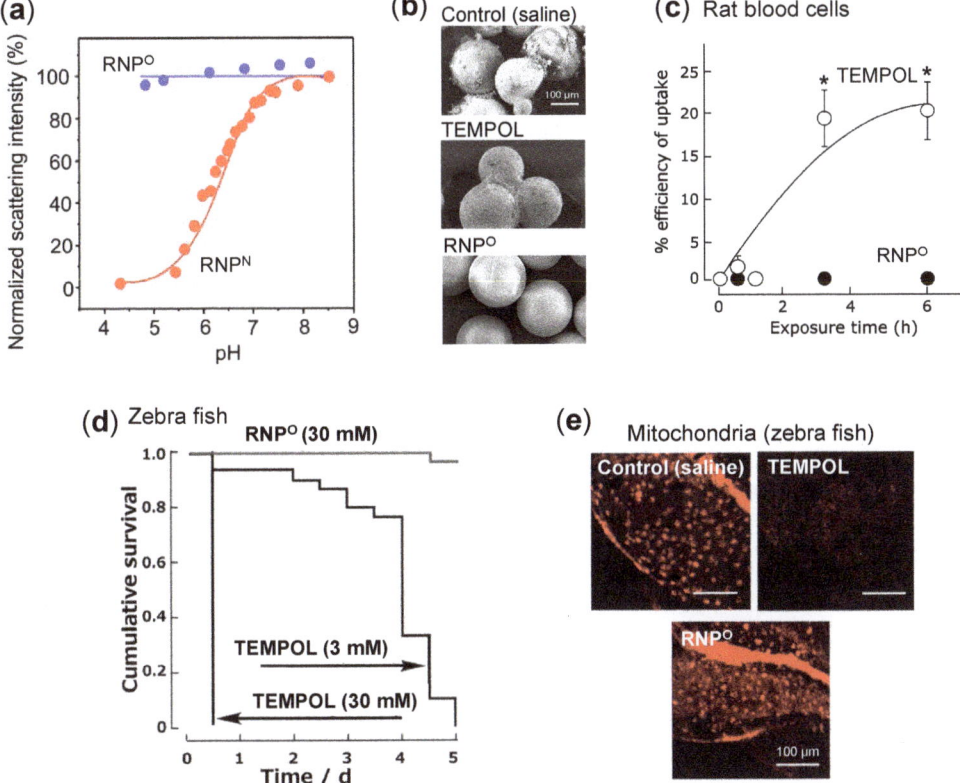

Figure 3. Characterization and non-toxicity of RNPs. (**a**) Laser light scattering intensity of RNP^O and RNP^N as a function of pH, assessed by dynamic light scattering [77]. (**b**) SEM images of glass beads spiked in rat whole blood with saline, TEMPOL, and RNP^O (5 mM) for 30 min [85]. (**c**) The cellular uptake of TEMPOL and RNP^O by rat whole blood cells evaluated by ESR [85]. (**d**) Cumulative survival of zebrafish embryo maintained in RNP^O (30 mM) and TEMPOL (3 and 30 mM) [88]. (**e**) Microscopic images of the mitochondrial damage in zebrafish larva after 12 h of treatment, assessed by mitotracker and analyzed using a fluorescent confocal microscope system, scale bar 100 µm [88]. * $p < 0.05$ was considered significant. This figure is reproduced with permission from References [77,85,88]. Copyright 2011, Elsevier; Copyright 2014, JCBN; Copyright 2016, American Chemical Society.

4.3. Pharmacokinetic Properties of RNPs

TEMPOL, a low molecular weight compound with an exposed reactive nitroxide radical, has poor pharmacokinetics, which excretes rapidly after the administration. Thus, to suppress the rapid excretion and avoid the unwanted adverse effects, we covalently conjugated TEMPO to the amphiphilic block copolymer backbone with self-assembling characteristics, forming nanoparticle with several tends nanometer in size and accumulation tendency in the target inflamed site, such as a tumor. We confirmed this improvement of the pharmacokinetic property of RNPs in the renal ischemia-reperfusion induced acute kidney injury mice model [77]. In this study, an equal dose of RNP^O, RNP^N, and TEMPOL (TEMPO: 75 mmol/kg) were administered to ICR mice, after which TEMPO concentration was measured in the blood and kidneys by ESR. As shown in Figure 4a, TEMPOL cleared from the blood within 0.1 h of the administration, whereas RNP^O and RNP^N remained in the blood for more than 10 h. In the injured kidney (Figure 4b), TEMPOL was excreted within 0.5 h of administration, whereas RNP^O remained for 24 h and RNP^N managed to stay more than 10 h. This data confirmed that the kidneys, a major clearance organ, do not remove the RNPs as fast as LMW TEMPO due to their suitable structure and size. It is known that after reperfusion in the ischemic kidney, ROS level is significantly elevated, causing inflammation and decreased pH via acidosis [90]. As shown in Figure 4a, RNP^O and RNP^N in the blood are observed as intact micelles, assessed through a broader ESR signal than TEMPOL radical. In kidneys with acidic lesions, RNP^O integrity remains intact. In contrast, the ESR signal of RNP^N resembles to that of free TEMPOL radical (Figure 4b), implying the micelle collapse in response to acidic pH in the injured kidneys. This data confirms the pH sensitivity of RNPs in the diseased condition and their stability during systemic circulation compared to LMW TEMPOL.

We also confirmed the pharmacokinetics of RNP^N in a mice model of colon cancer, by intravenous administration of RNP^N and TEMPOL (40 mg/kg of TEMPO), which was assessed by ESR measurement [82]. As shown in Figure 4c, RNP^N remains in the blood even until 24 h (AUC, 769.49). In contrast, the LMW TEMPOL signal decreases drastically within 2 h (AUC, 19.2), which may be attributed to their diffusion into the normal cells and preferential renal clearance. The total accumulation of RNP in the tumor tissues (AUC, 39.6) was at least 6–7 fold higher than LMW-TEMPOL (AUC, 6.5). After 24 h of administration, RNP^N in tumor tissues was 8–9 fold higher (3.3% ID/g tumor tissue) compared to TEMPOL (0.4% ID/g tumor tissue) (Figure 4d). Interestingly, RNP^N remained intact as micelle in the blood and collapsed in a low pH tumor area, as assessed by ESR spectra. The reports mentioned above confirm that the covalent conjugation of TEMPO with amphiphilic copolymer and their self-assembling core-shell structure significantly suppresses their adverse effect and prolongs their presence in the systemic circulation. Due to the long blood circulation of RNP, they gradually accumulate in the target site via the EPR effect with negligible diffusion in the normal cells compared to LMW highly reactive TEMPO radical. With such favorable pharmacokinetics and negligible toxicity compared to LMW antioxidants, we evaluated the therapeutic efficacy of RNPs in various cancer models. The next section will discuss the application of RNPs in breast cancer, colon cancer, prostate cancer, and resistant epidermoid cancers as stand-alone or as adjuvants with conventional anti-cancer drugs.

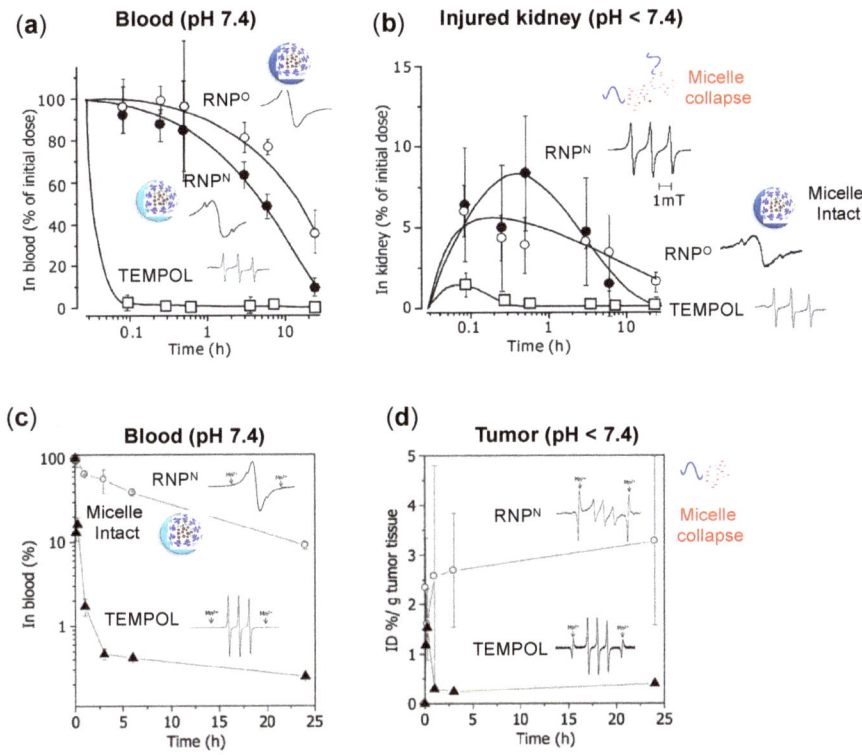

Figure 4. (**top**) Pharmacokinetic property of RNP^N and RNP^O in the blood and diseased organs. Time profile changes in the concentration of RNP^O, RNP^N, and TEMPOL; (**a**) blood and (**b**) injured kidney, after intravenous administration (75 mmol/kg of TEMPO concentration) in a renal ischemia-reperfusion induced acute kidney injury mice model [75,77]. The graph also displays ESR spectra of TEMPO radical of RNPs and TEMPOL. The ESR spectra of RNPs are broad under the physiological pH conditions (7.4), confirming their micelle integrity, in contrast with the sharp triplet peak of free TEMPOL. Under the decreased pH conditions, a typical diseased state, the pH-sensitive RNP^N group shows sharp triplet ESR signals, indicating the micelle collapse as compared to pH-insensitive RNP^O, whose micelle integrity is unaffected. (**bottom**). Biodistribution of RNP^N and TEMPOL in a colon tumor (C-26 colon cancer cell line) bearing mice after intravenous administration with 40 mg/kg of TEMPO concentration; (**c**) blood and (**d**) tumor [82]. These data confirm that RNP^N is stable in the blood (broad ESR signal), while it is collapsed in the tumor environment due to the reduced pH (sharp ESR peaks). This figure is reproduced with permission from References [75,77,82]. Copyright 2011, Elsevier; Copyright 2014, WILEY-VCH Verlag GmbH & Co. KGaA, Weinheim; Copyright, 2013 Elsevier B.V.

4.4. RNPs for Cancer Therapy

4.4.1. RNPs Inhibit the Tumorigenic Potential of Triple-Negative Breast Cancer

As stated above, we have succeeded in developing novel self-assembling antioxidants, which is less toxic and do not cause intracellular disturbance to the redox homeostasis of the normal cells. With these characteristics, the functionality of RNP as an anti-cancer drug was investigated in breast cancer. Breast cancer is the most common cancer occurring in women worldwide, with 2 million new cases diagnosed in 2018 (American Institute for Cancer Research). Due to the increase in the mortality rate of breast cancer patients, an alternative treatment is needed [91]. It was reported that breast cancer patients have significantly higher ROS levels such as superoxide and hydrogen peroxide in plasma, which correlated with the severity of the disease and altered antioxidant enzyme levels such as SOD in the tumor cells [92,93]. Copper, a potent oxidant, was also significantly elevated in the serum and tumor of cancer patients than the healthy subjects [94]. It is reported that copper induces HIF-1α and VEGF expression through the activation of the EGFR/ERK/c-fos transduction pathway promoting breast tumor angiogenesis and progression, which were reversed upon the addition of copper chelating agent and antioxidant NAC [95]. Menon et al. reported that the loss of redox control of the cell cycle might contribute to the aberrant proliferation of breast cancer cells [96]. Another report suggested that sublethal oxidative stress by H_2O_2/hypoxanthine and xanthine oxidase inhibited tumor cell adhesion to laminin and fibronectin and enhanced lung tumors of murine mammary carcinoma in an experimental metastasis model [97]. Based on these critical roles of oxidative stress in breast cancer survival, we evaluated the efficacy of our antioxidant self-assembled nanoparticle in a breast cancer model.

We investigated the anti-tumor and anti-metastatic effects of RNP^O and RNP^N using the triple-negative breast cancer cell line, MDA-MB231 (Figure 5a) [98,99]. Colony-forming assay was carried out in vitro using breast cancer cell lines, metastatic MDA-MB-231 and non-metastatic MCF-7. Treatment with IC_{50} values (RNP^O; MDA-MB-231 = 2.20 mM, MCF-7 = 1.14 mM, RNP^N; MDA-MB-231 = 3.00 mM, MCF-7 = 1.08 mM, and TEMPOL; MDA-MB-231 = 0.56 mM, MCF-7 = 0.46 mM), revealed that RNP^N showed the highest inhibition of colony-forming potential, followed by RNP^O and TEMPOL (Figure 5b). This data clearly indicates that the TEMPO-based antioxidants, RNP^N and RNP^O, exerted a long-term inhibitory effect on the breast cancer cell growth regardless of their metastasis tendency than LMW TEMPOL with less toxicity. We next investigated in vivo efficacy of RNPs in a mouse xenograft model of breast cancer cell line, MDA-MB231. Intravenous administration of RNP^O and RNP^N (TEMPO; 74.13 mg/kg, five times, three days interval) showed a significantly decreased tumor growth than the untreated control and TEMPOL (Figure 5c). The tumor growth profile graph clearly shows that RNPs inhibit tumor growth much higher than TEMPOL and comparable to the conventional anti-cancer drug paclitaxel (10 mg/kg, five times, three days interval), indicating the importance of ROS scavenging in breast cancer treatments. We also confirmed that RNPs showed anti-metastatic effect by inhibiting the growth of MDA-MB231 lung tumors in an experimental metastasis model, which was higher than TEMPOL (TEMPO: 18.53 mg/kg/mouse, 10 times, 3 days interval) and comparable to paclitaxel (5 mg/kg/mouse, 10 times, 3 days interval) (Figure 5d). This decrease in tumor size exerted by RNPs corroborated with decreased tumor ROS, which was negligibly reduced in the TEMPOL-treated group (Figure 5e).

NF-kB is a redox-sensitive transcriptional factor which regulates expression of metallomatrix protease (MMP-2) and α 2,6-sialyltransferae. MMPs function to degrade the extracellular matrix proteins and has been correlated with poor clinical outcome in breast cancer patients [10,100]. α 2,6-sialyltransferae catalyzes the addition of sialic acid to terminal oligosaccharides attached on the lipid or protein moieties of the tumor surface, which contributes to tumorigenesis, progression, and metastasis [101]. As shown in Figure 5f,g, both RNPs downregulate the expression of NF-kB, MMP-2, and α 2,6-sialyltransferae in MDA-MB231 tumors and cells, suggesting the mechanism of anti-tumor and anti-metastatic effect of RNPs. It should be noted that such high efficacy of our antioxidant nanoparticle was achieved with negligible adverse effects on the kidneys and livers, in contrast to LMW TEMPOL, and paclitaxel-treated group (Figure 5h,i). These reports suggest that our RNPs alone are more effective in inhibiting ROS-mediated tumorigenesis and metastasis of breast cancer as compared to LMW antioxidants.

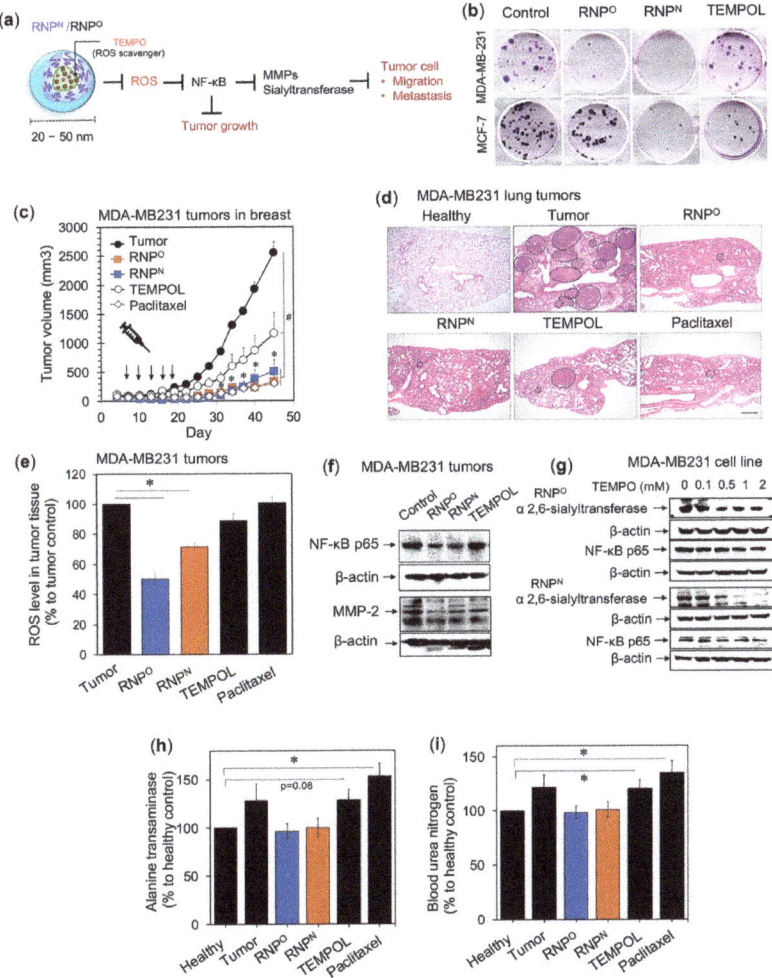

Figure 5. RNP^N and RNP^O inhibits the growth, proliferation, and metastatic potential of triple-negative breast cancer, MDA-MB231, with negligible adverse effects. (**a**) Schematic illustration of ROS-reduction mediated anti-tumor and anti-metastatic effect of RNPs. (**b**) Inhibition of colony-forming potential of breast cancer cell lines, MDA-MB231 and MCF-7 by RNP^N, RNP^O, and TEMPOL (IC_{50} value, 48 h). (**c**) Tumor growth profile of breast cancer cell line (MDA-MB231) in the mice xenograft model, intravenously administered with RNP^N, RNP^O, TEMPOL (74.13 mg/kg of TEMPO concentration), and conventional anti-cancer drug paclitaxel (10 mg/kg). (**d**) Representative histopathological H and E-stained lung sections of MDA-MB231 experimental metastasis model mice, intravenously administered with RNP^N, RNP^O, TEMPOL (18.5 mg/kg of TEMPO concentration) and paclitaxel (5 mg/kg). The encircled areas are representing MDA-MB231 tumors. Scale bar 500 μm. (**e**) ROS scavenging potential of RNPs in MDA-MB231 tumors detected by dihydroethidium compared to the untreated tumor as 100%. (**f**) Downregulation of MMP-2 and NF-kB expression by RNPs in MDA-MB231 tumors, as assessed by immunoblotting. (**g**) The ability of RNPs to suppress the expression of NF-kB and sialyltransferase, important enzymes assisting the metastasis of MDA-MB231 cell line, as assessed by immunoblotting [99]. Non-toxicity of RNPs as compared to LMW TEMPOL and paclitaxel after their intravenous administration, confirmed by liver and kidney damage markers: (**h**) alanine transaminase and (**i**) blood urea nitrogen, respectively. * $p < 0.05$ was considered significant [98]. This figure is reproduced with permission from References [98,99]. Copyright 2017, Elsevier Ltd.; Copyright 2018, Elsevier Ltd.

4.4.2. RNPs Inhibit the Tumor Growth and Progression of Colitis-Associated Cancer

An increase in oxidative stress and oxidative cellular damage promoting carcinogenesis has been observed in inflammatory bowel disease patients [102,103]. Ulcerative colitis (an inflammatory bowel disease) associated with colon cancer (CAC) is the third most common malignancy and one of the major causes of cancer-related death [104]. With these facts, we tested the efficacy of RNPs to suppress the oxidative stress-mediated tumor formation in the mice colon [105]. The pharmacokinetics of RNP^O by free drinking confirmed that RNP^O accumulates in the colon with negligible internalization in the blood (ESR measurement) (Figure 6a). The localization of rhodamine-labeled RNP^O further validated the colon accumulation of RNP^O after 4 h of administration. As shown in Figure 6b, the rhodamine-labeled RNP^O was strongly observed in the colon, especially in the colon's mucosa area. In contrast, no fluorescent was observed in rhodamine administered group, as it was excreted out sooner than RNP^O. This data confirmed that LMW antioxidants might not be suitable for CAC treatment due to their poor retentivity in the colon [106]. The effect of RNPs on colon cancer was investigated by a CAC mice model, which was prepared by intraperitoneal injection with azoxymethane (AOM) (10 mg/kg body weight) followed by two cycles of 7d-treatment of 3% dextran sodium sulfate (DSS) (Figure 6c). As shown in Figure 6d,e, the oral administration of RNP^O during DSS treatment significantly suppressed the tumor formation in the colon, which was confirmed by endoscopy and H and E stained colon tissues. In the RNP-treated group, no change in the body weight was observed compared to AOM/DSS control, which was significantly reduced during DSS treatment (data not shown).

It is worth noting that such an effect of RNP^O was supported with decreased colitis disease index and pro-inflammatory cytokine interferon-gamma (IFN-γ). These results indicate the potential of RNP^O to reduce colitis-induced inflammation, which is a major factor for the induction of colon cancer. Ad libitum drinking of RNP^O solution (5 mg/mL) after AOM and DSS treatment also significantly suppressed the tumor formation in the colon as assessed by endoscopy and histology (Figure 6f–h). These reports confirmed that RNP^O is an effective and suitable nano-antioxidant for the treatment of colon cancer.

4.4.3. Synergistic Effects of RNP and Fibrinolytic Tissue Plasminogen Activator for Colon Cancer Therapy

It is well known that the efficacy of drugs to inhibit tumor growth depends on whether the drug has sufficiently reached the target site or not, which depends on the blood perfusion status within the tumor vessels [107]. The tumor microenvironment is complex, comprising of extracellular matrix (ECM) components such as fibrin, elastin, laminin, collagen, platelet aggregation, etc. The ECM is known to obstruct the blood flow and perfusion to the tumor areas, limiting the effective delivery of drugs, contributing to inadequate drug response, and promoting drug resistance [108].

Degradation of ECM components from the tumor environment is a robust strategy to improve vascularization and blood supply to the tumors. Fibrinolytic tissue plasminogen activator (t-PA), is a member of the serine protease family, physiologically involved in the matrix regulation and homeostasis of the blood coagulation/fibrinolysis [109]. Zhang et al. reported on the use of t-PA for modulating the tumor microenvironment to improve the delivery efficiency of anti-cancer drug to the target site [110].

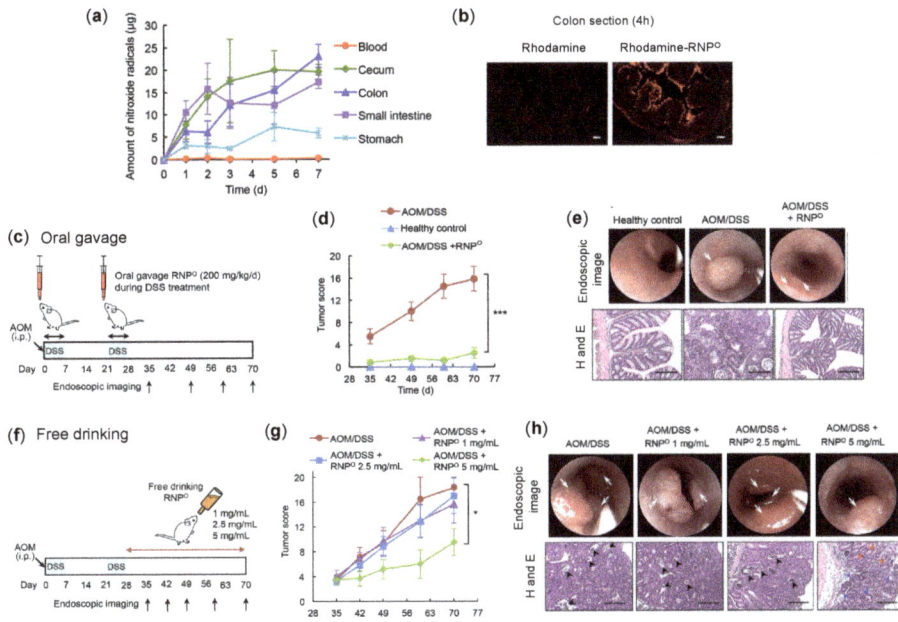

Figure 6. Anti-tumor effect of RNP^O in colitis-induced colon cancer (CAC) model. (**a**) Accumulation of RNP^O in the gastrointestinal tract by ad libitum drinking, assessed by ESR measurement [105]. (**b**) Localization of rhodamine-labeled RNP^O (rhodamine-RNP^O) in the colon section, 4 h after the oral administration with 5 mg/mL of rhodamine-RNP^O (1 mL), scale bar 200 μm [106]. (**c**) The scheme showing anti-tumor effect (protective) of orally administered RNP^O in azoxymethane (AOM) and dextran sodium sulfate (DSS) (AOM/CAC) induced colitis-associated cancer in mice. RNP^O (200 mg/kg/d) was administered by oral gavage during the two weeks of the DSS treatment period. (**d**) RNP^O inhibits the formation of colon tumor, confirmed by tumor score and assessed by endoscopy. (**e**) The endoscopic imaging of mice colon, displaying tumor shown by white arrows and H and E-stained colon tissues (scale bar 100 μm) at the experimental endpoint (day 70). (**f**) The scheme showing anti-tumor effect (therapeutic) of ad libitum drinking of RNP^O in AOM/CAC-induced colitis-associated cancer in mice. RNP^O (1, 2.5, and 5 mg/mL) was available as ad libitum drinking after AOM/DSS treatment. (**g**) The therapeutic effect of RNP^O to inhibit the formation of colon tumor as confirmed by tumor score, which was assessed by endoscopy. (**h**) The endoscopic imaging of mice colon, displaying tumor shown by white arrows and H and E stained colon tissues (scale bar 100 μm), at the experimental endpoint (day 70). Black arrows in H and E colon stained tissues indicate the necrotic cells surrounded by cancer cells, blue arrows indicate adenoma, and red arrows display normal crypts [105]. * $p < 0.05$ was considered significant. This figure is reproduced with permission from References [105,106]. Copyright 2018, Elsevier Ltd.; Copyright 2012, AGA Institute (Elsevier publisher).

Because the half-life of the naked t-PA is extremely short (<5 min), continuous and invasive intravenous administrations are required to show their effectiveness [111]. In this line, we employed RNP as a new delivery platform for t-PA, which not only acts as DDS with favorable pharmacokinetics but also contributes to the anti-tumor effect through ROS scavenging characteristic (Figure 7a) [112,113]. t-PA@iRNP (hereafter "i" in iRNP denotes the core composed of polyion complex) is a core-shell structured polyion complex (PIC) micelle consisting of three components: (i) ROS scavenging cationic PEG-b-PMNT diblock amphiphilic copolymers, (ii) anionic poly (acrylic acid) (PAAc) and (iii) fibrinolytic t-PA (Figure 7a). We found that t-PA@iRNP retained their enzymatic activity after 2 h ($t_{1/2}$ = 71 min) of intravenous administration, whereas the activity of naked t-PA decreased within 0.5 h ($t_{1/2}$ = 8 min) (Figure 7b) [113]. The prolonged enzymatic activity of t-PA@iRNP than naked t-PA is due to the stable encapsulation of t-PA in the iRNP matrix, which protected it from the enzymatic degradation. We have previously confirmed that t-

PA@iRNP had almost no enzymatic activity under the physiological pH (7.4). On the other hand, upon decreasing the pH, its enzymatic activity was significantly increased, indicating the pH responsive collapse of t-PA@iRNP. Intravenous administration of t-PA@iRNP (t-PA; 0.04mM and iRNP; 5.3 mM TEMPO, five times with interval of three days) to mouse xenograft model of C-26 colon cancer cell line, showed effective suppression of tumor growth as compared to control, t-PA@niRNP (no antioxidant capacity), naked t-PA, and iRNP, validating the synergistic effect of iRNP and t-PA (Figure 7c) [112]. Interestingly, iRNP alone also showed a significant anti-tumor effect on colon tumors. It should be noted that the pharmacokinetics of t-PA upon encapsulation by iRNP is favorably changed for in vivo application. This pattern can be seen in t-PA@niRNP, where a higher effect of t-PA could be observed when encapsulated in niRNP (no antioxidant capacity), than the naked t-PA itself, indicating the importance of delivery systems for the proteins (Figure 7c,d).

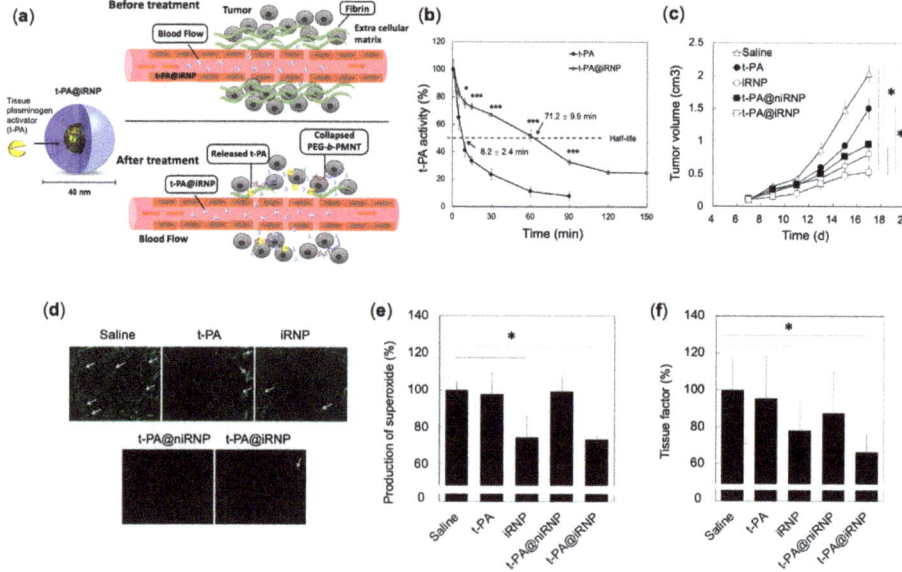

Figure 7. Anti-tumor effect of fibrinolytic tissue plasminogen activator installed in radical containing nanoparticles (t-PA@iRNP). (**a**) Schematic illustration of the delivery and therapeutic effect of t-PA@iRNP in tumors characterized by dense fibrin extracellular matrix [112]. (**b**) Ex vivo thrombolytic activity of t-PA enzyme, after intravenous administration in mice with equimolar dose of naked t-PA and t-PA@iRNP, measured using t-PA's ability to hydrolyze a tri-peptide chromogenic substrates of H-D-isoleucyl-L-prolyl-L-arginine-p-nitroanilide dihydrochloride to p-nitroaniline. Liberated p-nitroaniline was measured spectrophotometrically at 405 nm by using a UV-Vis spectrometer [113]. (**c**) Tumor growth profile in a C-26 colon murine cancer model, intravenously administered (5 times) with saline (control), t-PA (0.04 mM), and iRNP (TEMPO; 5.3 mM). (**d**) Representative images of fibrin immunofluorescence (white arrow) in the tumor tissues, scale bar 10 μm. (**e**) Superoxide level in tumor tissue homogenate measured by ROS sensitive dye, dihydroethidium. (**f**) Tissue factor in tumor lysates measured by ELISA [112]. * $p < 0.05$ was considered significant. This figure is reproduced with permission from References [112,113]. Copyright 2020, Elsevier Ltd.; Copyright 2019, Elsevier Ltd.

We also confirmed that the higher effect of t-PA@iRNP was due to higher fibrin degradation in the tumor area by t-PA (Figure 7d), decreased ROS (Figure 7e), and downregulated NF-kB by iRNP (data not shown). Both t-PA@iRNP and iRNP-treated group significantly reduced the expression of ROS-regulated tissue factor, which activates coagulation and platelets essential for tumor growth and metastasis increase (Figure 7f) [114,115]. Based on these results, it is clear that RNP possesses bidentate roles, viz., effective carriers for t-PA to target solid tumors and suitable anti-cancer drugs, which effectively scavenge overproduced ROS around the tumor environment.

4.4.4. RNPs Enhances the Therapeutic Efficiency of Pioglitazone on Prostate Cancer

Pioglitazone belongs to thiazolidinediones family that shows efficacy in type 2 diabetes mellitus and cancer, accompanied by several adverse effects such as hepatotoxicity, cardiac abnormalities, and weight gain due to fluid retention [116]. In addition to severe toxicity exerted by pioglitazone, poor solubility and low bioavailability due to extensive liver metabolism are also its drawbacks [117]. Several reports have confirmed that liver metabolism of pioglitazone forms reactive oxidative intermediates that potentially damages hepatocytes [118]. Considering this, we prepared RNP encapsulated with pioglitazone (Pio@RNP^N) to prevent premature metabolism of pioglitazone in the liver by modulating its pharmacokinetics property and decrease its ROS-mediated adverse effect by TEMPO radical of RNP (Figure 8a) [116]. Pharmacokinetic studies revealed that oral administration of Pio@RNP^N, enhanced systemic presence of pioglitazone (AUC: 113.2) to twice as compared to free pioglitazone (oral) (AUC: 51.2), whereas intravenous administration Pio@RNP^N showed the highest plasma concentration of pioglitazone (AUC: 723.9) (Figure 8b). In this study, free pioglitazone was administered orally in a CMC formulation due to its low solubility, whereas no such issue was observed in the encapsulation of pioglitazone in RNP. Biodistribution studies confirmed that Pio@RNP^N (intravenous; i.v.) accumulated highest in tumor tissues (10% ID/g tissue) followed by oral administration of Pio@RNP^N (3.8% ID/g tissue) and oral pioglitazone (1.2% ID/g tissue) (Figure 8c).

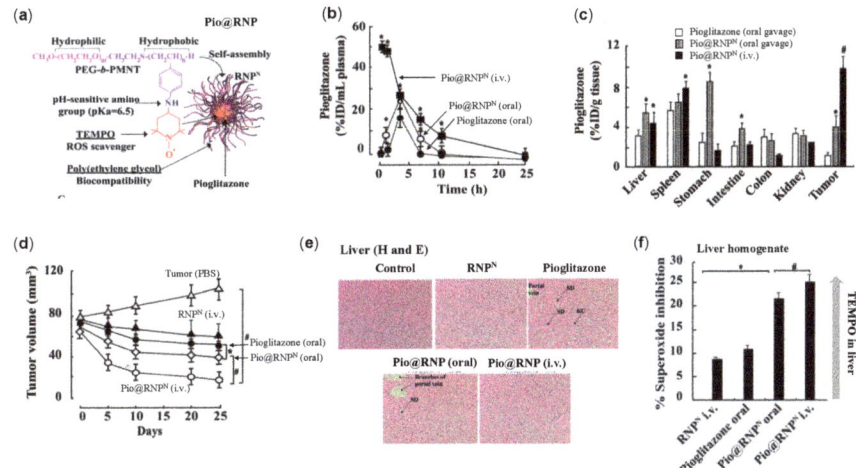

Figure 8. RNP increases the chemotherapeutic efficiency of pioglitazone (Pio) and suppresses its adverse effects. (**a**) Chemical structure of RNP^N's polymer (PEG-b-PMNT) and illustration of pioglitazone encapsulated in RNP^N. (**b**) Systemic bioavailability pioglitazone (oral), Pio@RNP^N (oral), and Pio@ RNP^N (i.v.) in mice administered with 15 mg/kg of pioglitazone. (**c**) Biodistribution of pioglitazone in various organs of mice after the treatment period of 25 days. (**d**) Tumor growth profile of prostate cancer (PC-3) in a mouse model, administered with PBS (control), free pioglitazone and Pio@ RNP^N (Pio: 15 mg/kg and RNP^N: 300 mg/kg). (**e**) RNP^N suppresses the adverse effect exerted by pioglitazone as assessed by liver histology stained by H and E (SD: sinusoidal dilatation, KC: Kupffer cells). (**f**) Superoxide inhibitory activity in liver homogenates administered with samples (from tumor xenograft studies) as evaluated by xanthine-xanthine oxidase assay [116]. * $p < 0.05$ was considered significant. This figure is reproduced with permission from Reference [116]. Copyright 2016, Elsevier Ltd.

With such favorable pharmacokinetic properties of Pio@RNP^N over free pioglitazone, its anti-cancer therapeutic efficacy was tested in a mouse xenograft model of prostate cancer (PC-3) (Figure 8d). At the experimental endpoint, orally administered pioglitazone reduced tumor volume by only 25%, Pio@RNP^N (oral) by 36%, while Pio@RNP^N (i.v.) showed the highest anti-tumor effect with 60% growth inhibition. In addition, intravenous administration of Pio@RNP^N largely protected the liver toxicity exerted by ROS induced by the pioglitazone treatment (Figure 8e). An ex vivo xanthine/xanthine oxidase (superoxide scavenging) assay was conducted to measure the ROS scavenging effect of the TEMPO in the liver homogenates of the treated mice. In this assay, the xanthine/xanthine oxidase system generates superoxide ion radicals detected by nitro blue tetrazolium. When liver homogenates from treated mice are spiked with xanthine/xanthine oxidase, the generated superoxide ions are scavenged by antioxidants in liver homogenates, in our case, nitroxide radical (TEMPO). Higher the TEMPO in the liver homogenates, the higher the superoxide inhibition/scavenging ability. Figure 8f shows that Pio@RNP^N (i.v.) exerts highest superoxide ion inhibition potential than orally administered Pio@RNP^N, and pioglitazone itself, suggesting the localization of RNP^N in liver which might have contributed to the inhibition of pioglitazone-mediated adverse effect. This data corroborated with the result of lipid peroxidation status in the liver. We confirmed that Pio@RNP^N (i.v.) treated group had a significantly lower lipid peroxidation level than pioglitazone (data not shown). These reports highlights the potential of RNP^N as a DDS that increases the therapeutic efficacy of pioglitazone and decreases its adverse effects.

4.4.5. RNPs Enhances the Therapeutic Efficiency of Doxorubicin on Colon Cancer and Epidermoid Cancers

The effectiveness of cancer chemotherapy is greatly limited due to the drug-resistant characteristics of tumor cells, attributed largely to their drug efflux system [119]. It is reported that P-glycoprotein (P-gp) and multi-drug resistance-associated protein-1 (MRP1), which belong to the ATP-binding cassette (ABC) transporter superfamily, are overexpressed in various cancers [120]. P-gp and MRP-1 both have been reported to confer resistance to various cancers against anti-cancer drugs [121]. With this fact in mind, several drug combination approaches have been applied that use ABC transporter inhibitors as adjuvants to overcome the drug resistance and potentiate the anti-cancer drug efficacy. For instance, administration of dofequidar, a P-gp inhibitor, with anti-cancer drugs such as cyclophosphamide, doxorubicin (Dox) and fluorouracil to patients with advanced or recurrent breast cancer, increased progression-free survival days from 241 (without P-gp inhibitor) to 366 [122]. However, several clinical trials have largely failed to manifest the therapeutic efficacy of such anti-cancer drugs/adjuvants. For instance, no improvement in the disease-free survival was observed in recurring or refractory multiple myeloma patients with and without P-gp inhibitor, valspodar, in conjunction with vincristine, Dox, and dexamethasone [123]. Although drug-efflux system inhibition for multi-drug resistance tumor therapy seems to be robust, these effects are not noteworthy. Binkhathlan et al. attributed the apparent failure of these adjuvants (drug efflux inhibitors) to demonstrate clinical efficacy to their non-specific action and distribution, causing toxicities due to their LMW [124]. Another possibility might be that the inhibitors themselves were not compelling enough. In this line, improved drug efflux inhibitors or the use of the delivery platform that specifically accumulates in the resistant tumors are highly desirable.

It was reported previously that oxidative stress is strongly related to this drug resistance. For example, ROS activates NF-kB, which increases drug efflux proteins such as P-gp and MRP-1, located in the cellular membrane [125]. It was also previously reported that P-gp and MRP-1 both are regulated independently by ROS in cancers [126,127]. Therefore, antioxidants are one of the candidates to suppress this drug resistance and increase the efficacy of anti-cancer drugs. Although pre-administration of LMW antioxidants such as edaravone and TEMPO have been evaluated to suppress the drug resistance of cancers, the results are not satisfactory [60,128]. Despite the fact that the antioxidant application for the chemoresistant cancer treatment may be in the right direction, however, they might not be effective due to the preferential clearance properties or low systemic retention as stated above. Therefore, in this line, we applied antioxidant RNPs to overcome the shortcoming of LMW drug efflux protein inhibitors/antioxidants by decreasing the ROS associated drug resistance.

Dox, is known to generate ROS in vivo, which results in severe adverse effects in the normal tissues and increases the drug resistance of tumors [129]. Thus, we evaluated the ability of our RNPs to sensitize cancer cells and potentiate the efficacy of Dox by scavenging ROS in the colon and epidermoid cancer models. We have previously shown that intravenous administration of RNP accumulates significantly higher in C-26 colon tumors, while LMW TEMPOL excretes faster (Figure 4c,d) [82]. To confirm the sensitizing effect of RNPs, in a C-26 colon cancer model, we pre-administered RNP^N (i.v.) for 4 days, followed by Dox administration (10 mg/kg) [82]. The RNP^N + Dox-treated group showed the highest tumor growth suppression, followed by the free Dox administration group, as shown in the tumor growth profile graph (Figure 9a). It is interesting to see that pre-administration of TEMPOL did not decrease any tumor growth at all as compared to Dox alone, which indicates the poor systemic and tumor presence of TEMPOL compared to RNP^N (Figure 4c,d and Figure 9a). As previously mentioned, Dox increases the ROS, which is one of the reasons for its off-target effects on the heart and several other organs. We confirmed that pre-administration of RNP^N decreases the ROS in the heart tissues (Figure 9b), which prevented Dox-induced cardiotoxicity as assessed by creatine phosphokinase, a marker for myocardial damage (Figure 9c). Such protective effect was not seen in the TEMPOL treated group. These data implied that RNP not only potentiate the efficacy of Dox against colon cancer but also decreases its adverse effects.

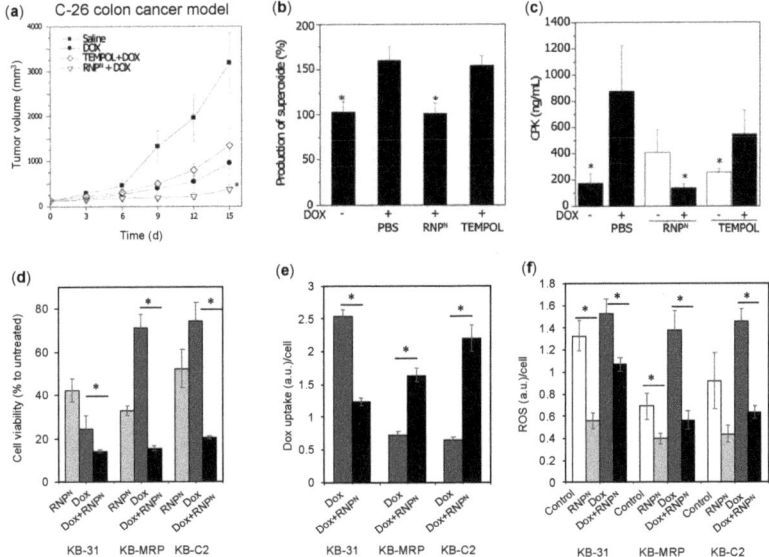

Figure 9. (top). RNP increases the therapeutic effect of doxorubicin (Dox) in a colon cancer model. (**a**) Tumor growth profile of subcutaneous colon tumor (C-26) pre-treated with RNP^N (i.v., 100 mg/day for 4 days, days−4 to −1), followed by a single injection of DOX (i.v., 10 mg/kg on day 0). The ability of RNP^N to inhibit the cardiotoxicity of Dox mediated by increased ROS [82]; (**b**) inhibition of superoxide level by RNP^N in the heart homogenates, (**c**) creatine phosphokinase (CPK) in plasma, a marker of heart damage. Mice were intravenously injected with RNP^N (25 mg/kg/day) and LMW-TEMPOL (4 mg/kg/day), followed by DOX (20 mg/kg, i.v.) 30 min later. 3 days post Dox administration, samples were analyzed. (**bottom**). RNPs increases the therapeutic effect of Dox by overcoming drug resistance in the epidermoid cancer cell lines. (**d**) Cytotoxicity of combination treatments: RNP^N (2 mg/mL) and Dox (5 μg/mL) for 48 h in epidermoid cancer cell lines-drug sensitive KB-31, drug-resistant KB-MRP overexpressing drug efflux transporter, MRP-1 and drug-resistant KB-C2 overexpressing drug efflux transporter, P-gp; (**e**) Dox uptake in epidermoid cancer cell lines after 2 h of treatment (RNP^N (2 mg/mL) and Dox (5 μg/mL)). (**f**) ROS level after 24 h of treatment with RNP^N (2 mg/mL) and Dox (5 μg/mL) in epidermoid cancer cell lines [130]. * $p < 0.05$ was considered significant. This figure is reproduced with permission from Reference [82] and adapted from [130]. Copyright 2013, Elsevier B.V.; Copyright 2017, Elsevier Ltd.

In our next study, we confirmed this effect by co-treatment of RNP^N with Dox in 3 different types of epidermoid cancer cells: Drug-sensitive KB-31, drug-resistant KB-C2 (overexpressing P-gp) and KB-MRP (overexpressing MRP-1) (Figure 9d–f) [130]. As shown in Figure 9d, the viability of resistant cancer cell lines with the combination treatment of RNP^N + Dox decreases significantly as compared to the Dox alone (48 h treatment). These significantly different efficiencies corroborated with Dox uptake tendencies; where in RNP^N treatment (2 h), a significantly higher Dox uptake was observed in contrast to cells without RNP^N (Figure 9e). Figure 9f shows that ROS is elevated in the resistant cancer cells that may further confer resistance to the cancer cells, which was significantly reduced upon RNP^N treatment. It should be noted that the drug-sensitive cell line, KB-31, was sensitive to RNP and Dox treatment, with high internalization of Dox, confirming negligible drug resistance level due to low drug efflux proteins. These data imply that the antioxidant activity of RNP is essential to modulate the drug efflux proteins by scavenging regulatory ROS, allowing the enhanced internalization and toxicity of Dox. Based on these data, it is concluded that RNP is a potential antioxidant to decrease the drug resistance of various cancers.

5. Conclusions

Cancers are characterized by persistent elevated intracellular ROS, critical for their survival, proliferation, angiogenesis, and metastasis. Therefore, the use of antioxidants is a suitable choice of therapeutic interventions to impede tumorigenesis. However, the failure of LMW antioxidants to inhibit tumors clinically accentuates the need for new therapeutic strategies to limit various cancers. In this line, our newly developed self-assembling antioxidants, RNP^O and RNP^N, both have shown effective ROS-reduction mediated anti-cancer effect in vitro and in vivo as stand-alone or as an adjuvant to reduce aggressiveness and/or sensitize several cancers for chemotherapy. Higher bioavailability, specific tumor accumulation, and negligible toxicity of RNPs make them more suitable antioxidant therapeutic intervention than LMW counterparts for the cancer treatment. Recently, several other groups have started antioxidant therapy based on their own design. For instance, Moriyama et al., prepared antioxidant micelles from poly (ethylene glycol)-b-poly (dopamine) block copolymers that inhibits angiogenesis in the chicken ex ovo chorioallantoic membrane assay [131]. Rocha et al., also developed epigallocatechin-3-gallate incorporated polysaccharide nanoparticles which inhibited Du145 prostate cancer cells in vitro [132]. Including their work, the authors hope to establish a new field for antioxidant-based cancer therapeutics.

Author Contributions: Original draft preparation, review and editing, B.S. and Y.N. All authors have read and agreed to the published version of the manuscript.

Funding: This research received no external funding.

Institutional Review Board Statement: Not applicable.

Informed Consent Statement: Not applicable.

Data Availability Statement: Not applicable.

Acknowledgments: We would like to thank Nguyen Le Bui Thao for her assistance in the literature search.

Conflicts of Interest: The authors declare no conflict of interest.

References

1. Mukherji, S.M.; Singh, S.P. *Reaction Mechanism in Organic Chemistry*; Macmillan India Press: Chennai, India, 1986.
2. Gomberg, M. An incidence of trivalent carbon trimethylphenyl. *J. Am. Chem. Soc.* **1900**, *22*, 757–771. [CrossRef]
3. Gerschman, R.; Gilbert, D.L.; Nye, S.W.; Dwyer, P.; Fenn, W.O. Oxygen poisoning and x-irradiation: A mechanism in common. *Science* **1954**, *119*, 623–626. [CrossRef]
4. McCord, J.M.; Fridovich, I. Superoxide dismutase. an enzymic function for erythrocuprein (hemocuprein). *J. Biol. Chem.* **1969**, *24*, 6049–6055. [CrossRef]

5. Halliwell, B. Free radicals and other reactive species in disease. In *Nature Encyclopedia of Life Sciences*; Nature Publishing Group: London, UK, 2001; pp. 1–7.
6. Phaniendra, A.; Jestadi, D.B.; Periyasamy, L. Free radicals: Properties, sources, targets, and their implication in various diseases. *Indian J. Clin. Biochem.* **2015**, *30*, 11–26. [CrossRef] [PubMed]
7. McCord, J.M.; Fridovich, I. Free radicals, antioxidants in disease and health. *Int. J. Biomed. Sci.* **2008**, *4*, 89–96.
8. Dreher, D.; Junod, A.F. Role of oxygen free radicals in cancer development. *Eur. J. Cancer* **1996**, *32*, 30–38. [CrossRef]
9. Fuchs-Tarlovsky, V. Role of antioxidants in cancer therapy. *Nutrition* **2013**, *29*, 15–21. [CrossRef]
10. Morry, J.; Ngamcherdtrakul, W.; Yantasee, W. Oxidative stress in cancer and fibrosis: Opportunity for therapeutic intervention with antioxidant compounds, enzymes, and nanoparticles. *Redox. Biol.* **2017**, *11*, 240–253. [CrossRef]
11. Perillo, B.; Di Donato, M.; Pezone, A.; Zazzo, E.D.; Giovannelli, P.; Galasso, G.; Castoria, G.; Migliaccio, A. ROS in cancer therapy: The bright side of the moon. *Exp. Mol. Med.* **2020**, *202052*, 192–203. [CrossRef]
12. Hsie, A.W.; Recio, L.; Katz, D.S.; Lee, C.Q.; Wagner, M.; Schenley, R.L. Evidence for reactive oxygen species inducing mutations in mammalian cells. *Proc. Natl. Acad. Sci. USA* **1986**, *83*, 9616–9620. [CrossRef]
13. Weiss, S.J. Tissue destruction by neutrophils. *N. Engl. J. Med.* **1989**, *320*, 365–376. [PubMed]
14. Terzić, J.; Grivennikov, S.; Karin, E.; Karin, M. Inflammation and colon cancer. *Gastroenterology* **2010**, *138*, 2101–2114. [CrossRef] [PubMed]
15. Ames, B.N.; Shigenaga, M.K.; Hagen, T.M. Oxidants, antioxidants, and the degenerative diseases of aging. *Proc. Natl. Acad. Sci. USA* **1993**, *90*, 7915–7922. [CrossRef] [PubMed]
16. Shigenaga, M.K.; Gimeno, C.J.; Ames, B.N. Urinary 8-hydroxy- 2-deoxyguanosine as a biological marker of in vivo oxidative DNA damage. *Proc. Natl. Acad. Sci. USA* **1989**, *86*, 9697–9701. [CrossRef]
17. Valko, M.; Rhodes, C.J.; Moncol, J.; Izakovic, M.; Mazur, M. Free radicals, metals and antioxidants in oxidative stress-induced cancer. *Chem. Biol. Interact.* **2006**, *160*, 1–40. [CrossRef]
18. Ames, B.N. Dietary carcinogens and anticarcinogens. Oxygen radicals and degenerative diseases. *Science* **1983**, *221*, 1256–1264. [CrossRef]
19. Lindahl, T. Instability and decay of the primary structure of DNA. *Nature* **1993**, *362*, 709–715. [CrossRef]
20. Marnett, L.J. Oxyradicals and DNA damage. *Carcinogenesis* **2000**, *21*, 361–370. [CrossRef]
21. Cooke, M.S.; Evans, M.D.; Dizdaroglu, M.; Lunec, J. Oxidative DNA damage: Mechanisms, mutation, and disease. *FASEB J.* **2003**, *17*, 1195–1214. [CrossRef]
22. Prior, I.A.; Lewis, P.D.; Mattos, C. A comprehensive survey of Ras mutations in cancer. *Cancer Res.* **2012**, *72*, 2457–2467. [CrossRef]
23. Xu, W.; Trepel, J.; Neckers, L. Ras, ROS and proteotoxic stress: A delicate balance. *Cancer Cell* **2011**, *20*, 281–282. [CrossRef]
24. Vousden, K.H.; Lane, D.P. p53 in health and disease. *Nat. Rev. Mol. Cell Biol.* **2007**, *8*, 275–283. [CrossRef] [PubMed]
25. Maillet, A.; Pervaiz, S. Redox regulation of p53, redox effectors regulated by p53: A subtle balance. *Antioxid. Redox Signal.* **2012**, *16*, 1285–1294. [CrossRef] [PubMed]
26. He, Z.; Simon, H.U. A novel link between p53 and ROS. *Cell Cycle* **2013**, *12*, 201–202. [CrossRef] [PubMed]
27. Perri, F.; Pisconti, S.; Della Vittoria Scarpati, G. P53 mutations and cancer: A tight linkage. *Ann. Transl. Med.* **2016**, *4*, 522. [CrossRef] [PubMed]
28. Vogelstein, B.; Kinzler, K.W. p53 function and dysfunction. *Cell* **1992**, *70*, 523–526. [CrossRef]
29. Amiri, K.I.; Richmond, A. Role of nuclear factor-kappa B in melanoma. *Cancer Metast. Rev.* **2005**, *24*, 301–313. [CrossRef]
30. Nakajima, S.; Kitamura, M. Bidirectional regulation of NF-κB by reactive oxygen species: A role of unfolded protein response. *Free Radic. Biol. Med.* **2013**, *65*, 162–174. [CrossRef]
31. Knight, J.A. Free radicals, antioxidants, and the immune system. *Ann. Clin. Lab. Sci.* **2000**, *30*, 145–158.
32. Xia, L.; Tan, S.; Zhou, Y.; Lin, J.; Wang, H.; Oyang, L.; Tian, Y.; Liu, L.; Su, M.; Wang, H.; et al. Role of the NFκB-signaling pathway in cancer. *OncoTargets Ther.* **2018**, *11*, 2063–2073. [CrossRef]
33. Larsson, R.; Cerutti, P. Translocation and enhancement of phosphotransferase activity of protein kinase C following exposure in mouse epidermal cells to oxidants. *Cancer Res.* **1989**, *49*, 5627–5632. [PubMed]
34. Gopalakrishna, R.; Anderson, W. Ca^{2+}-and phospholipid-independent activation of protein kinase C by selective oxidative modification of the regulatory domain. *Proc. Natl. Acad. Sci. USA* **1989**, *86*, 6758–6762. [CrossRef]
35. Lopez-Ilasaca, M.; Crespo, P.; Pellici, P.G.; Gutkind, J.S.; Wetzker, R. Linkage of G protein-coupled receptors to the MAPK signaling pathway through PI 3-kinase gamma. *Science* **1997**, *275*, 394–397. [CrossRef] [PubMed]
36. Gao, N.; Jiang, B.H.; Leonard, S.S.; Corum, L.; Zhang, Z.; Roberts, J.R.; Antonini, J.; Zheng, J.Z.; Flynn, D.C.; Castranova, V.; et al. p38 Signaling-mediated hypoxia-inducible factor 1 alpha and vascular endothelial growth factor induction by Cr (VI) in DU145 human prostate carcinoma cells. *J. Biol. Chem.* **2002**, *277*, 45041–45048. [CrossRef] [PubMed]
37. Hsu, T.C.; Young, M.R.; Cmarik, J.; Colburn, N.H. Activator protein 1 (AP-1)- and nuclear factor kappa B (NF-kappa B)- dependent transcriptional events in carcinogenesis. *Free Rad. Biol. Med.* **2000**, *28*, 1338–1348. [CrossRef]
38. Huang, C.; Li, J.; Costa, M.; Zhang, Z.; Leonard, S.S.; Castranova, V.; Vallyathan, V.; Ju, G.; Shi, X. Hydrogen peroxide mediates activation of nuclear factor of activated T cells (NFAT) by nickel sulfide. *Cancer Res.* **2001**, *61*, 8051–8057. [PubMed]
39. Mancini, M.; Toker, A. NFAT proteins: Emerging roles in cancer progression. *Nat. Rev. Cancer.* **2009**, *9*, 810–820. [CrossRef]
40. Um, H.D. Bcl-2 family proteins as regulators of cancer cell invasion and metastasis: A review focusing on mitochondrial respiration and reactive oxygen species. *Oncotarget* **2016**, *7*, 5193–5203. [CrossRef]

41. Sharma, M.; Rajappa, M.; Kumar, G.; Sharma, A. Oxidant-antioxidant status in Indian patients with carcinoma of posterior one-third of tongue. *Cancer Biomark.* **2009**, *5*, 253–260. [CrossRef]
42. Lee, Y.J.; Lee, D.M.; Lee, C.H.; Heo, S.H.; Won, S.Y.; Im, J.H.; Cho, M.K.; Nam, H.S.; Lee, S.H. Suppression of human prostate cancer PC-3 cell growth by N-acetylcysteine involves over-expression of Cyr61. *Toxicol. In Vitro* **2011**, *25*, 199–205. [CrossRef]
43. Lee, M.F.; Chan, C.Y.; Hung, H.C.; Chou, I.T.; Yee, A.S.; Huang, C.Y. N-acetylcysteine (NAC) inhibits cell growth by mediating the EGFR/Akt/HMG box-containing protein 1 (HBP1) signaling pathway in invasive oral cancer. *Oral Oncol.* **2013**, *49*, 129–135. [CrossRef] [PubMed]
44. Lv, H.; Wang, C.; Fang, T.; Li, T.; Lv, G.; Han, Q.; Yang, W.; Wang, H. Vitamin C preferentially kills cancer stem cells in hepatocellular carcinoma via SVCT-2. *NPJ Precis. Oncol.* **2018**, *2*, 1. [CrossRef] [PubMed]
45. Zeng, L.H.; Wang, Q.M.; Feng, L.Y.; Ke, Y.D.; Xu, Q.Z.; Wei, A.Y.; Zhang, C.; Ying, R.B. High-dose vitamin C suppresses the invasion and metastasis of breast cancer cells via inhibiting epithelial-mesenchymal transition. *OncoTargets Ther.* **2019**, *12*, 7405–7413. [CrossRef] [PubMed]
46. Turley, J.M.; Fu, T.; Ruscetti, F.W.; Mikovits, J.A.; Bertolette, D.C., 3rd; Birchenall-Roberts, M.C. Vitamin E succinate induces Fas-mediated apoptosis in estrogen receptor-negative human breast cancer cells. *Cancer Res.* **1997**, *57*, 881–890. [PubMed]
47. Weiping, Y.; Qiao, Y.L.; Feras, M.; Hantash, B.G. Sanders and Kimberly Kline. Activation of extracellular signal-regulated kinase and c-Jun-NH$_2$-terminal kinase but not p38 mitogen-activated protein kinases is required for RRR-α-Tocopheryl succinate-induced apoptosis of human breast cancer cells. *Cancer Res.* **2001**, *61*, 6569–6576.
48. Choi, J.A.; Kim, J.Y.; Lee, J.Y.; Kang, C.M.; Kwon, H.J.; Yoo, Y.D.; Kim, T.W.; Lee, Y.S.; Lee, S.J. Induction of cell cycle arrest and apoptosis in human breast cancer cells by quercetin. *Int. J. Oncol.* **2001**, *19*, 837–844. [CrossRef]
49. Pratheeshkumar, P.; Budhraja, A.; Son, Y.O.; Wang, X.; Zhang, Z.; Ding, S.; Wang, L.; Hitron, A.; Lee, J.C.; Xu, M.; et al. Quercetin inhibits angiogenesis mediated human prostate tumor growth by targeting VEGFR- 2 regulated AKT/mTOR/P70S6K signaling pathways. *PLoS ONE* **2012**, *7*, e47516. [CrossRef]
50. Richter, M.; Ebermann, R.; Marian, B. Quercetin-induced apoptosis in colorectal tumor cells: Possible role of EGF receptor signaling. *Nutr. Cancer* **1999**, *34*, 88–99. [CrossRef]
51. Wilcox, C.S. Effects of tempol and redox-cycling nitroxides in models of oxidative stress. *Pharmacol. Ther.* **2010**, *126*, 119–145. [CrossRef]
52. Münzel, T.; Afanas'ev, I.B.; Kleschyov, A.L.; Harrison, D.G. Detection of superoxide in vascular tissue. *Arter. Thromb. Vasc. Biol.* **2002**, *22*, 1761–1768. [CrossRef]
53. Soule, B.P.; Hyodo, F.; Matsumoto, K.; Simone, N.L.; Cook, J.A.; Krishna, M.C.; Mitchell, J.B. The chemistry and biology of nitroxide compounds. *Free Radic. Biol. Med.* **2007**, *42*, 1632–1650. [CrossRef] [PubMed]
54. Suy, S.; Mitchell, J.B.; Ehleiter, D.; Haimovitz-Friedman, A.; Kasid, U. Nitroxides tempol and tempo induce divergent signal transduction pathways in MDA-MB 231 breast cancer cells. *J. Biol. Chem.* **1998**, *273*, 17871–17878. [CrossRef] [PubMed]
55. Gariboldi, M.B.; Lucchi, S.; Caserini, C.; Supino, R.; Oliva, C.; Monti, E. Antiproliferative effect of the piperidine nitroxide TEMPOL on neoplastic and nonneoplastic mammalian cell lines. *Free Radic. Biol. Med.* **1998**, *24*, 913–923. [CrossRef]
56. Gariboldi, M.B.; Rimoldi, V.; Supino, R.; Favini, E.; Monti, E. The nitroxide tempol induces oxidative stress, p21(WAF1/CIP1), and cell death in HL60 cells. *Free Radic. Biol. Med.* **2000**, *29*, 633–641. [CrossRef]
57. Gariboldi, M.B.; Ravizza, R.; Petterino, C.; Castagnaro, M.; Finocchiaro, G.; Monti, E. Study of in vitro and in vivo effects of the piperidine nitroxide Tempol-a potential new therapeutic agent for gliomas. *Eur. J. Cancer* **2003**, *39*, 829–837. [CrossRef]
58. Schubert, R.; Erker, L.; Barlow, C.; Yakushiji, H.; Larson, D.; Russo, A.; Mitchell, J.B.; Wynshaw-Boris, A. Cancer chemoprevention by the antioxidant tempol in *Atm*-deficient mice. *Hum. Mol. Genetics* **2004**, *13*, 1793–1802. [CrossRef] [PubMed]
59. Mitchell, J.B.; Xavier, S.; DeLuca, A.M.; Sowers, A.L.; Cook, J.A.; Krishna, M.C.; Hahn, S.M.; Russo, A.A. A low molecular weight antioxidant decreases weight and lowers tumor incidence. *Free Rad. Biol. Med.* **2003**, *34*, 93–102. [CrossRef]
60. Suy, S.; Mitchell, J.B.; Samuni, A.; Mueller, S.; Kasid, U. Nitroxide tempo, a small molecule, induces apoptosis in prostate carcinoma cells and suppresses tumor growth in athymic mice. *Cancer* **2005**, *103*, 1302–1313. [CrossRef]
61. Klein, E.A.; Thompson, I.M.; Tangen, C.M., Jr.; Crowley, J.J.; Lucia, M.S.; Goodman, P.J.; Minasian, L.M.; Ford, L.G.; Parnes, H.L.; Gaziano, J.M.; et al. Vitamin E and the risk of prostate cancer: The selenium and vitamin E cancer prevention trial (SELECT). *JAMA* **2011**, *306*, 1549–1556. [CrossRef]
62. Lippman, S.M.; Klein, E.A.; Goodman, P.J.; Lucia, M.S.; Thompson, I.M.; Ford, L.G.; Parnes, H.L.; Minasian, L.M.; Gaziano, J.M.; Hartline, J.A.; et al. Effect of selenium and vitamin E on risk of prostate cancer and other cancers: The Selenium and Vitamin E Cancer Prevention Trial (SELECT). *JAMA* **2009**, *301*, 39–51. [CrossRef]
63. Neuhouser, M.L.; Barnett, M.J.; Kristal, A.R.; Ambrosone, C.B.; King, I.B.; Thornquist, M.; Goodman, G.G. Dietary supplement use and prostate cancer risk in the carotene and retinol efficacy trial. *Cancer Epidemiol. Biomark.* **2009**, *18*, 2202–2206. [CrossRef] [PubMed]
64. Blot, W.J.; Li, J.Y.; Taylor, P.R.; Guo, W.; Dawsey, S.; Wang, G.Q.; Yang, C.S.; Zheng, S.F.; Gail, M.; Li, G.Y.; et al. Nutrition intervention trials in Linxian, China: Supplementation with specific vitamin/mineral combinations, cancer incidence, and disease-specific mortality in the general population. *J. Natl. Cancer Inst.* **1993**, *85*, 1483–1492. [CrossRef] [PubMed]
65. Goodman, G.E.; Thornquist, M.D.; Balmes, J.; Cullen, M.R.; Meyskens, F.L., Jr.; Omenn, G.S.; Valanis, B.; Williams, J.H., Jr. The beta-carotene and retinol efficacy rrial: Incidence of lung cancer and cardiovascular disease mortality during 6-year follow-up after stopping beta-carotene and retinol supplements. *J. Natl. Cancer Inst.* **2004**, *96*, 1743–1750. [CrossRef] [PubMed]

66. Radak, Z.; Zhao, Z.; Koltai, E.; Ohno, H.; Atalay, M. Oxygen consumption and usage during physical exercise: The balance between oxidative stress and ROS-dependent adaptive signaling. *Antioxid. Redox Signal.* **2013**, *18*, 1208–1246. [CrossRef] [PubMed]
67. Bjelakovic, G.; Nikolova, D.; Gluud, L.L.; Simonetti, R.G.; Gluud, S. Mortality in randomized trials of antioxidant supplements for primary and secondary prevention. *JAMA* **2007**, *297*, 842–857. [CrossRef] [PubMed]
68. Gal, L.K.; Ibrahim, M.; Wiel, C.; Sayin, V.; Akula, M.; Karlsson, C. Antioxidants can increase melanoma metastasis in mice. *Sci. Transl. Med.* **2015**, *7*, 308re8. [CrossRef] [PubMed]
69. Porporato, P.E.; Payen, V.L.; Perez-Escuredo, J.; Saedeleer, C.J.; Danhier, P.A.; Copetti, T.; Suveera, D.; Tardy, M.; Vazeille, T.; Bouzin, C.; et al. Mitochondrial switch promotes tumor metastasis. *Cell Rep.* **2014**, *8*, 754–766. [CrossRef]
70. Matsumura, Y.; Maeda, H. A new concept for macromolecular therapeutics in cancer chemotherapy: Mechanism of tumoritropic accumulation of proteins and the antitumor agent smancs. *Cancer Res.* **1986**, *46*, 6387–6392.
71. Rezaei-Sadabady, R.; Eidi, A.; Zarghami, N.; Barzegar, A. Intracellular ROS protection efficiency and free radical-scavenging activity of quercetin and quercetin-encapsulated liposomes. *Artif. Cells Nanomed. Biotechnol.* **2016**, *44*, 128–134. [CrossRef]
72. Hijaz, M.; Das, S.; Mert, I.; Gupta, A.; Al-Wahab, Z.; Tebbe, C.; Sajad, D.; Chinna, J.; Giri, S.; Munkarah, A.; et al. Folic acid tagged nanoceria as a novel therapeutic agent in ovarian cancer. *BMC Cancer* **2016**, *16*, 220. [CrossRef]
73. Morry, J.; Ngamcherdtrakul, W.; Gu, S.; Reda, M.; Castro, D.J.; Sangvanich, T.; Gray, J.W.; Yantasee, W. Targeted treatment of metastatic breast cancer by PLK1 siRNA delivered by an antioxidant nanoparticle platform. *Mol. Cancer Ther.* **2017**, *16*, 763–772. [CrossRef] [PubMed]
74. Li, L.; Liu, T.; Fu, C.; Tan, L.; Meng, X.; Liu, H. Biodistribution, excretion, and toxicity of mesoporous silica nanoparticles after oral administration depend on their shape. *Nanomedicine* **2015**, *11*, 1915–1924. [CrossRef] [PubMed]
75. Yoshitomi, T.; Nagasaki, Y. Reactive oxygen species-scavenging nanomedicines for the treatment of oxidative stress injuries. *Adv. Healthc. Mater.* **2014**, *3*, 1149–1161. [CrossRef] [PubMed]
76. Yoshitomi, T.; Nagasaki, Y. Nitroxyl radical-containing nanoparticles for novel nanomedicine against oxidative stress injury. *Nanomedicine* **2011**, *6*, 509–518. [CrossRef]
77. Yoshitomi, T.; Hirayama, A.; Nagasaki, Y. The ROS scavenging and renal protective effects of pH-responsive nitroxide radical-containing nanoparticles. *Biomaterials* **2011**, *32*, 8021–8028. [CrossRef]
78. Yoshitomi, T.; Suzuki, R.; Mamiya, T.; Matsui, H.; Hirayama, A.; Nagasaki, Y. pH-Sensitive radical-containing-nanoparticle (RNP) for the L-Band-EPR imaging of low pH circumstances. *Bioconjugate Chem.* **2009**, *20*, 1792–1798. [CrossRef]
79. Francis, M.; Cristea, M.; Winnik, F. Polymeric micelles for oral drug delivery: Why and how. *Pure Appl. Chem.* **2004**, *76*, 1321–1335. [CrossRef]
80. Suk, J.S.; Xu, Q.; Kim, N.; Hanes, J.; Ensign, L.M. PEGylation as a strategy for improving nanoparticle-based drug and gene delivery. *Adv. Drug Deliv. Rev.* **2016**, *99*, 28–51. [CrossRef]
81. Sha, S.; Vong, L.B.; Chonpathompikunlert, P.; Yoshitomi, T.; Matsui, H.; Nagasaki, Y. Suppression of NSAID-induced small intestinal inflammation by orally administered redox nanoparticles. *Biomaterials* **2013**, *34*, 8393–8400. [CrossRef]
82. Yoshitomi, T.; Ozaki, Y.; Thangavel, S.; Nagasaki, Y. Redox nanoparticle therapeutics to cancer—Increase in therapeutic effect of doxorubicin, suppressing its adverse effect. *J. Control. Release* **2013**, *172*, 137–143. [CrossRef]
83. Choi, H.S.; Liu, W.; Misra, P.; Tanaka, E.; Zimmer, J.P.; Ipe, B.I.; Bawendi, M.G.; Frangioni, J. Renal clearance of nanoparticles. *Nat. Biotechnol.* **2017**, *25*, 1165–1170. [CrossRef] [PubMed]
84. Li, S.D.; Huang, L. Pharmacokinetics and biodistribution of nanoparticles. *Mol. Pharm.* **2008**, *5*, 496–504. [CrossRef] [PubMed]
85. Shimizu, M.; Yoshitomi, T.; Nagasaki, Y. The behavior of ROS scavenging nanoparticles in blood. *J. Clin. Biochem.* **2014**, *54*, 166–173. [CrossRef]
86. Nagasaki, Y. Design and application of redox polymers for nanomedicine. *Polym. J.* **2018**, *50*, 821–836. [CrossRef]
87. Monti, E.; Supino, R.; Colleoni, M.; Costa, B.; Ravizza, R.; Gariboldi, M.B. Nitroxide TEMPOL impairs mitochondrial function and induces apoptosis in HL60 cells. *J. Cell. Biochem.* **2001**, *82*, 271–276. [CrossRef] [PubMed]
88. Vong, L.B.; Kobayashi, M.; Nagasaki, Y. Evaluation of the toxicity and antioxidant activity of redox nanoparticles in Zebrafish (Danio rerio) embryos. *Mol. Pharm.* **2016**, *13*, 3091–3097. [CrossRef] [PubMed]
89. Hahn, S.M.; Tochner, Z.; Krishna, C.M.; Glass, J.; Wilson, L.; Samuni, A.; Sprague, M.; Venzon, D.; Glatstein, E.; Mitchell, J.B.; et al. Tempol, a stable free radical, is a novel murine radiation protector. *Cancer Res.* **1992**, *52*, 1750–1753.
90. Magalhães, P.A.; de Brito, T.S.; Freire, R.S.; da Silva, M.T.; dos Santos, A.A.; Vale, M.L.; de Menezes, D.B.; Martins, A.M.; Libório, A.B. Metabolic acidosis aggravates experimental acute kidney injury. *Life Sci.* **2016**, *146*, 58–65. [CrossRef]
91. Azamjah, N.; Soltan-Zadeh, Y.; Zayeri, F. Global trend of breast cancer mortality rate: A 25-Year Study. *Asian Pac. J. Cancer Prev.* **2019**, *20*, 2015–2020. [CrossRef]
92. Yeh, C.C.; Hou, M.F.; Tsai, S.M.; Lin, S.K.; Hsiao, J.K.; Huang, J.C.; Wang, L.H.; Wu, S.H.; Hou, L.A.; Ma, H.; et al. Superoxide anion radical, lipid peroxides and antioxidant status in the blood of patients with breast cancer. *Clin. Chim. Acta* **2005**, *361*, 101–111. [CrossRef]
93. Renschler, F. The emerging role of reactive oxygen species in cancer therapy. *Eur. J. Cancer* **2004**, *40*, 1934–1940. [CrossRef] [PubMed]
94. Kumaraguruparan, R.; Subapriya, R.; Kablimoorthy, J.; Nagini, S. Antioxidant profile in the circulation of patients with fibroadenoma and adenocarcinoma of the breast. *Clin. Biochem.* **2002**, *35*, 275–279. [CrossRef]

95. Rigiracciolo, D.C.; Scarpelli, A.; Lappano, R.; Pisano, A.; Santolla, M.F.; De Marco, P.; Cirillo, F.; Cappello, A.R.; Dolce, V.; Belfiore, A.; et al. Copper activates HIF-1alpha/GPER/VEGF signalling in cancer cells. *Oncotarget* **2015**, *6*, 34158–34177. [CrossRef] [PubMed]
96. Menon, S.G.; Coleman, M.C.; Walsh, S.A.; Spitz, D.R.; Goswami, P.C. Differential susceptibility of nonmalignant human breast epithelial cells and breast cancer cells to thiol antioxidant-induced G(1)-delay. *Antioxid. Redox Signal.* **2005**, *7*, 711–718. [CrossRef] [PubMed]
97. Kundu, N.; Zhang, S.; Fulton, A.M. Sublethal oxidative stress inhibits tumor cell adhesion and enhances experimental metastasis of murine mammary carcinoma. *Clin. Exp. Metastasis* **1995**, *13*, 16–22. [CrossRef]
98. Shashni, B.; Nagasaki, Y. Nitroxide radical-containing nanoparticles attenuate tumorigenic potential of triple negative breast cancer. *Biomaterials* **2018**, *178*, 48–62. [CrossRef]
99. Shashni, B.; Horiguchi, Y.; Kurosu, K.; Furusho, H.; Nagasaki, Y. Application of surface enhanced Raman spectroscopy as a diagnostic system for hypersialylated metastatic cancers. *Biomaterials* **2017**, *134*, 143–153. [CrossRef]
100. Duffy, M.J.; Maguire, T.M.; Hill, A.; McDermott, E.; Higgins, N.O. Metal-loproteinases: Role in breast carcinogenesis, invasion and metastasis. *Breast Cancer Res.* **2000**, *2*, 252–257. [CrossRef]
101. Bull, C.; Stoel, M.A.; Brok, M.H.D.; Adema, G.J. Sialic acids sweeten a tumor's life. *Cancer Res.* **2014**, *74*, 3199–3204. [CrossRef]
102. Coussens, L.M.; Werb, Z. Inflammation and cancer. *Nature* **2002**, *420*, 860–867. [CrossRef]
103. Gommeaux, J.; Cano, C.; Garcia, S.; Gironella, M.; Pietri, S.; Culcasi, M.; Gommeaux, J.; Pébusque, M.J.; Malissen, B.; Dusetti, N.; et al. Colitis and colitis-associated cancer are exacerbated in mice deficient for tumor protein 53-induced nuclear protein 1. *Mol. Cell. Biol.* **2007**, *27*, 2215–2228. [CrossRef] [PubMed]
104. Tenesa, A.; Dunlop, M.G. New insights into the aetiology of colorectal cancer from genome-wide association studies. *Nat. Rev. Genet.* **2009**, *10*, 353–358. [CrossRef] [PubMed]
105. Vong, L.B.; Yoshitomi, T.; Matsui, H.; Nagasaki, Y. Development of an oral nanotherapeutics using redox nanoparticles for treatment of colitis-associated colon cancer. *Biomaterials* **2015**, *55*, 54–63. [CrossRef] [PubMed]
106. Vong, L.B.; Tomita, T.; Yoshitomi, T.; Matsui, H.; Nagasaki, Y. An orally administered redox nanoparticle that accumulates in the colonic mucosa and reduces colitis in mice. *Gastroenterology* **2012**, *143*, 1027–1036. [CrossRef] [PubMed]
107. Minchinton, A.I.; Tannock, I.F. Drug penetration in solid tumours. *Nat. Rev.* **2006**, *6*, 583–592. [CrossRef]
108. Netti, P.A.; Berk, D.A.; Swartz, M.A.; Grodzinsky, A.J.; Jain, R.K. Role of extracellular matrix assembly in interstitial transport in solid tumors. *Cancer Res.* **2000**, *60*, 2497–2503.
109. Mars, W.M.; Zarnegar, R.; Michalopoulos, G.K. Activation of hepatocyte growth factor by the plasminogen activators uPA and tPA. *Am. J. Pathol.* **1993**, *143*, 949–958.
110. Zhang, B.; Jiang, T.; She, X.; Shen, S.; Wang, S.; Deng, J.; Shi, W.; Mei, H.; Hu, Y.; Pang, Z.; et al. Fibrin degradation by rtPA enhances the delivery of nanotherapeutics to A549 tumors in nude mice. *Biomaterials* **2016**, *96*, 63–71. [CrossRef]
111. Nilsson, T.; Wallen, P.; Mellbring, G. In vivo metabolism of human tissue-type plasminogen activator. *Scand. J. Haematol.* **1984**, *33*, 49–53. [CrossRef]
112. Mei, T.; Shashni, B.; Maeda, H.; Nagasaki, Y. Fibrinolytic tissue plasminogen activator installed redox-active nanoparticles (t-PA@iRNP) for cancer therapy. *Biomaterials* **2020**, *259*, 120290. [CrossRef]
113. Mei, T.; Kim, A.; Vong, L.B.; Marushima, A.; Puentes, S.; Matsumaru, Y.; Matsumura, A.; Nagasaki, Y. Encapsulation of tissue plasminogen activator in pH-sensitive self-assembled antioxidant nanoparticles for ischemic stroke treatment-Synergistic effect of thrombolysis and antioxidant. *Biomaterials* **2019**, *215*, 119209. [CrossRef] [PubMed]
114. Fernandez, P.M.; Patierno, S.R.; Rickles, F.R. Tissue factor and fibrin in tumor angiogenesis. *Semin. Thromb. Hemost.* **2004**, *30*, 31–44. [PubMed]
115. Cadroy, Y.; Dupouy, D.; Boneu, B.; Plaisancié, H. Polymorphonuclear leukocytes modulate tissue factor production by mononuclear cells: Role of reactive oxygen species. *J. Immunol.* **2000**, *164*, 3822–3828. [CrossRef] [PubMed]
116. Thangavel, S.; Yoshitomi, T.; Sakharkar, M.K.; Nagasaki, Y. Redox nanoparticle increases the chemotherapeutic efficiency of pioglitazone and suppresses its toxic side effects. *Biomaterials* **2016**, *99*, 109–123. [CrossRef] [PubMed]
117. Floyd, J.S.; Barbehenn, E.; Lurie, P.; Wolfe, S.M. Case series of liver failure associated with rosiglitazone and pioglitazone. *Pharmaco epidemiol. Drug Saf.* **2009**, *18*, 1238–1243.
118. Rabbani, S.I.; Devi, K.; Khanam, S. Role of pioglitazone with metformin or glimepiride on oxidative stress-induced nuclear damage and reproductive toxicity in diabetic rats. *Malays. J. Med. Sci.* **2010**, *17*, 3–11.
119. Fojo, T.; Menefee, M. Mechanisms of multidrug resistance: The potential role of microtubule-stabilizing agents. *Ann. Oncol.* **2007**, *18*, v3–v8. [CrossRef]
120. Holohan, C.; Schaeybroeck, S.V.; Longley, D.B.; Johnston, P.G. Cancer drug resistance: An evolving paradigm. *Nat. Rev.* **2013**, *13*, 714–726. [CrossRef]
121. Housman, G.; Byler, S.; Heerboth, S.; Lapinska, K.; Longacre, M.; Snyder, N.; Sarkar, S. Drug resistance in cancer: An overview. *Cancers* **2014**, *6*, 1769–1792. [CrossRef]
122. Saeki, T.; Nomizu, T.; Toi, M.; Ito, Y.; Noguchi, S.; Kobayashi, T.; Asaga, T.; Minami, H.; Yamamoto, N.; Aogi, K.; et al. Dofequidar fumarate (MS-209) in combination with cyclophosphamide, doxorubicin, and fluorouracil for patients with advanced or recurrent breast cancer. *J. Clin. Oncol.* **2007**, *25*, 411–417. [CrossRef]

123. Friedenberg, W.R.; Rue, M.; Blood, E.A.; Dalton, W.S.; Shustik, C.; Larson, R.A.; Sonneveld, P.; Greipp, P.R. Phase III study of PSC-833 (valspodar) in combination with vincristine, doxorubicin, and dexamethasone (valspodar/VAD) versus VAD alone in patients with recurring or refractory multiple myeloma (E1A95): A trial of the Eastern Cooperative Oncology Group. *Cancer* **2006**, *106*, 830–838. [CrossRef] [PubMed]
124. Binkhathlan, Z.; Lavasanifar, A. P-glycoprotein inhibition as a therapeutic approach for overcoming multidrug resistance in cancer: Current status and future perspectives. *Curr. Cancer Drug Targets* **2013**, *13*, 326–346. [CrossRef] [PubMed]
125. Bentires-Alj, M.; Barbu, V.; Fillet, M.; Chariot, A.; Relic, B.; Jacobs, N.; Gielen, J.; Merville, M.P.; Bours, B. NF-κB transcription factor induces drug resistance through MDR1 expression in cancer cells. *Oncogene* **2003**, *22*, 90–97. [CrossRef] [PubMed]
126. Szakacs, G.; Paterson, J.K.; Ludwig, J.A.; Booth-Genthe, C.; Gottesman, M.M. Targeting multidrug resistance in cancer. *Nat. Rev. Drug Discov.* **2006**, *5*, 219–234. [CrossRef] [PubMed]
127. Rivera, E. Implications of anthracycline-resistant and taxane-resistant meta- static breast cancer and new therapeutic options. *Breast J.* **2010**, *16*, 252–263. [CrossRef]
128. Kokura, S.; Yoshida, N.; Sakamoto, N.; Ishikawa, T.; Takagi, T.; Higashihara, H.; Nakabe, N.; Handa, O.; Naito, Y.; Yoshikawa, T. The radical scavenger edaravone enhances the anti-tumor effects of CPT-11 in murine colon cancer by increasing apoptosis viainhibition of NF-kappaB. *Cancer Lett.* **2005**, *229*, 223–233. [CrossRef] [PubMed]
129. DeAtley, S.M.; Aksenov, M.Y.; Aksenova, M.V.; Jordan, B.; Carney, J.M.; Butterfield, D.A. Adriamycin-induced changes of creatine kinase activity in vivo and in cardiomyocyte culture. *Toxicology* **1999**, *134*, 51–62. [CrossRef]
130. Shashni, B.; Alshwimi, A.; Minami, M.; Furukawa, T.; Nagasaki, T. Nitroxide radical-containing nanoparticles as potential candidates for overcoming drug resistance in epidermoid cancers. *Polymer* **2017**, *116*, 429–438. [CrossRef]
131. Moriyama, M.; Metzger, S.; van der Vlies, A.J.; Uyama, H.; Ehrbar, M.; Hasegawa, U. Inhibition of angiogenesis by antioxidant micelles. *Adv. Healthc. Mater.* **2015**, *4*, 569–575. [CrossRef]
132. Rocha, S.; Generalov, R.; Pereira Mdo, C.; Peres, I.; Juzenas, P.; Coelho, M.A. Epigallocatechin gallate-loaded polysaccharide nanoparticles for prostate cancer chemoprevention. *Nanomedicine* **2011**, *6*, 79–87. [CrossRef]

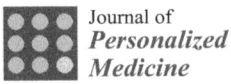

Review

Harnessing Extracellular Matrix Biology for Tumor Drug Delivery

Nithya Subrahmanyam [1,2] and Hamidreza Ghandehari [1,2,3,*]

1. Department of Pharmaceutics and Pharmaceutical Chemistry, University of Utah, Salt Lake City, UT 84112, USA; nithya.subrahmanyam@utah.edu
2. Utah Center for Nanomedicine, University of Utah, Salt Lake City, UT 84112, USA
3. Department of Biomedical Engineering, University of Utah, Salt Lake City, UT 84112, USA
* Correspondence: hamid.ghandehari@utah.edu

Abstract: The extracellular matrix (ECM) plays an active role in cell life through a tightly controlled reciprocal relationship maintained by several fibrous proteins, enzymes, receptors, and other components. It is also highly involved in cancer progression. Because of its role in cancer etiology, the ECM holds opportunities for cancer therapy on several fronts. There are targets in the tumor-associated ECM at the level of signaling molecules, enzyme expression, protein structure, receptor interactions, and others. In particular, the ECM is implicated in invasiveness of tumors through its signaling interactions with cells. By capitalizing on the biology of the tumor microenvironment and the opportunities it presents for intervention, the ECM has been investigated as a therapeutic target, to facilitate drug delivery, and as a prognostic or diagnostic marker for tumor progression and therapeutic intervention. This review summarizes the tumor ECM biology as it relates to drug delivery with emphasis on design parameters targeting the ECM.

Keywords: extracellular matrix; drug delivery; tumor; cancer; targeting

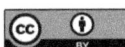

1. Introduction

Targeted drug delivery capitalizes on biological aspects of the tumor ECM, and can thus be informed by an understanding of the intricate dynamics that affect the tumor microenvironment. Many drug carriers are modified to target specific upregulated biomarkers, proteins, receptors, and other epitopes within the tumor ECM in order to increase localization by capitalizing on a biological change in the tumor microenvironment compared to healthy tissue. Here we summarize both drug delivery and cancer biology literature to understand the local dynamics that influence drug delivery.

The ECM, the complex non-cellular environment, is essential to cell processes [1]. It has a reciprocal relationship with cells, providing signaling cues that influence nearly all aspects of cell life [2]. Once thought to be merely a structural support, the ECM is now well-recognized to have a homeostatic relationship with cells maintained through biochemical and mechanotransducive interactions [3]. Homeostasis is maintained through a tightly structured enzymatic processing of ECM components. In cancer, this homeostasis is disrupted in favor of promoting excessive growth of cells and an invasive phenotype [4]. The ECM presents opportunities to target, treat, and modulate the stroma, as well as epitope targets and biological mechanisms that can be harnessed for therapeutic intervention [5]. For example, the contribution of various ECM enzymes to tumor growth and invasion has led to development of therapeutics based on enzyme inhibition strategies. Additionally, the biochemical and morphological changes in the ECM can be interpreted as diagnostic and prognostic markers [6,7].

In this review, we take a comprehensive look at the many ways that the ECM can be used as a tool for cancer treatment. To this end, we first discuss the complex biology of the ECM, its function and composition, and the changes it undergoes in cancer. We then examine efforts to employ it as a therapeutic target and as a diagnostic and prognostic marker, as well as strategies to prime the ECM to improve drug delivery through small molecule approaches and mechanical or enzymatic strategies. Finally, we examine efforts to further improve delivery through the use of drug carriers by ECM targeting or modulation.

2. Extracellular Matrix: Structure, Function, and Involvement in Cancer Etiology

In this section, we provide background for ECM-based therapeutic strategies by presenting an overview of the biology of the healthy ECM, its components, and its structure. We then discuss the changes induced by cancer in the ECM, which present epitopes for targeting and pathways to hijack for therapeutic intervention. Finally, we highlight some of the differences between healthy and tumor ECM. These ideas together provide a basis for a biological platform that can be leveraged for ECM-based strategies.

2.1. Function and Role of the ECM

The ECM firstly serves as a physical scaffold that helps to maintain the structure of organs [8]. It delineates tissue boundaries, preventing unnecessary cell migration and abnormal proliferation, and provides elasticity for organs [8,9]. Providing elasticity is particularly important during development and morphogenesis [10].

Next, the extracellular matrix serves as an adhesive substrate to facilitate cell migration. The mechanisms of cell adhesion are carried out through a set of molecules and receptors collectively known as the adhesome [11]. The adhesion sites help connect cells with their neighboring cells [12]. Additionally, with respect to the ECM, these adhesion molecules are important for environmental sensing, including for both chemical and physical properties [12]. Adhesion interactions occur through both integrin and non-integrin receptors. Integrins are transmembrane proteins composed of an α subunit and a β subunit. They interact with molecules in the ECM. There are 18 different α chain subunits and 8 different β chain subunits, which give many possible heterodimeric integrins [12]. The adhesome molecules are substrates for attachment, as well as mediators involved in the growth and remodeling of the ECM [11,13,14]. Integrins are stimulated by both mechanical (detecting stiffness of the ECM) and biochemical cues which instigate a conformational change, leading to downstream biochemical responses that modulate cell behavior [15–17]. Specific integrins on cells sense corresponding proteins and epitopes from the ECM [16]. Several matricellular proteins (including fibronectin [18], collagen, and others) are recognized by integrins and participate in the ECM–cell communication. These proteins are then further connected by a web of interactions with cells and other ECM components. Integrins and adhesion dynamics offer many opportunities for drug development and targeting [19–21].

Related to this environmental sensing that facilitates cell migration, an interesting and complex role that the ECM plays is in ECM–cell signaling, which is facilitated through multiple mechanisms. Fibrous proteins and glycosaminoglycans in the ECM bind growth factors and serve as a repository of embedded molecules which then get released in a regulated fashion through enzymatic processing [22]. These molecules are presented to the cell surface and in turn activate cellular pathways, in addition to direct ECM molecular interactions with cell surface receptors, facilitating intracellular signaling [22,23]. Examples of the ECM molecules that serve as reservoirs include heparan sulfate and heparan, collagen, and others. Examples of bound growth factors include vascular endothelial growth factor (VEGF), fibroblast growth factors (FGF), and others [24]. Remodeling of ECM molecules is facilitated predominantly by matrix metalloproteinases (MMPs) [25]. In some cases, the ECM molecule instead serves as a cofactor in the binding of growth factors to their cognate receptors [26].

In addition to the biochemical dynamics of these components, biomechanics also plays an important role in the ECM, both in terms of maintaining homeostasis as well as ECM–cell signaling [3]. The ECM communicates with cells through mechanotransduction [3]. In this process, the fibrous structure of the ECM exerts a mechanical pressure on the cell surface, where the tensile strength conveys signals [3]. The density and alignment of the fibrous structures both play an important role in this process [6].

The mechanical and dynamic homeostasis of the ECM is critical [3]. Homeostasis is maintained through effector cells and sensing. In the case of fibrous collagen, fibroblasts are important as effector cells in this process, as they secrete both collagen and proteases such as matrix metalloproteinases that can break down collagen in response to cues [3]. This breakdown maintains homeostasis within the ECM and with respect to cells and cellular function [27]. Disruptions to this homeostasis matter because they are both symptomatic and causative of pathological conditions, and often promote disease progression.

2.2. Composition of the ECM

The composition of the ECM varies depending on the type of ECM and the location. There are approximately 300 proteins in the mammalian ECM [9]. ECM material is secreted by fibroblasts, and it is in general made up of proteins (such as collagen, elastin, and fibronectin), glycosaminoglycans (largely hyaluronic acid), and proteoglycans (heparan sulfate and others). It interacts with cells and organs and maintains a tensile and compressive force [2]. It is also comprised of growth factors and signaling molecules, and it houses various immune and other cells, such as fibroblasts. The most abundant constituent is collagen, with the interstitium containing primarily collagen type I [28]. Fibroblasts secrete collagen and help organize its structure [29]. Elastin is secreted as tropoelastin, assembled into fibers, and tightly associated with the collagen, providing elasticity [2]. Fibronectin is involved in organizing the ECM, mediating cell functions and interaction, and its unfolding is mediated by mechanical forces [2]. Proteoglycans, which are made up of proteins covalently attached to glycosaminoglycans, are involved in interactions with growth factors and other signaling molecules, playing a role in the organization of the ECM structure [1]. Hyaluronan, a glycosaminoglycan, is involved in mediating several functions through binding to cell receptors [1]. Additionally there is a milieu of enzymes, which continually remodel the ECM and maintain homeostasis. Some examples of these include MMPs, a disintegrin and metalloproteases (ADAMs), a disintegrin and metalloproteases thrombospondin motifs (ADAMTs), heparanase, and many others [1]. The interstitium is connected to a basement membrane which separates it from blood vessels [30]. The basement membrane is predominantly composed of collagen type IV and laminin [30]. All of these molecules have receptors with which they interact in order to facilitate communication between cells and the ECM. Specific components of the ECM that are important targets for delivery are described in more detail later.

2.3. Pathological ECM

Hanahan and Weinberg famously described the hallmarks of cancer [31], and Pickup et al. extended this concept to how the extracellular matrix contributes to each of these hallmarks [32]. Cues from the ECM play a role in influencing each of these hallmarks, attesting to the integrative nature of cancer with its environment, and these are in fact essential to the development of malignancies [32]. In cancer, the ECM processes are dysregulated to collectively promote tumor growth and metastasis.

2.3.1. Enzyme Upregulation

Numerous enzymes (such as MMPs and cathepsins) are upregulated in the tumor ECM, which promote degradation and weakening of the basement membrane (although the relationship with these enzymes is more complex, with some enzymes showing both pro- and anti- tumor effects [33,34]). A summary of ECM enzymes is given in Table 1. Additionally, it is important to consider the distribution of enzymes and molecules within the tumor microenvironment, particularly in the context of targeting. Figure 1, adapted from Isaacson et al. [25], summarizes the distribution of MMP enzyme subtypes within a tumor microenvironment. Enzyme inhibition is a common disease therapy, and Table 2 gives examples of enzyme inhibitors with corresponding enzymes. The list is by no means exhaustive, but highlights some of the more studied examples of small molecules, drugs, and others and their associated matrix components. Increased enzymatic remodeling of various constituents primes the microenvironment for cancer through breakdown of the matrix to allow cell migration, weakening of the basement membrane to permit escape, increased growth, and increased presentation and release of pro-tumor cues [4]. Additionally, enzymatic remodeling leads to exposing cryptic domains within ECM protein structures, which enables binding of signaling factors that promote growth and angiogenesis [30]. This includes largely MMPs as well as cathepsins. Cathepsin K, for example, is responsible for bone resorption [35], and it is upregulated in breast cancer tumors that metastasize to the bone. Cathepsin B is involved in weakening of the basement membrane, promoting metastasis [36]. These also vary by tumor type and subtype. The differences attest to the heterogeneity of tumor stroma profiles. Another example, tissue-type plasminogen activator (tPA), is known to be secreted by cancer cells, and it is associated with several proteolytic channels, including fibrin degradation, and coagulation and complement systems [1]. This can lead to fibrin clots, leading to a restriction of tumor vascular permeability. Fibrin blood clots are degraded by plasmin, which is produced through the digestion of plasminogen via tPA [1]. These various enzymatic changes and processes are essential to cancer progression and metastasis.

Table 1. Extracellular matrix enzymes.

Enzyme Family	Enzyme	Substrate	Ref
MMPs	MMP-1	Type I and II collagen	[37]
	MMP-2	Gelatin, Type IV collagen	[38]
	MMP-3	E-cadherin, laminin, Type IV collagen; activates cytokines and growth factors; activates MMP-1, -8, -13, -9	[39]
	MMP-7	Type IV collagen, fibronectin, vitronectin, elastin, aggrecan	[40]
	MMP-8	Type I, II, and III collagens, gelatin, aggrecan, fibronectin	[34,41,42]
	MMP-9	Gelatin, Type IV collagen	[38]
Cathepsins	Cat B	Type IV collagen, laminin, fibronectin	[36]
	Cat K	Type I collagen, particularly bone	[35]
	Cat L	Type I and IV collagen, laminin, fibronectin, and elastin	[43]
	Cat S	Collagen, Elastin, E-cadherin	[44]
ADAMs	ADAMTS-18	Chondroitin sulfate	
Other Proteinases	Lysyl oxidase	Crosslinks elastins and collagens through conversion of lysines	[45]

2.3.2. Weakening of Basement Membrane

The basement membrane is thinner in invasive tumors due to remodeling, and it contains significantly lower levels of laminin (the key structural component of the basement membrane along with collagen type IV) [16]. The basement membrane serves as a barrier between the epithelial cells and the interstitium, and weakening it promotes escape [46]. Invasion is triggered by interactions (degradation) between membrane-bound matrix metalloproteinases (MT-MMPs) and basement membrane. This physical interaction triggers a cross-talk between several factors which then facilitate the process [46].

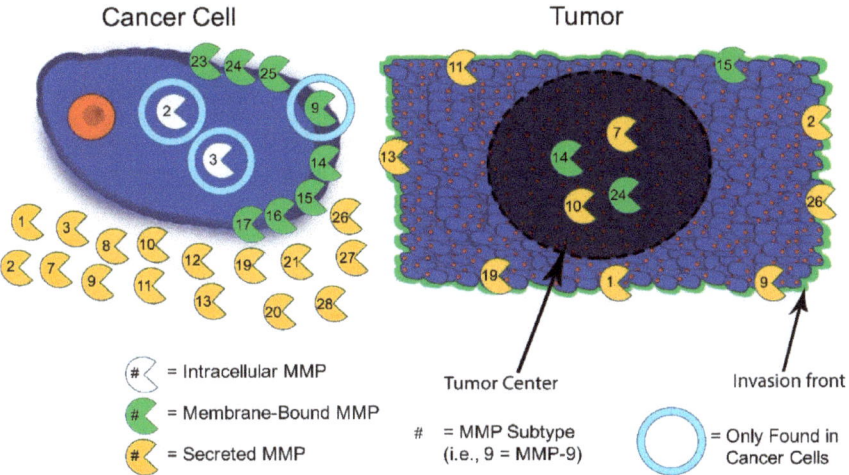

Figure 1. Schematic depicting the distribution of matrix metalloproteinase (MMP) subtypes within the tumor microenvironment. The cancer cell on the left, depicts intracellular MMPs (shown to the right of the nucleus, represented in red), membrane-bound MMPs, and secreted MMPs. Additionally, the light blue circle indicates those MMPs that are found in that particular location only in cancer cells (e.g., MMP-2 is found intracellularly in cancer cells, but not in healthy cells). The tumor microenvironment on the right (depicted with a background of cancer cells for schematic representation) shows the distribution of MMPs within the tumor microenvironment, indicating those present near the tumor interior versus near the periphery. Image adapted with permissions from Isaacson et al., 2017 [25].

2.3.3. Increased ECM Deposition and Stiffness

Next, there is an increased deposition of ECM material. One example is an increased deposition of collagen (desmoplasia) [7]. There is also increased alignment of collagen and increased cross-linking. Cross-linking is due to lysyl oxidase activity [47]. This leads to a higher level of mechanical rigidity and stress [2]. These changes are correlated with and further promote tumor growth and invasion, by mechanotransducive signaling (through density, cross-linked stiffness, and fiber alignment) on the cells [3]. Collagen is an integral component of the ECM landscape and it plays an important role in the biophysical communication between ECM and cells, and it has been shown to be highly involved in metastasis [17].

2.3.4. Causative Factors and Pathways

Much of the tumor ECM is synthesized and secreted by cancer-associated fibroblasts (CAFs) [48]. Additionally, stromal cells produce enzymes that digest the basement membrane, which contributes to invasion [48]. Signaling molecules and growth factors play a role as well. For example, TGF-β is particularly important in this cascade in activating fibroblasts [48]. Other important pathways include FAK, ERK, and FGF [49]. Similarly, proteoglycan changes also influence these processes [49]. There are higher levels of proteoglycans, such as chondroitin sulfate and heparan sulfate, as well as variations in enzyme expression. Ultimately, when considering the ECM in tumor progression, it is necessary to consider the effect of the cells on the stroma and the effect of the stroma on the cells [48].

2.4. In Summary

The involvement of the matrix in causing invasive phenotype is being analyzed at the most fundamental level: the interactions between a cell's local environment and physical cues, and the physical forces translated to biochemical signals, attesting to its complexity and importance [50]. Different cancers (such as breast cancer and prostate cancer for instance) display different stroma profiles [46]. The literature sometimes shows varying conclusions about the stroma profiles in different studies, suggesting heterogeneity. A comprehensive and detailed picture of stroma profiles is important because it is common to make conclusions and generalize about upregulated enzymes in the context of drug delivery, while specifics about the site of the enzyme within the microenvironment and the quantity of the enzyme are not always specified.

Ultimately these changes in the tumor ECM are important because they present new targets and avenues in the treatment of cancer. By targeting the mechanisms and components that play a supportive and causative role in tumor progression and metastasis, we can address the complex integration of cancer with its environment, modulating the ECM in conjunction with cytotoxic approaches. Furthermore, understanding the local architecture and interactions is not only important in the context of ECM-based strategies, but in any tumoral drug delivery, as these local dynamics influence migration of drugs and carriers to cells.

Table 2. Inhibitors of extracellular matrix enzymes.

Inhibitor Family	Inhibitor	Type of Inhibitor	Enzyme	Clinical Use/Translation	Ref.
MMP Inhibitors	Batimastat	Small molecule	Broad spectrum	Ended at Phase III	[51,52]
	Marimastat	Small molecule	Broad spectrum	Ended at Phase III	[53]
	Tanomastat	Small molecule	MMP-2, -3, -9	Ended at Phase III	[54]
	Doxycycline	Small molecule	Broad spectrum	Ongoing	[54]
	TIMP-1, -2, -3, -4	Endogenous inhibitor	Broad spectrum	n/a	[55,56]
	SDS3	Antibody	MMP-2, MMP-9	n/a	[55,57,58]
	Prinomastat	Small molecule	Broad spectrum	Ended at Phase III	[59]
Cathepsin Inhibitors	L-235	Small molecule	Cat K	n/a	[60]
	Relacatib	Small molecule	Cat K, B, L, S V	Ended at Phase I	[35,61]
	Odanacatib	Small molecule	Cat K, B, L, S, V	Ended at Phase III	[35,62,63]
	E64	Small molecule	Cat B, Cat L	n/a	[64]

3. Harnessing ECM Biology

With an understanding of matrix biology, research efforts are underway to exploit this information for cancer treatment. This includes enhancing drug delivery to tumor cells by priming the ECM, as well as designing drugs that act on ECM targets and mechanisms. Additionally, upregulated matrix components are used as prognostic and diagnostic markers. The strategies which focus on either small molecule, enzyme-based, or other modalities are discussed in this section. The section following it discusses drug delivery approaches to further improve targeting.

3.1. Priming the ECM to Enhance Drug Delivery

Because the matrix poses a barrier to the migration of drugs and is often cited as the reason for the failure of many treatments, there have been approaches to enhance drug delivery through breaking down the ECM using enzymes such as hyaluronidase. Clinical trials have explored the use of PEGylated hyaluronidase (PEGPH20) in combination with the chemotherapeutic eribulin mesylate, as a means to break down the hyaluronic acid barrier in the ECM [65,66]. Hyaluronidase digests the ECM allowing facile diffusion of the drug molecules to the target. These are particularly relevant in cancers such as pancreatic cancer which have an especially dense stromal matrix. Similarly, it has been shown that administering collagenase improves penetration [67].

In addition to enzyme-based strategies, mechanical strategies are also employed to facilitate drug delivery. An example of priming the matrix to enhance drug delivery is in the use of pulsed high intensity focused ultrasound (HIFU) to alter the collagen structure of the ECM to allow for better penetration of chemotherapeutic drugs [68]. HIFU can be used to induce localized hyperthermia [69], and it can also disrupt collagen structure [68]. Mice inoculated with A549 tumors and administered pulsed-HIFU exhibited increased penetration of chitosan nanoparticles, due to disruption of the ECM. The porosity of the ECM was shown to be increased with higher intensity of the administered ultrasound.

Another strategy is the direct modulation of the cancer-associated fibroblasts (which deposit ECM material) to reduce ECM deposition. An example is the use of all-*trans* retinoic acid (ATRA), which induces quiescence in pancreatic stellate cells (PSCs) of pancreatic ductal adenocarcinoma (PDAC) [70]. Inducing quiescence in PSCs restores homeostasis in the PDAC ECM, resulting in less ECM deposition. This allows for better penetration and delivery of drugs. Lysyl oxidase inhibition has also been shown to improve delivery, as lysyl oxidase, discussed earlier, is responsible for cross-linking the ECM proteins and thus increasing the tumor stiffness [71]. Inhibiting lysyl oxidase showed the ability to potentiate the delivery of other treatments [71].

3.2. ECM Molecules as a Therapeutic Target

The ECM can be modulated using small molecules as a therapeutic strategy. Many of these rely on either the signaling pathways between the ECM and cells or on enzyme inhibition. Some examples of ECM therapeutic targets include thrombospondins [72], osteopontins [72], periostins [72], tenascins [72], matrix metalloproteinases [73,74], and cathepsins [75]. Inhibitors are often based on epitopes and binding motifs that are inspired by endogenous substrates.

One example is cathepsin K (Cat K), a cysteine protease responsible for osteoclast-mediated bone resorption. Cat K degrades collagen type I by cleaving the triple helices at different sites, and it has been implicated in cancers with skeletal (bone) metastases [60]. It is found to be upregulated in several tumor types (including bone, lung, prostate, and breast cancer), and specifically more expressed in cancers that are more invasive and metastasize to the bone [75–78]. Modulation of Cat K activity using Cat K inhibitors influences osteolysis [60]. Though cathepsin K inhibitors have predominantly found their home in the treatment of osteoporosis, they have also gone through clinical trials to treat metastatic bone disease [75]. They have been shown to reduce osteolytic lesions (indicative of metastasis) in breast cancer [60,75].

Another example is matrix metalloproteinases (MMPs), a zinc-dependent family of proteinases which is most implicated in matrix degradation, which plays an important role in invasion and metastasis in the context of cancer [79]. These are located either bound to cell surfaces, within the interstitium, or near the periphery [25]. MMP inhibitors have gone through clinical trials, albeit with limited success towards cancer treatment [80]. Some notable examples include batimastat [51], marimastat [79], and several others. Many of these are broad spectrum inhibitors which coordinate with sites on the enzyme (mimicking the enzyme's endogenous peptide substrate) and act through chelation of the essential zinc, most classically through a hydroxamic acid moiety [79]. The first generation of MMP inhibitors largely failed due to lack of specificity and off-target toxicities [55].

Proteins, glycoproteins, and proteoglycans additionally are therapeutic targets. Osteopontin (OPN) is a matricellular phosphoglycoprotein that binds to integrins to facilitate ECM–cell communication. Its upregulation promotes tumor progression through several interactions and cascades [81,82]. Osteopontin interacts with several integrins (both with and without its RGD motif), as well as with CD44 receptors [82]. It plays a structural role in the ECM, and it binds to collagen and other proteins [83]. Osteopontin has been shown to be upregulated in several types of cancer, and it is thought to be involved in tumor proliferation, metastasis, induction of angiogenesis, and potentially chemoresistance [82,84]. Osteopontin inhibitors are investigated for cancer treatment, at the level of gene delivery as well as small molecule inhibitors [72,81,82,84].

Thrombospondin is another example that has been explored as a target. Thrombospondins are a family of proteins that regulate cell phenotype and ECM structure [85]. They are suggested to have both supportive and suppressive roles in metastasis, complicated by the fact that they have interactions with numerous other proteins [85]. Thrombospondin-1 regulates angiogenesis, and inhibiting it leads to enhanced vasculature formation, which creates a leakier vasculature in order to enhance extravasation and delivery. However, it is also an inhibitor of tumor growth, making the interaction more complicated [86]. Additionally, thrombospondins are thought to activate TGF-β in some tumor types but not others, further complicating its influence on tumor progression [86]. Inhibitors of thrombospondin have had more progress associated with inhibiting fibrosis [87].

Heparan sulfate proteoglycans have also been explored as a target in breast cancer therapy, because they participate in signaling pathways involved in tumor progression [88]. Heparan sulfate binds growth factors that are involved in signaling angiogenesis, metastasis, and tumor proliferation [89]. However, heparan sulfate also contains growth factors that are cancer inhibitory, so its role is complex [89]. Furthermore, heparan itself is also explored as a therapeutic molecule [89].

In summary, the complexity of the ECM interactions offers many opportunities that are very complicated since many proteins have both pro- and anti- tumor properties, emphasizing the importance of homeostasis.

3.3. ECM as a Prognostic and Diagnostic Biomarker

The ECM has also been utilized as a biomarker for its tight correlation with cancer stage. One well-established example is collagen [90]. Collagen radial alignment has been recognized as a prognostic signature for tumor advancement [6]. This has been termed TACS (tumor associated collagen signature) [6]. Increased radial alignment and direction with respect to tumor cells has been associated with local invasion and transition to metastasis.

Osteopontin is also an important biomarker in cancer [84]. Osteopontin is secreted as a glycophosphoprotein, and then post-translationally modified [91]. Osteopontin is overexpressed in several cancers including breast, lung, skin, and ovarian cancer [91]. It has shown potential as a biomarker for treatment and prognosis in osteosarcoma, as patient survival and therapeutic efficacy in osteosarcoma is correlated with osteopontin overexpression [91]. Similarly, fibronectin has also shown promise as an ECM marker for malignancy [92]. Researchers have developed antibody fragments to help detect fibrin as a tumor marker [92]. Additionally, fibronectin targeting has been used along with MRI to detect micrometastases [93].

3.4. In Summary

Given the development of drugs and drug-like molecules that inhibit and generally act on ECM components (through harnessing biology), drug carriers can take this a step further in a few ways. First we can improve delivery of these small molecules, which are subject to rapid wash, to the tumor ECM, by complexing them to nanocarriers. Furthermore, the upregulated ECM components have potential as targets to improve localization to the tumor. In terms of priming the ECM, we can recapitulate some of the approaches described earlier. The next section discusses ways to utilize drug carriers to further the ideas discussed so far.

4. ECM Targeting and Drug Delivery

Macromolecular drug carriers have been employed to improve the pharmacokinetics of small molecule drugs. Both passive targeting by the enhanced permeability and retention effect (EPR) and active targeting through use of targeting ligands have been proposed for tumor targeting. A subset of active targeting is targeting the matricellular components. In this section we first describe the advantages and limitations of ECM targeting, followed by examples of targeted ECM components. We then summarize the ECM-based strategies to improve drug delivery for cancer treatment. The strategies include the use of nanocarriers to modulate the ECM to improve drug penetration, to create a drug depot within the

ECM, and to directly modulate the ECM. Finally, we include a brief discussion of some immunomodulatory factors that are involved in ECM delivery approaches.

4.1. ECM Targeting

4.1.1. Advantages of ECM Targeting

Targeting the ECM carries several advantages. The dense stromal barrier as well as the inefficient lymphatic drainage results in a higher interstitial pressure that favors intravasation and limits diffusion [94,95]. There is a limitation in the diffusion of macromolecules to the cell surface, which can result in a gradient of drug localization [94,95]. Passive accumulation via the enhanced permeability and retention (EPR) effect does not affect the migration and diffusion upon extravasation. Furthermore, diffusion can be limited not only by pore size through the matrix but may also be influenced by electrostatic interactions [96]. Thus it is influenced not only by the size of nanocarriers but the surface charge of the carrier. This has been shown through in vitro models which simulate ECM interactions [97]. Targeting the matrix itself can limit the need to traverse this barrier, resulting in more accumulation at the target site. Targeting the ECM and extracellular drug activity may allow for evasion of a common mode of drug resistance: cellular efflux pumps [98].

4.1.2. Limitations and Barriers to ECM Targeting

ECM targeting faces some problems of heterogeneity, a problem associated with tumors in general. It is also important to be cognizant of the site-specificity of different ECM components (i.e., their proximity to blood vessels, gradients within the ECM, etc.). Finally, the ubiquity of ECM processes and targeting sites leads to non-specific localization and action, a problem inherent in most cancer treatments. Targeting ECM components with greater upregulation in the ECM can help to improve tumor selectivity.

4.1.3. ECM Components as Targeting Peptides and as Delivery Targets

Interactions between ECM components and with cell surface receptors have provided information on specific epitopes that are involved in integrin binding [99]. Here we look at some of the matrix components that can serve as delivery targets. Table 3 lists a selection of ECM proteins and targeting peptides known to bind to them. Some examples of matrix targets include collagen, laminin, fibronectin, chondroitin sulfate, tenascin-C, heparan sulfate, and aggrecan [99,100].

Table 3. Extracellular matrix components and associated targeting moieties.

Matrix Targets	Targeting Peptides/Antibodies	Reference
Fibronectin	CREKA	[101]
	CLT1	[101]
	CLT2	[101]
	F8 antibody	[102]
	L19 antibody	[102]
Collagen	CNA35	[103]
	WYRGRL	[104]
	Collagen mimetic peptides	[105]
	TKKTLRT	[106]
	WREPSFMALS	[107]
Tenascin-C	FHKHKSPALSPVGGG	[108]
	F16 antibody	[108]
Hyaluronan	CKRDLSRRC (IP3)	[109]
Heparan Sulfate	NT4	[110]
	CGKRK	[100]

Fibronectin as a Target

Fibronectin is a glycoprotein that is abundant in the ECM and upregulated in tumors. It regulates a wide range of processes in the ECM. Upregulated fibronectin is an indicator of epithelial-to-mesenchymal transition. Fibronectin has been explored as a binding target, in complex with fibrin [101,102]. The structure of fibronectin contains two domains that are frequently used for targeting: extra domain A (EDA) and extra domain B (EDB), with most methods targeting the latter [102]. Extra domain B is particularly important for tumor angiogenesis. Targeting methods for fibronectin employ either antibodies or peptides [102].

A commonly studied example is CREKA (Cys-Arg-Glu-Lys-Ala), a 5-mer peptide which binds to the fibrin-fibronectin complex and is employed as a targeting moiety [101]. PEGylated liposomes modified to incorporate CREKA, and loaded with doxorubicin, had a higher retention in 4T1 breast tumor inoculated mice, owing to CREKA's stable binding to fibrinogen [111]. Additionally, an invasion assay demonstrated that binding of CREKA to fibrinogen had an inhibitory effect on cell motility through the invasion chamber [111]. Importantly, CREKA shows negligible binding to fibrin-fibronectin complexes in healthy tissue [93].

Collagen as a Target

Collagen has also been explored for ECM targeting. Collagen is the most abundant protein in the human body and in the extracellular matrix, and there are both fibrillar and non-fibrillar (network-forming) types [106]. There are 28 different known subtypes of collagen, with collagen type I being the most prevalent. All collagen types display a signature triple helix structure [106]. There are several collagen binding peptides which are inspired by various ECM motifs, and which bind both to intact and denatured collagen [106]. Some examples are given in Table 3. One well-known example of a collagen binding peptide is the collagen binding domain from the A3 domain of the von Willebrand factor [112]. For example, albumin modified with this collagen binding domain has been utilized as a drug carrier for delivery of doxorubicin in a subcutaneous MC38 colon cancer mouse model, and it showed an increase in accumulation [113].

Hyaluronan as a Target

Hyaluronan, a non-sulfated glycosaminoglycan in the ECM, is also a common target, due to the CD-44-hyaluronan interaction's influence on tumor progression [114,115]. CD-44 is a transmembrane protein, and this interaction plays a role in cell motility [115]. Approximately a quarter of tumors overexpress HA [116]. Reducing hyaluronan reduces CD-44 expression [115,117]. Targeting CD-44 receptors to inhibit HA signaling is a common approach related to hyaluronan, as harnessing the interaction between hyaluronan and the cell surface receptors can modulate tumor growth [114]. Hyaluronan itself has also been employed as a targeting moiety for tumor targeting, and it has been used to modify nanoparticles to improve delivery [114].

Tenascin-C as a Target

Tenascin C has been targeted using peptides as well as antibodies [100]. Tenascin-C is a large glycoprotein that is upregulated in tumor ECM, and it plays a supportive role in tumor growth, angiogenesis, and metastasis [100]. Interestingly there is little expression of tenascin in healthy ECM [100]. Using nanoparticle delivery (including liposomes and extracellular release strategies), tenascin-C targeting has been used to deliver drugs towards tumor cells as well as cancer-associated fibroblasts [100].

Heparan Sulfate as a Target

Heparan sulfate is a glycosaminoglycan that is expressed in the ECM, cell surface, and basement membrane [118]. It is also significantly upregulated in the tumor ECM and has served as a target [100]. Targeting peptides have been employed to direct nanoparticles (often liposomes) to heparan sulfate for tumor localization [100].

4.2. ECM Strategies to Improve Drug Delivery and Modulate Tumor Growth and Invasion

ECM-based strategies carry different approaches to facilitate drug delivery, and here we divide them into three broad categories. The first is breaking down the ECM to improve drug penetration. The second is targeting to an epitope within the matrix generally upregulated in order to create a depot for drug delivery to the tumor cells. The third is to target to an epitope in the tumoral ECM to modulate the ECM itself in order to directly impact the tumor. These are depicted schematically in Figure 2.

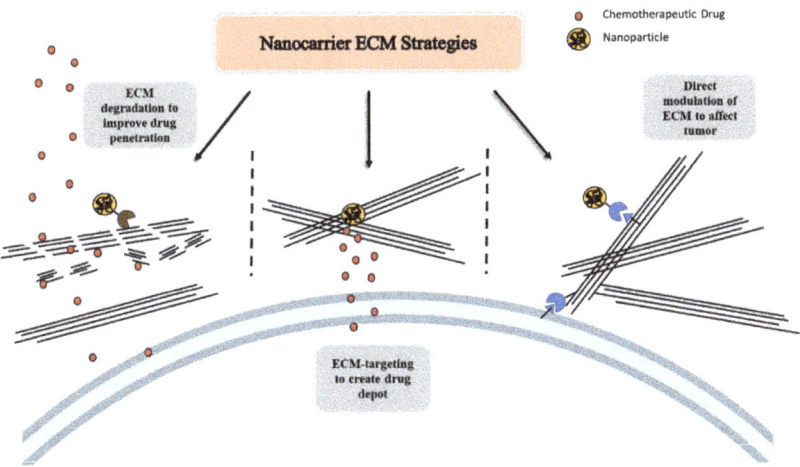

Figure 2. Schematic of extracellular matrix (ECM)-based strategies to improve drug delivery and modulate tumor growth and invasion, with the aid of nanoparticles, through ECM degradation to improve drug delivery, ECM-targeting to create a local drug depot, and direct modulation of the ECM.

4.2.1. ECM-Based Strategies to Enhance Drug Penetration through Stroma Modulation

Some cancers are particularly known for their highly desmoplastic stroma, such as pancreatic cancer and some types of breast cancer. Treatment inefficacy is often attributed to an inability to penetrate the ECM. As mentioned earlier, efforts have been made to improve delivery by reducing the ECM barrier. Employing nanocarriers can improve this. One strategy of employing the ECM and nanocarrier targeting to improve drug delivery focuses on reducing the ECM material (which poses a barrier to drug penetration and delivery). Pancreatic ductal adenocarcinoma (PDAC) is often the most utilized application [119]. Many examples of these strategies have found their niche in PDAC, due to the impact of the ECM on its drug exposure. As mentioned earlier PSCs are responsible for ECM deposition in PDAC [120], and the tumor microenvironment is known for its dense desmoplasia and its hypoxic and acidic extracellular environment [121,122]. A greater collagen content in many of these cancers is also correlated with poorer outcomes [123]. Breaking down the stroma also poses the risk of tumor cell escape and metastasis becoming more likely with increased pathways for migration.

Nanoparticles are employed to enhance this strategy through improving the delivery of drugs to tumor ECM with the purpose of downregulating the production of ECM material. This has been done through encapsulating either degradative enzymes (to directly break down ECM) or drug molecules (to downregulate the production of ECM material). These methods further capitalize on ECM biology, by employing an ECM enzyme-responsive aspect to trigger payload release or incorporating binding motifs that bind to upregulated ECM components. For example, MMP-2 responsive peptide-hybrid liposomes (liposome-like particles that incorporate MMP-2 cleavable peptides) designed to encapsulate and release pirfenidone (to down-regulate ECM production) at the site of the pancreatic tumors were able to down-regulate ECM material production and increase penetration of small molecules in a model of PDAC [124]. Gemcitabine was delivered with improved penetration and delivery. Delivery of the ECM-altering drug relied on improved targeting of delivery, which was aided by the nanoparticle. In a similar study, collagenase was encapsulated in liposomes (to afford enzyme protection and encourage localization at the tumor) and delivered similarly to break down the ECM in pancreatic cancer [125]. Following this, paclitaxel micelles were delivered resulting in improved delivery. Interestingly, breaking down the ECM in this study did not seem to increase metastasis [125]. Another study used PEGylated polyethyleneimine-coated gold nanoparticles to deliver all-*trans* retinoic acid (ATRA) [126]. ATRA is used to inhibit pancreatic stellate cells, which reduces deposition of ECM material in pancreatic tumors. The nanosystem is pH-responsive, capitalizing on the slightly acidic tumor extracellular pH, generally cited as being between pH 6–7. This strategy led to the inhibition of PSCs in order to restore homeostasis in the ECM. Following this gemcitabine is delivered, and drug penetration is increased due to a decreased barrier function.

Photothermal agents have also been incorporated into nanoparticles for delivery to the tumor ECM, in order to then break down the ECM for drug delivery. Bioinspired lipoprotein nanoparticles loaded with a photothermal agent that can be triggered by near-infrared light irradiation were delivered to a 4T1 orthotopic mouse breast tumor model [127]. The photothermal agent used was DiOC18 (7) (DiR), and its purpose was to remodel the tumor microenvironment to allow for better penetration of the drug mertansine, also loaded into the particles. The nanoparticle allowed for increased accumulation at the target site, and administration of near infrared light irradiation allowed for the activation of photothermal effects to remodel the ECM in favor of promoting penetration. The improved drug delivery was effective in killing cancer-associated fibroblasts and tumor-associated macrophages. This study represents another important concept because it addresses these supportive cells present in the ECM which contribute to tumor proliferation, strategically combining aspects of the ECM's contribution to tumors.

These examples demonstrate that the enzymes that break down the ECM can improve delivery using nanocarriers, and this in turn improves small molecule delivery through the ECM for treatment. Furthermore, nanocarriers can deliver other ECM degraders to help prime the ECM.

4.2.2. Utilizing the ECM as an Attachment Site for a Drug Delivery System

Another often employed strategy utilizing the ECM is in targeting sites within the matrix for localization, and then releasing drugs for delivery to the cells. In this fashion nanoparticles targeted to the ECM serve as a localized depot. The value of doing this is to improve penetration into the tumor microenvironment, reducing the need for a drug to diffuse across this barrier. Utilizing the ECM for targeting and as a drug depot is further beneficial compared to targeting cell surface receptors, as intratumoral heterogeneity may result in targeting some cells while leaving others. Furthermore, it will also directly affect cancer-associated cells, which may not display the same upregulations. Lastly an active targeting strategy to the ECM may also see a greater differential in upregulation compared to one targeting cell surface receptors [100].

Researchers have applied this concept to treat epithelial ovarian cancer, using for example the single chain antibody GD3G7, which binds to chondroitin sulfate, incorporated into a lyophilisome. Chondroitin sulfate is highly expressed in ovarian cancer. The lyophilisomes were loaded with doxorubicin. It was validated that the lyophilisome was bound to chondroitin sulfate and the drug load released extracellularly, demonstrating the ability to create a depot within the ECM [128]. Another study similarly used a triple negative breast tumor 3D spheroid model and demonstrated that liposomes targeted to the ECM could serve as a depot releasing cisplatin to alter the distribution of drug molecules within the matrix [129]. On the premise that many ECM components are negatively charged, they used a positively charged nanoparticle to be attracted to the ECM. An in vivo study showed that this nanoparticle reduced growth rate in tumors. A similar study used pH-sensitive liposomes designed to be triggered to release cisplatin load in an acidic environment [130]. They found that cell viability decreased with delivery using these pH-sensitive liposomes, and that the distribution increased. Again targeting the matrix here addressed the purpose of improving drug distribution within the tumor microenvironment.

These examples illustrate the utility of the ECM as a target, some of which are noted in Table 3. They also illustrate pH-mediated extracellular drug release in the mildly acidic tumor ECM. Finally, they illustrate the idea of delivering drugs to cells, but the concept can be extrapolated to non-cellular targets as well, as is exemplified in the next section.

4.2.3. Modulating the ECM to Reduce Tumor Growth and Invasion

Another important strategy involves direct modulation of the ECM. This addresses the important influence that the ECM has on cancer growth and especially invasion and metastasis. As discussed earlier in this review, the ECM contributes significantly to delivering cues to cells, and modulating it can have a direct result on growth and invasion, as separate from priming the ECM for other drug delivery to cells. Modulation of the ECM in conjunction with cytotoxic approaches may prove to have additional advantages. Here we present examples that either directly modulate the ECM or deliver small molecule drugs that modulate the ECM.

PLGA nanoparticles incorporating batimastat (first generation MMP inhibitor) were delivered to treat hepatocellular carcinoma (HCC) [52]. Batimastat inhibits MMPs, in order to directly modulate the ECM remodeling, and this results in slowing of angiogenesis. Treatment was done in conjunction with transarterial chemoembolization (TACE), which is the primary treatment for HCC and often results in stimulating angiogenesis to compensate for the embolized blood vessels. The strategy employed here is that by using batimastat to inhibit MMPs, angiogenesis could be slowed, supporting the TACE treatment. Thus a combination of nanoparticles and ECM modulation is used to aid another treatment hampered by angiogenesis. Nanoparticles can also be used to deliver ECM-modulating drugs. For example, a study demonstrated the use of lysolipid-containing thermosensitive liposomes to deliver marimastat (an MMP inhibitor) to the breast tumor ECM in order to suppress the ECM remodeling which contributes to metastasis, demonstrating suppression of lung metastasis [131].

These studies exemplify the use of nanocarriers to modulate the ECM, as well to play a supportive role in another form of treatment (TACE), which would be a fruitful use of ECM tools. Table 4 provides a summary of ECM-based strategies.

Finally, it is important to note the immunomodulatory factors that may be associated with ECM targeting and modulation. The tumor microenvironment fosters immune suppression through many pathways. For example, collagen deposition is associated with immune modulation, specifically through functioning as a receptor in immune inhibitory signaling [132]. Disruption of these pathways may have unintended consequences in immune suppression. For example, suppression of the CAFs associated with the aforementioned collagen deposition has also been shown to contribute to immune suppression through other pathways [132].

Table 4. Strategies Employing the Tumor ECM.

	Types of Nanocarrier Delivery Systems	Examples and Remarks
Targeting ECM Components	Polymer nanoparticles [52]	Matricellular targets include: Collagen [112,113], Fibronectin [101,102]. Laminin, Hyaluronan [114], Tenascin-C [114], Heparan sulfate [100]
	Antibodies [114]	
	Liposomes [114]	
Modulating ECM to reduce barrier to delivery	Liposomes [124]	Breakdown of matrix through direct breakdown or reduction of matrix expression
	Gold nanoparticles [126]	
	Lipoprotein nanoparticles [127]	
Using ECM as a local drug depot	Liposomes [128–130]	
	Lyophilosomes [129]	
Modulating ECM to directly alter tumor growth and invasion	Liposomes [131]	MMP inhibitors [131]
	Polymer nanoparticles [52]	

5. Discussion and Future Directions

At this time, clinical studies employing ECM-based approaches are very limited. While some examples of ECM-acting drugs have progressed to clinical trials (with many obstacles to their success, particularly delivery), there is not a wealth of information on the translatability of these delivery strategies. Furthermore, the heterogeneity of the tumor microenvironment poses a significant obstacle. Many of the biomarkers and epitopes targeted in these strategies have varying levels of overexpression in different patients and at different stages, underscoring the need for a personalized approach. A key merit of ECM-based approaches is that they move away from oversimplifying the tumor microenvironment, by considering the specific location of different ECM components as well as the limits to migration and diffusion within the site. It also takes into consideration the supportive and responsive nature of the tumor environment, including for example pancreatic stellate cells, which critically limit the efficacy of drugs. The drug delivery field has advanced to incorporate and adapt many of its strategies (polymers, antibody-drug conjugates, inorganic nanoparticles, etc.) to address the ECM. Furthermore, strategies have been appropriately applied to cancers in which the ECM is the most significant barrier, notably pancreatic cancer, ovarian cancer, and breast cancer. The ECM provides ample opportunity as a battlefront in the treatment of cancer, and a solid biological understanding is key to harnessing its potential. Furthermore, an understanding of the local stromal biology can aid even other delivery strategies, which sometimes oversimplify the tumor to a homogenous site immediately presenting itself after drug extravasation. There are many elegant approaches to harnessing the ECM's contribution to tumor biology to aid in treatment, both direct and indirect methods. This includes priming the ECM, directly modulating the ECM, delivery to matrix targets, therapeutically targeting the ECM, and other combinations which can facilitate treatment, and these methods are further enhanced through the wealth of information on nanocarriers. The ECM's most important role is in invasion and metastasis, and addressing the ECM to slow metastasis can be done in conjunction with cytotoxic approaches. Nanocarrier approaches can greatly benefit from a knowledge of the ECM's biology and influence, and similarly ECM approaches can greatly benefit from improvements in carrier technology to improve delivery and targeting.

Author Contributions: N.S.: substantial contribution to the conception, analysis, figure design, and writing of this work; H.G.: discussion, advice, editing, and final approval. All authors have read and agreed to the published version of the manuscript.

Funding: This work was funded by the Ruth L. Kirschstein NIH National Research Service Award (NRSA), award number #5F31CA213901.

Institutional Review Board Statement: Not applicable.

Informed Consent Statement: Not applicable.

Conflicts of Interest: The authors have no conflicts of interest to declare.

References

1. Theocharis, A.D.; Skandalis, S.S.; Gialeli, C.; Karamanos, N.K. Extracellular matrix structure. *Adv. Drug Deliv. Rev.* **2016**, *97*, 4–27. [CrossRef] [PubMed]
2. Frantz, C.; Stewart, K.M.; Weaver, V.M. The extracellular matrix at a glance. *J. Cell Sci.* **2010**, *123*, 4195–4200. [CrossRef] [PubMed]
3. Humphrey, J.D.; Dufresne, E.R.; Schwartz, M.A. Mechanotransduction and extracellular matrix homeostasis. *Nat. Rev. Mol. Cell Biol.* **2014**, *15*, 802–812. [CrossRef] [PubMed]
4. Insua-Rodriguez, J.; Oskarsson, T. The extracellular matrix in breast cancer. *Adv. Drug Deliv. Rev.* **2016**, *97*, 41–55. [CrossRef] [PubMed]
5. Stylianopoulos, T.; Munn, L.L.; Jain, R.K. Reengineering the Physical Microenvironment of Tumors to Improve Drug Delivery and Efficacy: From Mathematical Modeling to Bench to Bedside. *Trends Cancer* **2018**, *4*, 292–319. [CrossRef] [PubMed]
6. Conklin, M.W.; Eickhoff, J.C.; Riching, K.M.; Pehlke, C.A.; Eliceiri, K.W.; Provenzano, P.P.; Friedl, A.; Keely, P.J. Aligned collagen is a prognostic signature for survival in human breast carcinoma. *Am. J. Pathol.* **2011**, *178*, 1221–1232. [CrossRef] [PubMed]
7. Walker, R.A. The complexities of breast cancer desmoplasia. *Breast Cancer Res.* **2001**, *3*, 143–145. [CrossRef]
8. Hoshiba, T.; Yamaoka, T. Chapter 1: Extracellular Matrix Scaffolds for Tissue Engineering and Biological Research. In *Decellularized Extracellular Matrix: Characterization, Fabrication and Applications*; The Royal Society of Chemistry: London, UK, 2019; pp. 1–14. [CrossRef]
9. Bonnans, C.; Chou, J.; Werb, Z. Remodelling the extracellular matrix in development and disease. *Nat. Rev. Mol. Cell Biol.* **2014**, *15*, 786–801. [CrossRef]
10. Rozario, T.; DeSimone, D.W. The extracellular matrix in development and morphogenesis: A dynamic view. *Dev. Biol.* **2010**, *341*, 126–140. [CrossRef]
11. Geiger, B.; Yamada, K.M. Molecular architecture and function of matrix adhesions. *Cold Spring Harb. Perspect. Biol.* **2011**, *3*, a005033. [CrossRef]
12. Zaidel-Bar, R.; Geiger, B. The switchable integrin adhesome. *J. Cell Sci.* **2010**, *123*, 1385–1388. [CrossRef] [PubMed]
13. Costa, P.; Parsons, M. Chapter Two—New Insights into the Dynamics of Cell Adhesions. In *International Review of Cell and Molecular Biology*; Jeon, K., Ed.; Academic Press: Cambridge, MA, USA, 2010; Volume 283, pp. 57–91.
14. Worth, D.C.; Parsons, M. Adhesion dynamics: Mechanisms and measurements. *Int. J. Biochem. Cell Biol.* **2008**, *40*, 2397–2409. [CrossRef] [PubMed]
15. Filipe, E.C.; Chitty, J.L.; Cox, T.R. Charting the unexplored extracellular matrix in cancer. *Int J. Exp. Pathol* **2018**, *99*, 58–76. [CrossRef] [PubMed]
16. Kai, F.; Drain, A.P.; Weaver, V.M. The Extracellular Matrix Modulates the Metastatic Journey. *Dev. Cell* **2019**, *49*, 332–346. [CrossRef] [PubMed]
17. Walker, C.; Mojares, E.; Del Rio Hernandez, A. Role of Extracellular Matrix in Development and Cancer Progression. *Int. J. Mol. Sci.* **2018**, *19*, 3028. [CrossRef]
18. Humphries, J.D.; Chastney, M.R.; Askari, J.A.; Humphries, M.J. Signal transduction via integrin adhesion complexes. *Curr. Opin. Cell Biol.* **2019**, *56*, 14–21. [CrossRef] [PubMed]
19. Dunehoo, A.L.; Anderson, M.; Majumdar, S.; Kobayashi, N.; Berkland, C.; Siahaan, T.J. Cell Adhesion Molecules for Targeted Drug Delivery. *J. Pharm. Sci.* **2006**, *95*, 1856–1872. [CrossRef]
20. Raab-Westphal, S.; Marshall, J.F.; Goodman, S.L. Integrins as Therapeutic Targets: Successes and Cancers. *Cancers* **2017**, *9*, 110. [CrossRef]
21. Goodman, S.L.; Picard, M. Integrins as therapeutic targets. *Trends Pharmacol. Sci.* **2012**, *33*, 405–412. [CrossRef]
22. Sainio, A.; Järveläinen, H. Extracellular matrix-cell interactions: Focus on therapeutic applications. *Cell. Signal.* **2020**, *66*, 109487. [CrossRef]
23. Hastings, J.F.; Skhinas, J.N.; Fey, D.; Croucher, D.R.; Cox, T.R. The extracellular matrix as a key regulator of intracellular signalling networks. *Br. J. Pharmacol.* **2019**, *176*, 82–92. [CrossRef] [PubMed]
24. Taipale, J.; Keski-Oja, J. Growth factors in the extracellular matrix. *Faseb J.* **1997**, *11*, 51–59. [CrossRef] [PubMed]
25. Isaacson, K.J.; Martin Jensen, M.; Subrahmanyam, N.B.; Ghandehari, H. Matrix-metalloproteinases as targets for controlled delivery in cancer: An analysis of upregulation and expression. *J. Control. Release* **2017**, *259*, 62–75. [CrossRef] [PubMed]
26. Hynes, R.O. The extracellular matrix: Not just pretty fibrils. *Science* **2009**, *326*, 1216–1219. [CrossRef] [PubMed]
27. Naba, A.; Clauser, K.R.; Ding, H.; Whittaker, C.A.; Carr, S.A.; Hynes, R.O. The extracellular matrix: Tools and insights for the "omics" era. *Matrix Biol.* **2016**, *49*, 10–24. [CrossRef]
28. Ricard-Blum, S. The collagen family. *Cold Spring Harb. Perspect. Biol.* **2011**, *3*, a004978. [CrossRef]
29. Karsdal, M.A.; Nielsen, S.H.; Leeming, D.J.; Langholm, L.L.; Nielsen, M.J.; Manon-Jensen, T.; Siebuhr, A.; Gudmann, N.S.; Rønnow, S.; Sand, J.M.; et al. The good and the bad collagens of fibrosis—Their role in signaling and organ function. *Adv. Drug Deliv. Rev.* **2017**, *121*, 43–56. [CrossRef]

30. Kalluri, R. Basement membranes: Structure, assembly and role in tumour angiogenesis. *Nat. Rev. Cancer* **2003**, *3*, 422–433. [CrossRef]
31. Hanahan, D.; Weinberg, R.A. The hallmarks of cancer. *Cell* **2000**, *100*, 57–70. [CrossRef]
32. Pickup, M.W.; Mouw, J.K.; Weaver, V.M. The extracellular matrix modulates the hallmarks of cancer. *EMBO Rep.* **2014**, *15*, 1243–1253. [CrossRef]
33. Decock, J.; Thirkettle, S.; Wagstaff, L.; Edwards, D.R. Matrix metalloproteinases: Protective roles in cancer. *J. Cell Mol. Med.* **2011**, *15*, 1254–1265. [CrossRef] [PubMed]
34. López-Otín, C.; Palavalli, L.H.; Samuels, Y. Protective roles of matrix metalloproteinases: From mouse models to human cancer. *Cell Cycle* **2009**, *8*, 3657–3662. [CrossRef] [PubMed]
35. Duong, L.T.; Leung, A.T.; Langdahl, B. Cathepsin K Inhibition: A New Mechanism for the Treatment of Osteoporosis. *Calcif. Tissue Int.* **2016**, *98*, 381–397. [CrossRef] [PubMed]
36. Ruan, H.; Hao, S.; Young, P.; Zhang, H. Targeting Cathepsin B for Cancer Therapies. *Horiz. Cancer Res.* **2015**, *56*, 23–40. [PubMed]
37. Vincenti, M.P.; Brinckerhoff, C.E. Transcriptional regulation of collagenase (MMP-1, MMP-13) genes in arthritis: Integration of complex signaling pathways for the recruitment of gene-specific transcription factors. *Arthr. Res. Ther.* **2001**, *4*, 157. [CrossRef]
38. Li, H.; Qiu, Z.; Li, F.; Wang, C. The relationship between MMP-2 and MMP-9 expression levels with breast cancer incidence and prognosis. *Oncol. Lett.* **2017**, *14*, 5865–5870. [CrossRef]
39. Mirastschijski, U.; Lupše, B.; Maedler, K.; Sarma, B.; Radtke, A.; Belge, G.; Dorsch, M.; Wedekind, D.; McCawley, L.J.; Boehm, G.; et al. Matrix Metalloproteinase-3 is Key Effector of TNF-α-Induced Collagen Degradation in Skin. *Int. J. Mol. Sci.* **2019**, *20*, 5234. [CrossRef]
40. Han, J.-C.; Li, X.-D.; Du, J.; Xu, F.; Wei, Y.-J.; Li, H.-B.; Zhang, Y.-J. Elevated matrix metalloproteinase-7 expression promotes metastasis in human lung carcinoma. *World J. Surg. Oncol.* **2015**, *13*, 5. [CrossRef]
41. Balbín, M.; Fueyo, A.; Tester, A.M.; Pendás, A.M.; Pitiot, A.S.; Astudillo, A.; Overall, C.M.; Shapiro, S.D.; López-Otín, C. Loss of collagenase-2 confers increased skin tumor susceptibility to male mice. *Nat. Genet.* **2003**, *35*, 252–257. [CrossRef]
42. Jabłońska-Trypuć, A.; Matejczyk, M.; Rosochacki, S. Matrix metalloproteinases (MMPs), the main extracellular matrix (ECM) enzymes in collagen degradation, as a target for anticancer drugs. *J. Enzyme Inhib. Med. Chem.* **2016**, *31*, 177–183. [CrossRef]
43. Sudhan, D.R.; Siemann, D.W. Cathepsin L targeting in cancer treatment. *Pharmacol. Ther.* **2015**, *155*, 105–116. [CrossRef] [PubMed]
44. Richard, D.A.W.; Rich, W.; Christopher, J.S.; Roberta, E.B. Cathepsin S: Therapeutic, diagnostic, and prognostic potential. *Biol. Chem.* **2015**, *396*, 867–882. [CrossRef]
45. Smith-Mungo, L.I.; Kagan, H.M. Lysyl oxidase: Properties, regulation and multiple functions in biology. *Matrix Biol.* **1998**, *16*, 387–398. [CrossRef]
46. Planche, A.; Bacac, M.; Provero, P.; Fusco, C.; Delorenzi, M.; Stehle, J.-C.; Stamenkovic, I. Identification of prognostic molecular features in the reactive stroma of human breast and prostate cancer. *PLoS ONE* **2011**, *6*, e18640. [CrossRef]
47. Cox, T.R.; Gartland, A.; Erler, J.T. Lysyl Oxidase, a Targetable Secreted Molecule Involved in Cancer Metastasis. *Cancer Res.* **2016**, *76*, 188–192. [CrossRef]
48. Miles, F.L.; Sikes, R.A. Insidious changes in stromal matrix fuel cancer progression. *Mol. Cancer Res.* **2014**, *12*, 297–312. [CrossRef]
49. Reiland, J.; Kempf, D.; Roy, M.; Denkins, Y.; Marchetti, D. FGF2 binding, signaling, and angiogenesis are modulated by heparanase in metastatic melanoma cells. *Neoplasia* **2006**, *8*, 596–606. [CrossRef]
50. Mierke, C.T. The matrix environmental and cell mechanical properties regulate cell migration and contribute to the invasive phenotype of cancer cells. *Rep. Prog. Phys.* **2019**, *82*, 064602. [CrossRef]
51. Giavazzi, R.; Garofalo, A.; Ferri, C.; Lucchini, V.; Bone, E.A.; Chiari, S.; Brown, P.D.; Nicoletti, M.I.; Taraboletti, G. Batimastat, a synthetic inhibitor of matrix metalloproteinases, potentiates the antitumor activity of cisplatin in ovarian carcinoma xenografts. *Clin. Cancer Res.* **1998**, *4*, 985.
52. Xiao, L.; Wang, M. Batimastat Nanoparticles Associated with Transcatheter Arterial Chemoembolization Decrease Hepatocellular Carcinoma Recurrence. *Cell Biochem. Biophys.* **2014**, *70*, 269–272. [CrossRef]
53. Sinno, M.; Biagioni, S.; Ajmone-Cat, M.A.; Pafumi, I.; Caramanica, P.; Medda, V.; Tonti, G.; Minghetti, L.; Mannello, F.; Cacci, E. The matrix metalloproteinase inhibitor marimastat promotes neural progenitor cell differentiation into neurons by gelatinase-independent TIMP-2-dependent mechanisms. *Stem Cells Dev.* **2013**, *22*, 345–358. [CrossRef] [PubMed]
54. Cathcart, J.; Pulkoski-Gross, A.; Cao, J. Targeting matrix metalloproteinases in cancer: Bringing new life to old ideas. *Genes Dis.* **2015**, *2*, 26–34. [CrossRef] [PubMed]
55. Levin, M.; Udi, Y.; Solomonov, I.; Sagi, I. Next generation matrix metalloproteinase inhibitors—Novel strategies bring new prospects. *BBA Mol. Cell Res.* **2017**, *1864*, 1927–1939. [CrossRef] [PubMed]
56. Murphy, G. Tissue inhibitors of metalloproteinases. *Genome Biol.* **2011**, *12*, 233. [CrossRef] [PubMed]
57. Sela-Passwell, N.; Kikkeri, R.; Dym, O.; Rozenberg, H.; Margalit, R.; Arad-Yellin, R.; Eisenstein, M.; Brenner, O.; Shoham, T.; Danon, T.; et al. Antibodies targeting the catalytic zinc complex of activated matrix metalloproteinases show therapeutic potential. *Nat. Med.* **2012**, *18*, 143–147. [CrossRef] [PubMed]
58. Fields, G.B. Mechanisms of Action of Novel Drugs Targeting Angiogenesis-Promoting Matrix Metalloproteinases. *Front. Immunol.* **2019**, *10*, 1278. [CrossRef] [PubMed]

59. Bissett, D.; O'Byrne, K.J.; Von Pawel, J.; Gatzemeier, U.; Price, A.; Nicolson, M.; Mercier, R.; Mazabel, E.; Penning, C.; Zhang, M.H.; et al. Phase III Study of Matrix Metalloproteinase Inhibitor Prinomastat in Non–Small-Cell Lung Cancer. *J. Clin. Oncol.* **2005**, *23*, 842–849. [CrossRef]
60. Duong, L.T.; Wesolowski, G.A.; Leung, P.; Oballa, R.; Pickarski, M. Efficacy of a cathepsin K inhibitor in a preclinical model for prevention and treatment of breast cancer bone metastasis. *Mol. Cancer Ther.* **2014**, *13*, 2898–2909. [CrossRef]
61. Kumar, S.; Dare, L.; Vasko-Moser, J.A.; James, I.E.; Blake, S.M.; Rickard, D.J.; Hwang, S.M.; Tomaszek, T.; Yamashita, D.S.; Marquis, R.W.; et al. A highly potent inhibitor of cathepsin K (relacatib) reduces biomarkers of bone resorption both in vitro and in an acute model of elevated bone turnover in vivo in monkeys. *Bone* **2007**, *40*, 122–131. [CrossRef]
62. Jensen, A.; Wynne, C.; Ramirez, G.; He, W.; Song, Y.; Berd, Y.; Wang, H.; Mehta, A.; Lombardi, A. The Cathepsin K Inhibitor Odanacatib Suppresses Bone Resorption in Women With Breast Cancer and Established Bone Metastases: Results of a 4-Week, Double-Blind, Randomized, Controlled Trial. *Clin. Breast Cancer* **2010**, *10*, 452–458. [CrossRef]
63. Alberca, L.N.; Chugunansky, S.R.; Álvarez, C.L.; Talevi, A.; Salas-Sarduy, E. In silico Guided Drug Repurposing: Discovery of New Competitive and Non-competitive Inhibitors of Falcipain-2. *Front Chem.* **2019**, *7*, 534. [CrossRef] [PubMed]
64. Wilder, C.L.; Walton, C.; Watson, V.; Stewart, F.A.A.; Johnson, J.; Peyton, S.R.; Payne, C.K.; Odero-Marah, V.; Platt, M.O. Differential cathepsin responses to inhibitor-induced feedback: E-64 and cystatin C elevate active cathepsin S and suppress active cathepsin L in breast cancer cells. *Int. J. Biochem. Cell Biol.* **2016**, *79*, 199–208. [CrossRef] [PubMed]
65. Fleming, J.M.; Yeyeodu, S.T.; McLaughlin, A.; Schuman, D.; Taylor, D.K. In Situ Drug Delivery to Breast Cancer-Associated Extracellular Matrix. *ACS Chem. Biol.* **2018**, *13*, 2825–2840. [CrossRef] [PubMed]
66. Doherty, G.J.; Tempero, M.; Corrie, P.G. HALO-109-301: A Phase III trial of PEGPH20 (with gemcitabine and nab-paclitaxel) in hyaluronic acid-high stage IV pancreatic cancer. *Future Oncol.* **2018**, *14*, 13–22. [CrossRef] [PubMed]
67. Goodman, T.T.; Olive, P.L.; Pun, S.H. Increased nanoparticle penetration in collagenase-treated multicellular spheroids. *Int. J. Nanomed.* **2007**, *2*, 265–274.
68. Lee, S.; Han, H.; Koo, H.; Na, J.H.; Yoon, H.Y.; Lee, K.E.; Lee, H.; Kim, H.; Kwon, I.C.; Kim, K. Extracellular matrix remodeling in vivo for enhancing tumor-targeting efficiency of nanoparticle drug carriers using the pulsed high intensity focused ultrasound. *J. Control. Release* **2017**, *263*, 68–78. [CrossRef] [PubMed]
69. Frazier, N.; Payne, A.; De Bever, J.; Dillon, C.; Panda, A.; Subrahmanyam, N.; Ghandehari, H. High intensity focused ultrasound hyperthermia for enhanced macromolecular delivery. *J. Control. Release* **2016**, *241*, 186–193. [CrossRef] [PubMed]
70. Chronopoulos, A.; Robinson, B.; Sarper, M.; Cortes, E.; Auernheimer, V.; Lachowski, D.; Attwood, S.; García, R.; Ghassemi, S.; Fabry, B.; et al. ATRA mechanically reprograms pancreatic stellate cells to suppress matrix remodelling and inhibit cancer cell invasion. *Nat. Commun.* **2016**, *7*, 12630. [CrossRef] [PubMed]
71. Röhrig, F.; Vorlová, S.; Hoffmann, H.; Wartenberg, M.; Escorcia, F.E.; Keller, S.; Tenspolde, M.; Weigand, I.; Gätzner, S.; Manova, K.; et al. VEGF-ablation therapy reduces drug delivery and therapeutic response in ECM-dense tumors. *Oncogene* **2017**, *36*, 1–12. [CrossRef] [PubMed]
72. Sawyer, A.J.; Kyriakides, T.R. Matricellular proteins in drug delivery: Therapeutic targets, active agents, and therapeutic localization. *Adv. Drug Deliv. Rev.* **2016**, *97*, 56–68. [CrossRef] [PubMed]
73. Winer, A.; Adams, S.; Mignatti, P. Matrix Metalloproteinase Inhibitors in Cancer Therapy: Turning Past Failures Into Future Successes. *Mol. Cancer Ther.* **2018**, *17*, 1147–1155. [CrossRef] [PubMed]
74. Liu, H.-Y.; Gu, W.-J.; Wang, C.-Z.; Ji, X.-J.; Mu, Y.-M. Matrix metalloproteinase-9 and -2 and tissue inhibitor of matrix metalloproteinase-2 in invasive pituitary adenomas: A systematic review and meta-analysis of case-control trials. *Medicine* **2016**, *95*, e3904. [CrossRef] [PubMed]
75. Liu, H.; Wang, G.; Gu, W.; Mu, Y. Cathepsin K: The association between Cathepsin K expression and sphenoid sinus invasion of pituitary adenomas. *Med. Hypotheses* **2016**, *97*, 88–89. [CrossRef] [PubMed]
76. Lu, J.; Wang, M.; Wang, Z.; Fu, Z.; Lu, A.; Zhang, G. Advances in the discovery of cathepsin K inhibitors on bone resorption. *J. Enzyme Inhib. Med. Chem.* **2018**, *33*, 890–904. [CrossRef] [PubMed]
77. Yamashita, K.; Iwatake, M.; Okamoto, K.; Yamada, S.-I.; Umeda, M.; Tsukuba, T. Cathepsin K modulates invasion, migration and adhesion of oral squamous cell carcinomas in vitro. *Oral Diseases* **2017**, *23*, 518–525. [CrossRef] [PubMed]
78. Le Gall, C.; Bellahcène, A.; Bonnelye, E.; Gasser, J.A.; Castronovo, V.; Green, J.; Zimmermann, J.; Clézardin, P. A Cathepsin K Inhibitor Reduces Breast Cancer–Induced Osteolysis and Skeletal Tumor Burden. *Cancer Res.* **2007**, *67*, 9894–9902. [CrossRef]
79. Wojtowicz-Praga, S.M.; Dickson, R.B.; Hawkins, M.J. Matrix metalloproteinase inhibitors. *Invest. New Drugs* **1997**, *15*, 61–75. [CrossRef]
80. Rasmussen, H.S.; McCann, P.P. Matrix Metalloproteinase Inhibition as a Novel Anticancer Strategy: A Review with Special Focus on Batimastat and Marimastat. *Pharmacol. Ther.* **1997**, *75*, 69–75. [CrossRef]
81. Shevde, L.A.; Samant, R.S. Role of osteopontin in the pathophysiology of cancer. *Matrix Biol.* **2014**, *37*, 131–141. [CrossRef]
82. Zhao, H.; Chen, Q.; Alam, A.; Cui, J.; Suen, K.C.; Soo, A.P.; Eguchi, S.; Gu, J.; Ma, D. The role of osteopontin in the progression of solid organ tumour. *Cell Death Disease* **2018**, *9*, 356. [CrossRef]
83. Ramadan, A.; Afifi, N.; Yassin, N.Z.; Abdel-Rahman, R.F.; Abd El-Rahman, S.S.; Fayed, H.M. Mesalazine, an osteopontin inhibitor: The potential prophylactic and remedial roles in induced liver fibrosis in rats. *Chem. Biol. Interact.* **2018**, *289*, 109–118. [CrossRef] [PubMed]

84. Wei, R.; Wong, J.P.C.; Kwok, H.F. Osteopontin—A promising biomarker for cancer therapy. *J. Cancer* **2017**, *8*, 2173–2183. [CrossRef] [PubMed]
85. Yee, K.O.; Connolly, C.M.; Duquette, M.; Kazerounian, S.; Washington, R.; Lawler, J. The effect of thrombospondin-1 on breast cancer metastasis. *Breast Cancer Res. Treat.* **2009**, *114*, 85–96. [CrossRef] [PubMed]
86. Daubon, T.; Léon, C.; Clarke, K.; Andrique, L.; Salabert, L.; Darbo, E.; Pineau, R.; Guérit, S.; Maitre, M.; Dedieu, S.; et al. Deciphering the complex role of thrombospondin-1 in glioblastoma development. *Nat. Commun.* **2019**, *10*, 1146. [CrossRef] [PubMed]
87. Xie, X.-S.; Li, F.-Y.; Liu, H.-C.; Deng, Y.; Li, Z.; Fan, J.-M. LSKL, a peptide antagonist of thrombospondin-1, attenuates renal interstitial fibrosis in rats with unilateral ureteral obstruction. *Arch. Pharmacal Res.* **2010**, *33*, 275–284. [CrossRef] [PubMed]
88. Chuay-Yeng, K.; Yin-Ping, S.; Boon-Huat, B.; George, W.Y. Targeting Heparan Sulfate Proteoglycans in Breast Cancer Treatment. *Recent Pat. Anti Cancer Drug Discov.* **2008**, *3*, 151–158. [CrossRef]
89. Knelson, E.H.; Nee, J.C.; Blobe, G.C. Heparan sulfate signaling in cancer. *Trends Biochem. Sci.* **2014**, *39*, 277–288. [CrossRef]
90. Xu, S.; Xu, H.; Wang, W.; Li, S.; Li, H.; Li, T.; Zhang, W.; Yu, X.; Liu, L. The role of collagen in cancer: From bench to bedside. *J. Transl. Med.* **2019**, *17*, 309. [CrossRef]
91. Han, X.; Wang, W.; He, J.; Jiang, L.; Li, X. Osteopontin as a biomarker for osteosarcoma therapy and prognosis. *Oncol. Lett.* **2019**, *17*, 2592–2598. [CrossRef]
92. Obonai, T.; Fuchigami, H.; Furuya, F.; Kozuka, N.; Yasunaga, M.; Matsumura, Y. Tumour imaging by the detection of fibrin clots in tumour stroma using an anti-fibrin Fab fragment. *Sci. Rep.* **2016**, *6*, 23613. [CrossRef]
93. Zhou, Z.; Qutaish, M.; Han, Z.; Schur, R.M.; Liu, Y.; Wilson, D.L.; Lu, Z.-R. MRI detection of breast cancer micrometastases with a fibronectin-targeting contrast agent. *Nat. Commun.* **2015**, *6*, 7984. [CrossRef] [PubMed]
94. Jain, R.K. Transport of molecules in the tumor interstitium: A review. *Cancer Res.* **1987**, *47*, 3039–3051. [PubMed]
95. Jain, R.K.; Stylianopoulos, T. Delivering nanomedicine to solid tumors. *Nat. Rev. Clin. Oncol.* **2010**, *7*, 653–664. [CrossRef] [PubMed]
96. Stylianopoulos, T.; Poh, M.-Z.; Insin, N.; Bawendi, M.G.; Fukumura, D.; Munn, L.L.; Jain, R.K. Diffusion of particles in the extracellular matrix: The effect of repulsive electrostatic interactions. *Biophys. J.* **2010**, *99*, 1342–1349. [CrossRef] [PubMed]
97. Tomasetti, L.; Breunig, M. Preventing Obstructions of Nanosized Drug Delivery Systems by the Extracellular Matrix. *Adv. Healthcare Mater.* **2018**, *7*, 1700739. [CrossRef] [PubMed]
98. Chen, S.; Yang, K.; Tuguntaev, R.G.; Mozhi, A.; Zhang, J.; Wang, P.C.; Liang, X.-J. Targeting tumor microenvironment with PEG-based amphiphilic nanoparticles to overcome chemoresistance. *Nanomedicine* **2016**, *12*, 269–286. [CrossRef]
99. Hwang, J.; Sullivan, M.O.; Kiick, K.L. Targeted Drug Delivery via the Use of ECM-Mimetic Materials. *Front. Bioeng. Biotechnol.* **2020**, *8*, 69. [CrossRef]
100. Raavé, R.; Van Kuppevelt, T.H.; Daamen, W.F. Chemotherapeutic drug delivery by tumoral extracellular matrix targeting. *J. Control. Release* **2018**, *274*, 1–8. [CrossRef]
101. Han, Z.; Lu, Z.-R. Targeting Fibronectin for Cancer Imaging and Therapy. *J. Mater. Chem. B* **2017**, *5*, 639–654. [CrossRef]
102. Kumra, H.; Reinhardt, D.P. Fibronectin-targeted drug delivery in cancer. *Adv. Drug Deliv. Rev.* **2016**, *97*, 101–110. [CrossRef]
103. Mees, G.; Dierckx, R.; Mertens, K.; Vermeire, S.; Van Steenkiste, M.; Reutelingsperger, C.; D'Asseler, Y.; Peremans, K.; Van Damme, N.; Van de Wiele, C. 99mTc-Labeled Tricarbonyl His-CNA35 as an Imaging Agent for the Detection of Tumor Vasculature. *J. Nucl. Med.* **2012**, *53*, 464–471. [CrossRef] [PubMed]
104. Rothenfluh, D.A.; Bermudez, H.; O'Neil, C.P.; Hubbell, J.A. Biofunctional polymer nanoparticles for intra-articular targeting and retention in cartilage. *Nat. Mater.* **2008**, *7*, 248–254. [CrossRef] [PubMed]
105. Bennink, L.L.; Li, Y.; Kim, B.; Shin, I.J.; San, B.H.; Zangari, M.; Yoon, D.; Yu, S.M. Visualizing collagen proteolysis by peptide hybridization: From 3D cell culture to in vivo imaging. *Biomaterials* **2018**, *183*, 67–76. [CrossRef] [PubMed]
106. Wahyudi, H.; Reynolds, A.A.; Li, Y.; Owen, S.C.; Yu, S.M. Targeting collagen for diagnostic imaging and therapeutic delivery. *J. Control. Release* **2016**, *240*, 323–331. [CrossRef] [PubMed]
107. Goldbloom-Helzner, L.; Hao, D.; Wang, A. Developing Regenerative Treatments for Developmental Defects, Injuries, and Diseases Using Extracellular Matrix Collagen-Targeting Peptides. *Int. J. Mol. Sci.* **2019**, *20*, 4072. [CrossRef] [PubMed]
108. Kim, M.Y.; Kim, O.R.; Choi, Y.S.; Lee, H.; Park, K.; Lee, C.-T.; Kang, K.W.; Jeong, S. Selection and characterization of tenascin C targeting peptide. *Mol. Cells* **2012**, *33*, 71–77. [CrossRef]
109. Ikemoto, H.; Lingasamy, P.; Anton Willmore, A.-M.; Hunt, H.; Kurm, K.; Tammik, O.; Scodeller, P.; Simón-Gracia, L.; Kotamraju, V.R.; Lowy, A.M.; et al. Hyaluronan-binding peptide for targeting peritoneal carcinomatosis. *Tumour. Biol.* **2017**, *39*, 1010428317901628. [CrossRef]
110. Depau, L.; Brunetti, J.; Falciani, C.; Scali, S.; Riolo, G.; Mandarini, E.; Pini, A.; Bracci, L. Coupling to a cancer-selective heparan-sulfate-targeted branched peptide can by-pass breast cancer cell resistance to methotrexate. *Oncotarget* **2017**, *8*, 76141–76152. [CrossRef]
111. Jiang, K.; Song, X.; Yang, L.; Li, L.; Wan, Z.; Sun, X.; Gong, T.; Lin, Q.; Zhang, Z. Enhanced antitumor and anti-metastasis efficacy against aggressive breast cancer with a fibronectin-targeting liposomal doxorubicin. *J. Control. Release* **2018**, *271*, 21–30. [CrossRef]
112. Romijn, R.A.P.; Bouma, B.; Wuyster, W.; Gros, P.; Kroon, J.; Sixma, J.J.; Huizinga, E.G. Identification of the Collagen-binding Site of the von Willebrand Factor A3-domain. *J. Biol. Chem.* **2001**, *276*, 9985–9991. [CrossRef]

113. Sasaki, K.; Ishihara, J.; Ishihara, A.; Miura, R.; Mansurov, A.; Fukunaga, K.; Hubbell, J.A. Engineered collagen-binding serum albumin as a drug conjugate carrier for cancer therapy. *Sci. Adv.* **2019**, *5*, eaaw6081. [CrossRef] [PubMed]
114. Platt, V.M.; Szoka, F.C. Anticancer Therapeutics: Targeting Macromolecules and Nanocarriers to Hyaluronan or CD44, a Hyaluronan Receptor. *Mol. Pharm.* **2008**, *5*, 474–486. [CrossRef] [PubMed]
115. Shuster, S.; Frost, G.I.; Csoka, A.B.; Formby, B.; Stern, R. Hyaluronidase reduces human breast cancer xenografts in SCID mice. *Int. J. Cancer* **2002**, *102*, 192–197. [CrossRef] [PubMed]
116. Kultti, A.; Li, X.; Jiang, P.; Thompson, C.B.; Frost, G.I.; Shepard, H.M. Therapeutic Targeting of Hyaluronan in the Tumor Stroma. *Cancers* **2012**, *4*, 873–903. [CrossRef] [PubMed]
117. Stern, R.; Shuster, S.; Wiley, T.S.; Formby, B. Hyaluronidase can modulate expression of CD44. *Exp. Cell Res.* **2001**, *266*, 167–176. [CrossRef]
118. Simon Davis, D.A.; Parish, C.R. Heparan Sulfate: A Ubiquitous Glycosaminoglycan with Multiple Roles in Immunity. *Front. Immunol.* **2013**, *4*. [CrossRef]
119. Neesse, A.; Michl, P.; Frese, K.K.; Feig, C.; Cook, N.; Jacobetz, M.A.; Lolkema, M.P.; Buchholz, M.; Olive, K.P.; Gress, T.M.; et al. Stromal biology and therapy in pancreatic cancer. *Gut* **2011**, *60*, 861–868. [CrossRef]
120. Pothula, S.P.; Xu, Z.; Goldstein, D.; Pirola, R.C.; Wilson, J.S.; Apte, M.V. Key role of pancreatic stellate cells in pancreatic cancer. *Cancer Lett.* **2016**, *381*, 194–200. [CrossRef]
121. Looi, C.-K.; Chung, F.F.-L.; Leong, C.-O.; Wong, S.-F.; Rosli, R.; Mai, C.-W. Therapeutic challenges and current immunomodulatory strategies in targeting the immunosuppressive pancreatic tumor microenvironment. *J. Exp. Clin. Cancer Res.* **2019**, *38*, 162. [CrossRef]
122. Feig, C.; Gopinathan, A.; Neesse, A.; Chan, D.S.; Cook, N.; Tuveson, D.A. The pancreas cancer microenvironment. *Clin. Cancer Res.* **2012**, *18*, 4266–4276. [CrossRef]
123. Dolor, A.; Szoka, F.C. Digesting a Path Forward: The Utility of Collagenase Tumor Treatment for Improved Drug Delivery. *Mol. Pharm.* **2018**, *15*, 2069–2083. [CrossRef] [PubMed]
124. Ji, T.; Lang, J.; Wang, J.; Cai, R.; Zhang, Y.; Qi, F.; Zhang, L.; Zhao, X.; Wu, W.; Hao, J.; et al. Designing Liposomes To Suppress Extracellular Matrix Expression To Enhance Drug Penetration and Pancreatic Tumor Therapy. *ACS Nano* **2017**, *11*, 8668–8678. [CrossRef] [PubMed]
125. Zinger, A.; Koren, L.; Adir, O.; Poley, M.; Alyan, M.; Yaari, Z.; Noor, N.; Krinsky, N.; Simon, A.; Gibori, H.; et al. Collagenase Nanoparticles Enhance the Penetration of Drugs into Pancreatic Tumors. *ACS Nano* **2019**, *13*, 11008–11021. [CrossRef] [PubMed]
126. Han, X.; Li, Y.; Xu, Y.; Zhao, X.; Zhang, Y.; Yang, X.; Wang, Y.; Zhao, R.; Anderson, G.J.; Zhao, Y.; et al. Reversal of pancreatic desmoplasia by re-educating stellate cells with a tumour microenvironment-activated nanosystem. *Nat. Commun.* **2018**, *9*, 3390. [CrossRef] [PubMed]
127. Tan, T.; Hu, H.; Wang, H.; Li, J.; Wang, Z.; Wang, J.; Wang, S.; Zhang, Z.; Li, Y. Bioinspired lipoproteins-mediated photothermia remodels tumor stroma to improve cancer cell accessibility of second nanoparticles. *Nat. Commun.* **2019**, *10*, 3322. [CrossRef]
128. Van der Steen, S.C.; Raavé, R.; Langerak, S.; Van Houdt, L.; Van Duijnhoven, S.M.; Van Lith, S.A.; Massuger, L.F.; Daamen, W.F.; Leenders, W.P.; Van Kuppevelt, T.H. Targeting the extracellular matrix of ovarian cancer using functionalized, drug loaded lyophilisomes. *Eur. J. Pharm. Biopharm.* **2017**, *113*, 229–239. [CrossRef]
129. Stras, S.; Howe, A.; Prasad, A.; Salerno, D.; Bhatavdekar, O.; Sofou, S. Growth of Metastatic Triple-Negative Breast Cancer Is Inhibited by Deep Tumor-Penetrating and Slow Tumor-Clearing Chemotherapy: The Case of Tumor-Adhering Liposomes with Interstitial Drug Release. *Mol. Pharm.* **2020**, *17*, 118–131. [CrossRef]
130. Stras, S.; Holleran, T.; Howe, A.; Sofou, S. Interstitial Release of Cisplatin from Triggerable Liposomes Enhances Efficacy against Triple Negative Breast Cancer Solid Tumor Analogues. *Mol. Pharm.* **2016**, *13*, 3224–3233. [CrossRef]
131. Lyu, Y.; Xiao, Q.; Yin, L.; Yang, L.; He, W. Potent delivery of an MMP inhibitor to the tumor microenvironment with thermosensitive liposomes for the suppression of metastasis and angiogenesis. *Signal. Transduct. Target. Ther.* **2019**, *4*, 26. [CrossRef]
132. Mushtaq, M.U.; Papadas, A.; Pagenkopf, A.; Flietner, E.; Morrow, Z.; Chaudhary, S.G.; Asimakopoulos, F. Tumor matrix remodeling and novel immunotherapies: The promise of matrix-derived immune biomarkers. *J. Immunother. Cancer* **2018**, *6*, 65. [CrossRef]

MDPI
St. Alban-Anlage 66
4052 Basel
Switzerland
Tel. +41 61 683 77 34
Fax +41 61 302 89 18
www.mdpi.com

Journal of Personalized Medicine Editorial Office
E-mail: jpm@mdpi.com
www.mdpi.com/journal/jpm

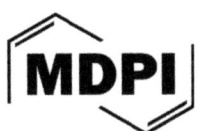

www.ingramcontent.com/pod-product-compliance
Lightning Source LLC
LaVergne TN
LVHW070049120526
838202LV00101B/1898